a **LANGE** medical book

Clinical
Anatomy

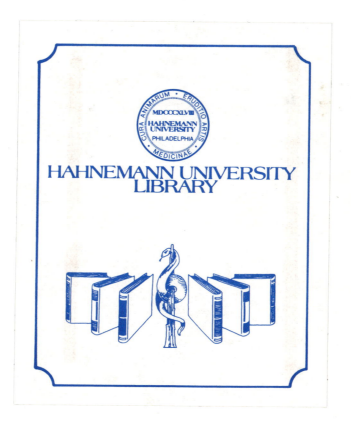

a **LANGE** medical book

Clinical Anatomy

Harold H. Lindner, MD
Clinical Professor of Surgery and Topographic Anatomy
University of California, San Francisco

Illustrated by **Laurel V. Schaubert**

APPLETON & LANGE
Norwalk, Connecticut/San Mateo, California

0-8385-1259-3

89 90 91 92 / 10 9 8 7 6 5 4 3 2 1

Prentice-Hall International (UK) Limited, *London*
Prentice-Hall of Australia, Pty. Limited, *Sydney*
Prentice-Hall Canada, Inc., *Toronto*
Prentice-Hall Hispanoamericana, S.A., *Mexico*
Prentice-Hall of India Private Limited, *New Delhi*
Prentice-Hall of Japan, Inc., *Tokyo*
Simon & Schuster Asia Pte. Ltd., *Singapore*
Editora Prentice-Hall do Brasil Ltda., *Rio de Janeiro*
Prentice Hall, *Englewood Cliffs, New Jersey*

ISBN: 0–8385–1259–3
ISSN: 0891–2238

Library of Congress Cataloging-in-Publication Data
Lindner, Harold H., b. 1908.
    Clinical anatomy.
    "A Lange medical book."
    1. Anatomy, Human. I. Title. [DNLM: 1. Anatomy.
QS 4 L747c]
QM23.2.L55—1989   611   88-24167
ISBN 0–8385–1259–3

Cover: M. Chandler Martylewski

PRINTED IN THE UNITED STATES OF AMERICA

Table of Contents

Preface

A course in clinical anatomy was developed over many years by Professor Harold Lindner at UCSF. Dr Lindner's outstanding success in teaching anatomy to two generations of medical students was due to his ability to make anatomy understandable and meaningful by emphasizing its relationship and importance to medicine and surgery. CLINICAL ANATOMY evolved out of Dr Lindner's experience in teaching this course. It is designed to teach anatomy and its relationship to clinical medicine and surgery in a way that makes the subject valid and clear to students.

CLINICAL ANATOMY is designed to achieve the following goals:

- To be a reliable basic anatomy text that helps the student learn the material presented in first-year anatomy;
- To serve as a concise clinically oriented reference and review text for the clinical courses in the third and fourth years of medical school; and
- To serve as a rapid review text in preparing for examinations and particularly for the National Boards.

The important elements that facilitate learning with CLINICAL ANATOMY are as follows:

- Complete coverage by organ system or regions of the body in a concise, consistently organized, and simply presented manner
- A clear and easy-to-follow format
    - Highlights of embryology
    - Concise description of organ or region
    - Relationship to other organs
    - Details of blood supply, lymphatics, and nerves
- Helpful clinical considerations
    - Many important clinical facts
    - Relates anatomy to actual clinical practice
- Outstanding illustrations
    - Numerous illustrations of anatomy and clinical problems by Laurel Schaubert, an outstanding medical artist
    - Careful integration of illustrations and text for optimal learning
    - Selected radiographic images to enhance anatomic detail

One of Dr Lindner's students had this to say: "I really didn't understand anatomy until I had taken his course. All the bits and pieces fell together and became meaningful." It is our hope that the readers of CLINICAL ANATOMY will benefit similarly from this book.

Many people have contributed to the refinement of CLINICAL ANATOMY, and some of them participated in its original development. Julien Goodman greatly assisted in the early development of the book. Those who helped in the polishing include both clinicians and students. A few of the chapters were written by specialists, and many of Dr Lindner's friends have looked at chapters dealing with their own areas of interest and made contributions. Particular mention must be made recognizing the great efforts of Drs Lorraine Day, Donald Grant, Kan Gill, Jeremy Lieberman, Kent Olson, Lawrence Way, and Jack McAninch, each refining the text from his or her own specialty point of view.

The beautiful illustrations are the work of Laurel Schaubert, our principal artist for almost 30 years. Though most of the illustrations were newly made, a number by the same artist have been taken from our other clinical books, most importantly *Current Surgical Diagnosis & Treatment*, *Current Obstetric & Gynecologic Diagnosis & Treatment*, *General Urology*, *Correlative Neuroanatomy & Functional Neurology*, *Current Emergency Diagnosis & Treatment*, *Clinical Cardiology*, and *General Ophthalmology*.

The author died before completion of this book. We are grateful for the contribution he made to teaching and for his great effort in putting this teaching into book form.

The Publishers

San Mateo, California
June, 1988

Authors

Joseph G. Chusid, MD

Professor of Neurology Emeritus, New York Medical College, New York City. Director of Department of Neurology Emeritus, St. Vincent's Hospital and Medical Center, New York City.

Jack deGroot, MD, PhD

Professor of Anatomy and Radiology, University of California School of Medicine, San Francisco.

Harold H. Lindner, MD[†]

Clinical Professor of Surgery and Topographic Anatomy, University of California School of Medicine, San Francisco.

Robert A. Schindler, MD

Professor and Vice-Chairman, Ear, Nose, & Throat, Department of Otolaryngology, University of California School of Medicine, San Francisco.

Khalid F. Tabbara, MD

Professor of Ophthalmology and Chairman of Department of Ophthalmology, King Khaled Eye Specialist Hospital, Riyadh, Saudi Arabia.

[†] Deceased.

The Scalp, the Skull, & the Cerebral Meninges

1

Jack deGroot, MD, & Joseph G. Chusid, MD

EMBRYOLOGY OF THE SKULL

The skull may be divided into 2 parts: the neurocranium, which encases the brain; and the viscerocranium, which forms the skeleton of the face (see Chapter 3).

1. EMBRYOLOGY OF THE NEUROCRANIUM

The neurocranium is divided into 2 portions: (1) membranous, consisting of the flat bones that form the cranial vault; and (2) cartilaginous, consisting of the bones of the base of the skull.

The Base of the Skull

Chondrification of the mesenchyme surrounding the notochord plus the bodies of the occipital sclerotomes forms the basal plate. This plate forms the base of the skull and the occipital bone.

Anomalies. Platybasia, a deformity of occipital bone and the atlas, results from abnormal growth of the basal plate. Meningocele (herniation of the meninges through a defect protruding through the squamous portion of the occipital bone) results from failure of growth of the median plate. Malformations of the craniocerebral junction may also occur.

Sphenoid & Ethmoid Bones

Hypophyseal cartilages, trabeculae cranii, and parachordal cartilages join to form the median plate of cartilage extending from the nasal region to the anterior border of the foramen magnum. These anlagen give rise to the central portion of the sphenoid and ethmoid bones.

Mesenchymal condensations on either side of the median plate give rise to the greater and lesser wings of the sphenoid.

Anomalies are uncommon.

Temporal Bone

A mesenchymal mass lying lateral to the parachordal plate becomes the periotic capsule from which is derived the petrous and mastoid portions of the temporal bone.

Anomalies are uncommon.

Skull: Roof & Sides

Dense mesenchyme in the sides and roof of the embryonic skull undergoes membranous ossification to form the frontal and parietal bones and parts of the sphenoid, temporal, and occipital bones.

Cranioschisis (large or small skull defects)—chiefly anencephalus (failure of vault to form)—can occur. Craniostenosis (premature closure of one or more sutures) results in microcephalus, from abnormal growth of the sides and roof, when the sutures between the flat bones close prematurely. Oxycephaly (tower skull) results from bilateral premature closure of the coronal suture. Plagiocephaly (asymmetric skull) results when there is premature unilateral closure of the coronal suture.

2. EMBRYOLOGY OF THE VISCEROCRANIUM

The skeleton of the face is formed mainly from the mesenchyme of the first pharyngeal arches. (See Chapters 3 and 4.)

GROSS ANATOMY

The skull has 2 major components: the **cranium,** which houses the brain and consists of 8 bones; and the **skeleton of the face,** which is composed of 14 bones. The bones of the face are flattened, irregular, and immovably joined at their junctional areas (sutures) except for the mandible, which is movable at the temporomandibular joints.

THE SCALP

The scalp is the soft tissue covering of the calvaria (skullcap). Posteriorly, it begins at the upper border of the neck and then proceeds superiorly and anteriorly as far as the inferior border of the forehead. Laterally, it descends to the upper border of the zygomatic arches.

The scalp is made up of 5 layers. The superficial 3 layers are closely knit together and are difficult to separate. The 5 layers of the scalp are the skin, connective tissue, the epicranial aponeurosis, a layer of loose connective tissue, and the pericranium, or periosteal tissue.

The **skin** of the scalp is quite thick, especially posteriorly, where it borders the upper neck. It contains multiple sebaceous and sweat glands and has an extensive arterial and venous network and abundant lymphatic drainage. In most persons, the scalp is covered with hair.

➠ *Sebaceous cysts. The skin of the scalp is often the site of freely movable and often infected sebaceous cysts (wens) that occur as a result of plugging of a duct of a sebaceous gland. Unless they are removed completely, they tend to recur, and a second or third removal is usually more difficult.*

The **connective tissue** of the scalp is a thick, extremely vascular layer whose fibers attach the skin to the epicranial aponeurosis. There is usually a fair amount of fat within its fibrous lobules as well as in the arteries and veins.

The **epicranial aponeurosis** (galea) is a solid fibrous layer that covers the calvaria. Inserted into it are the occipitalis and frontalis muscles. The aponeurosis joins laterally with the fascia covering the temporalis muscle. The **occipitalis muscle** arises from the lateral two-thirds of the highest nuchal line and from the mastoid prominence of the temporal bones. The fibers ascend to terminate in the epicranial aponeurosis. The aponeurosis fills in the space between the medial borders of the 2 occipitalis muscles. The 2 **frontalis muscles** are wider than the occipitalis and have no bony sites of origin. Their fibers take origin from the corrugator and orbicularis oculi muscles and, more superiorly and posteriorly, meet and insert into the epicranial aponeurosis just inferior to the coronal suture. Together, the occipitofrontalis muscles raise the eyebrows and wrinkle the forehead. If the frontalis acts alone, it raises the eyebrows. The frontalis is supplied by the temporal branches of the facial nerve, while the occipitalis is supplied by the posterior auricular branch of the facial nerve.

➠ *Scalp hemorrhage. Because of the rich blood supply to the outer 3 layers of the scalp, incised wounds of the area bleed briskly, and large amounts of blood may be lost if such wounds are not treated early. Scalp wounds seldom become infected. Spread of a scalp infection into the underlying cranial bones and the meninges is rare.*

➠ *Repair of scalp wounds. Because of the frontal and occipital muscular pull upon the epicranial aponeurosis, a gaping wound results when the aponeurosis is incised. Scalp wounds must be carefully inspected, and if the aponeurosis is incised, sutures must be placed deep to it in order to properly close the wound. If the wound is superficial to the aponeurosis, sutures may be placed superficial to the aponeurosis, as such wounds will not gape.*

Loose connective tissue lies between the epicranium and the pericranium, the deepest layer of scalp tissue. It is a potential space upon which the 3 external layers of the scalp can move easily in response to contractions of the frontalis and occipitalis muscles.

➠ *Trauma to loose connective tissue. The deep loose connective tissue layer becomes involved in deep scalp lacerations. In blunt trauma to the scalp, it can become the seat of an extensive subgaleal hematoma. Secondary to deep incised scalp wounds, blood or pus may accumulate within its space. The connective tissue layer of the scalp, just superficial to the pericranium, has definite limits that prevent the spread of blood or pus to adjacent areas of the body. Posteriorly, the occipitalis and the aponeurosis are tightly fixed to the occipital bone. Laterally, the aponeurosis is fixed to the zygomatic arch and the temporal fascia. Anteriorly, because the frontalis muscle is fixed only to subcutaneous tissue, the fluids may invade the upper eyelids and the superior portion of the bridge of the nose. Spread of infection to the intracranial area is rare, but infection may on occasion use the pathway of the emissary veins to reach the brain tissue or meninges.*

The **pericranium,** the deepest layer of the scalp, is the periosteum of the cranial bones. It is held somewhat tightly to the underlying bone by connective tissue fibers. It strips easily from the bone except over the area of the cranial sutures.

➠ *Closure of cranial defects. The pericranium has very poor osteogenic potential. Consequently, when cranial bone has been lost or devitalized, there is little or no chance for bony regeneration. In such cases, a metal or Marlex type of mesh must be used to protect the brain and prevent herniation of brain tissue.*

SKULL EXTERIOR

The superior portion of the skull is called the **calvaria,** or skullcap. The shape of the skull varies in different individuals. Some display brachycephaly (broad skull), others dolichocephaly (elongated skull). These variations are readily seen on horizontal CT or MRI scans of the head. The calvaria is crossed by 3 sutures: (1) the **coronal suture,** approximately transverse in direction, between the frontal and parietal bones; (2) the **sagittal suture,** situated medially between the 2 parietal bones and deeply serrated in its anterior two-thirds; and (3) the superior portion of the **lambdoidal suture,** which lies between the 2 parietal bones and the occipital bones.

The point of juncture of the sagittal and coronal sutures is called the **bregma** and the sagittal and lambdoidal sutures the **lambda.** The bregma indicates the position of the fetal anterior fontanelle and the lambda the position of the fetal posterior fontanelle.

The **glabella** lies in the midline anteriorly. Lateral to it are the superciliary arches. Superior to the arches are the frontal eminences of the forehead. Just superior to the glabella, remnants of the frontal suture may persist and extend as the **metopic suture** to the bregma.

The temporal lines, the upper limits of the temporal fossa, may be seen passing superiorly and posteriorly from the zygomatic process of the frontal bone.

➠ *Effect of intracranial tumors on skull markings. Changes in skull markings may suggest the presence of an intracranial space-occupying lesion such as a tumor. In children, such changes include suture diastasis or separation, sella turcica changes, and increased convolutional markings of the cranial vault. In adults, intracranial tumors may cause sella turcica changes ranging from demineralization and thinning of the dorsum sellae to actual erosion or fracture. Increased vascular markings may be associated with intracranial vascular malformation. Locally increased diploic markings often occur with angioma or meningioma.*

➠ *Chronic pyogenic osteomyelitis. Chronic pyogenic osteomyelitis of the skull may simulate tumors or fibrous dysplasia. It may appear without a preceding acute infection and characteristically is an indolent process. Local manifestations are variable, ranging from no symptoms to continuous severe pain over the involved area. There is on occasion a cutaneous discharge of pus.*

FRONTAL (ANTERIOR) VIEW OF THE SKULL
(Figs 1–1 and 1–2)

The skull is roughly oval when seen from the anterior (frontal) position. The superior segment of the frontal area of the skull is formed by the squama of the frontal bone and is convex and smooth. The inferior segment of the frontal area is made up of the facial bones and contains the orbital cavities and the external nasal apertures.

The frontal eminences are joined in the midline at the glabella. Inferior to the glabella is the frontonasal suture, the midpoint of which is called the **nasion.** Lateral to the frontonasal suture, the frontal bone joins with the frontal process of the maxilla and with the lacrimal bone.

Inferior to the superciliary arch is the superior margin of the orbit, with its supraorbital notch or foramen for the passage of the supraorbital nerve and vessels. The central supraorbital border merges into the frontal zygomatic process, which articulates with the zygomatic bone.

Nasal Bones

Inferior to the frontonasal suture is the bridge of the nose, formed by the 2 nasal bones and supported in the midline by the perpendicular plate of the ethmoid and farther laterally by the frontal process of the maxilla.

Inferior to the nasal bones between the maxillas are the external apertures of the nose. Laterally, these apertures are bounded by well-defined margins to which are attached the lateral and alar nasal cartilages. The nasal apertures thicken inferiorly and curve medially to terminate in the anterior nasal spine.

Inferior and lateral to the anterior nasal apertures are the anterior surfaces of the maxillas, perforated by the infraorbital foramen just inferior to the caudal border of the orbit for passage of the infraorbital nerve and vessels. Below and medial to the infraorbital foramen is the canine eminence, which separates the incisive from the canine fossa. Deep to these fossae are the alveolar processes of the maxilla, containing the upper teeth.

The zygomatic bone forms the lateral swelling of the cheek, the inferolateral segment of the orbital cavity, and the medial segment of the zygomatic arch. It joins medially with the maxilla and with the zygomatic process of the frontal bone. It is perforated by the zygomaticofacial foramen, through which passes the zygomaticofacial nerve.

Lying in the anterior midline of the body of the mandible is a median ridge that denotes the position in fetal life of the mandibular symphysis (symphysis menti). Lying on the anterior surface of the body of the mandible beneath the second premolar tooth is the mental foramen, through which passes the mental nerve and vessels.

The Orbits
(Fig 1–2)

The orbits are 2 pyramid-shaped cavities in the upper anterior face. Their superficial borders are quadrilateral. The bases of the pyramids are superficial and directed anteriorly and laterally, while their apexes are directed posteriorly and medially. Thus, the axes of the 2 orbits, if prolonged in a dorsal direction, would meet near the center of the skull.

The roof of the orbit is formed anteriorly by the orbital plate of the frontal bone and posteriorly by the lesser wing of the sphenoid. Medially in the orbital roof is the trochlear fovea for attachment of the fibrocartilaginous pulley of the superior oblique muscle.

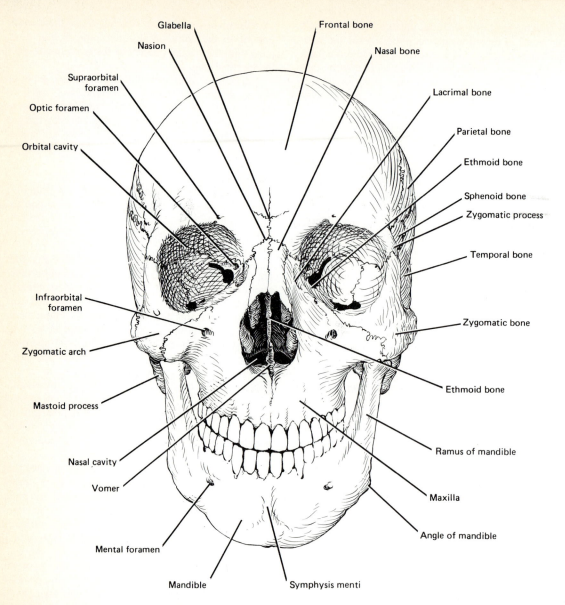

Figure 1–1. Anterior view of the skull. (Reproduced, with permission, from Chusid JG: *Correlative Neuroanatomy & Functional Neurology,* 19th ed. Lange, 1985.)

Laterally, the orbit presents the lacrimal fossa for lodgment of the lacrimal gland. Posteriorly, the orbit presents the suture that lies between the maxilla and the lesser wing of the sphenoid bone.

The area of the floor of the orbit presents as smaller than that of the roof and is directed superiorly and laterally. It is composed of the orbital surface of the maxilla, the orbital processes of the zygomatic bone, and the palatine bone. At its medial angle is the superior orifice of the nasolacrimal canal. Laterally on the orbital floor is the suture between the maxilla and zygomatic bone; posteriorly is the suture that lies between the maxilla and the orbital process of

the palatine bone. Running anteriorly in the midline of the orbital floor is the infraorbital groove, which terminates in the infraorbital canal, from which the infraorbital nerve and vessels exit onto the face.

The medial wall of the orbit is almost vertical. It is composed of the frontal process of the maxilla, the lacrimal bone, the orbital lamina of the ethmoid, and a small segment of the body of the sphenoid.

The lateral wall of the orbit is directed medially and anteriorly. It is composed of the orbital process of the zygomatic bone and the orbital surface of the great wing of the sphenoid. Near the apex of the orbit, between its roof and its lateral wall, lies

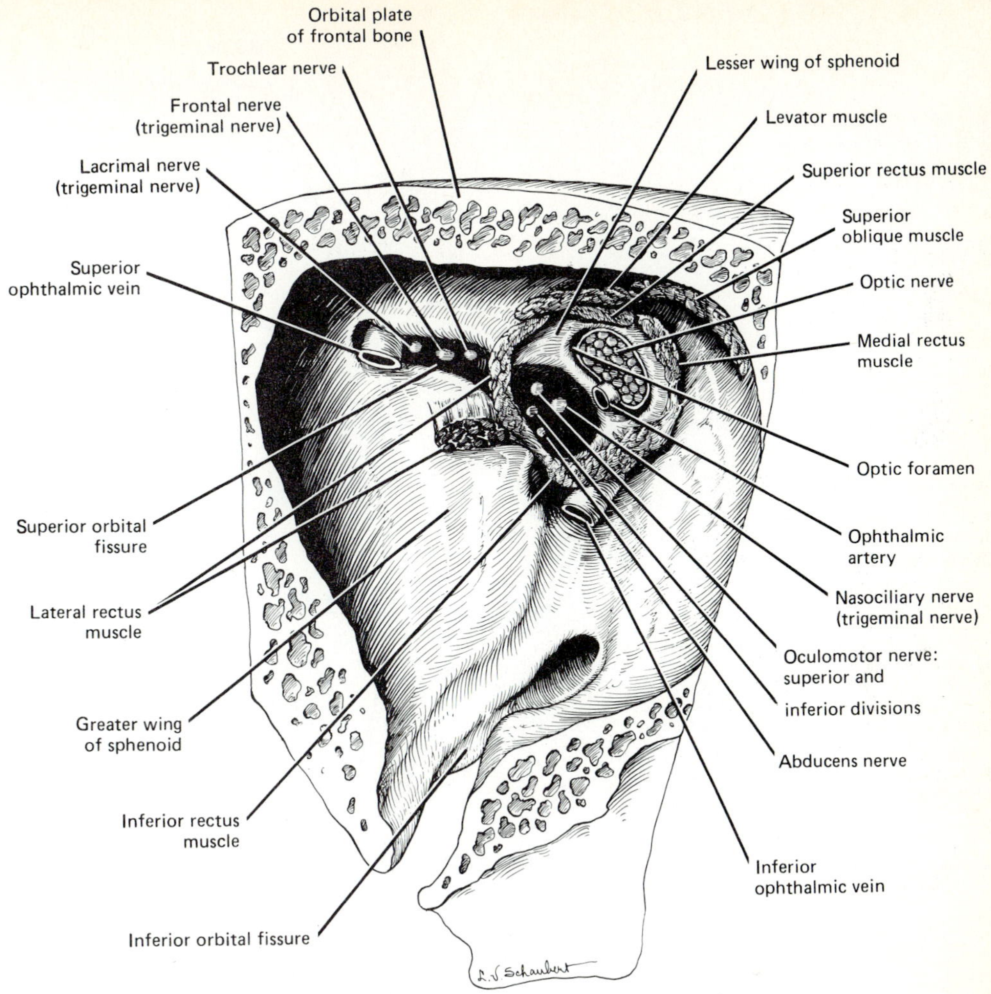

Figure 1–2. Anterior view of right orbit. (Reproduced, with permission, from Chusid JG: *Correlative Neuroanatomy & Functional Neurology,* 19th ed. Lange, 1985.)

the superior orbital fissure, through which pass the oculomotor nerve, the trochlear nerve, the ophthalmic division of the trigeminal nerve, the abducens nerve, filaments of the cavernous plexus of the sympathetic nervous system, the orbital branches of the middle meningeal artery, the superior ophthalmic vein, and the recurrent branch from the lacrimal artery, which runs to the dura mater. The lateral wall and the floor of the orbit are separated by the inferior orbital fissure.

The anterior margin of the orbit is quadrilateral, with its superior margin formed by the supraorbital arch of the frontal bone. The posterior margin or apex of the orbit continues posteriorly as the optic foramen, a short cylindric passage that transmits the optic nerve and the ophthalmic artery.

There are 9 foramens in each orbit: the optic foramen, the superior and inferior orbital fissures, the supraorbital foramen, the infraorbital canal, the anterior and posterior ethmoidal foramens, the zygomatic foramen, and the canal for the nasolacrimal duct.

➠ *Fractures about the orbit. Facial fractures in and around the orbit may exert pressure upon the optic nerve that must be relieved to prevent loss of vision.*

2. LATERAL VIEW OF THE SKULL (FIG 1–3)

The lateral aspect of the skull consists of the cranium superiorly and posteriorly and the face inferiorly and anteriorly. The principal bones of the lateral skull are the frontal, parietal, occipital, and temporal bones and the greater wing of the sphenoid. The mandible also forms part of the lateral skull.

Sutures visible in the lateral view are the zygomaticofrontal and zygomaticotemporal sutures and those that surround the greater wing of the sphenoid: sphenozygomatic, sphenofrontal, sphenoparietal, and sphenosquamosal. The pterion is the point marking the posterior end of the sphenoparietal suture.

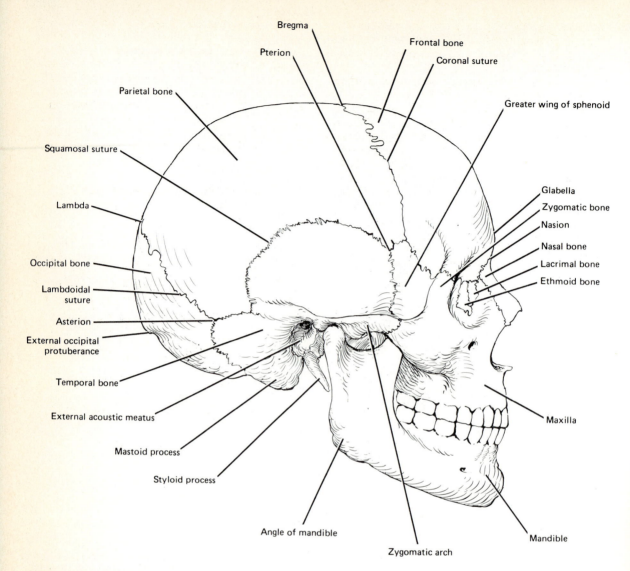

Figure 1–3. Lateral view of the skull. (Reproduced, with permission, from Chusid JG: *Correlative Neuroanatomy & Functional Neurology*, 19th ed. Lange, 1985.)

The zygomatic arch is formed by the zygomatic process of the temporal bone and the temporal process of the zygomatic bone. The tendon of the temporalis muscle passes deep to the arch in order to insert into the coronoid process of the mandible. The upper border of the arch gives attachment to the temporal fascia. The lower border and the medial surface of the arch serve as origin for the masseter muscle. Just inferior to the posterior root of the zygomatic arch is the almost circular opening of the external acoustic meatus.

➧ *Zygomatic fractures. The zygomatic arch protrudes laterally from the face and is often fractured. Depression of the fragments must be corrected in order to prevent facial deformity.*

The **mandibular fossa** lies between the tympanic portion of the temporal bone and the articular tubercle. The anterior (larger) segment of the fossa is related to the condyle of the mandible; the posterior segment usually accommodates a portion of the parotid gland. The styloid process extends inferiorly and anteriorly from the tympanic part of the temporal bone and gives attachment to the styloglossus, stylohyoid, and stylopharyngeus muscles and to the stylohyoid and stylomandibular ligaments. The mastoid process of the temporal bone projects inferiorly posterior to the external acoustic meatus; to its external surface are attached the sternocleidomastoid, splenius capitis, and longissimus capitis muscles.

The **infratemporal fossa** inferior and deep to the zygomatic arch contains the lower segment of the temporalis muscle, the pterygoid (medial and lateral) muscles, the internal maxillary vessels, and mandibular and maxillary nerves. The foramen ovale and foramen spinosum open on its roof and the alveolar canals on its anterior wall.

The **inferior orbital fissure** opens into the lateral and posterior part of the orbit. By means of the inferior orbital fissure, the orbit joins with the temporal, infratemporal, and pterygopalatine fossae. The fissure transmits the maxillary nerve and its zygomatic branch, ascending branches from the sphenopalatine ganglion, and a vein connecting the inferior ophthalmic vein with the pterygoid venous plexus.

The **pterygomaxillary fissure** is a triangular slit. It descends at right angles to the medial end of the inferior orbital fissure. It joins the infratemporal and pterygopalatine fossae, and through it pass the terminal segment of the internal maxillary veins and the internal maxillary artery.

The **pterygopalatine fossa** is a small triangular space placed at the juncture of the inferior orbital and pterygomaxillary fissures. It lies at the apex of the orbit. Five foramens open into it: 3 on its posterior wall—the foramen rotundum, the pterygoid canal, and the pharyngeal canal; and 2 on the medial wall—the pterygopalatine canal and the sphenopalatine opening. The pterygopalatine fossa contains the maxillary nerve, the pterygopalatine ganglion, and the terminal portion of the internal maxillary artery.

3. OCCIPITAL (POSTERIOR) VIEW OF THE SKULL (Fig 1–4)

Posteriorly, the cranium presents an almost circular outline. Superiorly in the midline is placed the poste-

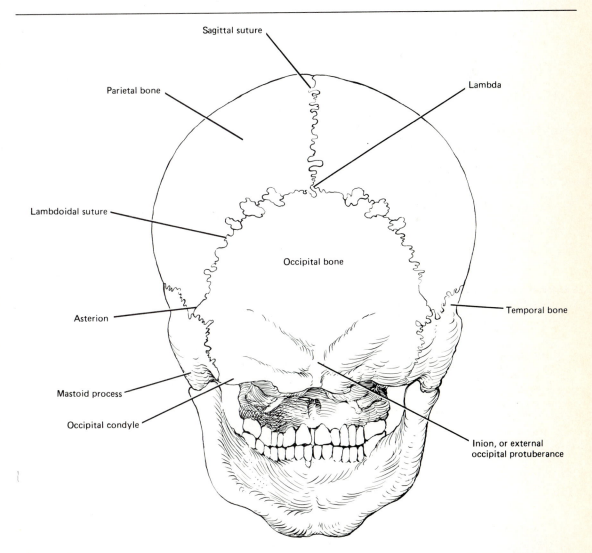

Figure 1–4. Posterior view of the skull. (Reproduced, with permission, from Chusid JG: *Correlative Neuroanatomy & Functional Neurology,* 19th ed. Lange, 1985.)

rior segment of the sagittal suture, which connects the parietal bones. The serrated lambdoidal suture joining the parietal and occipital bones extends inferiorly and laterally from the posterior end of the sagittal suture and is continuous with the parietomastoid and occipitomastoid sutures.

Close to the middle of the occipital squama is the external occipital protuberance (inion), and moving laterally from either side of it is the superior nuchal line. The occipitalis muscle covers that part of the occiput superior to the inion and the superior nuchal line.

The segment of the squama of the occipital bone that lies below the inion is called the planum nuchale. It is divided by the median nuchal line, which runs caudally and anteriorly from the inion to the foramen magnum. The ligamentum nuchae inserts into the median nuchal line.

Inferior and anterior to the occiput are the mastoid processes, which are convex laterally and grooved medially by the mastoid notches. Close to the occipito-mastoid suture is the mastoid foramen, through which passes the mastoid emissary vein.

4. BASAL (INFERIOR) VIEW OF THE SKULL (FIG 1–5)

With the mandible removed, the inferior surface of the base of the skull is seen to be formed by the palatine process of the maxillas, the palatine bones, the vomer, the pterygoid processes, the inferior sur-

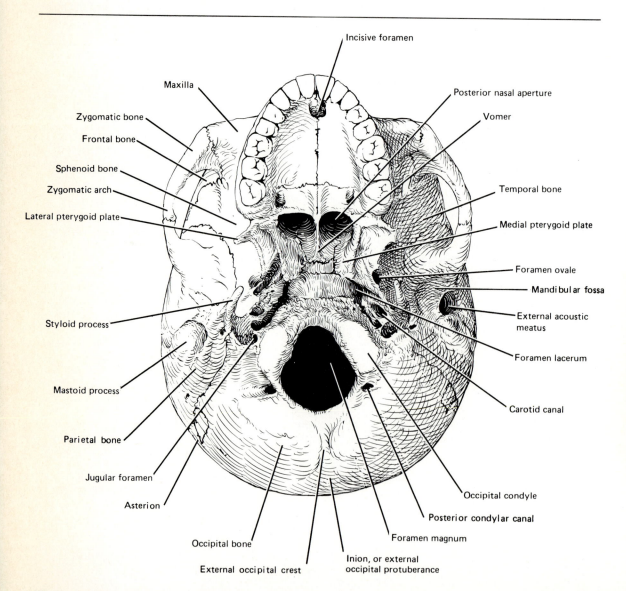

Figure 1–5. Basal view of the skull (external aspect, inferior view). (Reproduced, with permission, from Chusid JG: *Correlative Neuroanatomy & Functional Neurology*, 19th ed. Lange, 1985.)

faces of the greater wings of the sphenoid, the spinous processes, portions of the body of the sphenoid, the inferior surfaces of the squamae and the petrous portions of the temporal bone, and the inferior surface of the occipital bone.

5. BASE OF THE SKULL: FOSSAE & FORAMENS (Fig 1–6)

The anterior portion of the base of the skull, the **hard palate,** lies on a plane inferior to the level of the remainder of the inferior skull surface. It is bounded ventrally and laterally by the alveolar arch, which contains the 16 teeth of the maxillas. The hard palate is crossed by a cruciate suture formed by the junction of the 4 bones that compose the structure. At each posterior angle of the hard palate is the greater palatine foramen for the exit of the greater palatine vessels and nerves. Dorsal to this foramen is the pyramidal process of the palatine bone, perforated by several lesser palatine foramens. Projecting posteriorly from the midline of the hard palate's dorsal border is the posterior nasal spine, to which attach

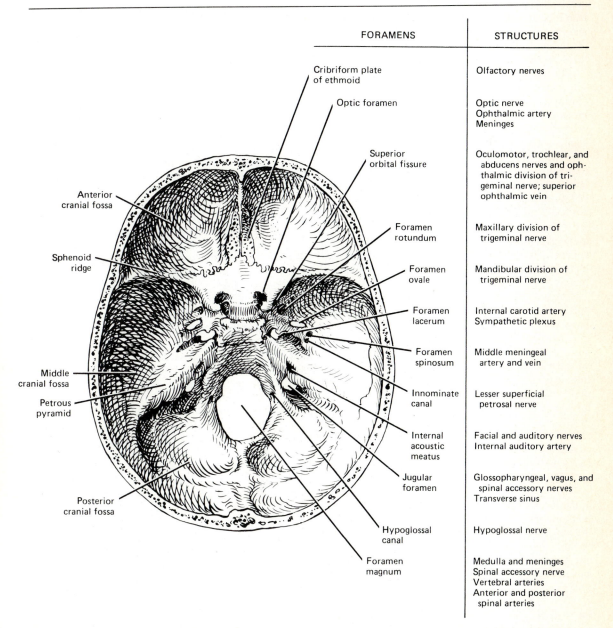

FORAMENS	STRUCTURES
Cribriform plate of ethmoid	Olfactory nerves
Optic foramen	Optic nerve, Ophthalmic artery, Meninges
Superior orbital fissure	Oculomotor, trochlear, and abducens nerves and ophthalmic division of trigeminal nerve; superior ophthalmic vein
Foramen rotundum	Maxillary division of trigeminal nerve
Foramen ovale	Mandibular division of trigeminal nerve
Foramen lacerum	Internal carotid artery, Sympathetic plexus
Foramen spinosum	Middle meningeal artery and vein
Innominate canal	Lesser superficial petrosal nerve
Internal acoustic meatus	Facial and auditory nerves, Internal auditory artery
Jugular foramen	Glossopharyngeal, vagus, and spinal accessory nerves, Transverse sinus
Hypoglossal canal	Hypoglossal nerve
Foramen magnum	Medulla and meninges, Spinal accessory nerve, Vertebral arteries, Anterior and posterior spinal arteries

(Figure labels: Anterior cranial fossa; Sphenoid ridge; Middle cranial fossa; Petrous pyramid; Posterior cranial fossa)

Figure 1–6. Base of the skull showing the fossal and principal foramens (superior view). (Reproduced, with permission, from Chusid JG: *Correlative Neuroanatomy & Functional Neurology,* 19th ed. Lange, 1985.)

the muscles controlling the movement of the uvula (musculi uvulae).

6. BASE OF THE SKULL DORSAL TO THE HARD PALATE

The choanae, the posterior openings into the nasal cavities, lie dorsal and superior to the hard palate. The medial pterygoid plate is a long, thin segment of bone. Close to the lateral side of its bone is the scaphoid fossa, from which the tensor muscle of the soft palate takes origin. At the inferior extremity of the medial pterygoid plate is the hamulus, the point at which the tendon of the tensor muscle turns. The lateral pterygoid plate is wider than the medial plate, and its lateral surface forms the medial boundary of the infratemporal fossa. This plate provides an attachment for the external pterygoid muscle.

The basilar portion of the occipital bone lies posterior to the nasal cavities. Close to its center is the pharyngeal tubercle for attachment of the central fibrous raphe of the pharynx. Onto this portion of the occiput attach the musculi longus capitis and rectus capitis anterior.

At the base of the lateral pterygoid plate is the foramen ovale for transmission of the mandibular nerve (the third branch of the trigeminal nerve), the accessory meningeal artery, and occasionally the superficial petrosal nerve. Posterior to the foramen ovale are the foramen spinosum, which transmits the middle meningeal vessels, and the well-marked sphenoidal spine (spina angularis), to which attach the sphenomandibular ligament and the tensor veli palatini muscle.

The mandibular fossa is lateral to the sphenoidal spines and divided into 2 segments by the petrotympanic fissure.

The styloid process projects from between the laminae of the tympanic part of the temporal bone. At the base of the styloid process is the stylomastoid foramen for exit of the facial nerve and entrance of the stylomastoid artery. Lateral to the stylomastoid foramen is the tympanomastoid fissure for passage of the auricular branch of the vagus. On the medial side of the mastoid process is the mastoid notch for attachment of the posterior belly of the digastric muscle, while medial to the notch is placed the occipital groove for reception of the occipital artery.

The foramen lacerum is a large triangular aperture at the base of the medial pterygoid plate. Its inferior portion is closed by a fibrocartilaginous plate. Within the superior aspect of the foramen lacerum is the opening of the carotid canal. The internal carotid artery as it leaves the carotid canal crosses only the superior opening of the foramen lacerum.

➠ *Pathologic enlargements of skull foramens. Local erosions or enlargements of the skull foramens occur with some intracranial neo-*plasms. *An acoustic neuroma causes enlargement of the internal auditory meatus, usually resulting in a funnel-shaped deformity. An optic nerve glioma may enlarge the optic foramen. The superior orbital fissure may be enlarged by a retro-orbital aneurysm or meningioma. The foramen spinosum may be enlarged by an ipsilateral meningioma near the foramen because of the increase in size of the middle meningeal vessel.*

Lateral to the foramen lacerum is a groove, the sulcus tubae auditivae, in which lies the cartilaginous part of the auditory (eustachian) tube. This segment of the tube is continuous posteriorly with the canal in the temporal bone that forms the bony segment of the auditory tube. Situated in the deep surface of the sulcus is the petrosphenoidal fissure, and posterior to the fissure is a quadrilateral rough surface for attachment of the tensor veli palatini. Lateral to this rough surface is the opening of the carotid canal, which transmits the internal carotid artery and the carotid plexus of nerves derived from the sympathetic plexus of the autonomic nervous system.

Posterior to the carotid canal is the large jugular foramen, bounded laterally by the petrous portion of the temporal bone and medially by the occipital bone. The jugular foramen may be subdivided into 3 compartments: The anterior compartment contains the inferior petrosal sinus; the middle compartment contains the glossopharyngeal, the vagus, and the cranial part of the spinal accessory nerves; and the posterior compartment contains the transverse sinus and minor meningeal branches from both the occipital and ascending pharyngeal arteries.

Dorsal to the basilar portion of the occipital bone is the **foramen magnum,** which transmits the medulla oblongata and its covering membranes, the spinal segment of the spinal accessory nerves, the vertebral arteries, the anterior and posterior spinal arteries, and the ligaments that join the occipital bone to the axis (C2). The foramen magnum is bounded laterally by the occipital condyles.

Posterior to each occipital condyle is the condyloid fossa, perforated on one or both sides by the posterior condyloid canal, transmitting a vein that is a branch of the transverse sinus. Anterior to the occipital condyles is an anterior canal for the hypoglossal nerve and a minor meningeal artery. Dorsal to the foramen magnum is the median nuchal line, which terminates superiorly at the external occipital protuberances. On either side of the foramen are the superior and inferior nuchal lines.

SKULL INTERIOR

INNER SURFACE OF THE CALVARIA

The inner concave surface of the calvaria, or skull-cap, has multiple depressions into which fit the convolutions of the cerebrum. It also presents numerous furrows in which run branches of the meningeal vessels. In the midline is a groove that is narrow anteriorly and widens as it runs posteriorly. This groove contains the superior sagittal sinus, and its lateral edges provide attachment for the falx cerebri. On either side of the groove are a few depressions for the arachnoidal granulations. The superior sagittal sinus is crossed anteriorly by the coronal suture and posteriorly by the lambdoidal suture.

Internal Surface of the Base of the Skull

The internal surface of the base of the skull forms the floor of the cranial cavity and is composed of 3 fossae: anterior, middle, and posterior (Fig 1–6).

1. ANTERIOR CRANIAL FOSSA

The base of the anterior cranial fossa is composed of the orbital plates of the frontal bone, the cribriform plate of the ethmoid, and the lesser wings and the smooth anterior segment of the sphenoid—the jugum or planum sphenoidale. It is bounded posteriorly by the posterior borders of the lesser wings of the sphenoid and by the anterior border of the optic chiasmal groove. It is crossed by the frontoethmoidal and sphenofrontal sutures.

The lateral segments of the anterior cranial fossa form the roof of the orbital cavity, and upon them rest the frontal lobes of the cerebrum. Its medial segments lie on either side of the crista galli and act as the roof of the nasal cavity.

The olfactory groove of the cribriform plate of the ethmoid bone, lying on either side of the crista galli, supports the olfactory bulb. It shows multiple small openings for passage of the olfactory nerves. It is also perforated by a slit for the passage of the nasociliary nerve. The crista galli, between the cribriform plates, forms the inferior attachment of the falx cerebri.

➠ *Cerebrospinal fluid rhinorrhea. Cerebrospinal fluid rhinorrhea (leakage of spinal fluid from the nose) may follow fracture of the frontal bone associated with tearing of the dura mater and the arachnoid over the cribriform plate of the ethmoid. Erect posture and straining and coughing usually cause an increase in the amount of fluid flow. Replacement of lost fluid by air entering the cranial vault through the same or a similar pathway may lead to aerocele.*

Infection and meningitis are hazards in cerebrospinal fluid rhinorrhea and may be prevented by the early use of prophylactic antibiotics. Surgical repair of the dural tear may be necessary to stop the flow of fluid and prevent infection.

2. MIDDLE CRANIAL FOSSA

The middle cranial fossa is deeper than the anterior cranial fossa and is narrow centrally and wide peripherally. It is bounded ventrally by the posterior borders of the lesser wings of the sphenoid and the anterior clinoid processes of the sella turcica and by the elevation that forms the anterior margin of the groove for the optic chiasm. It is bounded dorsally by the superior angles of the petrous portion of the temporal bones and by the dorsum of the sella turcica, and laterally by the squamae of the temporal bones, the sphenoidal angles of the parietal bones, and the greater wings of the sphenoid bone.

Anteriorly, the mid segment of the fossa presents a groove for the optic chiasm and the tuberculum sellae. The groove for the optic chiasm terminates at the optic foramen, which serves to convey the optic nerve and the ophthalmic artery as well as the meninges to the orbital cavity.

Dorsal to the optic foramen lies the anterior clinoid process, which is directed dorsally and medially and gives attachment to the tentorium cerebelli.

Posterior to the tuberculum sellae lies a deep depression, the sella turcica, which contains the hypophysis (pituitary gland).

The sella turcica is bounded posteriorly by a square plate of bone, the dorsum sellae, whose posterior angles are crowned by the posterior clinoid processes, which give attachment to the tentorium cerebelli. Inferior to each posterior clinoid is a notch for the abducens nerve.

Lateral to the sella turcica is the carotid groove, which is wide and shallow. This groove extends from the foramen lacerum to the medial side of the anterior clinoid process. Here it often becomes the caroticoclinoid foramen as a result of the union of the anterior and middle clinoid processes. The cavernous sinus is covered by dura that attaches to the lateral border of the carotid groove. The carotid groove lodges the cavernous sinus and the internal carotid artery, which at this point is surrounded by a profuse plexus of nerves.

The lateral segments of the middle cranial fossa are quite deep, and the temporal lobes of the brain rest upon them. They are marked by depressions for the brain convolutions and show multiple furrows for the anterior and posterior branches of the middle meningeal vessels. From a point close to the foramen spinosum, the anterior branch of the middle meningeal artery runs to the sphenoidal angle of the parietal bone. The posterior branch of the same artery runs laterally across the temporal squama and proceeds onto the parietal bone near the center of the bone's inferior border.

⬛➡ *Middle meningeal artery hemorrhage. Extradural hemorrhage classically follows traumatic rupture of the posterior branch of the middle meningeal artery and is often difficult to detect early. Transient loss of consciousness followed by apparent recovery usually occurs. The patient then starts to develop signs of increasing intracranial pressure as a result of accumulation of blood in the extradural space from the ruptured vessel. Untreated, the condition progresses rapidly to death in a few hours. Any temporal bone fracture that on skull x-ray appears to cross the middle meningeal groove should alert the clinician to the possibility of this so-called middle meningeal arterial rupture syndrome. CT scan is used to show both the hemorrhage and the fracture. MRI readily demonstrates the location and extent of the epidural hematoma and the fracture.*

The superior orbital fissure lies in the anterior portion of the middle fossa, bounded superiorly by the lesser wing of the sphenoid, inferiorly by the greater wing of the sphenoid, medially by the body of the sphenoid, and laterally by the orbital plate of the frontal bone. It transmits to the orbital cavity the oculomotor nerve, the trochlear nerve, the ophthalmic division of the trigeminal nerve, the abducens nerve, some filaments from the cavernous autonomic plexus, and the orbital branch of the middle meningeal artery. Leaving the orbital cavity via the fissure is a recurrent branch of the lacrimal artery, which supplies the dura mater. The ophthalmic veins also leave by this portal.

Dorsal to the medial wall of the superior orbital fissure lies the **foramen rotundum,** which allows for passage of the maxillary nerve. Dorsal and lateral to the foramen rotundum is the **foramen ovale,** which transmits the mandibular nerve, the accessory meningeal artery, and the lesser superficial petrosal nerve.

The foramen ovale lies just lateral to the **foramen spinosum.** It allows for passage of the middle meningeal vessels and a recurrent branch from the mandibular nerve.

Medial to the foramen ovale is the foramen lacerum. The internal carotid artery passes through the superomedial portion of the foramen lacerum. The inferior portion of the foramen is closed by fibrocartilage and pierced by the small nerve of the pterygoid canal and by a meningeal branch arising from the ascending pharyngeal artery.

On the ventral projection of the petrous portion of the temporal bone is the arcuate eminence, a projection of the superior semicircular canal. Ventral to and slightly lateral to this projection is a hollowed area that corresponds to the roof of the tympanic cavity. Medial to the arcuate eminence is the groove leading to the hiatus of the facial canal for transmission of the greater superficial petrosal nerve and the petrosal branch of the middle meningeal artery. Inferior to the arcuate eminence is a small groove for passage of the lesser superficial petrosal nerve, and near the apex of the petrous bone is the depression containing the semilunar ganglion and the orifice of the carotid canal.

3. POSTERIOR CRANIAL FOSSA

The posterior cranial fossa is the deepest and most capacious of the 3 cranial fossae. It is composed of the dorsum sellae; the clivus of the sphenoid; the occipital, petrous, and mastoid segments of the temporal bones; and the mastoid angles or portions of the parietal bones. The occipitomastoid and parietomastoid sutures cross it.

The posterior fossa contains the cerebellum, pons, and medulla oblongata. It is separated from the middle cranial fossa by the dorsum sellae of the sphenoid bone and by the superior angles of the petrous portion of the temporal bone. This angle provides attachment for the tentorium cerebelli and contains in a groove the superior petrosal sinus.

Located centrally in the posterior fossa is the foramen magnum. On each side of the foramen is a rough tubercle for attachment of the alar ligaments. Just superior to the tubercle is the hypoglossal canal, which transmits the hypoglossal nerve and a meningeal branch of the ascending pharyngeal artery.

Anterior to the foramen magnum, the basilar segment of the occipital bone and the dorsal segment of the body of the sphenoid bone form a grooved surface for support of the adjacent brain stem (medulla and pons). In children, the 2 bones in this position are joined by a synchondrosis. On either side, the petrooccipital fissure is continuous dorsally with the jugular foramen. The edges of the fissure are grooved for passage of the inferior petrosal sinus.

The jugular foramen lies between the lateral segment of the occipital bone and the petrous portion of the temporal bone. The ventral segment of the foramen permits passage of the inferior petrosal sinus; the posterior segment permits passage of the transverse sinus and meningeal branches from the occipital and ascending pharyngeal arteries. The central segment of the foramen passes the glossopharyngeal, vagus, and spinal accessory nerves. Superior and lateral to the jugular foramen is the internal acoustic meatus for passage of the facial and acoustic nerves and the internal auditory artery.

⬛➡ *Cerebrospinal fluid otorrhea. Leakage of cerebrospinal fluid from the ear is usually caused by injuries to the posterior cranial fossa close to the internal acoustic meatus. It is a serious prognostic sign because it is caused by injuries to vital areas of the base of the brain.*

The squamous portion of the occipital bone supports the hemisphere of the cerebellum. A midline internal occipital crest serves for attachment of the falx cerebelli. The occipital sinus lies on this crest.

The posterior fossa is surrounded by deep grooves containing the transverse sinuses and sigmoid sinuses. Each of these depressions, in passing to and ending at the jugular foramen, grooves the occipital bone, the mastoid angle of the parietal bone, the mastoid portion of the temporal bone, and the jugular portion of the occipital bone.

THE CEREBRAL MENINGES
(Fig 1–7)

1. DURA MATER

The dura mater, or pachymeninx, is a dense fibrous structure that serves as the outer layer of the covering of the brain and spinal cord. It is made up of an inner meningeal and an outer periosteal layer. Over the brain, the 2 dural layers generally are fused except where they separate to provide space for the intervening venous sinuses.

The outer layer of the dura attaches firmly to the inner surface of the cranial bones and sends vascular and fibrous extensions into the bone itself. The subdural space lies between the dura mater and the arachnoid.

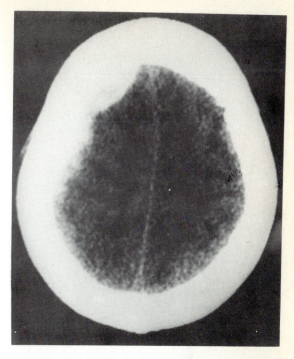

Figure 1–8. Horizontal CT image high through the head; a high-density irregular layer covers the right hemisphere. This image is compatible with an acute subdural hemorrhage.

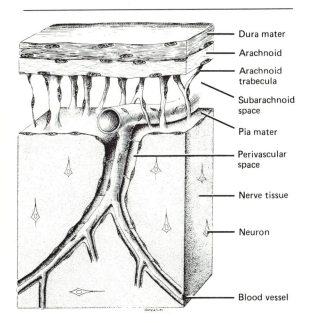

Figure 1–7. Schematic drawing of the meninges. The blood vessel initially located in the subarachnoid space penetrates the nerve tissue and is partly enveloped by the pia mater. (Reproduced, with permission, from Junqueira LC, Carneiro J, Long JA: *Basic Histology*, 5th ed. Appleton & Lange, 1986.)

Labels for Figure 1–7:
- Dura mater
- Arachnoid
- Arachnoid trabecula
- Subarachnoid space
- Pia mater
- Perivascular space
- Nerve tissue
- Neuron
- Blood vessel

➠ *Bleeding into the subdural space. (Figs 1–8 and 1–9.) Bleeding into the subdural space may follow relatively minor head injuries. The subdural space is ordinarily filled with small amounts of lymph-like material and has little or no capacity to absorb blood. Bleeding into the space usually follows rupture of a subdural vein. The hematoma gradually increases in size and later may be enveloped by a mesothelial membrane. Signs of increasing intracranial pressure, focal neurologic deficits, and personality changes may appear early or weeks, months, or even years after injury. CT scan, MRI, or angiography is diagnostic. Acute subdural bleeding of minor degree may not require operative management. However, a massive subdural hematoma usually requires surgical treatment. Evacuation of the hematoma through trephine openings usually gives rapid relief.*

The inner layer of the dura encloses the venous sinuses and forms partitions between the brain segments. These partitions are as follows:

(1) The **falx cerebri,** which extends inferiorly into the longitudinal fissure between the right and left cerebral hemispheres. It attaches to the inner surface of the skull bones along the midline, reaching from the crista galli to the internal occipital protuberance,

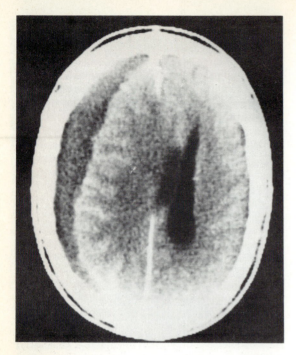

Figure 1–9. Horizontal CT image through the head; a low-density crescent covers the right hemisphere, causing a right to left shift of the brain and ventricles. This image represents a chronic subdural hematoma.

from which point it continues as the tentorium cerebelli.

(2) The **tentorium cerebelli,** which separates the occipital lobes of the cerebrum from the cerebellum. It is a sloping transverse dural membrane that attaches posteriorly and laterally to the transverse sinuses and anteriorly to the petrous portion of the temporal bone and to both anterior and posterior clinoid processes of the sphenoid bone. Toward the midline, it slopes upward and joins with the falx cerebri. Its free border curves laterally and in so doing leaves a sizable oval opening, the incisura tentorii, through which the midbrain passes.

(3) The **falx cerebelli,** a dural sheet that projects into the posterior cerebellar notch between the cerebellar hemispheres via its free border. It extends from the inner surface of the occipital bone as a small triangular process.

(4) The **diaphragma sellae,** which forms a ceiling over the hypophysis, which lies within the sella turcica. It joins the clinoidal attachments of the 2 sides of the tentorium cerebelli.

2. ARACHNOID

The arachnoid is a thin avascular membrane between the dura mater and pia mater. It is separated from the overlying dura mater by the subdural space and from the underlying pia mater by the subarachnoid space, which contains the cerebrospinal fluid. Together, the arachnoid and the pia are called the leptomeninges.

The inner surface of the arachnoid is connected to the pia mater by the arachnoid trabeculae. The cranial arachnoid lies in close apposition to the inner surface of the dura mater, separated from it only by the subdural space, which contains a thin film of fluid. The arachnoid does not dip into the fissures and sulci of the brain except where it follows the course of the falx and the tentorium. The subarachnoid space is quite narrow where it covers the surface of the cerebral hemispheres. However, at the base of the brain the arachnoid becomes thicker, and in some areas there is a group of dilated spaces called the subarachnoid cisterns. These derive their names from their anatomic positions.

The **cisterna magna** (cisterna cerebellomedullaris) is present between the medulla and the inferior surface of the cerebellar hemispheres. It is continuous with the spinal subarachnoid space and is shaped like a pyramid when seen in sagittal section. The **cisterna pontis** is related to the mid portion of the ventral surface of the pons and contains the basilar artery. The **cisterna basalis** (cisterna interpeduncularis) is the wide cavity that lies between the 2 temporal lobes. It includes the interpeduncular fossa and extends rostrally over the optic chiasm, where it forms the **cisterna chiasmatis.**

Arachnoid granulations are villose or berrylike areas of arachnoid that protrude into the superior sagittal sinus or its associated venous lacunae. With advancing age, these villi increase in size and number, on occasion pushing against the overlying dura and causing bone absorption and depressions of the inner table of the calvaria.

➠ *Bleeding into the subarachnoid space.* (Fig 1–10.) Bleeding into the subarachnoid space may occur spontaneously or secondary to cranial injury. In either case, the clinical diagnostic features are similar and consist of sudden severe headache, often with impairment or loss of consciousness, painful neck stiffness (Kernig's sign), and the presence of fresh blood in the cerebrospinal fluid on lumbar spinal tap or on CT scan or MRI. Massive hemorrhage is often fatal; lesser hemorrhages often resolve with few or no residual neurologic deficits. In patients with spontaneous hemorrhage, the possibility of an underlying aneurysm or vascular malformation must be excluded by arteriography and treated surgically if feasible.*

3. PIA MATER

The thin inner connective tissue layer of the meninges, the pia mater, is the closest to the brain and spinal cord of the 3 meningeal layers and carries to

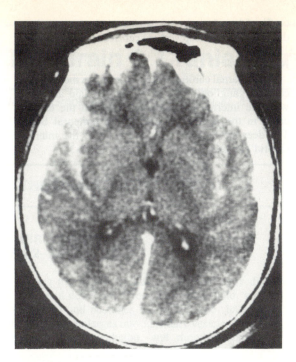

Figure 1–10. Horizontal CT image through the head; high-intensity contents of the fissures and sulci, especially on the right side, represent a subarachnoid hemorrhage probably from a right middle cerebral trifurcation aneurysm.

the brain and cord the blood vessels that supply them. The pia mater covers the entire brain surface, extending down into the divisional sulci and fissures. In extending into the transverse cerebral fissure, it forms the tela choroidea of the third ventricle and combines with the ependyma to form the choroid plexuses of the lateral and third ventricles. The pia mater passes over the roof of the fourth ventricle and forms its tela choroidea and choroid plexus.

BLOOD VESSELS, LYMPHATICS, & NERVES

Arteries

The skull and meninges are supplied by branches of the external carotid and vertebral arteries and by intracranial branches of the internal carotid artery.

A. External Carotid Artery: The following are some of the branches that supply the skull and meninges.

1. Ascending pharyngeal artery–Branches of this artery include the inferior tympanic artery, which supplies the medial wall of the tympanic cavity. Meningeal branches of the ascending pharyngeal artery enter the skull through the jugular foramen, hypoglossal canal, and foramen lacerum to supply the dura mater.

2. Occipital artery–The auricular branch of this artery may enter the skull through the mastoid foramen to supply the dura mater, the diploë, and the mastoid cells of the temporal bone. A meningeal branch enters the skull through the jugular foramen and the condylar canal to supply the dura mater of the posterior fossa. The terminal branches of the occipital artery on occasion send a branch to the pericranium and also give off a small meningeal branch.

3. Maxillary artery–This vessel, through its multiple branches, supplies chiefly the deep facial structures. However, the following branches supply the skull and meninges: (1) The middle meningeal artery enters the skull through the foramen spinosum of the sphenoid bone. The vessel divides into an anterior and a posterior branch, each of which supplies the inner cranial surface of the temporal bone and the neighboring dura mater. (2) The accessory meningeal branch enters the skull via the foramen ovale and supplies the neighboring dura mater.

B. Internal Carotid Artery: Both the cavernous branches and the meningeal branches of the petrous segment of the internal carotid supply the walls of the cavernous and inferior petrosal sinuses and the dura mater of the anterior cranial fossa, as well as the tentorium cerebelli.

The ophthalmic artery has branches as follows: (1) The lacrimal artery, which sends a recurrent branch dorsally through the superior orbital fissure to supply the dura mater of the anterior cranial fossa. (2) The posterior ethmoidal artery, which sends twigs to the dura.

C. Vertebral Artery: Several arterial twigs from the multiple intracranial branches of the vertebral artery supply the dura of the posterior cranial fossa.

Veins

The **sinuses of the dura mater** form a venous pathway lined by endothelium along which blood from the brain passes on its way to the internal jugular vein. They contain no valves and lie between 2 layers of dura mater. They are generally listed as 2 separate but communicating groups—a posterosuperior group and an anteroinferior group. The posterosuperior group consists of the superior and inferior sagittal sinuses, the straight and transverse sinuses, the occipital sinus, and the confluence of the sinuses. The anteroinferior group is composed of the cavernous, circular, superior, and inferior petrosal sinuses and the basilar plexus, which anastomoses with the epidural vertebral plexus.

The **diploic veins** are found in the diploic spaces of the cranial bones. They join both with the meningeal veins and the dural sinuses and with the pericranial veins.

The **emissary veins** are communications between the intracranial dural sinuses and the venous channels on the exterior of the skull. They form potential pathways for spread of infection. The major emissary veins are the mastoid emissary vein, the parietal emissary vein, a group of very small veins that pass out

Anomalies. The prosencephalon may present the following anomalies: (1) exencephaly, in which the brain protrudes from the cranium; (2) anencephaly, wherein the rostral part of the neural tube fails to close; (3) hydranencephaly, in which the cerebral hemispheres are absent and the cranium is intact; (4) agenesis of the corpus callosum; and (5) encephalocele, in which brain structures extrude through an opening in the cranium.

Mesencephalon

The mesencephalon (midbrain) forms the quadrigeminal plate and the cerebral peduncles, and within it is the cerebral aqueduct.

Anomalies. In hydrocephalus, all or part of the ventricular system is enlarged. The usual developmental cause is aqueductal stenosis.

Rhombencephalon

The rhombencephalon (hindbrain) develops into (1) the metencephalon and (2) the myelencephalon. The metencephalon forms the cerebellum and the pons, while the myelencephalon forms the medulla oblongata. The fourth ventricle lies within the pons and the medulla.

Anomalies. In **Arnold-Chiari malformation,** a tonguelike projection of the medulla and cerebellum herniates through the foramen magnum. This anomaly is often associated with meningomyelocele or spina bifida.

GROSS ANATOMY

The brain is enclosed within the cranial cavity of the skull and covered by 3 protective membranes, the meninges. The brain is grossly divided into the cerebrum, the cerebellum, and the brain stem (midbrain, pons, and medulla).

CEREBRUM
(Figs 2–1 and 2–2)

The cerebrum is divided into 2 cerebral hemispheres, which make up the largest portion of the brain. Each cerebral hemisphere is made up of the frontal, parietal, temporal, and occipital lobes and the insula.

The Frontal Lobe

The frontal lobe of the cerebrum extends from the frontal pole to the central sulcus posteriorly and as far as the lateral fissure laterally.

➠ *Focal brain dysfunction. Irritative lesions of the motor centers in the frontal lobe may cause convulsive seizures, beginning as contralateral focal twitchings and spreading to involve large muscle groups according to their representations in the central cortex (jacksonian epilepsy). This type of seizure may or may not be associated with alterations of consciousness and is frequently followed by postictal weakness or paralysis.*

Irritative lesions elsewhere in the frontal lobe may cause seizures characterized by repetitive, stereotyped ideational disturbances, vocalizations, hallucinations, impairment of external awareness, and repetitive motor activity (complex partial seizures).

➠ *Destructive lesions of the motor cortex. Acute destructive lesions of the motor cortex produce contralateral flaccid paresis or paralysis of affected muscle groups.*

➠ *Destructive lesions of the frontal lobe. The portion of the frontal lobe anterior to the precentral gyrus is associated with higher intellectual and psychic functions. Classically, destructive lesions of this area may produce personality changes, facetiousness, changes in moral and social attitudes, disinterest in the environment and in former interests, mental slowing, intellectual deterioration, and easy distractibility.*

➠ *Frontal lobe tumors. Brain tumors involving the frontal lobe tend to produce a disturbed mental state marked by defective memory, impaired judgment, irritability, mood changes, facetiousness, and contralateral hemiplegia. Convulsive seizures may also occur. In right-handed individuals, frontal lobe tumors may produce expressive aphasia and agraphia if located in the left hemisphere (the dominant hemisphere). Anosmia may occur secondary to a tumor at the base of the frontal lobe.*

➠ *Aphasia and speech defects. Aphasia (speech defects) resulting from the cortical lesions illustrate the significance of association areas. In right-handed persons, aphasia is produced by lesions in the left (dominant) hemisphere. Motor aphasia may result from destruction of the triangular and opercular portions of the inferior frontal gyrus. The individual can move his or her lips and tongue but is unable to formulate speech. Agraphia (inability to write words) is associated with motor aphasia.*

The Parietal Lobe

The parietal lobe extends from the central sulcus to the parieto-occipital fissure and laterally to the level of the lateral cerebral fissure (fissure of Sylvius).

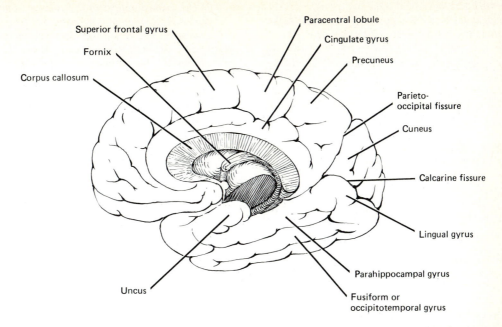

Figure 2–2. Medial view of right cerebral hemisphere. (Reproduced, with permission, from Chusid JG: *Correlative Neuroanatomy & Functional Neurology,* 19th ed. Lange, 1985.)

⟫ *Irritative lesions of the postcentral gyrus. Irritative lesions of the postcentral gyrus produce contralateral paresthesias, eg, numbness, formication, and sensations of electric shock or pins and needles. Destructive lesions produce objective impairment in sensibility, eg, inability to localize or gauge the intensity of painful stimuli, a diminution in the various forms of cutaneous sensation, or sensory neglect.*

⟫ *Lesions of the parietal lobe association areas. The parietal lobe association centers are necessary for correlation of cutaneous sensations and thus make it possible with the eyes closed to recognize familiar objects placed in the hands. This skill is called stereognosis; its loss (astereognosis) may be due to lesions of the parietal cortex.*

⟫ *Parietal lobe tumors.* (*Fig 2–3.*) *Sensory and motor abnormalities are common in parietal lobe tumors. The abnormalities may include motor or sensory focal seizures, contralateral hemiparesis, hyperreflexia, impaired sensory perception, astereognosis, and extensor plantar responses. Aphasia, agraphia, acalculia, alexia, and agnostic components may also be present when the dominant side is involved, and anosognosia and dressing apraxia with lesions of either side.*

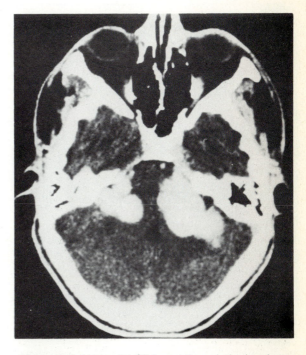

Figure 2–3. Horizontal CT image through the head; an irregular mass with surrounding edema lies in the left parietal lobe (pathology: glioblastoma).

Occipital Lobe

The occipital lobe is the pyramid-shaped posterior lobe behind the parieto-occipital fissure.

⟾ **Lesions of the occipital cortex.** *Irritative lesions of the occipital cortex may produce visual hallucinations, eg, flashes of light, rainbows, brilliant stars, or bright lines. Destructive lesions of the occipital cortex may cause contralateral homonymous defects in the visual fields; if they involve all of the calcarine cortex, there is destruction of macular vision contralaterally.*

⟾ **Occipital lobe tumors.** *Visual defects and seizures preceded by an aura of lights or by visual hallucinations are characteristic of tumors in the occipital lobe. In addition, contralateral homonymous hemianopia occurs; whether there is sparing of the macular area depends on the site of the tumor. Agnosia may be present.*

Temporal Lobe

The temporal lobe is inferior to the lateral cerebral fissure and extends posteriorly to the level of the parieto-occipital fissure.

⟾ **Sensory aphasia secondary to temporal lobe lesions.** *Sensory aphasia results from lesions in the posterior part of the superior temporal gyrus in the dominant hemisphere. The patient may hear the spoken word or see the written word but cannot comprehend its meaning. Word blindness—the inability to understand written words although vision is unimpaired—may result from* parieto-*occipital lesions.*

⟾ **Seizures secondary to temporal lobe tumors.** *Complex partial (psychomotor) seizures and automatisms may occur with temporal lobe tumors. If the dominant side is involved, sensory aphasia may be marked. A contralateral homonymous field defect may occur.*

In summary, the frontal lobe contains the principal motor area and the parietal lobe the primary sensory area; the occipital lobe contains the primary visual cortex; and the temporal lobe contains the primary auditory cortex.

The Insula
(Figs 2–4 and 2–5)

The insula (island of Reil) lies deep within the lateral cerebral fissure and can be exposed by separating the upper and lower lips of the fissure. Electrical stimulation of the posterior part of the orbital surface and of the contiguous anterior half of the insula produces marked autonomic effects. Inhibition of respira-

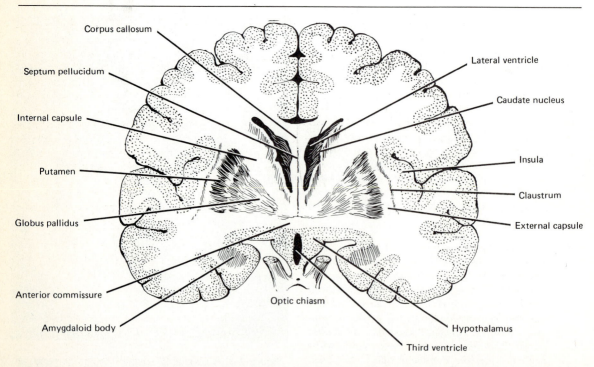

Figure 2–4. Coronal section through cerebrum at levels of anterior commissure. (Reproduced, with permission, from Chusid JG: *Correlative Neuroanatomy & Functional Neurology,* 19th ed. Lange, 1985.)

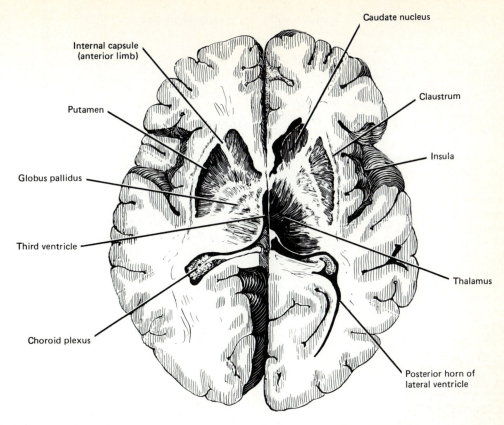

Figure 2–5. Horizontal sections through cerebrum at 2 levels to show basal ganglia. (Reproduced, with permission, from Chusid JG: *Correlative Neuroanatomy & Functional Neurology*, 19th ed. Lange, 1985.)

tion and alteration of blood pressure may also be readily induced by such stimulation.

White Substance

The white substance (white matter) of the cerebral hemisphere contains neuroglia and medullated (myelinated) nerve fibers. Three types of medullated nerve fibers make up the central portion of the cerebral hemisphere: (1) **transverse (commissural)** fibers, which connect the 2 cerebral hemispheres; (2) **projection fibers,** which connect the cerebral cortex with the lower portion of the brain and the spinal cord; and (3) **association fibers,** which connect the various portions of the same cerebral hemisphere.

➠ *Cerebral palsy. Infantile spastic hemiplegia is the most common form of cerebral palsy, accounting for about one-third of all cases. Prenatal spastic hemiplegia is uncommon (< 5%) and is caused by brain malformations or prenatal "stroke" due to toxemia. Of the types of infantile spastic hemiplegia, natal spastic hemiplegia is the most common (65%). Predisposing factors include prematurity and low birth weight and perhaps bleeding diathesis. Forceps trauma may injure the brain, and physiologic*

hazards of birth may cause injury to the fetal head, which acts as a battering ram during labor; pelvic disproportion, dystocia, or oxytocin induction may aggravate physiologic trauma. Postnatal infantile spastic hemiplegia is common (> 30%). It comprises over 90% of all postnatal cerebral palsies.

Mental retardation and convulsive seizures are common in all forms of infantile spastic hemiplegia. The upper extremity is more often involved than the lower. The sensory handicap may be more disabling than the motor handicap because proprioception and form discrimination are lost. Failure of growth may be of cerebral origin owing to involvement of the postcentral gyrus. Hemianopia may follow damage to the occipital lobe.

Basal Ganglia
(Figs 2–4 and 2–5)

The basal ganglia are masses of gray matter situated deep within the cerebral hemispheres. The corpus striatum includes the caudate and lentiform nuclei and a band of white fibers separating them, the internal capsule. The gray putamen and the thalamus are also separated by the internal capsule. In horizontal section, the internal capsule presents a V shape with the angle of the V directed medially.

The **caudate nucleus,** an elongated gray mass whose pear-shaped head is contiguous to the anterior perforated substance, is adjacent to the lower border of the anterior horn of the lateral ventricle. The slender end of the caudate nucleus continues inferiorly and posteriorly as the tail, entering the roof of the temporal horn of the lateral ventricle to end at the level of the amygdala.

The **lenticular (lentiform) nucleus** is situated between the insula, the caudate nucleus, and the thalamus and is divided into 2 parts by the external medullary lamina. The **putamen** is the larger, convex gray segment lateral and just inferior to the insular cortex. The **globus pallidus** is the smaller, median triangular segment whose numerous myelinated fibers make it lighter in color than the putamen. The corpus striatum sends efferent projections to the globus pallidus and receives fibers from the frontal lobe, thalamus, and hypothalamus. A major efferent route passes from the globus pallidus via the ansa lenticularis to the thalamic nuclei and brain stem nuclei.

The basal ganglia are a part of the extrapyramidal system, whose principal functions are concerned with associated movements, postural adjustments, and autonomic integrations. Three important syndromes associated with dysfunction of the extrapyramidal system are described below.

➧ *Parkinsonism. Parkinsonism is a syndrome due to a lesion of the dopaminergic nigrostriatal pathway in which rest tremors, bradykinesia, postural instability, and rigidity occur. The onset is usually insidious, and dysfunction progresses slowly. The patient may complain of increasing rigidity and tremor, loss of facial expression, and slowness of movements and may be aware of diminished swinging of the arms and a feeling of heaviness in the limbs when walking. Posture is usually stooped, and the arms hang close to the sides, with elbows and fingers slightly flexed. Tremors of any or all limbs and about the mouth may occur. The voice is soft and poorly modulated.*

➧ *Lesions of the caudate nucleus. Involuntary movements such as athetosis, chorea, and torsion spasm are frequently associated with degeneration and atrophy of this nucleus, as occurs in Huntington's disease.*

➧ *Vascular accidents involving the internal capsule. Lesions of the internal capsule frequently occur as sequelae of cerebrovascular accidents, such as thrombosis or hemorrhage of a lenticulostriate artery. Such an accident usually results in spastic hemiplegia of the contralateral side.*

DIENCEPHALON
(Fig 2–6)

The diencephalon encloses the third ventricle and includes the thalamus, epithalamus, subthalamus, and hypothalamus.

Thalamus

The embryology of the thalamus is outlined on p 17.

Each thalamus is an ovoid gray mass situated on either side of the third ventricle and lying obliquely across the rostral end of the cerebral peduncle. The rostral end of the thalamus is narrow, close to the midline, and forms the posterior limit of the interventricular foramen. The posterior end of the thalamus is broader; its prominent medial portion is called the **pulvinar,** overlying the **medial and lateral geniculate bodies.** The dorsal surface of the thalamus is separated from the more laterally situated caudate nucleus by the **stria terminalis** and the **terminal vein.** The medial surface of the thalamus forms the lateral wall of the third ventricle and is connected with the corresponding surface of the opposite thalamus by the **massa intermedia,** or interthalamic adhesion, a short communicating bar of gray matter (not always present).

The term **thalamic radiation** denotes the tracts that emerge from the lateral surface of the thalamus, enter the internal capsule, and terminate in the cerebral cortex. The **external medullary lamina** is the layer of myelinated fibers on the lateral surface of the thalamus close to the internal capsule. The **internal medullary lamina** is a vertical sheet of white matter that bifurcates anteriorly and thus divides the gray matter of the thalamus into lateral, medial, and anterior portions.

The thalamus—rather than the sensory cortex—is probably the crucial structure for perception of some types of sensation (especially pain), while the sensory cortex may function to give finer detail to these sensations.

Subthalamus

The subthalamus is a zone of brain tissue between the tegmentum of the midbrain and the dorsal thalamus. The hypothalamus lies medial and rostral to it and the internal capsule lateral to it. The **subthalamic nucleus,** or **body of Luys,** is a cylindric mass of gray substance dorsolateral to the upper end of the substantia nigra and extending posteriorly as far as the lateral aspect of the red nucleus. It receives fibers from the globus pallidus, forming part of the efferent descending path from the corpus striatum.

Epithalamus
(Fig 2–6)

The epithalamus consists of the habenular trigone, the pineal body, and the habenular commissure. The **habenular trigone** is a small depressed triangular

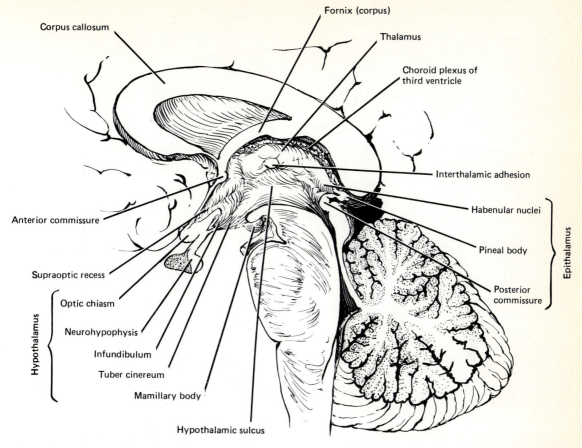

Figure 2–6. Sagittal section through brain showing the diencephalon. (Reproduced, with permission, from Chusid JG: *Correlative Neuroanatomy & Functional Neurology,* 19th ed. Lange, 1985.)

area anterior to the superior colliculus and containing the habenular nuclei.

The **pineal body** is a small midline mass lying in the depression between the superior colliculi. Its base is attached by a stalk. The ventral lamina of the stalk is continuous with the posterior commissure and the dorsal lamina with the habenular commissure. At their proximal ends, the laminae of the stalk are separated, forming the **pineal recess** of the third ventricle.

➟ *Pineal shift with intracranial tumors. The pineal body usually calcifies by middle age and becomes visible in most x-rays or CT and MR images of the adult skull. Deviation from the midline suggests a space-consuming lesion on the contralateral side.*

Hypothalamus
(Fig 2–6)

The hypothalamus lies inferior and anterior to the thalamus and forms the floor and a segment of the inferior lateral walls of the third ventricle. It includes the following structures: (1) the **mamillary bodies,** 2 adjacent pea-sized masses inferior to the gray matter of the floor of the third ventricle and rostral to the posterior perforated space; (2) the **tuber cinereum,** an eminence anterior to the mamillary bodies; (3) the **infundibulum,** a hollow process extending downward from the undersurface of the tuber cinereum to the posterior lobe of the hypophysis; and (4) the optic chiasm.

The lower portion of the infundibulum is continuous with the neural lobe of the hypophysis. The enlarged upper portion of the infundibulum, the median eminence, the infundibular stem, and the neural lobe of the hypophysis constitute the neurohypophysis.

➟ *Lesions of the hypothalamus. The hypothalamus has multiple functions. Lesions may produce a variety of symptoms, including diabetes insipidus, obesity, sexual dystrophy, somnolence, loss of libido, and loss of temperature control. Visual defects, such as bitemporal hemianopia, frequently result from involvement of the nearby optic chiasm.*

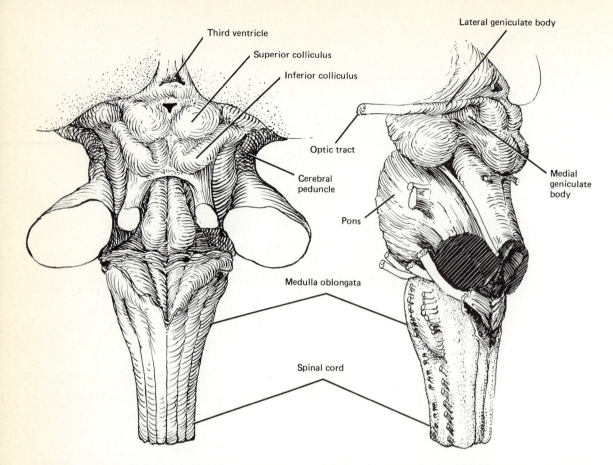

Figure 2–7. External anatomy of the brain stem. *Left:* dorsal view; *right:* dorsolateral view. (Reproduced, with permission, from Chusid JG: *Correlative Neuroanatomy & Functional Neurology,* 19th ed. Lange, 1985.)

BRAIN STEM
(Figs 2–7 and 2–8)

The brain stem is the portion of the brain connecting the cerebral hemispheres with the spinal cord and containing the midbrain, pons, and medulla oblongata. It is partially obscured by the cerebral hemispheres and cerebellum. The gray matter in the brain stem is scattered in numerous small masses called nuclei, many of which are motor or sensory nuclei of the cranial nerves.

➠ ***Brain stem lesions.*** *Lesions of the brain stem produce symptoms referable to involvement of the motor and sensory pathways passing through it and particularly to involvement of the nuclei of the cranial nerves that lie within it.*

MIDBRAIN
(Fig 2–9)

The midbrain (mesencephalon) is the short portion of the brain between the pons and the cerebral hemi-

spheres. The dorsal segment of the midbrain, called the **tectum,** comprises the 4 **corpora quadrigemina** (colliculi); the ventrolateral segments contain the 2 **cerebral peduncles.** The corpora quadrigemina are 4 rounded eminences arranged in pairs, the superior and inferior colliculi, separated from each other by a cruciate sulcus. The **superior colliculi** are larger than the inferior colliculi and are associated with the optic system. The superior quadrigeminal brachium extends laterally from the superior colliculus and connects with the **lateral geniculate body.** The **inferior colliculi** are associated with the auditory system. The inferior quadrigeminal brachium extends laterally from the inferior colliculus and passes to the **medial geniculate body.**

The cerebral peduncles converge toward the midline from the lower surface of the cerebral hemispheres, entering the ventral portion of the pons at its superior surface. The interpeduncular fossa is the depressed area between the peduncles and contains in its inferior portion the interpeduncular ganglion. The **substantia nigra** is a broad layer of pigmented gray substance that separates the ventral portion, or **base,** of the cerebral peduncle from the more central

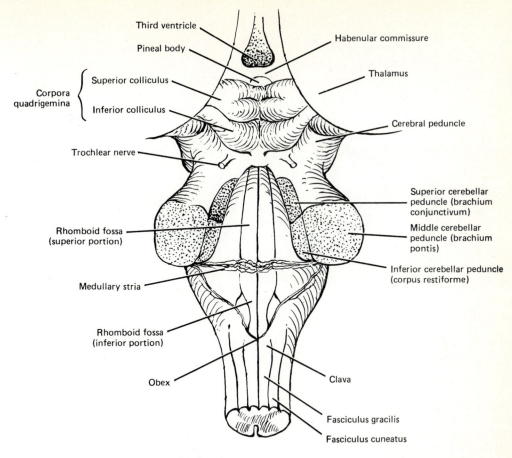

Figure 2–8. Dorsal aspect of the brain stem. (Reproduced, with permission, from Chusid JG: *Correlative Neuroanatomy & Functional Neurology,* 19th ed. Lange, 1985.)

portion of the midbrain, the **tegmentum.** The substantia nigra extends from the upper surface of the pons to the hypothalamus.

⟹ *Destructive lesions of the midbrain. Clinical findings in cases of destructive lesions of the midbrain usually reflect the structure involved. Destruction of the superior colliculi, as with pineal tumor, is associated with paralysis of upward movements of the eyes. Destruction of the third and fourth cranial nerve nuclei causes paralysis of the muscles supplied by these nerves. Destruction of the red nucleus, the substantia nigra, or the reticular substance (as in encephalitis) is associated with rigidity and involuntary movements. Destruction of the cerebral peduncle causes spastic paralysis of the contralateral side.*

PONS

The pons lies anterior to the cerebellum and superior to the medulla, from which it is separated by a groove through which the abducens, facial, and acoustic nerves emerge.

The anterior limits of the pons are marked by 2 cerebellar peduncles, one on each side of the midline. The brachium pontis, also known as the **middle cerebellar peduncle,** connects the bulging ventral portion of the pons with the cerebellum. The triangular posterior surface of the pons is concealed by the mass of the cerebellum.

The basilar (ventral) portion of the pons contains a thick superficial layer, the **superficial transverse fibers,** which give rise to the **brachium pontis;** the **deep transverse fibers,** which lie dorsal to the corticospinal tract, also contribute to the brachium pontis. The pons contains the nuclei of the abducens and facial nerves, the motor and sensory nuclei of the trigeminal nerve, and the nuclei of the vestibular and cochlear nerves.

⟹ *Lesions of the ventral and lateral segments of the pons. Lesions of the more ventral portion of the pons may cause abducens paralysis. Lesions of the lateral pons, often associated with*

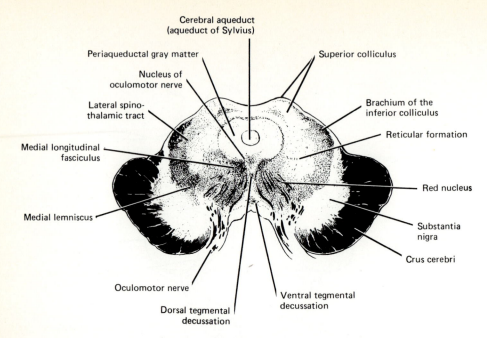

Figure 2–9. Cross section through the midbrain at the level of the superior colliculus. (Reproduced, with permission, from Chusid JG: *Correlative Neuroanatomy & Functional Neurology,* 19th ed. Lange, 1985.)

tumors of the pontocerebellar angle, may cause persistent tinnitus, progressive deafness, and vertigo; they may also result in ipsilateral ataxia and contralateral hemiplegia.

MEDULLA OBLONGATA

The medulla oblongata is the pyramid-shaped segment of the brain stem between the spinal cord and the pons. The lower half contains the remnants of the central canal; the posterior portion of the superior half forms the floor of the body of the fourth ventricle.

The **anterior median fissure** extends along the ventral surface of the medulla to terminate at the pontine border in the foramen cecum. In its inferior portion, the anterior median fissure is crossed by the obliquely decussating pyramidal tracts. The **posterior median fissure,** a shallow groove along the postero-inferior half of the medulla, ends at the dorsal limit of the fourth ventricle. The **median sulcus** is a longitudinal groove in the midsagittal portion of the floor of the fourth ventricle. The **anterolateral sulcus** is a shallow furrow through which the fibers of the hypoglossal nerve emerge from the medulla. The **posterolateral sulcus** is a furrow through which the spinal accessory, vagus, and glossopharyngeal nerves emerge from the medulla.

⟹ *Lesions of the medulla. Lesions of the ventral portion of the superior medulla may produce hypoglossal nerve palsy and crossed hemiple-*

gia, whereas lesions of the dorsolateral area of the superior medulla may produce the lateral medullary syndrome (of Wallenberg), often associated with posteroinferior cerebellar or vertebral artery disease. Involvement of the more central area of the upper medulla may produce a variety of clinical pictures depending upon the cranial nuclei and other structures involved.

CEREBELLUM
(Fig 2–10)

The cerebellum is located in the posterior fossa of the skull, behind the pons and the medulla. It is separated from the overlying cerebrum by an extension of dura mater, the tentorium cerebelli. It is oval in form, with its widest diameter along the transverse axis.

The cerebellum is composed of a small unpaired central portion, the vermis, and 2 large lateral masses, the cerebellar hemispheres, sometimes called the neocerebellum. The flocculonodular lobe includes the nodulus of the posterior vermis and the attached flocculi and is sometimes referred to as the archicerebellum. Descriptive subdivisions are shown in Fig 2–10.

⟹ *Lesions of the archicerebellum. The archicerebellum has the function of keeping the individual oriented in space. Lesions in this area are manifested by trunk ataxia, swaying, and staggering*

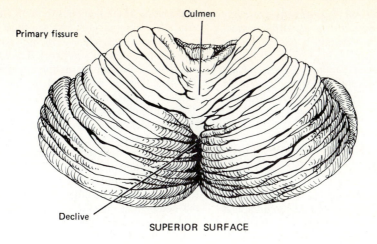

SUPERIOR SURFACE

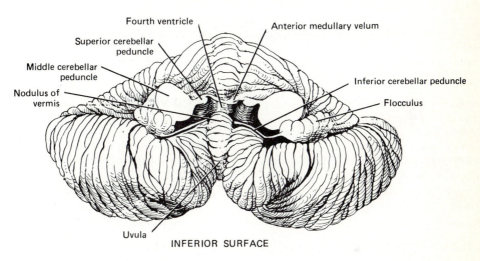

INFERIOR SURFACE

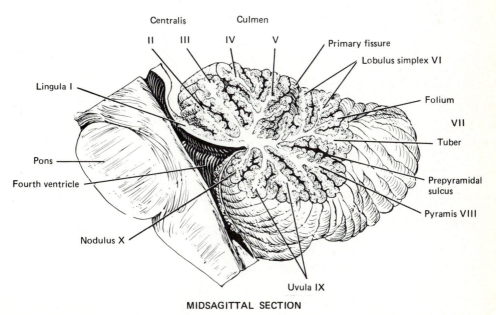

MIDSAGITTAL SECTION

Figure 2–10. The cerebellum. (Modified and reproduced, with permission, from Chusid JG: *Correlative Neuroanatomy & Functional Neurology,* 19th ed. Lange, 1985.)

that are not made worse by closing the eyes, and by diminished or absent responses to thermal or rotational stimulation of the labyrinths.

➠ **Lesions of the neocerebellum.** *Lesions of the neocerebellum produce dysmetrias, intention tremors, and inability to perform rapidly alternating movements.*

VENTRICLES
(Figs 2–11 and 2–12)

Within the brain substance is a communicating system of cavities filled with circulating cerebrospinal fluid: the 2 lateral, the third, and the fourth ventricles. The ventricles and subarachnoid spaces can be visualized by CT scan and MR imaging.

The irregularly shaped **lateral ventricles** are the largest and are lined with ependyma continuous with the ependyma of the third ventricle. The **anterior horn** lies anterior to the interventricular foramen. The **posterior horn** extends into the occipital lobe; its roof is formed by fibers of the corpus callosum. The **inferior (temporal) horn** traverses the temporal lobe. The body lies between the anterior horn, the lateral horn, and the trigone, or atrium, which forms the posterior and inferior horns.

The **interventricular (Monro) foramens** are oval apertures between the column of the fornix and the anterior end of the thalamus through which the lateral ventricle communicates with the third ventricle.

The **third ventricle** is a narrow vertical cleft lying between the 2 lateral ventricles. The roof of the third ventricle is formed by a thin layer of ependyma. The lateral walls are formed mainly by the medial surfaces of the 2 thalami.

Three openings communicate with the third ventricle. The interventricular foramens communicate with the lateral ventricles anteriorly, while the cerebral aqueduct (aqueduct of Sylvius) opens into the caudal end of the third ventricle.

The **fourth ventricle** is a cavity bounded ventrally by the pons and medulla oblongata and dorsally by the cerebellum. It is continuous with the cerebral aqueduct superiorly and the central canal of the medulla inferiorly. The fourth ventricle communicates with the subarachnoid space surrounding the spinal cord through the lateral apertures (foramens of Luschka) and a medial aperture (foramen of Magendie). The cerebrospinal fluid flows into the dorsal cisterna magna and surrounds the spinal cord.

BLOOD VESSELS

Arteries
(Figs 2–13, 2–14, and 2–15)

The **internal carotid arteries** are the major suppliers of blood to the brain. It begins at the common

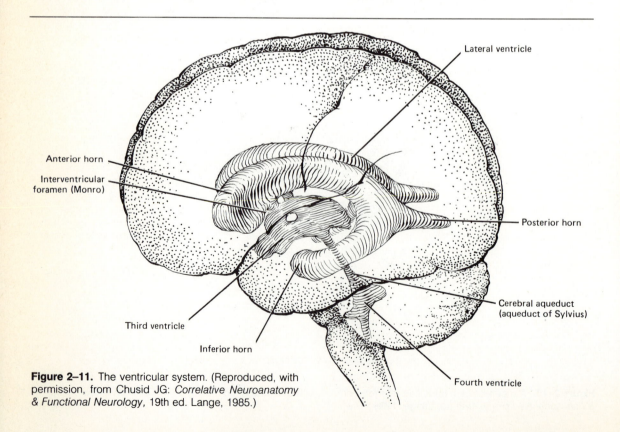

Figure 2–11. The ventricular system. (Reproduced, with permission, from Chusid JG: *Correlative Neuroanatomy & Functional Neurology,* 19th ed. Lange, 1985.)

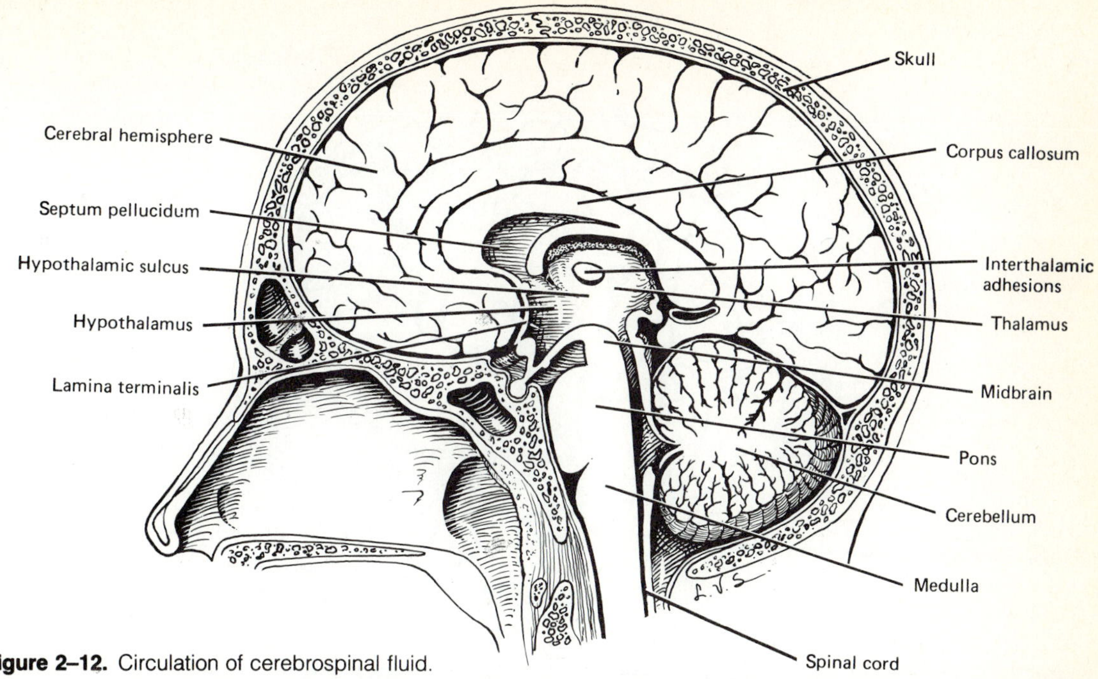
Skull
Cerebral hemisphere
Corpus callosum
Septum pellucidum
Hypothalamic sulcus
Interthalamic adhesions
Hypothalamus
Thalamus
Lamina terminalis
Midbrain
Pons
Cerebellum
Medulla
Spinal cord

Figure 2–12. Circulation of cerebrospinal fluid.

carotid bifurcation at about the level of the greater cornu of the hyoid bone and runs cephalad toward the inferior surface of the petrous segment of the temporal bone. The artery enters the carotid canal of the skull and runs anteriorly and medially to the foramen lacerum. It enters the middle cranial fossa, runs between the layers of dura mater that form the cavernous sinus, and extends toward the posterior clinoid process, where it makes an S curve (siphon). The artery then perforates the roof of the cavernous sinus, passes between the optic and oculomotor nerves, and extends to the medial end of the lateral cerebral fissure, where it gives off its terminal branches.

The internal carotid artery gives off no branches from its cervical portion as it passes through the neck. Within the petrous portion of the temporal bone, it variably gives off 4 branches: the caroticotympanic branch, the artery of the pterygoid canal, the cavernous branches, and the hypophyseal branches. Within the cavernous sinus, it gives off 5 branches: the ganglionic branches, the meningeal branch, the ophthalmic artery, and the anterior and middle cerebral arteries. The internal carotid artery gives off 4 branches in its cerebral course: the middle cerebral artery, the anterior cerebral artery, the posterior communicating artery, and the anterior choroidal artery.

Other major arteries supplying the brain are the **vertebral arteries,** branches of the subclavian artery. They run to the transverse process of C6 and extend superiorly through the foramens in the transverse processes of the other cervical vertebrae to the base of the skull. The vertebral artery enters the cranial cavity through the foramen magnum, gives off the posterior inferior cerebellar artery, and almost immediately joins the vertebral artery from the contralateral side to form the **basilar artery.** This large vessel gives off the pontine, labyrinthine, anteroinferior cerebellar, superior cerebellar, and posterior cerebral branches.

At the base of the brain, arterial branches from the internal carotid and vertebral arteries form an anastomosis called the **circle of Willis,** formed anteriorly by the anterior cerebral arteries and posteriorly by the posterior cerebral arteries. The circle of Willis is formed by the joining of the posterior cerebral arteries with the posterior communicating arteries, and then through the internal carotid and middle cerebral arteries to the 2 anterior cerebral arteries which are joined by the anterior communicating artery to complete the circle.

True end arteries do not exist within the brain tissue, for all arterial vessels have some connection with adjacent arteries. Anastomoses are small and sparse, however, so that sudden occlusion of an artery may not be compensated for by neighboring arteries. Thus, the arteries of the brain tissue function like end arteries.

➡ ***Onset of stroke.*** *The acute onset of stroke ("apoplexy") is usually associated with disease of the intracranial vascular tree, blood dyscrasia, or trauma. The commonest causes of generalized or focal disturbance of brain function are cerebrovascular lesions. The main types of spontaneous cerebrovascular accidents are cerebral thrombosis, cerebral hemorrhage, cerebral embolism, subarachnoid hemorrhage,*

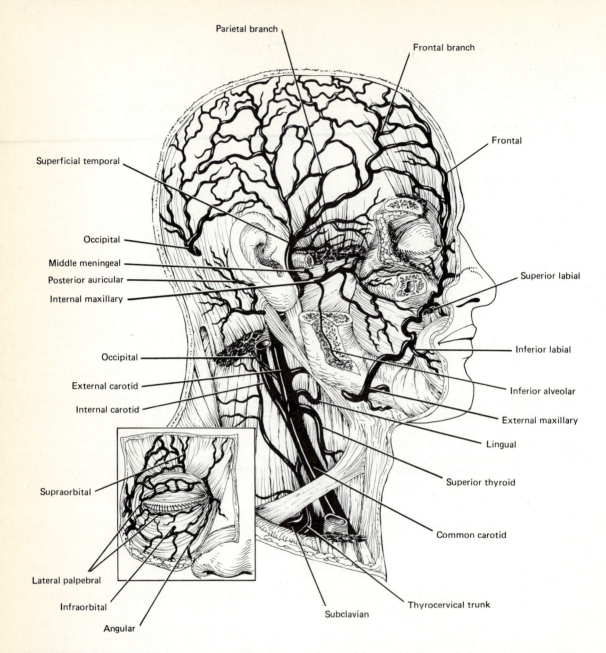

Figure 2–13. Arterial supply to head and brain. (Reproduced, with permission, from Chusid JG: *Correlative Neuroanatomy & Functional Neurology*, 19th ed. Lange, 1985.)

and transient cerebral ischemia. Cerebrovascular accidents may occur at any age, but intracerebral hemorrhage and thrombosis usually occur in adulthood.

➤ ***Internal carotid and vertebral artery stenosis.*** *Cerebral angiographic as well as postmortem studies have disclosed that in patients with cerebrovascular insufficiency there is a high incidence of occlusion or stenosis of extracranial portions of arteries supplying the brain, particularly of the internal carotid and vertebral arteries.*

➤ ***Intracranial aneurysms.*** *Aneurysmal dilatation of intracranial blood vessels usually results from arteriosclerosis or congenital abnormalities. Intracranial aneurysms vary from the size of a pea to that of an orange, and individual aneurysms may change in size. Larger aneu-*

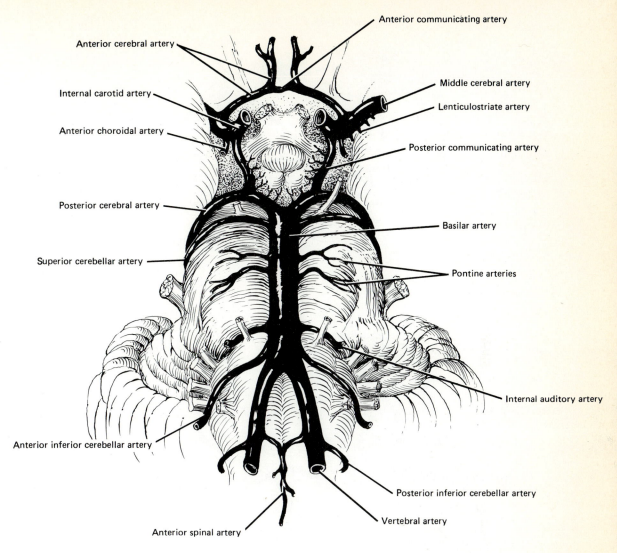

Figure 2–14. Circle of Willis and principal arteries of the brain. (Reproduced, with permission, from Chusid JG: *Correlative Neuroanatomy & Functional Neurology,* 19th ed. Lange, 1985.)

rysms may erode the bones of the skull and sella turcica and compress adjacent cerebral tissue and cranial nerves. Most intracranial aneurysms are located near the base of the skull, and almost half arise from the internal carotid or middle cerebral arteries. They are usually single but often multiple. An association of congenital intracranial aneurysms, polycystic kidneys, and coarctation of the aorta has been noted.

Prior to rupture, aneurysms may be asymptomatic or may cause focal symptoms, depending upon their size and proximity to functional areas. Following rupture, the symptoms are those of acute subarachnoid hemorrhage (severe headache, nausea, vomiting, depressed level of consciousness, and nuchal rigidity).

Veins
(Fig 2–16)

Venous drainage from the brain flows chiefly into the **dural sinuses,** vascular channels lying within the tough dural envelope. The dural sinuses contain no valves and, for the most part, are triangular in shape.

Superficial cortical veins drain mainly into the medially situated **superior sagittal sinus.** These cortical veins are the anastomotic vein, which drains into the superior sagittal sinus, and the inferior anastomotic vein, which drains into the transverse sinus. The deep cerebral veins drain the basal ganglia. The junction of the 2 internal cerebral veins forms the great cerebral vein, a short midline vein, and the basal veins, which enter the straight sinus.

In the falx cerebri lies the superior sagittal sinus.

LATERAL SURFACE

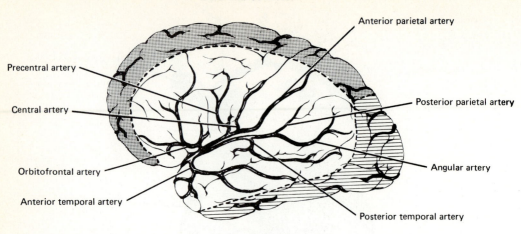

MEDIAN SURFACE

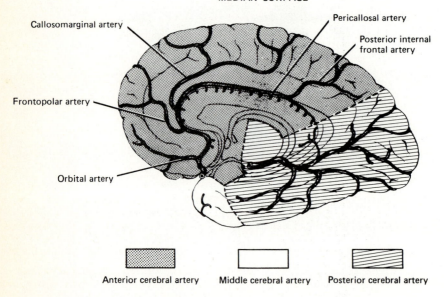

Figure 2–15. Arterial supply of cerebral cortex.

The **straight sinus,** a posterior continuation of the great cerebral vein, joins the superior sagittal sinus to form the **confluence of the sinuses.** The **transverse sinuses,** each divided into a lateral and a sigmoid portion, conduct blood received from the superior sagittal sinus and straight sinus into the internal jugular veins. The 2 **cavernous sinuses** receive blood from the middle cerebral veins and the ophthalmic veins and drain into the internal jugular veins and the transverse sinuses. The cavernous sinuses are joined across the midline by 2 **intercavernous sinuses,** one of which is anterior and the other posterior to the hypophysis; the 2 veins thus form a venous circle about the hypophysis, the **circular sinus.** The **inferior petrosal sinus** drains from the cavernous sinus into

the internal jugular vein. The **superior petrosal sinus** drains from the cavernous sinus into the transverse sinus. Emissary veins connecting extracranial veins with the intracranial venous sinuses are frequently present in the skull.

⟱   ***Brain abscesses.*** *Brain abscesses are usually caused by staphylococci or anaerobes, although any of the common pyogenic bacteria may be found upon culture. The organism may gain access to the brain by direct extension from otitis media, mastoiditis, sinusitis, and infected head injuries, or via the bloodstream as a result of pulmonary infection and bacter-*

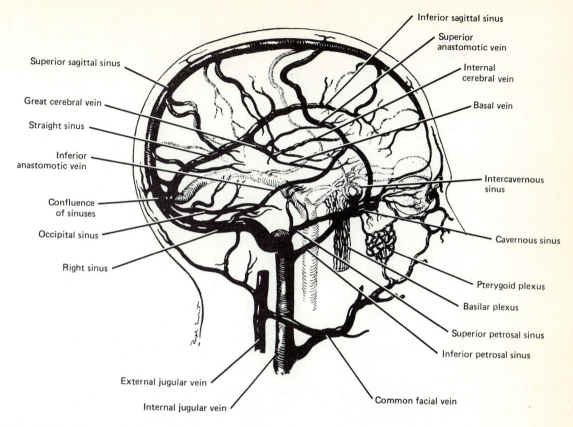

Figure 2–16. The venous drainage of the brain (semidiagrammatic). (Reproduced, with permission, from Shenkin, Harmel, and Kety: *Arch Neurol Psychiatry* 1948; **60:**245.)

emia. Abscesses lead to signs of increased intracranial pressure and focal neurologic deficits. Mild meningeal irritative signs may be present, such as rigidity of the neck and a positive Kernig sign. Somnolence and slowing of mental processes are common. The temperature may be mildly elevated but rarely exceeds 39 °C unless complications such as meningitis occur.

II. THE CRANIAL NERVES
(Fig 2–17)

Attached to the base of the brain are 12 pairs of cranial nerves that leave the cranial cavity through various foramens in the skull and, together with the spinal nerves and autonomic nervous system, make up the peripheral nervous system.

The cranial nerves are conventionally designated by roman numerals as well as by name. Cranial nerve I (olfactory nerve) is the most anterior of the nerves and cranial nerve XII (hypoglossal nerve) the most caudad. Cranial nerves I and II (optic nerve) are not true nerves but terminations of fiber tracts of the brain. Except for a part of cranial nerve XI (accessory nerve), which is derived from the upper cervical segments of the spinal cord, the posterior 10 pairs of cranial nerves emerge from the brain stem, in which lie their nuclei of origin.

The superficial origin of a cranial nerve is the area of the brain where the nerve appears or attaches. Cranial nerves with motor function originate from collections of cells deep within the brain stem (motor nuclei), which are analogous to the anterior horn cells of the spinal cord. Sensory cranial nerves originate from collections of cells outside the brain stem, usually in ganglia that may be considered analogous to the dorsal root ganglia of the spinal nerves.

CRANIAL NERVE I
(Olfactory Nerve)

The olfactory nerve fibers begin in the nasal cavity, coalesce into about 20 bundles, penetrate the foramens in the cribriform plate of the ethmoid bone, and end in the glomeruli of the olfactory bulb. Each olfactory

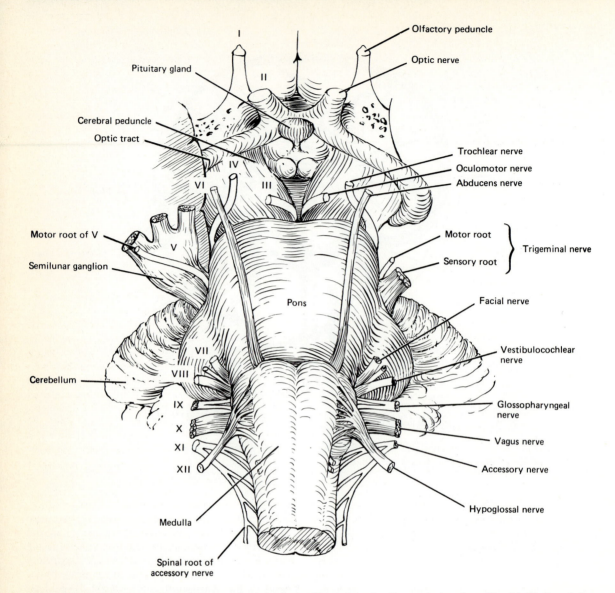

Figure 2–17. Emergence of cranial nerves from the brain. (Reproduced, with permission, from Chusid JG: *Correlative Neuroanatomy & Functional Neurology,* 19th ed. Lange, 1985.)

tract begins in an olfactory bulb and continues posteriorly to end just lateral to the optic chiasm, where it penetrates the cerebrum.

■➡ ***Olfactory nerve lesions.*** *Disorders of olfaction may be caused by traumatic injury to the anterior fossa of the skull, tumors of the frontal and temporal lobes or pituitary area, meningitis, hydrocephalus, posttraumatic cerebral syndrome, cerebrovascular accidents, drug intoxications, psychoses, neuroses, congenital defects, and inflammatory lesions of the nasal cavity.*

CRANIAL NERVE II
(Optic Nerve)

The optic nerve contains fibers arising from the inner (ganglionic) layer of the retina and proceeding posteriorly to enter the cranial cavity via the optic foramen. Some fibers cross to the contralateral side via the **optic chiasm.** After leaving the chiasm, the fibers diverge into the right and left **optic tracts,** which reach the base of the brain near the cerebral peduncle.

➠ *Optic nerve lesions. The optic nerve is involved in retrobulbar neuritis. The most common cause is multiple sclerosis. Other causes include syphilis, diabetes, and ischemic, traumatic, toxic, and nutritional disorders. It leads typically to a central scotoma.*

Papilledema (choked disk) is usually secondary to increased intracranial pressure and often due to brain tumor, brain abscess, and intracranial hemorrhage, or to hypertension.

Optic atrophy results in decreased visual acuity and a change in the color of the optic disk from light pink to white or gray. Primary optic atrophy is caused by diseases that involve the optic nerve but do not produce papilledema. It may result from tabes dorsalis or multiple sclerosis. Secondary optic atrophy may be due to neuritis, glaucoma, a late result of papilledema, or increased intracranial pressure.

Tumors at the base of the frontal lobe may cause ipsilateral blindness (due to optic atrophy), anosmia, and contralateral papilledema (Foster Kennedy syndrome).

CRANIAL NERVE III
(Oculomotor Nerve)

The oculomotor nerve leaves the brain from the medial side of the cerebral peduncle, where it lies between the posterior and the superior cerebellar arteries. It continues anteriorly into the cavernous sinus and leaves the skull through the superior orbital fissure. The oculomotor nerve supplies the levator palpebrae, all of the extrinsic eye muscles except the superior oblique and lateral rectus, and all of the intrinsic eye muscles except the dilator of the pupil. **Parasympathetic fibers** go to the sphincter muscle of the iris and to the ciliary muscle, whose contraction thickens the lens.

➠ *Oculomotor nerve lesions. Ophthalmoplegia (paralysis) due to lesions of nerve III may be acute, chronic, or progressive and central or peripheral. External ophthalmoplegia is manifested by divergent strabismus, diplopia, and ptosis. Internal ophthalmoplegia is characterized by a dilated pupil and loss of the light and accommodation reflexes. Paralysis of the levator palpebrae muscle results in marked ptosis of the upper lid.*

CRANIAL NERVE IV
(Trochlear Nerve)

The trochlear nerve is the smallest cranial nerve. It takes its superficial origin from the dorsal surface of the brain stem, then curves ventrally between the posterior cerebral and superior cerebellar arteries, lateral to the oculomotor nerve. It continues anteriorly

in the lateral well of the cavernous sinus between the oculomotor nerve and the ophthalmic branch of the trigeminal nerve and enters the orbit via the superior orbital fissure. The trochlear nerve supplies the superior oblique muscle of the orbit.

➠ *Trochlear nerve lesions. Superior oblique muscle paralysis is a rare disorder; it is characterized by mild convergent strabismus and diplopia when the patient looks down and in. This may be the first sign of trochlear palsy. Tilting of the head usually occurs as a compensatory adjustment to the effect of the paralysis.*

CRANIAL NERVE V
(Trigeminal Nerve)

The trigeminal nerve is composed of a large sensory root—the major segment—and a smaller motor root. The sensory segment arises from cells in the large trigeminal or semilunar (gasserian) ganglion in the lateral portion of the cavernous sinus, passes posteriorly under the superior petrosal sinus and the tentorium, and penetrates the lateral pons. Fibers of the ophthalmic division enter the skull via the superior orbital fissure. Fibers of the maxillary division penetrate via the foramen rotundum. Sensory fibers of the mandibular division of the nerve, joined by the motor or masticator portion (which leaves the pons ventromedial to the sensory rootlets), enter the cranial cavity through the foramen ovale.

The ophthalmic division is sensory. It supplies the bulb of the eye, the conjunctiva, and the lacrimal glands; part of the nasal mucosa; the paranasal sinuses; and the cutaneous areas of the forehead, eyelids, and nose. The maxillary division is also sensory. It supplies the skin of the mid face and lower eyelid, the side of the nose, and the upper lip; the mucous membranes of the nasopharynx, maxillary sinus, soft palate, tonsil, and roof of the mouth; and the upper gingiva and teeth. The mandibular division, the largest of the 3 divisions, is a mixed motor and sensory nerve. The sensory division supplies the temporal area, ear, cheek, lower lip, and lower face; the mucous membranes of the cheek and tongue; and the mastoid air cells, lower teeth and gums, mandible, temporomandibular joint, and parts of the dura and skull. The motor division supplies the muscles of mastication (masseter, temporalis, pterygoids), the mylohyoid, the anterior digastric, and, via the otic ganglion, the tensor tympani and tensor veli palatini.

➠ *Trigeminal nerve lesions. Trigeminal neuralgia (tic douloureux) is a syndrome characterized by severe pain along the distribution of one or more branches of the trigeminal nerve. The cause is unknown, but the disorder is sometimes associated with an anomalous vessel lying in close relation to the nerve roots; this is the basis of modern operative treatment for it.*

Auriculotemporal nerve (Frey's) syndrome consists of flushing and sweating of the ipsilateral side of the face along the distribution of the auriculotemporal nerve. Episodes are triggered by eating or tasting, and the syndrome usually follows injury to or infection of the parotid gland.

Symptoms of trigeminal nerve involvement include pain along one or more branches; loss of sensation over sensory distribution; corneal anesthesia; occasional loss of pain but not touch sensation (dissociate anesthesia); paresthesia; paralysis of muscles of mastication; impaired hearing due to paralysis of the tensor tympani; and occasional trismus (lockjaw) due to spasm of the muscles of mastication.

CRANIAL NERVE VI
(Abducens Nerve)

The abducens nerve emerges from the ventral surface of the brain stem in the groove between the pyramid of the medulla and the caudal end of the pons. It passes through the cavernous sinus, exits from the cranial cavity via the superior orbital fissure, and supplies the lateral rectus muscle. The abducens nerve runs the longest intracranial course and is thus the nerve most liable to undergo early compression secondary to a rise in intracranial pressure.

➠ *Gradenigo's syndrome. Gradenigo's syndrome, which usually appears as a complication of purulent otitis media, is characterized by facial pain and lateral rectus palsy. Internal strabismus and diplopia occur frequently. The syndrome is sometimes secondary to osteomyelitis of the tip of the petrous portion of the temporal bone.*

CRANIAL NERVE VII
(Facial Nerve)

The motor root of the facial nerve emerges from the posterior border of the pons, just lateral to the inferior olive, through the medial side of the cerebellopontine angle. It leaves the cranium by way of the internal acoustic meatus and the bony skull via the stylomastoid foramen. The facial nerve supplies motor fibers to the superficial muscles of facial expression, the muscles of the external ear and scalp, and the platysma, posterior digastric, stapedius, and stylohyoid muscles. The sensory component of the facial nerve arises from unipolar cells in the geniculate ganglion. Peripheral branches supply taste sensation to the anterior two-thirds of the tongue via the lingual nerve and chorda tympani and sensation for parts of

the soft palate, external auditory meatus, and pharynx adjacent to the soft palate.

➠ *Bell's palsy. Bell's palsy, or peripheral facial paralysis, is idiopathic facial paralysis. The symptoms and signs depend on the location of the lesion. If the lesion is distal to the stylomastoid foramen, the mouth droops and deep facial sensation is lost, along with ability to wink the eyes and wrinkle the forehead. If the lesion occurs in the facial canal and involves the chorda tympani nerve, the same signs are present, and taste is lost on the anterior two-thirds of the tongue. If the lesion is high in the facial canal, additional signs of hyperacusis occur.*

In so-called geniculate herpes, facial palsy is accompanied by a herpetic eruption behind the ear and on the eardrum (Ramsay Hunt syndrome).

CRANIAL NERVE VIII
(Vestibulocochlear Nerve)

The vestibulocochlear (statoacoustic) nerve enters the cranial cavity via the internal acoustic meatus along with the facial nerve and enters the brain stem behind the posterior edge of the middle cerebellar peduncle. The vestibular portion arises from cells of the vestibular ganglion (ganglion of Scarpa) located in the dorsal portion of the internal auditory meatus. The cochlear portion arises from the spiral ganglion. Both branches of the nerve are sensory. The cochlear root is the nerve of hearing; the vestibular root is the nerve of equilibration.

➠ *Vestibulocochlear nerve lesions. Peripheral lesions usually involve both the cochlear and vestibular divisions. Otitis media, meningitis, degenerative diseases, Meniere's syndrome, skull fractures, and otosclerosis are examples. Symptoms of cochlear nerve involvement are tinnitus, deafness, and hearing scotomas. The major vestibular symptoms are vertigo, nystagmus, diaphoresis, nausea, and vomiting.*

Central lesions of the nerve may involve either of the divisions independently. Tumors of the cerebellopontine angle frequently involve the eighth nerve (and indirectly the seventh). Drugs such as quinine and salicylates may affect the cochlear portion of the nerve, and streptomycin may cause vestibular nuclear degeneration.

CRANIAL NERVE IX
(Glossopharyngeal Nerve)

The glossopharyngeal nerve is a mixed nerve. It contains sensory fibers that originate in cells in the superior and petrous ganglia and pass through the jugular foramen along with nerves X and XI. The motor part arises in the nucleus ambiguus and leaves the lateral medulla to join the sensory part of the nerve. The sensory portion supplies the fauces, soft palate, tonsil, posterior tongue, auditory tube, tympanic membrane, and mucous membrane of the pharynx. The motor portion supplies the stylopharyngeus muscle.

➠ *Glossopharyngeal nerve lesions. The glossopharyngeal nerve is rarely involved alone. It is usually affected along with the vagus and accessory nerves as a result of compression, inflammation, or trauma. Nerve damage may be caused by bulbar disease, syphilis, basal tumors, tuberculosis, jugular vein thrombosis, or diphtheria. Symptoms include loss of the gag reflex, mild dysphagia, loss of taste over the posterior third of the tongue, deviation of the uvula to the unaffected side, and loss of sensation in the pharynx and on the base of the tongue.*

CRANIAL NERVE X
(Vagus Nerve)

The vagus nerve contains afferent fibers that originate in cells present in the jugular and nodose ganglia just inferior to the jugular foramen. It passes through the jugular foramen to enter the medulla behind the glossopharyngeal nerve. The vagus nerve pursues the longest extracranial course of all of the cranial nerves, with distribution to the neck, thorax, and abdomen. Its sensory fibers supply the skin of the posterior surface of the ear and the external auditory meatus as well as the mucous membranes of the pharynx, larynx, bronchi, and lungs. The nerve also sends fibers to the heart, esophagus, stomach, biliary tract, pancreas, small intestine, large intestine as far as the splenic flexure, and kidney. Motor fibers from the nucleus ambiguus leave the medulla to join the sensory part of the nerve.

➠ *Vagus nerve lesions. Lesions of the vagus nerve are intramedullary or peripheral. Intramedullary lesions are caused by hemorrhage, tumors, multiple sclerosis, syphilis, and rare neurologic diseases. Peripheral lesions may result from primary neuropathy (alcoholic, diphtheritic; due to poisoning with heavy metals), trauma, tumors of the mediastinum and bronchi, and aortic aneurysm.*

Motor disturbances of the vagus nerve include aphonia, dysphonia, change in vocal cord position, dysphagia, and loss of the gag reflex. Sensory disturbances include pain or paresthesias in the pharynx and larynx, anesthesia of the pharynx and larynx, and cough.

CRANIAL NERVE XI
(Accessory Nerve)

The **internal (medullary) branch** of the accessory nerve arises superficially from a series of filaments located behind the root filaments of the vagus nerve and from the lateral surface of the medulla and upper cervical spinal cord. This purely motor nerve leaves the cranial cavity through the jugular foramen and is distributed via the vagus nerve to the palate, pharynx, and larynx. The **external (spinal) branch** of nerve XI has motor fibers that arise from the lateral segments of the anterior horns of C1–5. They ascend into the skull through the foramen magnum, leave it via the jugular foramen, and supply the trapezius and sternocleidomastoid muscles.

➠ *Accessory nerve lesions. The accessory nerve may be affected by central nervous system syphilis, brain tumors, meningitis, trauma, cancer, etc. With accessory nerve palsy, the head may rotate with difficulty to the healthy side, and the sternocleidomastoid muscle atrophies. Atrophy of the trapezius muscle causes depression of the ipsilateral shoulder contour.*

CRANIAL NERVE XII
(Hypoglossal Nerve)

The hypoglossal nerve takes its superficial origin by way of several filaments in the ventrolateral sulcus of the medulla between the inferior olive and the pyramid; these filaments fuse and leave the posterior fossa of the skull by way of the hypoglossal canal in the occipital bone. Nerve XII is a motor nerve that supplies the inferior belly of the omohyoid, sternohyoid, and sternothyroid muscles via its descending hypoglossal branches. The nerve also supplies the superior belly of the omohyoid and the thyrohyoid, geniohyoid, styloglossus, genioglossus, hyoglossus, and intrinsic muscles of the tongue.

➠ *Hypoglossal nerve lesions. Peripheral lesions of nerve XII are usually caused by mechanical problems such as basal skull fractures and dislocations of the upper cervical vertebrae; the lesions are also caused by lead, arsenic, or alcohol poisoning. Nuclear and supranuclear lesions result from medullary hemorrhage, po-*

liomyelitis, bulbar palsy (*of all causes*), *and brain tumors and abscess. An intramedullary lesion may be characterized by contralateral hemiplegia and ipsilateral paralysis of the tongue. Peripheral paralysis is characterized by ipsilateral paralysis and wasting of the tongue, which deviates to the side of the lesion on protrusion. In bilateral lesions, the tongue is completely paralyzed, and dysphagia, dysarthria, and difficulty in chewing occur.*

The Face, Oral Cavity, & Nose

3

EMBRYOLOGY OF THE FACE, NOSE, & PALATE

The skeleton of the face, nose, and palate (viscerocranium) forms mainly from the mesodermal structures of the first pharyngeal arches (Fig 3–1).

Mouth

In the center of the developing face is an ectodermal depression, the stomodeum or future mouth. The maxillary swellings derived from the first arch begin to fuse with the frontonasal prominence to form the upper lip.

Anomalous development results in clefts of the hard and soft palates and face (median, oblique, and lateral fissures) and in the size of the mouth.

Mandible

The mandibular swellings associated with the first branchial arches lie inferior to the stomodeum and fuse early in the midline to form the lower jaw, the lower lip, and the lower cheek.

Maxilla

Maxillary swellings formed from first arch tissue lie lateral to the stomodeum and migrate medially to fuse with the frontonasal process. They form the cheeks, the lateral portions of the upper lip, and all of the palate and the upper jaw (maxilla) except for the premaxilla.

Anomalies. Defective formation results in clefts of the upper lip and the anterior part of the maxilla.

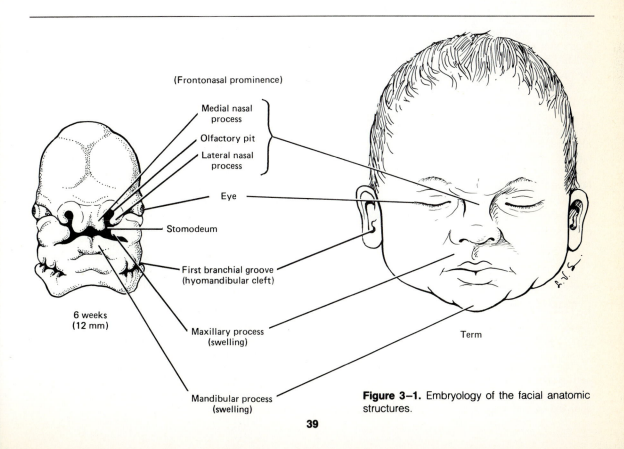

(Frontonasal prominence)

Medial nasal process

Olfactory pit

Lateral nasal process

Eye

Stomodeum

First branchial groove (hyomandibular cleft)

6 weeks (12 mm)

Maxillary process (swelling)

Term

Mandibular process (swelling)

Figure 3–1. Embryology of the facial anatomic structures.

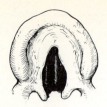

1. Partial division of palate involving both hard and soft palates. The premaxilla is not involved.

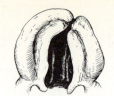

2. Unilateral type of complete cleft palate, with involvement of one side of the premaxilla.

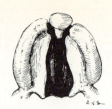

3. Bilateral type of complete cleft palate with cleavage of both sides of the premaxilla.

Figure 3–2. Types of cleft palate.

Nose & Forehead

The frontonasal prominence, superior to the stomodeum, projects caudally toward the stomodeum. It forms the dorsum and apex of the nose, the nasal septum, the philtrum (the infranasal depression on the upper lip), the premaxilla, and the forehead.

Anomalies. Remnants of the vomeronasal organs of the nasal septum may persist as cysts with wide orifices opening in the nasal vestibule on either side of the nasal septum. Other anomalies include absence of the nose, single nostril, and bifid nose.

Nose & Palate

Ectodermal islands (placodes) on each side of the frontonasal process form the nasal pits, the future nostrils. As the pits deepen cranial to the primitive palate, they come to open into the stomodeum. For a short time each pit is closed by a bucconasal membrane that eventually ruptures. When the secondary palatal processes unite with the nasal septum and the premaxilla, the nasal cavity is completely formed.

Anomalies. Palatal components may fail to unite or do so incompletely, producing varying degrees of cleft palate (Fig 3–2). In some cases they may be associated with cleft lip. Failure of the bucconasal membranes to break down may be a cause of choanal atresia.

Nasolacrimal Duct

The nasolacrimal duct develops from a thickening of the ectoderm of the floor of the nasolacrimal groove. It may fail to canalize.

I. THE FACE

The face is composed of the anterior skull bones and overlying soft tissue (muscles, cartilage, blood vessels, lymphatics, nerves, specialized glandular tissue, and special sense organs), which in the aggregate give the face its unique appearance and physiologic capabilities.

GROSS ANATOMY

Bony Landmarks
(Figs 3–3 and 3–4)

Facial bony landmarks may be visible or palpable.

The **superciliary ridge** is a portion of the frontal bone situated just above the orbit. The supraorbital notch is the central depression in the superciliary ridge.

The **orbital rim** encircles the hollow orbit. It is formed by fusion of the frontal, temporal, and zygomatic bones.

The **lateral projection of the mandible,** the chin, the inferior border of the transverse ramus, the mandibular angle, and the condyle of the ascending ramus can be easily seen and palpated.

If the jaws are opened wide, drawing the mandible inferiorly, a groove appears between the condyle of the mandible and the temporal fossa that lies just ventral to the tragus of the ear. The temporomandibular joint can be palpated in this groove.

The **frontal sinus** lies deep to the medial segment of the superciliary ridge.

The **maxilla,** whose cavity is occupied by the maxillary air sinus, is situated between the orbit, the nasal cavity, and the upper teeth.

The **infraorbital ridge** is easily palpated. Its central portion is just superior to the infraorbital foramen through which the infraorbital nerve exits.

Contour of Cheeks

The **masseter muscle** occupies the posterior cheek between the zygomatic arch superiorly and the angle of the mandible inferiorly. When the masseter is tensed by clenching the teeth together, one can palpate its anterior border. Just anterior to the masseter are the buccopharyngeal fat pad and the anterior facial muscles.

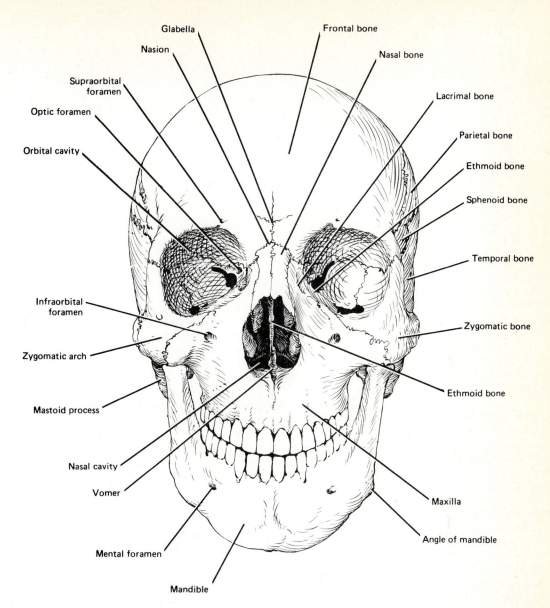

Figure 3–3. Anterior view of the skull. (Reproduced, with permission, from Chusid JG: *Correlative Neuroanatomy & Functional Neurology,* 19th ed. Lange, 1985.)

The **temporal muscle** fills the temporal fossa, the depression that lies deep to the zygoma. The temporalis muscle makes the superior edges of the zygomatic arch difficult to palpate.

The **facial artery** crosses the body of the transverse ramus of the mandible just medial to the masseter muscle. The arterial pulse can easily be palpated there.

Blood Supply & Nerves

The **anterior facial vein** accompanies the facial artery as it crosses the body of the mandible.

The **superficial temporal artery** can be palpated and on occasion seen pulsating perpendicular to the zygomatic arch, just anterior to the tragus.

The **supraorbital nerve** leaves the supraorbital foramen and can be compressed against the superciliary ridge.

The **infraorbital nerve** becomes superficial just below the inferior orbital rim.

The **middle meningeal artery** lies just deep to the thin squama of the temporal bone at the level of the mid segment of the zygomatic arch. It is vulnerable to trauma at this point.

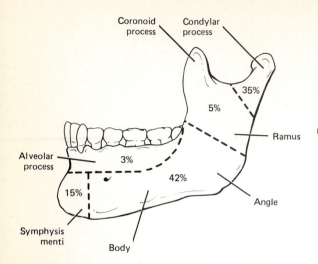

Figure 3–4. Regions of the mandible, showing fracture sites by frequency of involvement. (Redrawn and reproduced, with permission, from Dingman RO, Natvig P: *Surgery of Facial Fractures.* Saunders, 1964.)

THE MASSETER, MANDIBULAR, & TEMPORAL REGION

The masseter, mandibular, and temporal region contains the mandibular ramus and body; the temporomandibular joint; the masseter muscle, with its fascia; the parotid gland; the parotid duct; and those vessels and nerves which cross the body of the masseter muscle anteriorly.

The Mandible

The mandible, the bony framework of the lower jaw, consists of the body and an ascending ramus. The body of the mandible is U-shaped. Its anterior (external) surface is a poorly defined ridge, the mandibular symphysis, which represents the junction of the 2 fetal mandibular segments. The superior border of the body contains 16 sockets for the lower teeth. The buccinator muscle inserts into the superior border of the mandible near the first molar tooth. The rounded inferior border of the body of the mandible is thinner posteriorly than anteriorly. A groove between the body and the ascending ramus marks the site where the facial artery crosses the mandibular body. A portion of the platysma muscle interdigitates with the inferior facial muscles at the inferoanterior border of the body of the mandible. The inner surface bears a small spine on each side of the symphysis. The genioglossus muscles take their origin from the spines; the geniohyoid muscles take their origin just inferior to the spines.

➠ **Fractures of the mandible.** (Fig 3–4.) Mandibular fractures from external trauma often occur near the insertion of the lower canines.

Such fractures are usually compound, since the buccal mucous membrane and the alveolar periosteum are also disrupted. The body of the bone and the condyloid process are the areas most frequently fractured. Fractures may run through a cystic area of bone, which is often present in patients with hyperparathyroidism.

➠ **Malalignment of teeth following mandibular fractures.** Malalignment of the teeth following a blow to the jaw should suggest fracture of the mandible. Malalignment occurs when the anterior fragment of bone is drawn inferiorly and posteriorly by the geniohyoid, digastric, and hyoglossal muscles while the posterior fragment is drawn anteriorly and superiorly by the temporal, internal pterygoid, and masseter muscles.

The lateralmost surface of the body of the mandible is flattened and ridged at the insertion of the masseter. The thick inferior border of the transverse mandibular body meets the posterior border of the ascending mandibular ramus almost at a 90-degree angle, the angle of the mandible. The stylomandibular ligament inserts into its medial aspect.

The posterior border of the ascending ramus is almost totally covered by the parotid gland. The thin superior border of the ascending ramus is crowned by 2 elevations separated by the mandibular notch. The anterior elevation is the coronoid process, which is thin and roughly triangular. The temporal muscle inserts into both its medial and its lateral borders. The posterior thicker condylar process is made up of an articular condyle, inferior to which is a constricted neck. The articular surface of the condylar process is oval and articulates with the articular disk of the temporomandibular joint.

The zygomatic process of the temporal bone arches anteriorly as it leaves the temporal squama. It has a sharp superior border to which attaches the temporal fascia. The inferior border of the process is much shorter. The lateral surface of the zygoma is easily palpable and visible and gives attachment to the masseter. Anteriorly, the zygomatic arch joins the zygomatic bone. The posterior segment of the zygomatic process arises from the temporal squama by 2 roots: a long posterior root, which runs just superior to the external acoustic meatus; and a shorter anterior root, which runs anterior to the mandibular fossa and terminates in the articular tubercle, which is covered with cartilage. The mandibular (glenoid) fossa lies between the articular tubercle anteriorly and the external acoustic meatus posteriorly. The anterior portion of the mandibular fossa, which is covered with cartilage, articulates with the condyle of the mandible; the posterior segment of the fossa is nonarticular.

➠ **Fractures of the zygomatic arch.** Depressed fractures of the zygomatic arch result from *trauma to the protuberant subcutaneous zygomatic ridge. The fractured bone must be elevated to prevent a depressed facial deformity. This can usually be done easily using a towel clip, under local anesthesia.*

➡ ***Dislocation of the mandibular condyle with damage to the external auditory meatus.*** *A firm blow to the chin can push the condyle of the mandible superiorly and posteriorly, with resultant damage to the external auditory meatus. In reducing the dislocation, the condyle must be drawn anteriorly and inferiorly.*

The Temporomandibular Joint (Fig 3–5)

The temporomandibular joint lies between the articulating segment of the mandibular fossa of the temporal bone anteriorly and superiorly, the articular

tubercle posteriorly, and the condyle of the mandible inferiorly. The joint allows a combination of gliding and hingelike motions. The articular surfaces are covered with fibrocartilage. Within the joint is a fibrocartilaginous articular disk that divides the joint into superior and inferior synovial cavities. The strong articular capsule can support the joint alone. The joint is further supported by a lateral ligament, the sphenomandibular ligament, and by the stylomandibular ligament.

Movements of the joint result in depression and elevation, protrusion and retraction, and side-to-side movement of the lower jaw.

There are 2 segments in the articulation: one between the condyle of the mandible and the articular disk, and one between the articular disk and the mandibular fossa.

Opening of the jaw is accomplished by the lateral pterygoid, digastric, mylohyoid, and geniohyoid muscles; closure is accomplished by the masseter, tempo-

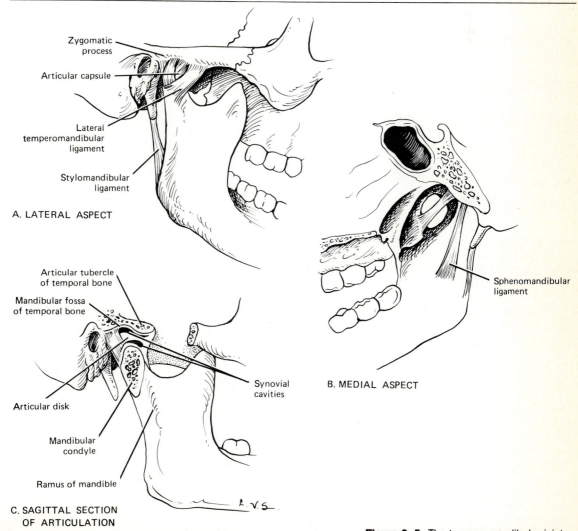

Zygomatic process
Articular capsule
Lateral temperomandibular ligament
Stylomandibular ligament

A. LATERAL ASPECT

Sphenomandibular ligament

B. MEDIAL ASPECT

Articular tubercle of temporal bone
Mandibular fossa of temporal bone
Articular disk
Mandibular condyle
Ramus of mandible
Synovial cavities

C. SAGITTAL SECTION OF ARTICULATION

Figure 3–5. The temporomandibular joint.

ral, and medial pterygoid muscles. Jaw protrusion is accomplished by the combined action of both lateral pterygoid muscles and the muscles of jaw closure. Jaw retraction is accomplished by the temporal muscle and lateral motion by the lateral pterygoid muscle of the opposite side.

⟹ *Dislocation of temporomandibular joint. This usually occurs when the mouth is opened too widely. The dislocation is always anterior. A strong muscular effort or downward force exerted against the chin throws the condyles farther anteriorly and out of their sockets. The condyles are held in the dislocated position by spasm of the temporal, masseter, and pterygoid muscles.*

A strong blow to the chin while the mouth is wide open will frequently dislocate the joint. In such cases, the dislocation is usually bilateral. The mouth then remains open, and the mandible projects anteriorly.

MUSCLES OF THE FACE
(Fig 3–6)

The **buccinator** is the major muscle of the cheek. It forms the deep lateral muscular boundary of the oral cavity. It takes origin from the alveolar processes of both the mandible and the maxilla and from the pterygomandibular raphe. Its fibers move toward the angle of the mouth, where they join with the fibers of the orbicularis oris to run to the upper and lower lips. The surface of the buccinator is related to the buccinator fat pad; its deep surface is related superficially to the buccal mucous membrane of the cheek. The parotid duct turns at a right angle and pierces the buccinator as it proceeds to its intraoral ostium. The buccinator is a cheek compressor and aids in mastication. It is innervated by the buccal branches of the facial nerve.

⟹ *Facial areolar tissues. The fatty areolar tissue of the deep lateral areas of the face is continu-*

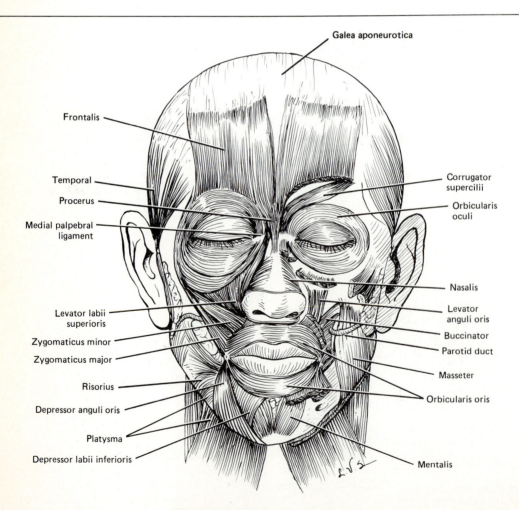

Figure 3–6. Muscles of the face.

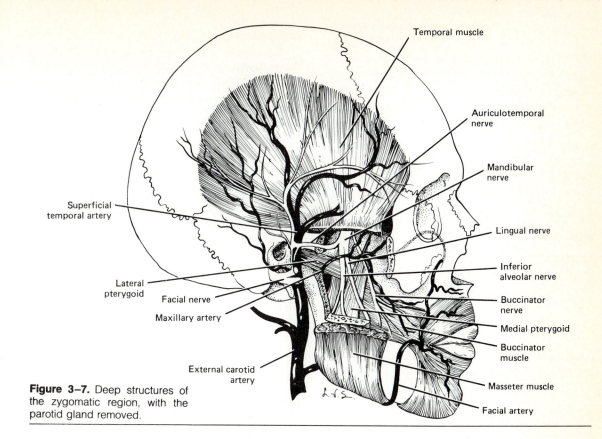

Figure 3–7. Deep structures of the zygomatic region, with the parotid gland removed.

ous and intimately connected with similar tissues of the tongue, the cheek, and the temporal region of the scalp. Consequently, infection spreads easily from one adjacent areolar area to the other.

The **temporal muscle** (Fig 3–7) is broad and fan-shaped on the lateral surface of the skull. It arises from the entire temporal fossa and the inner surface of the temporal fascia. It narrows as it descends, and its fibers finally terminate in a tendon that inserts into the coronoid process and the anterior border of the mandibular ramus. The temporal muscle participates in closing of the jaw and retraction of the mandible. It is innervated by the mandibular division of the trigeminal nerve.

The **masseter** is a bulky muscle that lies external to the ascending ramus of the mandible. The superficial segment arises from the zygomatic process of the maxilla and from the zygomatic arch, and its fibers insert into the angle and the ascending ramus of the mandible. The smaller deep segment arises from the zygomatic arch and inserts into the ascending mandibular ramus and the coronoid process of the mandible. The masseter participates in jaw closure and aids in retracting the mandible. It is supplied by branches from the mandibular division of the trigeminal nerve.

Tetanus. *In tetanus, the masseter muscle undergoes marked spasm (trismus). Tetanus must be suspected whenever a wound infection is associated with a history of early trismus.*

Myositis. *Myositis of the masseter with limitation of jaw motion can occur secondary to temporomandibular joint infection. Secondary permanent masseter fibrosis may follow acute myositis of the muscle.*

The **medial pterygoid** muscle (Fig 3–8) is a bulky muscle on the inner surface of the ascending ramus of the mandible. It arises from the pterygoid plate, the palatine bone, and the maxilla. Its fibers insert via a tendon into the medial surface of the ascending ramus of the mandible. The sphenomandibular ligament lies between the muscle and the inner surface of the mandible, as do also the maxillary vessels, the inferior alveolar vessels, the inferior alveolar nerve, and the lingual nerve. The muscle aids in jaw closure and is supplied by the mandibular division of the trigeminal nerve.

The **lateral pterygoid** (Fig 3–8) is a triangular muscle that arises from the great wing of the sphenoid and the pterygoid plate and inserts into the neck of the condyle of the mandible. It participates in opening of the jaw and protrusion and lateral movement of

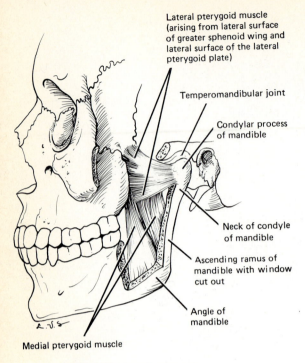

Lateral pterygoid muscle
(arising from lateral surface
of greater sphenoid wing and
lateral surface of the lateral
pterygoid plate)

Temperomandibular joint

Condylar process
of mandible

Neck of condyle
of mandible

Ascending ramus of
mandible with window
cut out

Angle of
mandible

Medial pterygoid muscle

Figure 3–8. The pterygoid muscles.

the mandible. It is supplied by the mandibular division of the trigeminal nerve.

BLOOD VESSELS, LYMPHATICS, & NERVES

Arteries & Veins
(Fig 3–9)

The external maxillary (facial) artery, the main vessel supplying the superficial areas of the face, is the third anterior branch of the external carotid artery. It enters the facial area by crossing the body of the mandible at the anteroinferior border of the masseter. It proceeds to the corner of the mouth, at which point it becomes the angular artery and ascends along the side of the nose to the medial canthus of the eye. The facial artery, gives off superior and inferior labial, lateral nasal, and facial muscular branches. The artery is accompanied by the anterior facial vein, which joins the ophthalmic veins near the lateral canthus of the eye; via this connection, blood enters the intracranial cavernous sinus.

Lymphatics

Lymph drainage from the superficial facial areas is into the submental and submandibular nodes and also directly into the superior group of the vertical chain of deep cervical nodes.

Nerves
(Figs 3–10 and 3–11)

The muscles of the cheek are supplied by the facial nerve; sensation to the skin of the face is supplied by the mandibular and maxillary divisions of the trigeminal nerve. The forehead, upper eyelid, and dorsum and tip of the nose are supplied by the ophthalmic division of the trigeminal nerve.

➠ *Blood supply to superficial areas of the face. The success of plastic procedures involving the skin and superficial tissues of the face is due to the vascularity of the facial tissues, which are supplied mainly by the facial artery. Incisions into the superficial facial tissues must be expected to bleed briskly and also to heal rapidly with a minimal risk of infection.*

THE PTERYGOMAXILLARY FOSSA

The pterygomaxillary fossa lies deep to the masseter and the mandible. It is bounded posteriorly by the anterior border of the parotid gland and anteriorly by the anterolateral border of the cheek. The pterygomaxillary region is separated from the pharynx only by the parapharyngeal space, so that tumors or collections of blood or pus within the space may bulge directly into the pharynx. Because of the rigid mandible and the bulk of the masseter muscle, it is difficult to examine and explore the region from a facial approach. Within the pterygoid fossa are the 2 pterygoid muscles, the interpterygoid fascia, the internal maxillary vessels, and the maxillary and mandibular branches of the trigeminal nerve. The main artery of this deep area of the face is the maxillary, a terminal branch of the external carotid. The artery arises within the parotid gland deep to the neck of the condyloid process of the mandible and runs anteriorly between the ramus of the mandible and the sphenomandibular ligament, then deep to the lateral pterygoid muscle into the pterygopalatine fossa. It supplies all of the deep structures of the face through its mandibular, pterygoid, and pterygopalatine branches.

➠ *Approach to the pterygomaxillary fossa. Because the pterygomaxillary region is difficult to explore via a facial approach, it is usually examined, explored, and drained via the pharyngeal cavity.*

The pterygoid processes of the sphenoid bone project inferiorly from the point where the body and greater wings of the sphenoid meet. Each process is made up of a medial and a lateral plate. The 2 plates are fused superiorly and anteriorly but diverge inferiorly, forming the pterygoid fissure, whose borders join with the palatine bone. The plates also diverge

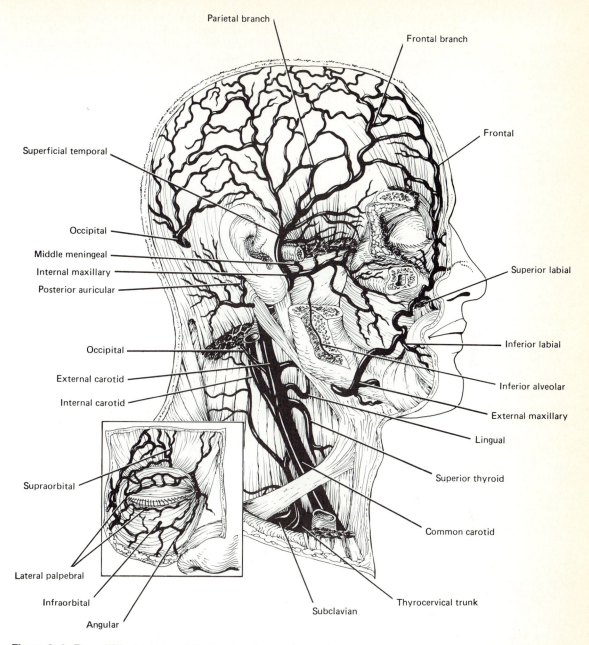

Figure 3–9. The principal arteries of the head and neck. (Reproduced, with permission, from Chusid JG: *Correlative Neuroanatomy & Functional Neurology,* 19th ed. Lange, 1985.)

posteriorly, forming a V-shaped fossa, the pterygoid fossa. Within the fossa are the medial pterygoid and the tensor veli palatini muscles. (See also section on Cranial Nerves for Motor and Sensory Supply to the Face in Chapter 2.)

THE RETROMANDIBULAR SPACE

The retromandibular space is bounded anteriorly by the ascending ramus of the mandible, the masseter muscle, and the internal pterygoid muscle; posteriorly by the mastoid process of the temporal bone and the sternocleidomastoid muscle; superiorly by the temporomandibular joint and the external auditory meatus; and inferiorly by the posterior belly of the digastric muscle, the stylohyoideus muscle, and the stylomandibular ligament.

The retromandibular space is covered by the skin and superficial fascia of the face. Just deep to these structures lies the thick superficial fascia of the parotid gland. Deep to the superficial parotid fascia lies the

ONLY Californians ... make ?
mistake this big!

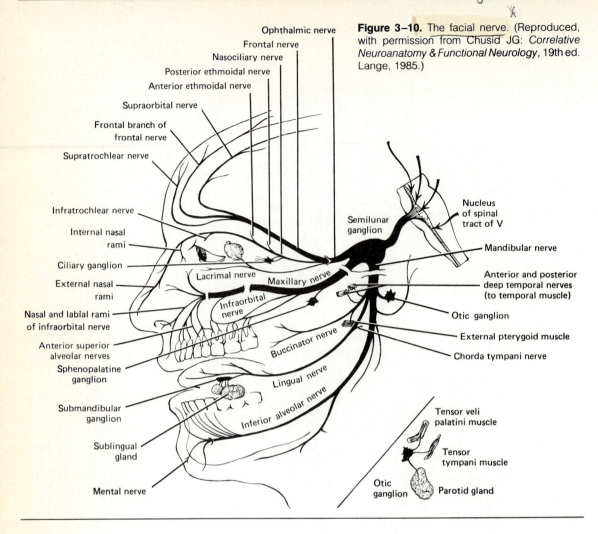

Ophthalmic nerve
Frontal nerve
Nasociliary nerve
Posterior ethmoidal nerve
Anterior ethmoidal nerve
Supraorbital nerve
Frontal branch of frontal nerve
Supratrochlear nerve
Infratrochlear nerve
Internal nasal rami
Ciliary ganglion
External nasal rami
Nasal and labial rami of infraorbital nerve
Anterior superior alveolar nerves
Sphenopalatine ganglion
Submandibular ganglion
Sublingual gland
Mental nerve
Lacrimal nerve
Maxillary nerve
Infraorbital nerve
Buccinator nerve
Lingual nerve
Inferior alveolar nerve
Semilunar ganglion
Nucleus of spinal tract of V
Mandibular nerve
Anterior and posterior deep temporal nerves (to temporal muscle)
Otic ganglion
External pterygoid muscle
Chorda tympani nerve
Tensor veli palatini muscle
Tensor tympani muscle
Otic ganglion
Parotid gland

Figure 3–10. The facial nerve. (Reproduced, with permission from Chusid JG: *Correlative Neuroanatomy & Functional Neurology,* 19th ed. Lange, 1985.)

parenchyma of the gland, its deep surface invested by the parotid fascia. The deep boundaries of the space are the styloid process of the temporal bone and the styloglossus, stylohyoid, and stylopharyngeus muscles and the stylomandibular ligament, all of which attach to the styloid process of the temporal bone. The lateral pharyngeal wall constitutes part of the deep boundary of the retromandibular space.

II. THE PAROTID GLAND (Fig 3–12)

The parotid gland occupies the major portion of the retromandibular space. It is the largest of the 3 major salivary glands (parotid, submandibular, and sublingual), which encircle the entrance to the oropharynx. Diffuse salivary gland tissue is found in the palate, cheeks, and lips.

GROSS ANATOMY

The outer surface of the parotid gland is an irregular structure; its deep surface is wedge-shaped and protrudes toward the lateral pharyngeal wall. The parotid weighs about 15–20 g. It fills most of the retromandibular space and protrudes anteriorly onto the ascending ramus of the mandible, where it lies upon the masseter muscle. A small deep segment lies between the 2 pterygoid muscles ("pterygoid lobe"). Just inferior to the zygomatic arch, superior to the parotid duct, a small segment of the gland lies upon the masseter muscle ("accessory lobe"). Two distinct processes take off from the deep surface of the gland. The first rests upon the styloid process, the digastric muscle, and the 3 muscles that attach to the styloid process. The second lies forward of the styloid process and thus is often found deep to the temporomandibular joint.

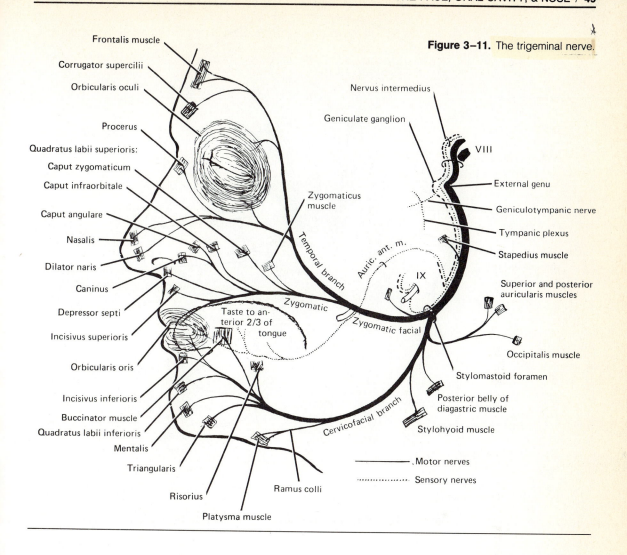

Figure 3–11. The trigeminal nerve.

CAPSULE OF THE PAROTID GLAND

The parotid gland is enclosed within a well-defined capsule which is an extension of the investing fascia of the neck. At the level of the inferior pole of the parotid, this fascia thickens to form the stylomandibular ligament. Just superior to this ligament, the investing fascia splits to enclose the parotid, and this forms the superficial and deep capsular structure of the gland. The superficial capsule is thick and unyielding and tightly affixed to the underlying glandular tissue by numerous fibrous septa. The deep capsule is quite thin and easily disrupted. As the superior pole of the parotid reaches the level of the zygomatic arch, its superficial and deep capsular layers attach firmly to the corresponding surfaces of the arch (Fig 3–12).

➠ *Pain in infectious parotitis. Mumps is a viral infection that presents clinically as an acute inflammation of the parotid gland and often of other salivary glands. Less frequently, there* may be accompanying inflammation of the pancreas, testes, ovaries, or central nervous system. Within the parotid, edema associated with inflammation compresses the nerves and engorged lymphatics against the unyielding superficial capsule of the gland. This pressure results in severe pain, often with radiation along the auriculotemporal nerve. Viral parotitis is associated with redness and swelling around the meatus of the parotid duct and sometimes exudate at the parotid papilla.*

➠ *Rupture of parotid abscesses through the thin, deep capsule of the gland. Parotid abscesses may develop secondary to breakdown of infected lymph nodes within the gland parenchyma, secondary to inflammation in the retropharyngeal space resulting from pharyngeal perforation by a sharp foreign body or instrument, or as a complication of blood-borne infection. An abscess deep within the parotid gland may rupture through the thin deep posterior*

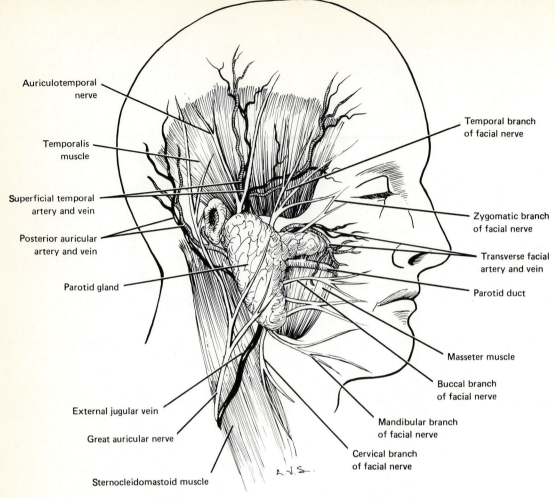

Figure 3–12. The parotid gland and the temporal muscle.

capsule to present in the retromandibular space. If large enough, such an abscess will bulge against the mucous membranes of the oral cavity. Drainage may be via the oral cavity or via an elevation of the parotid gland from its mandibular bed. Parotid abscesses on occasion follow infection secondary to calculi within the gland or in its ducts.

STRUCTURE OF THE PAROTID GLAND

The parotid, like the other salivary glands, is an exocrine gland. It is composed of a series of lobules bound together by thickened areolar tissue. Lying between the individual lobules is a thick network of blood vessels, lymphatics, and small ductules. The parotid is grossly divided into 2 major lobes: superficial and deep. This division is of great surgical significance, since the main trunk and the major branches of the facial nerve lie in the fascial plane that separates

the 2 lobes. This allows for complete removal of the superficial lobe of the gland with minimal trauma to the underlying facial nerve and its branches. The 2 major lobes of the gland are joined posteriorly by a stubby, thick isthmus of glandular tissue that lies just anterior to the stylomastoid foramen, where the facial nerve emerges from the skull.

➠ *Parotid neoplasms and their relationship to the parotid lobes. Parotid neoplasms may be benign or malignant. The most frequent benign tumors are the so-called mixed tumors. Warthin's tumor (papillary cystadenoma lymphomatosum), mucoepidermoid tumor, serous cell adenoma, acidophilic adenoma, basal cell adenoma, and oxyphilic adenoma occur less frequently. Most benign parotid tumors are found in the superficial lobe and consequently may be completely excised by superficial lobectomy, care being taken not to injure the underlying facial nerve. The major malignant parotid tu-*

mors are malignant mixed tumors, mucoepidermoid carcinoma, adenocarcinoma, and epidermoid carcinoma. The latter 2 types have a grave prognosis, particularly if resection is inadequate at the first operative procedure. The procedure of choice for parotid cancer is total parotidectomy with preservation of the facial nerve only if it does not appear to be involved in the malignant process.

The parotid excretory duct (Stensen's duct) averages about 7 cm in length. It is formed in the anterior portion of the superficial lobe of the gland by coalescence of multiple small ducts from the deep and superficial lobes. It emerges from the gland at its anterior border and runs forward in a transverse direction, superficial to the body of the masseter muscle. At the anterior border of the masseter muscle, the duct makes a right-angle turn and runs deeply toward the buccal surface of the cheek, piercing the buccinator fat pad and then the buccinator muscle. It then again changes direction and continues obliquely forward between the deep surface of the cheek and the mucous membrane of the oral cavity. It empties into the oral cavity via a prominent papilla located on the buccal surface of the cheek at the level of the upper second molar.

As the duct crosses the masseter muscle, it occasionally receives a small accessory duct that drains the anterior segment of the gland. The major parotid duct is generally palpable, since it lies upon the masseter muscle along a line running from the commissure of the mouth to the external auditory canal.

The duct wall is composed of a thick, dense layer of smooth muscle. The lumen of the duct averages about 3–4 mm but becomes markedly narrower as it approaches its orifice in the mouth and at sites where it changes direction. These anatomic narrowings make probing difficult and can be seen on sialograms.

➡ ***Probing of the parotid duct.*** *The parotid duct is difficult to probe because it changes direction 90 degrees as it passes through the buccinator fat pad and buccinator muscle.*

➡ ***Parotid sialography.*** *Parotid sialography is a means of visualizing the parotid gland and its ducts. It is used to investigate tumors of the gland and the possible presence of ductal or glandular calculi and as a means of identifying ductal deformities following facial trauma. The procedure involves cannulating the parotid duct and filling the ductal system with radiopaque contrast material.*

➡ ***Postoperative parotitis.*** *This occurs as a postoperative complication in elderly, dehydrated, or debilitated patients. It is less common now because of better oral hygiene and better management of fluid and electrolyte balance in surgical and in debilitated medical patients. The bacteria usually reach the parotid by retrograde invasion from the mouth along the excretory duct. Most cases respond well to specific antibiotic therapy.*

➡ ***Parotid fistulas.*** *Trauma to the cheek may result in disruption of the parotid duct, often followed by formation of a parotidofacial fistula. Surgical repair is often possible. When it is not, the proximal segment of the severed duct is usually ligated. The contralateral parotid gland delivers enough secretion to compensate for what is lost on the affected side.*

STRUCTURES RADIATING FROM THE PAROTID GLAND

Superiorly

The superficial temporal artery and vein, accompanied by the auriculotemporal nerve, are related to the mid superior surface of the parotid gland as they cross the posterior root of the zygoma. The superficial temporal artery is one of 2 terminal branches of the external carotid artery. The superficial temporal vein joins with the internal maxillary vein within the substance of the parotid gland to form the posterior facial vein. The auriculotemporal nerve is a branch of the third (mandibular) division of the trigeminal nerve. The temporal branch of the facial nerve, which supplies the frontal and orbicularis oculi muscles of the superior portion of the face, also issues from the anterosuperior surface of the gland.

Anteriorly

The following structures, from superior to inferior, issue from the anterior surface of the gland: the zygomatic branch of the facial nerve; the major parotid duct; and the buccal branch of the facial nerve, which pursues a course just inferior and parallel to the first segment of the parotid duct. The transverse facial vein enters the anterior border of the parotid and joins the posterior facial vein within the gland substance.

Inferiorly

Related to the inferior margin of the gland are the mandibular branch of the facial nerve, which supplies the facial muscles surrounding the labial commissure; the descending cervical branch of the facial nerve, which supplies the platysma muscle; the posterior facial vein, which serves as an excellent guide to the fascial plane between the superficial and deep lobes of the parotid gland; and the great auricular nerve, which enters the inferior margin of the parotid gland as it runs from the cervical plexus to join with the facial nerve within the substance of the gland.

Posteriorly

The posterior auricular artery, a posterior branch of the external carotid artery, leaves the posteroinferior margin of the gland and runs across the mastoid process of the temporal bone. The posterior auricular vein, just below the inferior margin of the gland, joins with the posterior branch of the posterior facial vein to form the external jugular vein. The posterior branch of the facial nerve supplies the occipitalis muscle and is the first branch given off the main facial trunk after the nerve exits from the stylomastoid foramen.

STRUCTURES LYING WITHIN THE SUBSTANCE OF THE PAROTID GLAND

The terminal segment of the **external carotid artery** lies close to the deep surface of the inferior third of the parotid gland. It enters the deep lobe and comes to lie just superficial to the deep capsule of the gland, the deepest structure within the upper half of the gland. Almost immediately upon entering the substance of the gland, the external carotid artery gives off the large maxillary branch, which runs anteriorly. The **maxillary artery** divides into 3 major branches: mandibular, pterygoid, and pterygopalatine. Smaller branchings issue from these branches to supply deep facial structures. An important nonfacial twig given off from the mandibular branch of the maxillary artery is the **middle meningeal artery.** This vessel enters the cranial cavity via the foramen spinosum. Within the cranial cavity, it supplies blood to the dura mater in the temporal region. As it courses superiorly after entering the cranium, the vessel occupies a vulnerable position as it lies on the inner surface of the exceedingly thin plate of the squama of the temporal bone.

After bifurcation, the external carotid artery continues superiorly within the deep lobe of the parotid gland as the **superficial temporal artery.** This vessel leaves the superior margin of the gland, crosses the posterior root of the zygoma, and supplies the temporal and parietal regions of the scalp.

⟹ *Trauma to the middle meningeal artery. The middle meningeal artery, as it runs just deep to the inner surface of the temporal bone, is quite vulnerable to trauma. Fracture of the temporal bone, with tearing of the artery, may lead to extradural hemorrhage with a rise in intracranial pressure followed by a lapse into unconsciousness within hours after the injury. The intracranial pressure must be relieved immediately to prevent permanent brain damage or death.*

The **posterior facial vein** lies within the substance of the deep lobe of the parotid gland, just superficial to the external carotid artery. The vein is formed by the junction of the superficial temporal, middle meningeal, and transverse facial veins. As it emerges from the parotid, the posterior facial vein divides into (1) an anterior branch, which continues to the suprahyoid area of the neck, to join the anterior facial vein and form the common facial vein; and (2) a posterior branch, which joins the posterior auricular vein to form the external jugular vein.

The **facial nerve** (Fig 3–10) emerges from the stylomastoid foramen in the temporal bone as a short, stubby trunk. It runs a short distance anteriorly in the retromandibular space toward the isthmus of the parotid gland. There it divides into a zygomatic facial branch, which passes superiorly to the isthmus, and a cervicofacial branch, which passes inferiorly to the isthmus. These 2 major divisions of the facial nerve both run anteriorly within the parotid substance in the plane between the superficial and deep lobes of the gland. The 2 nerves lie superficial to the external carotid artery and the posterior facial vein, both of which are within the deep lobe of the gland. Just before the main trunk of the facial nerve reaches the isthmus of the gland, it gives off (1) the posterior auricular branch, (2) the nerves to the stylohyoid muscle, and (3) the nerve to the posterior belly of the digastric muscle. Still within the parotid gland, the 2 major branches of the facial nerve give off multiple peripheral branches that supply the muscles of the face, the muscles of the sides of the scalp, and the platysma muscle. None of the facial nerve filaments lie within the superficial lobe of the gland, so that this segment may be operated on with small risk of injury to the facial nerve.

⟹ *Facial nerve lacerations. (Fig 3–13.) Laceration of the main trunk of the facial nerve or one of its major branchings within the parotid gland as a result of facial trauma is an uncommon injury requiring identification and microsurgical repair of the severed branches.*

⟹ *Parotid cancer involving the facial nerve. Malignant tumors of the parotid gland may involve branches of the facial nerve as they spread through the gland, with a resultant partial or total facial palsy. Benign tumors of the parotid seldom involve the facial nerve.*

⟹ *Localization of the facial nerve in surgical procedures upon the parotid. (Fig 3–14.) Most surgeons feel that in performing surgery on the parotid gland, the facial nerve should be identified early by establishing its relationship to the major structures described above. A few surgeons feel that tracing the peripheral branches of the facial nerve proximally into the parotid gland is the safest means of entering the fascial space between the 2 lobes of the gland. However, the best method of locating*

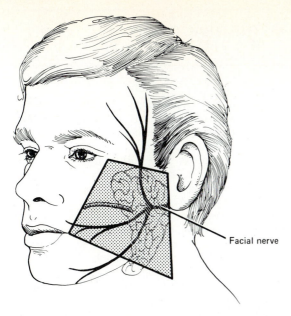

Figure 3–13. Area of the face where facial lacerations may injure the parotid gland, Stensen's duct, or the facial nerve. (Reproduced, with permission, from Way LW [editor]: *Current Surgical Diagnosis & Treatment,* 7th ed. Lange, 1985.)

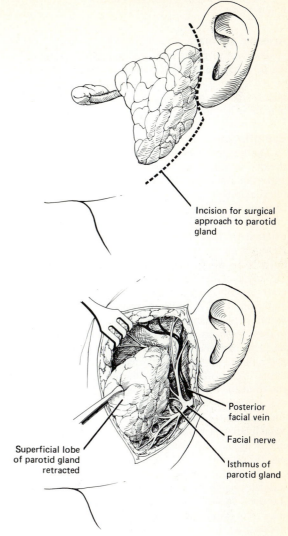

Figure 3–14. Surgical approach to the parotid gland.

the nerve is to use the mastoid process as a landmark. The facial nerve lies medial and deep to the mastoid process just as the nerve emerges from the stylomastoid foramen. At this point, the nerve is 2–3 mm in diameter and easily seen lying in the inverted V between the bony portion of the external auditory meatus and the mastoid process. This relationship of the nerve to the mastoid process is a constant and reliable one.

Lying in the retromandibular fossa beneath the thin, deep capsule of the parotid are the **internal jugular vein,** the **internal carotid artery,** and segments of the **glossopharyngeal, vagus, accessory,** and **hypoglossal nerves.** Deep within the retromandibular fossa are the bony styloid process of the temporal bone and the superior portions of the stylohyoideus, posterior digastric, stylopharyngeus, and styloglossus muscles as well as the superior segment of the stylomandibular ligament.

➡ ***Drainage of parotid abscesses.*** *(Fig 3–14.) Localized parotid abscesses are treated by incision and drainage, care being taken not to injure branches of the facial nerve. On occasion, a parotid abscess may rupture into the adjacent external auditory meatus or even into the tempo-*

romandibular joint. The usual incision for drainage of a parotid abscess is a vertical one placed just anterior to the external auditory meatus. The incision can easily be extended inferiorly and anteriorly around the angle of the mandible, taking care to avoid surgery to the mandibular branch of the facial nerve. If a deep retromandibular space abscess is to be drained, the posteroinferior segment of the parotid must be mobilized and partially lifted from its bed so that the deep surface of the gland and the retromandibular space can be adequately exposed.

BLOOD SUPPLY, LYMPHATICS, & NERVES

Arteries & Veins

The parotid gland receives its arterial supply primarily from the maxillary artery, a terminal branch of the external carotid artery. Venous drainage is mainly into the external jugular vein, via the posterior branch of the posterior facial vein.

Lymphatics

The lymph nodes related to the parotid gland are divided into 2 groups: superficial and deep. (1) The **superficial parotid lymph nodes** lie external to the thick external capsule of the gland and are placed between the capsule and the subcutaneous tissues of the cheek. These nodes receive afferents from the external ear, the eyelids, the forehead, and the temporal region of the scalp. The efferent lymphatics leaving these nodes run to deep cervical nodes that lie below the angle of the mandible. The superficial parotid nodes usually enlarge without causing significant facial pain. (2) The **deep parotid lymph nodes** lie within the substance of the parotid gland. Afferents to these nodes arrive from the middle ear, the auditory tube, the hard and soft palate, the nose, the pterygoid and palatine fossae, the external ear, and the parotid tissue itself. Efferents from the deep parotid nodes run to deep cervical nodes along the internal jugular vein where the vein is crossed by the accessory nerve. Enlargement of the deep nodes lying within the superficial lobe of the parotid, close to its unyielding superficial capsule, can cause considerable pain over the parotid gland.

A third group of nodes related to the parotid gland lies deep within the retromandibular space. They drain the deep fossae of the face, and their enlargement may result in symptoms of pharyngeal pressure. The nodes drain into the deep vertical chain of cervical nodes above the crossing of the omohyoid muscle.

Nerves

The nerve supply to the parotid is from the sympathetic plexus, which surrounds the external carotid artery. The parotid also receives some nerve supply from the auriculotemporal nerve, which contains cranial parasympathetics derived from the glossopharyngeal and facial nerves.

➠ *Frey's syndrome. A few patients who have undergone parotidectomy develop flushing and increased sweating over the parotid area following a meal. It is caused by abnormal regeneration of parasympathetic auriculotemporal nerve fibers following injury. Frey's syndrome usually appears 2–4 weeks following parotid surgery but may appear as late as a year after the operation. It can be treated by severing the tympanic plexus in the ear.*

III. THE ORAL CAVITY
(Fig 3–15)

The oral cavity is the beginning of the alimentary tract. It is an oval space divided into 2 segments, an outer vestibule and the inner oral cavity proper.

The **vestibule** is the space between the teeth, the lips, and the cheeks. Superiorly and inferiorly, it is contained by reflections of the mucous membranes from the cheeks and lips onto the upper and lower gums. The external secretion of the parotid gland empties into the vestibule via an ostium on the buccal surface just opposite the second upper molar.

The oral cavity proper is bounded anteriorly and laterally by the alveolar arches and the teeth. Posteriorly, it merges with the pharynx via a narrowed opening, the **isthmus faucium.** Superiorly, the oral cavity proper is contained by the hard and soft palates. The tongue forms the major segment of its floor. The oral cavity proper receives the secretions of the submandibular and sublingual salivary glands.

THE LIPS

The lips are 2 pouting folds of flesh that surround the entrance into the vestibule. Externally, the lips are covered with the skin of the face; internally, they are lined by mucous membrane. Between the skin and the mucous membrane are the orbicularis oris muscle and the vessels and nerves that supply the lips. Some areolar tissue and the labial glands also are between the 2 lip surfaces. The mucous membrane covering the inner surface of each lip is connected in the midline to the gum tissue covering the adjacent alveolar ridge by a fold, or frenulum.

➠ *Deformity of lips following lacerations. Because the lips have no bony attachment, severe lacerating injuries can result in contracture of underlying muscle and facial tissues, with a severe oral deformity unless primary repair includes meticulous building up of the supporting muscular and subcutaneous tissues and careful reestablishment of the vermilion border.*

➠ *Carcinoma of the lips. Carcinomas of the lip are usually of the squamous cell type and almost always involve the lower lip. Chronic irritation due to excessive heat, tobacco, or excessive exposure to actinic rays contributes to their occurrence. The cancer usually occurs in an area of previous chronic fissure or leukoplakia.*

Carcinoma of the lip is treated by chemotherapy when the lesion is early and limited. If the lesion is broad and deeper, excision is

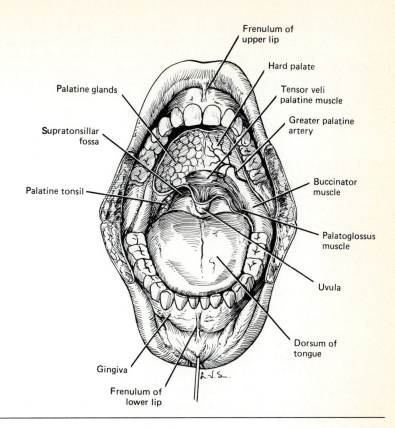

Figure 3–15. The oral cavity shown with the mucous membrane of the palate removed.

required along with plastic closure of the denuded lip area. Neck dissection or radiation therapy (or both) should follow excision if cervical node involvement is present or suspected.

The lips blend laterally into the cheeks. Superficially, the cheeks are covered by facial skin. Deep to skin is a layer of muscle, some fatty areolar tissue, vessels, nerves, and the buccal glands. The inner (buccal) surface of each cheek is covered with mucous membrane continuous with that covering the upper and lower gums. Posteriorly, the mucous membrane of the cheek joins with that of the soft palate. A papilla in the mucous membrane opposite the upper second molars contains the ostium of the parotid duct. The buccinator, risorius, zygomaticus, and platysma muscles contribute to the fullness of the cheeks and give expression to the face as they lie deep to the skin of the face and superficial to the mucous membrane of the oral cavity.

GLANDS OF THE MOUTH

The tiny **labial glands** encircle the lips as they lie between the orbicularis oris muscle and the mucous membrane of the inner surfaces of the lips. They are similar histologically to the salivary glands. They empty via minute orifices in the surfaces of the mucous membrane of the lips.

The small **buccal glands** lie between the mucous membrane of the cheek and the buccinator muscle. Histologically, they too resemble the salivary glands. They empty via small puncta in the mucous membrane of the cheek in the vicinity of the parotid papilla.

GUMS

The gums (gingivae) are composed of thick fibrous tissue that lies atop the alveolar processes close to the bases of the teeth. The gums are covered by a sensitive layer of mucous membrane.

THE ROOF OF THE MOUTH (PALATE)

The **anterior (hard) palate** is limited anteriorly and laterally by the alveolar margins of the upper teeth and posteriorly by the soft palate. Its vault is supported by the palatine plate of the maxilla and the horizontal plate of the palatine bone. The bony vault is covered by a closely adherent bony periosteum and the mucous membrane of the oral cavity. The midline of the hard palate is marked by a slight depression or raphe that terminates anteriorly in a small papilla. The covering mucous membrane is thrown up into thick rugal folds anteriorly; posteriorly, the membrane is smooth and flat. Deep to the mucous membrane are numerous small palatine glands.

⫸ *Tumors of the hard palate. Mucoepidermoid tumors and mixed tumors of salivary gland origin are occasionally found in the hard palate. They can become large enough to obstruct the oropharynx. The tumors have their origin either in the palatine glands or in islands of ectopic salivary gland tissue.*

The **posterior (soft) palate** hangs like a curtain from the posterior border of the hard palate and separates the nasopharynx from the posterior oropharynx. It is made up of a fold of mucous membrane between whose layers lie muscle fibers, nerves and blood vessels, mucous glands, and some lymphoid tissue. Attached to the midline of the posterior free border of the soft palate is the uvula. During swallowing and sucking, the soft palate is elevated, completely shutting off the nasal cavity and the nasopharynx from the oral cavity and from the intraoral pharynx.

The soft palate also has a median raphe. The lateral surfaces of the soft palate are bounded by the pharyngeal walls. From either side of the base of the uvula, 2 arching folds of mucous membrane, the arches of the fauces, fuse with the lateral pharyngeal walls. Fused with the posterior border of the hard palate and lying within the soft palate is a strong supporting sheet, the palatine aponeurosis.

⫸ *Paralysis of muscles of the soft palate. When a patient is unable to prevent food from entering the nose by way of the posterior nares, one must consider palsy of the muscles controlling the soft palate. This condition occurs secondary to diphtheritic neuropathy, in the late stages of degenerative diseases of the nervous system, and after intracranial hemorrhage.*

THE FAUCES

The fauces (throat) is the opening that connects the oral cavity with the pharyngeal cavity. The fauces is bounded superiorly by the soft palate, inferiorly by the dorsum of the tongue, and on both sides by the palatoglossal arch. The palatoglossal arch (the anterior pillar of the fauces) swings inferiorly from the lateral edge of the uvula and inserts into the lateral posterior surface of the tongue. The palatoglossus muscle lies just deep to the mucous membrane cover-

ing the arch. The palatopharyngeal arch (the posterior pillar of the fauces) leaves the posterior free border of the soft palate alongside the uvula and curves inferiorly and laterally to attach to the side of the base of the tongue posterior to the attachment of the anterior pillar. The palatopharyngeus muscle lies just deep to the covering mucous membrane of the posterior pillar. The 2 tonsillar pillars, which are close to each other superiorly, spread apart as they descend. A triangular interval (the tonsillar fossa) is thus formed. Within this interval lies the palatine tonsil.

THE MUSCLES OF THE PALATE

There are 5 palatine muscles.

The **levator veli palatini** arises from the petrous portion of the temporal bone and from the cartilaginous wall of the auditory tube. Its fibers run in the palatine velum until they reach the midline, where they blend with the fibers of the contralateral levator veli palatini.

The **tensor veli palatini** lies anterolateral to the levator veli palatini. It arises from the inner pterygoid plate from the sphenoidal spine and from the cartilaginous wall of the auditory tube; it ends in a tendon that inserts into both the palatine aponeurosis and the palatine bone.

The **musculus uvulae** arises from the posterior nasal spine of the palatine bone and the palatine fascial sheet and inserts into the uvula.

The **palatoglossus muscle** arises from the anterior surface of the soft palate and inserts into the side of the tongue. It forms the palatoglossal arch.

The **palatopharyngeus muscle,** with its covering mucous membrane, forms the palatopharyngeal arch. It arises from the soft palate, joins with the fibers of the stylopharyngeus, and inserts into the posterior border of the thyroid cartilage.

The tensor veli palatini is supplied by a branch from the trigeminal nerve; the other 4 palatine muscles are supplied by the accessory nerve via the pharyngeal plexus.

The palate receives its blood supply from the descending palatine branch of the maxillary artery, the palatine branch of the ascending pharyngeal artery, and the ascending palatine branch of the facial artery. Venous blood from the palate drains into the tonsillar and pterygoid plexuses. Lymphatic drainage from the palate is directly into the vertical deep cervical chain of nodes. Sensory innervation of the palate is from the nasopalatine, palatine, and glossopharyngeal nerves.

THE PALATINE TONSIL

The palatine tonsil is a protuberant mass of lymphoid tissue on either side of the fauces and lying between the palatoglossal and palatopharyngeal arches. The tonsil is covered by a fold of mucous membrane that stretches medially between the 2 arches. The size, shape, and degree of embedding of the tonsil are quite variable. On the medial surface, about 10–20 crypts extend deeply into the tonsillar structure. The lateral (deep) tonsillar surface is tightly adherent to a connective tissue capsule. The fibers of the superior constrictor of the pharynx lie just deep to the surface of the tonsil, separating the tonsil from the palatine and tonsillar branches of the facial artery. The internal carotid artery lies posterolateral to the tonsil, separated by a distance of 20–30 mm.

The palatine tonsils are part of Waldeyer's ring, which surrounds the oropharynx; the lingual, palatine, tubal, and pharyngeal tonsils form the circle of lymphoid tissue.

➡ *Lymphoid overgrowth of the palatine tonsil. A lymphoid enlargement of the palatine tonsils may close off the oropharynx and markedly obstruct the process of swallowing, especially of solids.*

➡ *Acute and chronic tonsillitis. Acute, subacute, and chronic tonsillitis are common diseases of childhood. Surgical removal of the tonsils is indicated if there are serious complications associated with tonsillitis.*

➡ *Tonsillar cancer. Tonsillar cancer is rare, with squamous cell cancer probably the most common type.*

➡ *Tonsillectomy. Tonsillectomy calls for the complete excision of the palatine tonsil, including its capsule. The capsule is separated easily from its pharyngeal bed except after chronic tonsillar infection, when there is a fibrous union between the capsule and the deep tonsillar bed. Dissection in such cases is apt to cause much bleeding, because so many small new blood vessels run into the posterior tonsillar capsule.*

➡ *Peritonsillar abscess. Peritonsillar abscess may develop external to the tonsillar capsule, usually following a bout of acute suppurative tonsillitis. The abscess may penetrate the wall of the pharynx or break through into the parapharyngeal spaces. It is usually drained by an incision about 1 cm above the free border of the anterior pillar into the peritonsillar space.*

The anterior surface of the palatine tonsil is covered with stratified squamous epithelium, which also lines the tonsillar crypts. The tonsillar substance is packed with discrete lymphoid nodules with prominent germinal centers. A thin connective tissue capsule surrounds the entire tonsil.

The palatine tonsil receives its blood supply from a branch of the lingual artery, the ascending palatine and tonsillar branches of the facial artery, the ascending pharyngeal branch of the external carotid, and the descending palatine branch of the maxillary artery. The rich blood supply makes tonsillectomy an extremely vascular procedure. Venous return from the tonsil reaches either the facial vein or the pterygoid venous plexus. Lymphatic drainage from the tonsils is via vessels that run through the pharyngeal wall into the deep vertical chain of cervical nodes. Nerve supply to the tonsil is from the glossopharyngeal nerve and from the posterior palatine branches of the maxillary division of the trigeminal nerve.

THE NASOPHARYNX
(Figs 3–16 and 3–17)

Posterior to the nose and superior to the soft palate lies the nasal segment of the pharynx. Unlike the oropharyngeal and laryngeal segments, the nasopharynx always remains open. It joins through the choanae with the 2 nasal cavities anterior to it. On each lateral wall of the nasopharynx is the opening of the auditory tube. The torus levatorius, an elevation that results when the pharyngeal termination of the auditory tube cartilage is thrust into the nasopharyngeal cavity, bounds the auditory ostium posteriorly. The salpingopharyngeal fold reaches inferiorly from the torus and encloses the salpingopharyngeus muscle. A deep depression (the pharyngeal recess or fossa of Rosenmüller) lies behind the pharyngeal ostium of the auditory tube. The pharyngeal tonsils lie on the posterior wall of the nasopharynx. Under the ciliated columnar epithelium lie racemose mucous glands. The salpingopharyngeus arises from the opening of the auditory tube to the soft palate, while the palatopharyngeus reaches from the torus to the palate. Both muscles are supplied by the pharyngeal plexus of nerves.

The **stylopharyngeus** is a long, thin muscle that arises from the base of the styloid process and passes inferiorly, paralleling the lateral pharyngeal wall. As it descends, some of its fibers join the middle and inferior constrictors of the pharynx to insert with them into the central posterior pharyngeal raphe. The remaining fibers of the stylopharyngeus insert into the posterior surface of the thyroid cartilage. The 2 stylopharyngeus muscles working together draw the pharynx superiorly and laterally, thus both raising it and widening its transverse diameter. The stylopharyngeus is supplied by the glossopharyngeal nerve.

➡ *Hypertrophy of adenoids. The mucous membrane lining the nasopharyngeal wall is extremely vascular. Just deep to the mucosa are large collections of lymphoid cells whose hypertrophy may block the opening of the auditory (eustachian) tube. When the opening of the auditory tube is occluded by lymphoid tissue overgrowth (adenoids), the air in the tympanic cavity is gradually absorbed, and serous otitis may result.*

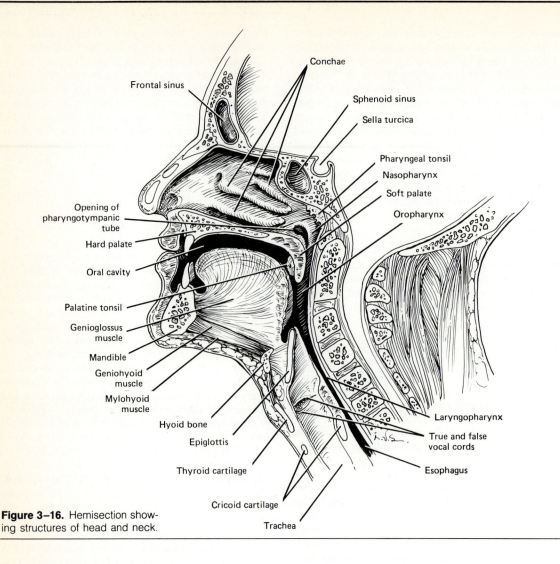

Figure 3–16. Hemisection showing structures of head and neck.

THE FLOOR OF THE MOUTH

The floor of the mouth is composed of the tongue and the 2 sublingual areas on either side of it.

THE SUBLINGUAL AREAS
(Figs 3–18 and 3–19)

Each sublingual area is a deep groove between the inner surface of the gingiva of the mandible and the root tissues of the tongue. The sublingual floor is formed by the mylohoid muscle anteriorly and the hyoglossus muscle posteriorly. The 2 muscles separate the floor of the mouth from the submandibular and submental areas of the neck. The posterior boundary of the sublingual area is the anterior tonsillar pillar; the anterior boundary is the inner surface of

the mandibular gingiva just posterior and lateral to the mandibular symphysis.

➡ *Ludwig's angina. Infection in the areolar tissue and lymphatics of the sublingual area passes rapidly to the neck either by direct extension through the cleft in the mylohoid and hyoglossus muscles or via lymphatic spread to the submental and submandibular lymph nodes. Ludwig's angina or frank abscess may develop in the upper anterior neck unless the infection is brought under rapid control with antibiotics.*

The sublingual compartment of the oral cavity contains (1) the sublingual salivary gland; (2) the anterior projection of the submandibular salivary gland; (3) the excretory duct of the submandibular salivary gland (Wharton's duct); (4) the excretory ducts of the sublingual gland; (5) the lingual and

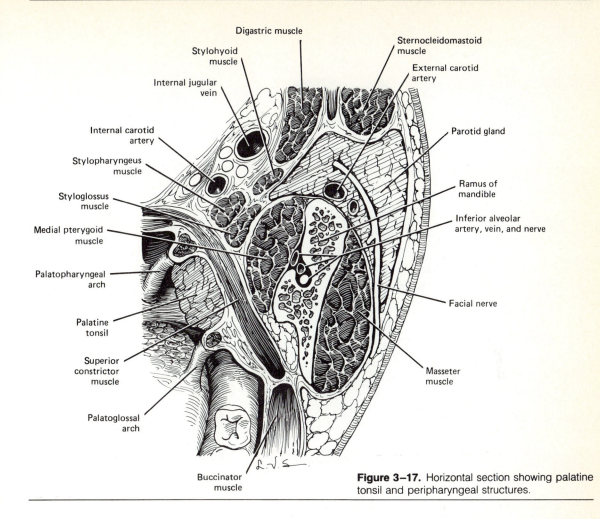

Figure 3–17. Horizontal section showing palatine tonsil and peripharyngeal structures.

hypoglossal nerves; and (6) the sublingual blood vessels and lymphatics.

The intraoral surface of the sublingual area is covered by the oropharyngeal mucous membrane, which is reflected medially from the lateral surface of the tongue and laterally onto the adjacent gingiva.

SURFACE ANATOMY

The frenulum of the tongue is a fold of mucous membrane whose concave surface presents anteriorly. At its base, the frenulum is attached to the underlying midline fusion of the 2 genioglossus muscles. A short, tight frenulum may hold the anterior segment of the tongue firmly against the floor of the mouth, hampering its physiologic function.

Lying on either side of the base of the frenulum is a papilla with an orifice at its tip through which empties the duct of the submandibular salivary gland. Just proximal to the papilla, the duct is joined by the principal duct of the sublingual salivary gland. Beginning at each of the papillae and running along-

side the lateral surface of the tongue is an elevated crest of mucous membrane called the sublingual fold or salivary ridge. The multiple tiny minor sublingual salivary ducts open into the oral cavity along this ridge.

➠ *Site of impaction of salivary gland calculi. Calculi often form in the parotid, submandibular, and sublingual salivary glands and in their excretory ducts. The calculi are usually accompanied by infection. Stones frequently become impacted in the narrowed area just proximal to the terminal oral ostium of the major salivary ducts.*

➠ *Extraction of submandibular calculi. Submandibular duct calculi, which present in the floor of the mouth, can sometimes be extracted through the ostium of the salivary duct, aided by manual or incisional dilatation of the ductal ostium. If the calculus cannot be extracted manually, it can be removed via a direct floor-of-*

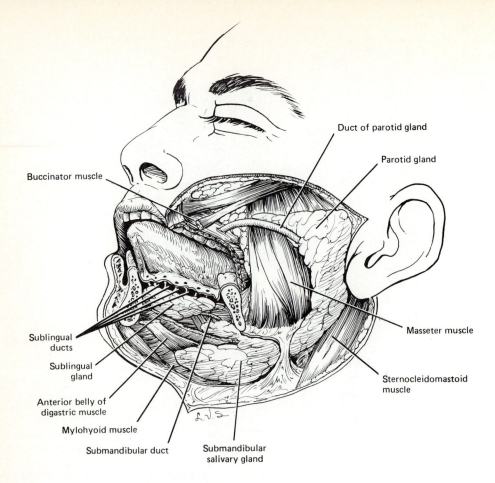

Figure 3–18. The large salivary glands.

the-mouth incision made over the course of the duct which lies deep to the salivary ridge. Occasionally, a submandibular gland has to be excised to prevent stone formation.

➠ ***Ranula.*** *A ranula is a cystic swelling in the submaxillary salivary duct secondary to ductal blockage. It often calls for salivary gland removal, particularly when it is associated with chronic glandular infection.*

The sublingual salivary gland (Fig 3–16) lies just deep to the mucous membrane of the lateral segment of the floor of the mouth. Deep to the gland is the mylohyoid muscle. The sublingual gland weighs 1.5–1.75 g and is almond-shaped. Its posterior pole lies at the level of the cleft between the mylohyoid and hyoglossus muscles. The sublingual gland raises the mucous membrane on either side of the frenulum of the tongue into the plica sublingualis, or salivary ridge. Posteriorly, the sublingual gland is in direct contact with a part of the submandibular salivary gland in the floor of the mouth. Medially, the sublin-

gual gland is in contact with the genioglossus muscle, separated from it only by the lingual nerve, the excretory duct of the submandibular salivary gland, the hypoglossal nerve, and the sublingual vessels. The close relationship of the posterior segment of the sublingual gland to the submandibular salivary gland makes for an almost solid mass of salivary tissue from the anterolateral segment of the floor of the mouth inferiorly to the suprahyoid region of the neck.

➠ ***Spread of intraoral infection.*** *The proximity of the sublingual area to the suprahyoid area of the neck favors the rapid spread of intraoral infection into the upper neck.*

The duct of the submandibular salivary gland is surrounded in its posterior course by the submandibular salivary gland. It lies medial to the sublingual gland under the salivary ridge. The submandibular duct is at first medial, then superior, and then lateral to the lingual nerve before it ends at the salivary papilla.

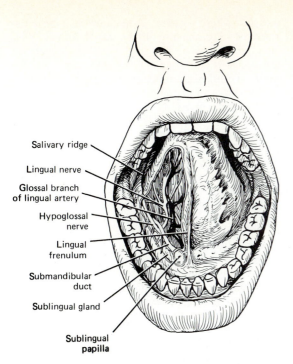

Salivary ridge

Lingual nerve

Glossal branch
of lingual artery

Hypoglossal
nerve

Lingual
frenulum

Submandibular
duct

Sublingual gland

Sublingual
papilla

Figure 3–19. The sublingual area and the inferior surface of the tongue. Mucous membrane has been removed from both areas on the left side of the tongue.

⟹ *Laceration of the floor of the mouth. Lacerations of the floor of the mouth may transect the superficially situated major salivary duct and result in a formation of intraoral salivary fistula.*

⟹ *Sialography via the submandibular ostium. Sialography performed through the ostium of the submandibular salivary duct can help in the diagnosis of disorders of the submandibular and sublingual salivary glands and their excretory ducts.*

⟹ *Palpation of ductal stones. The superficial position of the submandibular duct in the sublingual region permits palpation of intraductal stones. Pus issuing from the papilla of the duct suggests salivary calculi in the duct.*

The sublingual gland is drained by the smaller sublingual ducts and the major sublingual duct. The 6–8 smaller ducts empty either into the submandibular duct or directly into the floor of the mouth along the salivary ridge. Two—sometimes 3—of these smaller sublingual ducts join to form the major sublingual duct that opens directly into the terminal portion of the submandibular duct.

BLOOD VESSELS, LYMPHATICS, & NERVES

Arteries

The arteries that supply the sublingual area are branches of the lingual and facial arteries, both of which are anterior branches of the external carotid artery. The sublingual vessels are superficial in the floor of the mouth. The superficial position of these vessels makes floor-of-the-mouth surgery unusually vascular.

Veins

Venous return from the sublingual region is via multiple facial venous trunks leading to the facial vein, which eventually empties into the internal jugular vein.

Lymphatics

Lymphatic drainage from the sublingual area is into the submental and submandibular group of suprahyoid nodes. Efferents from these nodes empty into the superior deep cervical chain.

Nerves

Two major nerves present in the sublingual area are the lingual and the hypoglossal.

The **lingual nerve** is a branch of mandibular division of the trigeminal nerve. Before it reaches the sublingual area, it is joined by the chorda tympani nerve. In the suprahyoid region of the neck, the lingual nerve lies deep to the submandibular salivary gland and on the surface of the hyoglossus muscle. The nerve enters the floor of the mouth through the mylohyoid-hyoglossus cleft and runs anteriorly, lying at first lateral to the submandibular salivary duct. The nerve then passes under the submandibular duct to its medial side and continues in the floor of the mouth to the frenulum. The lingual nerve supplies sensation to the anterior two-thirds of the tongue and to the taste buds via its accompanying chorda tympani fibers. It also supplies sensation to the gingiva and to the mucous membrane of the anterior portion of the oral cavity. It also supplies the sublingual salivary glands.

The **hypoglossal nerve** enters the floor of the mouth through the mylohyoid-hyoglossus cleft. It lies at first lateral to the lingual nerve, then moves inferior to it, and finally comes to lie medial to the lingual nerve. The hypoglossal nerve lies deeper in the floor of the mouth than the lingual nerve and the submandibular salivary duct. It supplies the intrinsic muscles of the tongue.

THE TONGUE

The tongue is a muscular organ that occupies the central area of the floor of the mouth. It is used for tasting, speaking, masticating, and swallowing. It is important in the passage of foods and fluids into the pharynx and esophagus.

EMBRYOLOGY

The tongue is formed from the primitive pharynx and from the mandibular and the second, third, and fourth branchial arches. The anterior two-thirds of the tongue arises from the tuberculum impar, a small mass in the floor of the primitive pharynx, and from the adjacent regions of both mandibular arches. The tuberculum impar merges with elevations on either side of it that evolve from the first mandibular arch.

The posterior one-third of the tongue arises from the mesoderm of the second, third, and fourth branchial arches. It forms a median swelling—the copula, or hypopharyngeal eminence. Branchial arch mesenchyme forms the connective tissue and the lymphatic and blood vessels, and some muscle fibers of the tongue.

Anomalous development of these structures leads to congenital cysts and fistulas of the thyroglossal tract, ankyloglossia (tongue-tie), macroglossia or microglossia, cleft tongue, and bifid tongue.

GROSS ANATOMY

The 4 major areas of the tongue are the root, or base; the apex; the inferior surface (undersurface); and superior surface, or dorsum.

Root of the Tongue

The root (base) of the tongue is its only relatively fixed portion. Four anatomic structures help to anchor the base of the tongue: (1) The hyoid bone, which is attached to the base of the tongue by 2 muscles, the genioglossus and the hyoglossus. The hyoglossal membrane connects the undersurface of the root of the tongue to the hyoid bone. (2) Three folds of mucous membrane, which connect the base of the tongue to the epiglottis (glosso-epiglottic folds), tend to limit basilar tongue movement when these folds are put on stretch by the posterior movement of the epiglottis. (3) The glossopalatine arches (anterior tonsillar pillars), which connect the base of the tongue to the soft palate. (4) The superior constrictor muscles of the pharynx, which connect the base of the tongue to the superior segment of the pharynx.

Apex of the Tongue

The apex of the tongue is thin and narrow and lies anteriorly against the lingual surface of the anterior incisor teeth. It is attached to the floor of the mouth by the frenulum of the tongue.

Inferior Surface of the Tongue

The ventral surface of the tongue is fixed to both the mandible and the hyoid bone by the 2 genioglossus muscles, whose posterior fibers thrust the tongue forward and whose anterior fibers retract the organ. When all of the fibers of the genioglossi work together, the tongue is depressed. The mucous membrane that leaves the inferior surface of the tongue is reflected onto the floor of the mouth and then onto the lingual surface of the gums.

Dorsum of the Tongue
(Fig 3–20)

The dorsum of the tongue has a convex surface with a shallow median sulcus that divides the surface into 2 halves. The sulcus extends posteriorly to a shallow depression, the foramen cecum linguae, the site of the embryologic origin of the thyroglossal tract. From each side of the foramen cecum, furrows run laterally and anteriorly, not quite reaching to the middle of the tongue. These sulci terminales roughly divide the dorsum of the tongue into an anterior two-thirds and a posterior one-third. Anterior to the sulcus terminalis, the tongue faces superiorly and presents a rough surface with multiple papillae. The portion lying posterior to the sulcus terminalis faces posteriorly, is quite smooth, and contains in its depths multiple glands and lymph follicles. Nearly all the taste buds on the dorsal surface of the tongue are anterior to the sulcus terminalis, with only a few scattered taste buds on the base.

➠ *Leukoplakia of the tongue. Leukoplakia, common in heavy smokers and anyone with poor dental hygiene, is a premalignant tongue lesion. Pathologically, it consists of heavy whitish plaques composed of piled-up epithelium on the sides and dorsum of the tongue. Areas of leukoplakia must be observed over a period of time for signs of malignant degeneration (ulceration, increase in size and thickness).*

➠ *Syphilis and mycotic infection of the tongue. Primary and tertiary syphilis and some mycotic diseases can produce ulcerated lesions and solid tumor masses both on the surface and in the depths of the tongue. They must be considered in the differential diagnosis of tongue ulcerations.*

Tongue Musculature

The musculature of the tongue consists of extrinsic and intrinsic muscles. The extrinsic muscles take their origin at a distance from the tongue and insert into the tongue. The intrinsic muscles arise within the tongue itself and insert into its substance. The extrinsic muscles move the tongue in all directions; the intrinsic muscles serve only to alter the shape of the tongue.

A midline vertical fibrous **glossus septum** running almost the length of the tongue divides the organ into halves. The septum is fixed inferiorly to the hyoid bone. It runs from the undersurface of the

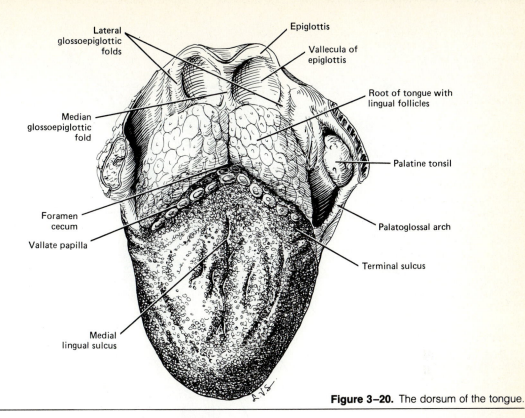

Lateral glossoepiglottic folds

Epiglottis

Vallecula of epiglottis

Root of tongue with lingual follicles

Median glossoepiglottic fold

Palatine tonsil

Foramen cecum

Vallate papilla

Palatoglossal arch

Terminal sulcus

Medial lingual sulcus

Figure 3–20. The dorsum of the tongue.

tongue to the mucous membrane on the dorsal surface. Little or no blood or lymph passes across the septum from one side of the tongue to the other except at the extreme anterior tip of the tongue and at the posterior border of the base.

A. Extrinsic Muscles: (Fig 3–21.)

1. Genioglossus–The genioglossus is a triangular paired muscle that parallels the median plane of the tongue. It arises by a short tendon from the mental spine just lateral to the mandibular symphysis. The wide insertion is into the tip of the tongue and into the whole of the undersurface. The muscle is separated from the genioglossus of the contralateral side by the median fibrous septum of the tongue. The genioglossus, supplied by the hypoglossal nerve, accomplishes protrusion of the tongue by contraction of its posterior fibers and retraction of the tongue by contraction of its anterior fibers.

➡ *Respiratory difficulty secondary to genioglossus relaxation. Under deep anesthesia, when the genioglossus is relaxed, the tongue may fall posteriorly into the central pharyngeal airway and cause complete respiratory obstruction.*

2. Hyoglossus–The hyoglossus is a thin muscle that takes origin from the greater cornu (horn) of the hyoid bone and inserts into the lateral surface

of the tongue, where it interlaces with fibers of the styloglossus and the inferior longitudinal tongue muscles. It forms the mid portion of the muscular diaphragm, which separates the oral cavity from the suprahyoid area. It draws the sides of the tongue inferiorly and, with the genioglossus, depresses the tongue. It is supplied by the hypoglossal nerve.

3. Styloglossus–The styloglossus arises from the apex of the styloid process of the temporal bone and the adjacent stylomandibular ligament. The muscle passes between the internal and external carotid arteries. It enters the substance of the tongue and interdigitates with the intrinsic tongue muscles. The styloglossus retracts and elevates the tongue and is supplied by the hypoglossal nerve.

4. Chondroglossus–The chondroglossus arises from the lesser horn and body of the hyoid bone and interdigitates with the intrinsic muscles of the tongue. Like the hyoglossus, it depresses the tongue. It is supplied by the hypoglossal nerve.

B. Intrinsic Muscles: (Fig 3–22.) The intrinsic muscles of the tongue are (1) the superior longitudinal muscle, which lies just inferior to the superior mucosal surface of the tongue; (2) the inferior longitudinal muscle, which lies just deep to the mucous membrane of the inferior surface; (3) the transverse muscle, made up of fibers that arise from the median fibrous septum and pass toward the lateral borders of the tongue; and (4) the vertical muscle, found only at the lateral borders of the forepart of the tongue, from the superior to the inferior surface.

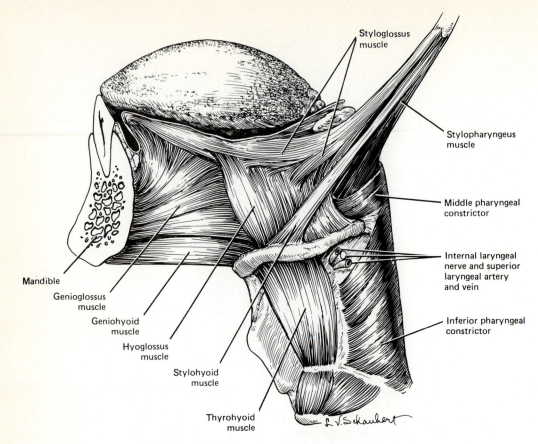

Figure 3–21. The extrinsic muscles of the tongue.

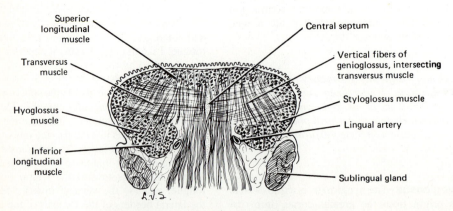

Figure 3–22. The intrinsic muscles of the tongue.

BLOOD VESSELS, LYMPHATICS, & NERVES

Arteries

The arterial supply to the tongue is mainly via 3 vessels: (1) The lingual artery, a branch of the external carotid, supplies most of the blood. It runs anteriorly in the suprahyoid area of the neck, deep to the fibers of the hyoglossus muscle, and in the floor of the mouth, where it breaks up into multiple glossal and lingual branches. (2) The facial or external maxillary artery sends small branches to the posterior and lateral surfaces of the tongue. (3) The ascending pharyngeal artery, a branch of the external carotid artery, supplies small branches to the base of the tongue.

Veins

Venous drainage from the tongue is via vessels that accompany the arterial supply. All of the venous channels eventually drain into the internal jugular venous system.

Lymphatics

Lymphatic drainage from the tongue is via lymph channels in 4 major groups.

A. Apical Lymph Channels: The apical channels drain the tip of the tongue toward submental or submandibular suprahyoid glands on both sides of the neck and directly to the supraomohyoid nodes of the deep cervical chain.

B. Marginal Lymph Channels: The marginal lymph channels drain the lateral surfaces of the tongue first to the submandibular nodes and then to the deep vertical chain of cervical nodes. Some vessels from the lateral margins of the tongue reach nodes that lie on the deep surface of the hyoglossus muscle. These lingual lymph glands may be palpated with a finger on the floor of the mouth while the other hand presses upward on the hyoglossus muscle from beneath the mandible.

C. Central Lymph Channels: The central lymphatics of the tongue drain the area alongside the central raphe. They pass vertically downward, close to the midline between the 2 genioglossus muscles. They then reach one or both deep cervical chains.

D. Basal Lymph Channels: The basal lymph channels drain the posterior segment of the tongue and reach the vertical chains of deep cervical nodes.

➠ *Lymphatic drainage in tongue cancer. Metastases from the tongue occur in the suprahyoid or the deep cervical lymphatic nodes on either or both sides of the neck.*

➠ *Treatment of carcinoma of the tongue. This presents 2 major problems: (1) treatment of the primary lesion and (2) treatment of the nodal areas into which it must be assumed that embolic or direct lymphatic spread may have occurred. Opinion is divided on how to best manage the primary malignant tongue lesion— by radiation or by surgical excision. Operation is made difficult by the great vascularity of the tongue and the floor of the mouth. The procedure is also a mutilating one, particularly if all or part of the transverse ramus of the mandible and its attached muscles are removed.*

➠ *Choice of operation for tongue carcinoma. The choice of the exact type of procedure for carcinoma of the tongue depends upon the nature of the lesion and general condition of the patient. Radical resection of the primary tumor with unilateral neck dissection on the dominant side is the most common procedure.*

Nerves
(Fig 3–23)

A. Motor Nerves: The hypoglossal nerve supplies motor power to all muscles of the tongue, both intrinsic and extrinsic, except the palatoglossus. If loss of motor nerve supply occurs, the entire tongue is pushed by the muscles of the uninvolved side toward the side with the motor nerve lesion.

➠ *Transection of the hypoglossal nerve. Severance or injury of the hypoglossal nerve as a result of a penetrating wound of the neck or the floor of the mouth, or iatrogenically incurred during neck dissection, leads to an ipsilateral hemiatrophy of the tongue manifested by a notching and a deviation toward the involved side.*

B. Sensory Nerves: There are 4 sensory nerves to the tongue.

The lingual branch of the mandibular division of the **trigeminal nerve** is distributed to the papillae of the anterior surface of the tongue to the sulcus terminalis. It supplies sensation to the anterior two-thirds of the tongue.

The chorda tympani branch of the **facial nerve,** which runs within the sheath of the lingual nerve, is the nerve of taste for the anterior two-thirds of the tongue. It is a continuation of the sensory root of the facial nerve and joins the lingual nerve close to the foramen ovale.

The lingual branch of the **glossopharyngeal nerve** is distributed to the mucous membrane of the base of the tongue and to its posterolateral surfaces. This nerve supplies both taste and sensation.

The superior laryngeal branch of the **vagus nerve** sends a few filaments to the base of the tongue.

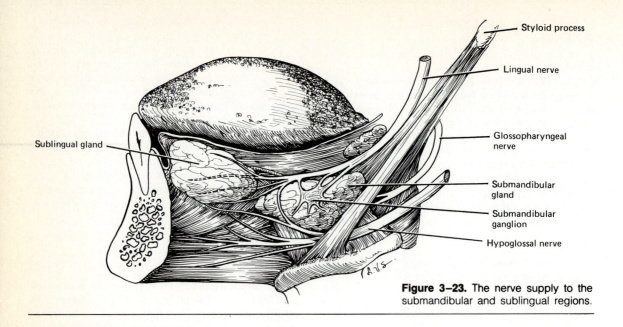

Figure 3–23. The nerve supply to the submandibular and sublingual regions.

IV. THE NOSE

THE EXTERNAL NOSE
(Fig 3–24)

The external nose (Fig 3–24) is roughly triangular in shape; its superior angle is called the nasal apex. The anterior margin (bridge) of the nose runs superiorly to its root at the forehead. The posterior nasal wall opens directly into the nasal cavity, or fossa.

The base of the nose presents 2 oval openings, the nares or nostrils, separated by a central septum, the columna nasi. Hairs in the nostrils help prevent inhalation of small foreign particles. The lateral walls of the nose separate to form the alae nasi, the smoothly rounded inferior termination of the lateral nasal walls.

➠ *Cosmetic importance of the nose. Many ingenious plastic procedures have been devised to repair nasal congenital and traumatic defects. They are also used to change what are perceived as unattractive natural configurations.*

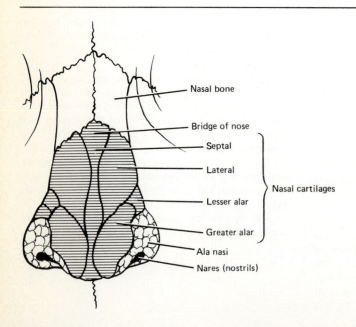

Figure 3–24. The external structures of the nose.

The skeletal portion of the external nose is composed of bones and cartilages, which are covered by skin externally and by mucous membrane internally. The skin over the anterior and lateral segments of the nose is thin and loosely applied to the subcutaneous tissues. However, in the region of the nasal tip and about the nostrils, the skin is thicker, contains many sebaceous follicles, and is closely applied to the underlying tissues.

➡ ***Nasal skin disorders.*** *The skin of the nose is frequently the site of basal cell cancer. Hypertrophy of the superficial connective tissue of the nose secondary to acne rosacea leads to a disfiguring rhinophyma.*

NASAL BONES
(Figs 3–24 and 3–25)

The bony support of the nose consists of the nasal bones and the frontal processes of the maxillae. The 2 nasal bones are small quadrilateral structures placed side by side to form the bridge of the nose. The external surfaces of the nasal bones are convex, and their superior borders are serrated for junction with the frontal bone. The inferior borders of the nasal bones give attachment to the lateral cartilage of the nose. The lateral borders of the nasal bones articulate with the frontal processes of the maxillae. The medial borders not only join with the contralateral nasal bones but are prolonged posteriorly, forming a vertical spine that contributes to the nasal septum and joins with the spine of the frontal bone, the perpendicular plate of the ethmoid, and the nasal septal cartilage.

➡ ***Nasal bone trauma.*** *The lower ends of the nasal bones are broad and thin and easily fractured by external trauma. Such fractures tend to be compound, since the nasal mucous membrane is usually torn. Nasal hemorrhage is common in nasal bone fracture. Healing is usually excellent, because of the great vascularity of the area. Trauma to the nose, even without fracture, may fracture the neighboring lacrimal bones. A blow high on the bridge of the nose may fracture the cribriform plate of the ethmoid bone or may involve the frontal sinuses.*

NASAL CARTILAGES

There are 5 nasal cartilages. They are joined by bands of strong fibrous tissue.

Septal Cartilage

The septal cartilage divides the interior of the nose into 2 cavities. Anteriorly, it connects with the 2 nasal bones and joins with the anterior border of the 2 lateral cartilages. Inferiorly, fibrous tissue joins

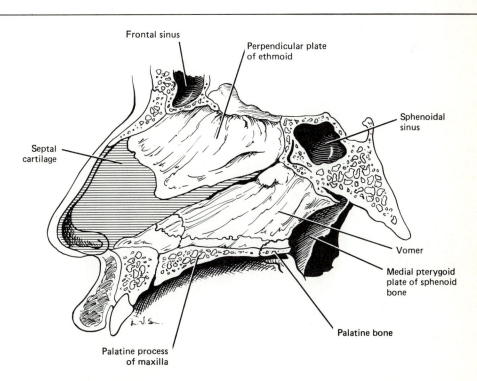

Figure 3–25. Hemisection of the nasal cavity to show nasal septum.

the septal cartilage to the alar cartilages. Superiorly, the septal cartilage joins with the perpendicular plate of the ethmoid bone. Posteriorly, it connects with the palatine and vomer processes of the maxilla. The most inferior segment of the nasal septum is formed not by the septal cartilage but by alar cartilages.

Lateral Cartilages

The 2 lateral cartilages lie inferior to the nasal bones. They are thick anteriorly and firmly united with the septal cartilage superiorly, but inferiorly a narrow crevice separates them from the septal cartilage. Superiorly, the lateral cartilage joins with the nasal bone and the frontal process of the maxilla; inferiorly it is joined to the greater alar cartilage by connective tissue.

Alar Cartilages

The 2 greater alar cartilages are thin and lie just inferior to the lateral cartilages. They form the medial and lateral boundaries of the ipsilateral nares. The lateral portion of the alar cartilage follows the curve of the nares; the medial portion joins with the medial segment of the opposite greater alar cartilage and with skin and subcutaneous tissue to form the septum mobile nasi (movable tip of the nose).

BLOOD VESSELS & NERVES

Arteries & Veins

The alae and septum of the nose are supplied by the septal and alar branches of the facial artery. The dorsum (bridge) and sides of the nose are supplied by branches of the ophthalmic and maxillary arteries.

Venous blood from the external nose is returned to either the ophthalmic or the anterior facial veins. The ophthalmic veins pass to the intracranial area, so that paranasal venous blood may carry infection into the cranium and its venous sinuses.

Nerves

The 3 small muscles that move the nose are supplied by the facial nerve; the nasal skin is supplied by branches of the ophthalmic and maxillary divisions of the trigeminal nerve. The 3 nasal muscles wrinkle the bridge of the nose (procerus), enlarge the nasal aperture (nasalis), and constrict the aperture of the nares (depressor septi).

THE NASAL CAVITY*
(Figs 3–25 and 3–26)

The nasal cavity is divided by the nasal septum into 2 spaces (nasal fossae). They open externally via the nostrils and internally into the nasopharynx via the choanae. The horizontal roof of the nasal cavity is formed anteriorly by the nasal bones and the spine of the frontal bone, centrally by the cribriform plate, and posteriorly by the sphenoid bone, the ala of the vomer, and the sphenoidal process of the palatine bones. The posterior roof of the cavity opens into the sphenoidal sinus.

* This section contributed by Robert A. Schindler, MD.

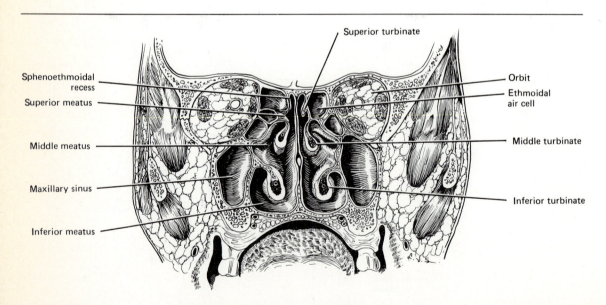

Figure 3–26. Coronal section through the nasal cavities.

GENERAL ANATOMY

Anterior Nasal Aperture

The bony borders of the anterior nasal aperture are formed superiorly by the nasal bones; laterally by the ridges that separate the anterior and nasal surfaces of the maxilla; and inferiorly by the same 2 ridges, which curve medially to form the anterior nasal spine.

Choanae

The bony borders of the choanae are formed superiorly by the undersurface of the body of the sphenoid and the ala of the vomer, inferiorly by the posterior border of the transverse segment of the palatine bone, and laterally by the medial pterygoid plate. The posterior border of the vomer separates the 2 choanae.

➠ *Posterior rhinoscopy. Posterior rhinoscopy to visualize the choanae is performed with a mirror placed behind the soft palate and illuminated orally to permit inspection of the choanal opening, the middle meatus, the auditory tube, and most of the inferior meatus.*

Vestibule

The vestibule of the nasal cavity is the area just within the nares. It is lined with skin with stiff hairs (vibrissae) and many sebaceous glands.

The Nasal Fossae

The bony floor of the nasal fossa is composed of the palatine process of the maxilla and the transverse portion of the palatine bone. The medial bony wall (septum nasi) is formed anteriorly by the ethmoidal crest, posteriorly by the vomer and the rostrum of the sphenoid, and inferiorly by the maxillary crest and the palatine bones. The lateral bony wall is formed anteriorly by the maxilla and the lacrimal bone; centrally by the ethmoid, the maxilla, and the lowest concha; and posteriorly by the medial pterygoid plate of the sphenoid and the vertical plate of the palatine bone.

Nasal Septum

The medial wall of each nasal fossa is formed by the nasal septum, which is a composite of the ethmoidal perpendicular plate, the vomer, and the septal cartilage. The septum is covered with mucous membrane of the ciliated, columnar epithelial type containing large numbers of goblet cells. The anteroinferior portion of the septum is membranous and freely movable. The septum normally presents some degree of deviation, usually at the junction of the ethmoid and vomer.

➠ *Septal deviation. Severe deviation of the nasal septum usually causes nasal airway obstruction and occasionally blocks the openings of the paranasal sinuses, leading to secondary infection in the sinus cavities. Trauma and errors in septal development are the most common causes of marked septal deviation.*

Lateral Nasal Wall
(Fig 3–27)

The lateral nasal wall has 3 anteroposterior canals known as the superior, middle, and inferior meatus of the nasal cavity. The superior meatus lies between the superior and middle nasal turbinates, and into it open the posterior ethmoidal cells. The middle meatus lies between the middle and inferior turbinates, and into it open the anterior ethmoidal cells and the frontonasal duct draining the frontal sinus. The inferior meatus lies between the inferior turbinate and the floor of the nasal cavity. The nasolacrimal duct opens into it.

The lateral walls of the nasal fossae show the 3 nasal turbinates situated one above the other. They appear as ledges projecting from the lateral nasal walls, their free edges pointing medially and inferiorly. The superior and middle turbinates derive their bony support from the ethmoid. The inferior turbinate is a separate bone. The free edges of the turbinates overlie the nasal meatus.

➠ *Improper drainage of ducts opening into the nasal chambers. Since the nasal chambers are very close to the openings of the paranasal sinuses, the tear ducts, and the auditory tubes, swelling of the nasal mucous membranes can plug the ostia of these ducts and can give rise to sinus disease, middle ear disease, and nasolacrimal duct obstruction.*

➠ *Hypertrophy of the middle turbinate. Hypertrophy of the middle turbinate may block free drainage from the maxillary sinus, causing severe facial pain over the anterior part of the maxillary sinus. This may require submucous resection of the nasal septum to allow swelling of the turbinate without interfering with sinus drainage.*

➠ *Chronic infection of the inferior nasal turbinate. Chronic swelling, redness, and edema of the inferior nasal turbinate suggest the presence of maxillary sinus infection, the pus from the sinus irritating the turbinate as it passes over it.*

➠ *Nasal bleeding from the turbinates. Since a large venous plexus lies just deep to the mucous membrane covering the turbinates, nosebleed (epistaxis) is a frequent consequence of nasal trauma. Bleeding from the anterior segment of the nasal cavity can usually be controlled*

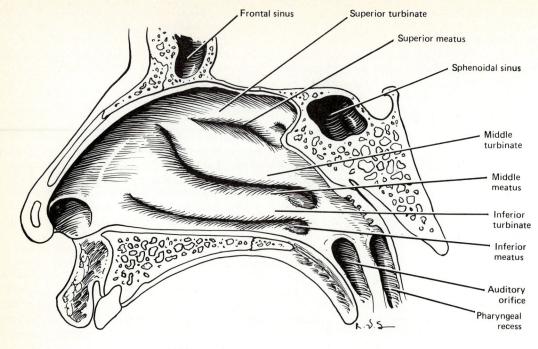

Figure 3–27. View of lateral nasal canal wall.

by firm packing of the anterior nares. If the bleeding point is in the posterior nasal cavity or if it cannot be localized, pressure packing of both the anterior and posterior nares may be necessary.

Lying above the superior turbinate—the smallest of the 3 turbinates—is the sphenoethmoidal recess, into which opens the sphenoid sinus. The middle turbinate extends farther anteriorly than the superior turbinate, reaching almost to the anterior extension of the cribriform plate. The posterior tip of the inferior turbinate lies about 0.5–0.75 cm anterior to the pharyngeal orifice of the auditory tube.

Cribriform Plate of the Ethmoid Bone

The cribriform plate of the ethmoid bone supports the olfactory lobe of the brain. The plate separates the nasal cavity from the intracranial cavity. The cribriform plate is easily fractured both because it is thin and because it contains many openings through which pass the fibers of the olfactory tract along with their covering meninges on their way from the cranial cavity to the nasal cavity.

➡ *Trauma to the nose with fracture of the cribriform plate of the ethmoid. A blow to the apex of the nose may fracture the cribriform plate and tear the overlying dura and arachnoid*

membranes. The consequent leak of cerebrospinal fluid through the nasal passages may lead to an ascending meningeal infection.

➡ *Meningocele. Care must be taken to distinguish a meningocele pushing down through the roof of the nasal cavity from a nasal polyp, since failure to do so will result in a spinal fluid leak when the pseudopolyp is removed.*

Mucous Membranes of the Nasal Cavity

The mucous membrane lining the nasal cavity is continuous with that of the pharynx, the paranasal sinuses, and the lacrimal sac. There are 2 separate types of nasal mucosa: respiratory and olfactory.

A. Respiratory Mucosa: The respiratory epithelium covers the lower two-thirds of the nasal cavity. It is made up of ciliated columnar epithelium and contains many mucus-producing glands. It is tightly attached to the underlying bone. Where it covers the 2 inferior turbinates, the blood vessels form a pseudoerectile tissue that becomes distended with blood when the mucous membrane is irritated.

B. Olfactory Mucosa: The mucosa covering the tissues of the olfactory region covers only the superior concha and the immediately adjacent area of the central nasal septum. It is of the columnar epithelial type, and scattered throughout it are modified epithelial cells containing the olfactory cells. The olfactory cells are bipolar, with a large circular nucleus. At the epithelial surface, each olfactory cell projects a group of fine filaments, the olfactory hairs. The subepithelial tissues of the olfactory area contain many branched tubular glands (Bowman's glands) that secrete a serous discharge which serves to keep the epithelium moist.

BLOOD VESSELS, LYMPHATICS, & NERVES

Arteries
The nasal cavity is supplied by the anterior and posterior ethmoidal branches of the ophthalmic artery, the sphenopalatine branch of the maxillary artery, and the labial branch of the facial artery. These vessels ramify to form a massive arterial network lying both deep to and within the mucous membrane of the nasal cavity.

Veins
Venous drainage from the nasal cavity is into the sphenopalatine, anterior facial, and ophthalmic veins. Since the ethmoidal veins open into the superior sagittal sinus and since the nasal veins empty into the ophthalmic veins, which in turn empty into the cavernous sinuses, a dual system of communication exists between the intracranial and intranasal venous circulations. This imposes a continuing risk of brain and meningeal infection secondary to nasal infection.

Lymphatics
Lymph drainage from the anterior nasal cavity and the skin of the nose is primarily into the submandibular nodes and then into the vertical deep cervical chain of nodes. Drainage from the posterior nasal cavity and from the paranasal sinuses is either into the retropharyngeal nodes or directly into the vertical deep cervical nodes.

Nerves
Individual nerve filaments that leave the olfactory nerve pass through the cribriform plate and supply the mucous membrane of the upper third of the nasal cavity. The lower two-thirds of the nasal cavity receives sensation from the ethmoidal branch of the ophthalmic nerve and branches of the maxillary nerve, which reach the nasal cavity via the sphenopalatine ganglion.

THE ACCESSORY SINUSES OF THE NOSE
(Paranasal Sinuses)

There are 4 paired accessory nasal sinuses lying on each side of the nasal passages: frontal, ethmoidal,

sphenoidal, and maxillary. There is great individual variation in their size and shape. Each sinus is lined with ciliated squamous epithelium, which is continuous with the lining epithelium of the nasal cavity.

FRONTAL SINUSES

The frontal sinuses lie behind the superciliary arches of the frontal bone. They are absent at birth and small in children, reaching adult size after the age of 14–15 years. In adults they are 2.5–3.5 cm wide, about 1 cm deep, and 3 cm in height. The septum that separates the frontal sinuses is often eccentrically placed. The frontal sinuses empty into the ipsilateral middle nasal meatus via the frontonasal duct.

➤ *Frontal sinus suppuration. To improve frontal sinus drainage, removal of nasal obstructions and cleaning out the anterior air cells both tend to promote resolution of suppurative processes involving the frontal sinuses.*

THE ETHMOIDAL AIR CELLS

The ethmoidal air cells occupy the labyrinth of the ethmoid and are an aggregate of small, thin-walled air sacs. They are surrounded by the frontal, maxillary, lacrimal, sphenoidal, and palatine bones. They are divided into 3 groups: anterior, middle, and posterior. The anterior and middle groups drain into the middle meatus of the nasal cavity; the posterior group drains into the superior meatus. The superior group of cells lies inferior to and on either side of the cribriform plate of the ethmoid, separated by the thin ethmoidal bony plate from the frontal lobes of the brain.

At birth, the ethmoidal air cells are very small. They do not develop fully until after age 14.

➤ *Intracranial extension of ethmoid disease. Since the relationship of the ethmoid sinuses to the cranial cavity is intimate, meningeal and cerebral extensions of ethmoid disease occur occasionally. Such intracranial complications are meningitis, brain abscess, subdural abscess, and intracranial venous sinus thrombosis.*

THE SPHENOIDAL SINUSES

The sphenoidal air cells lie within the sphenoidal body. They vary greatly in size in different individuals, and in people with marked nasal septal deviation they tend to show considerable asymmetry. They present an opening in the superior segment of the anterior wall that leads into the sphenoethmoidal recess, which

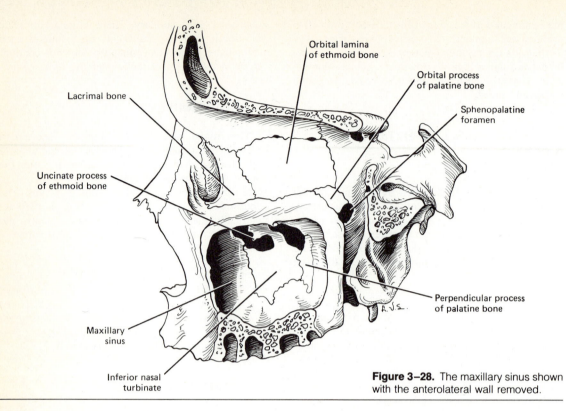

Figure 3–28. The maxillary sinus shown with the anterolateral wall removed.

lies above the level of the superior concha of the nasal cavity. The sphenoidal cells measure about 2 × 2 × 1 cm. They reach adult size by 12–14 years.

⮞ *Drainage of the sphenoidal sinus. Drainage of the sphenoidal sinus calls for as complete a removal as possible of the anterior wall of the sinus and of the neighboring ethmoid.*

⮞ *Hypophysectomy via the sphenoidal sinus. The intracranial hypophysis is exposed by removal of the roof and front wall of the sphenoidal sinus. The septal mucous membrane is elevated on both sides, and a portion of the septal bone and cartilage is removed. The turbinates are flattened against the lateral nasal walls, and the unroofing of the sphenoid and the removal of its anterior wall then exposes the floor of the sella turcica, which contains the pituitary gland. This approach to the pituitary is commonly used for removal of pituitary tumors.*

THE MAXILLARY SINUSES
(Figs 3–26 and 3–28)

The maxillary sinuses occupy the body of the maxilla. They are the largest of the nasal accessory sinuses, being about 3 cm in height, 3.5 cm in width,

and 2.5 cm in depth. The orbital wall forms the roof of the sinus. The alveolar process of the maxilla forms the sinus floor. Extending toward the floor of the maxillary sinus are the roots of the first and second molar teeth. These roots occasionally extend through the sinus floor and appear as small triangular elevations within the sinus. The maxillary sinus is large enough to hold 13–20 mL of fluid. Lying in the superior segment of the medial wall of the sinus is an opening that connects with the middle meatus. On occasion, an accessory opening empties into the middle meatus. The maxillary sinus does not reach adult size until the secondary dentition has erupted.

⮞ *Tumors of the maxillary antrum. The maxillary antrum is a frequent site of benign and malignant tumor formation. For unknown reasons, malignant tumors of the maxillary antrum are particularly common among ethnic Chinese.*

⮞ *Dental relationships of the maxillary antrum. Since the roots of the upper 3 molars and the neighboring 2 bicuspids bulge into the floor of the maxillary sinus and are separated from its cavity only by a thin layer of bone, maxillary sinusitis may occur as a consequence of apical abscesses in these teeth. It may also follow extraction of these teeth.*

⟾ ***Complications of maxillary sinus disease.*** *Disease of the maxillary sinus may cause blockage of the nasolacrimal duct, marked by excessive tearing; pressure on the orbit, with resultant diplopia; pressure on the infraorbital nerve, causing facial pain and a facial area of anesthesia; bulging in the roof of the palate; and involvement of the palatine nerves with pain referred to the teeth of the upper jaw.*

⟾ ***Fractures of the maxillary sinus.*** *So-called eggshell fractures of the maxillary sinuses follow severe injuries to the anterior mid portion of the face. Such fractures are common in deceleration automobile injuries when the face hits the dashboard or steering wheel.*

⟾ ***Drainage of the maxillary sinus.*** *Construction of a nasoantral window is the commonest method for drainage of the maxillary sinus. Such a resection usually includes a portion of the lateral wall of the inferior meatus and partial resection of the inferior concha.*

The Ear

Robert A. Schindler, MD

EMBRYOLOGY
(Fig 4–1)

The 3 portions of the adult ear (external, middle, and inner) have separate origins.

External Ear

The external ear structures—the external auditory meatus, the external surface of the eardrum (tympanic membrane), and the auricle (pinna)—arise from the dorsal segment of the first pharyngeal cleft and 6 surrounding mesenchymal swellings. Ectodermal cells grow inward as a plug which reaches to the entodermal cells of the tympanic membrane. In the seventh month, the meatal ectodermal plug is absorbed except for those cells which remain as the outer epithelial surface of the eardrum. The auricle develops from 6 swellings called the auricular hillocks, which arise around the margins of the first branchial groove. The swellings result from proliferation of the underlying mesenchyme of the first and second branchial arches.

Anomalies include atresia of the pinna, defects of the auricular helix (small preauricular appendage, microtia, preauricular sinus), and complete or partial atresia of the external auditory canal.

Middle Ear

The middle ear structures are the tympanic cavity, the tympanic (mastoid) antrum, the inner surface of the tympanic membrane, the auditory (eustachian) tube, and the tympanic ossicles. During the fourth week, an extension of the entodermal first pharyngeal pouch grows dorsolaterally to reach the floor of the first ectodermal cleft. Its distal part forms the tympanic cavity and the tympanic antrum; its proximal part, the auditory tube. Ear ossicles develop from the dorsal segments of the first and second pharyngeal arch cartilages.

Anomalies of middle ear development include congenital ossicle deformities often associated with mandibular defects (Treacher Collins syndrome).

Inner Ear

The inner ear structures include the membranous labyrinth, the cochlear duct, and the semicircular canals. It begins at the end of the third week as the otic placode, a thickening of the surface ectoderm opposite the rhombencephalon. The placode sinks inwards forming a pit which then separates from the surface epithelium as the otic vesicle. The latter develops ventral and dorsal enlargements, of which the former gives rise to the saccule, the cochlear duct, and the organ of Corti, and the latter to the utricle and the 3 semicircular canals.

Anomalies of the inner ear include (1) Michel's anomaly—total absence of the cochlea and vestibular labyrinth, with total deafness; (2) Mondini's malformation—arrested development of the membranous labyrinth and bony otic capsule; and (3) cochlear saccular dysplasia with malformed cochlear duct, collapse of Reissner's membrane, and malformation of the organ of Corti.

GROSS ANATOMY

The ear is composed of 3 parts: the external ear, the middle ear, and the inner ear.

The **external ear** funnels sound waves into the external auditory meatus. From the meatus, the external auditory canal passes inward to the tympanic membrane, or eardrum.

The **middle ear** is an air-filled cavity medial to the tympanic membrane in the temporal bone that opens via the auditory tube into the nasopharynx.

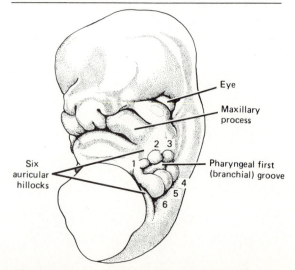

Figure 4–1. Embryologic development of the ear at the 14-mm stage.

The 3 auditory ossicles, the malleus, incus, and stapes, are located in the middle ear.

The **inner ear,** or labyrinth, is made up of 2 parts, one within the other. The bony labyrinth is a series of channels in the petrous portion of the temporal bone. Inside these channels, surrounded by a fluid called perilymph, is the membranous labyrinth. The cochlear portion of the labyrinth is a coiled tube, 35 mm long.

EXTERNAL EAR
(Fig 4–2)

The external ear is composed of the auricle (pinna), the external acoustic (auditory) canal (meatus), and the outer surface of the tympanic membrane. The auricle projects laterally from the head, gathers sound vibrations, and channels them through the external auditory meatus to the tympanic membrane.

The **auricle** is roughly ovoid, the superior curve being slightly larger than the inferior curve. The posterior surface is roughly concave. The **helix** forms the posterior ridge of the auricle and ends inferiorly in the **lobule.** Anterior and parallel to the helix, a second curved ridge, the **anthelix,** divides superiorly into a **triangular fossa.** The anthelix forms the posterior ridge of the **concha** that extends to the external acoustic meatus. Anterior to the concha, a small eminence, the **tragus,** partially overlies the external acoustic meatus. The inner surface of the tragus usually has multiple hair tufts. The auricle consists of a single thin plate of cartilage covered by a tightly applied layer of skin; the lobule consists mainly of fat, with scant fibrous areolar tissue.

➠ *Site of incisions for surgery on the temporal bone. The deep cleft behind the auricle (the postauricular sulcus) is the preferred site of cutaneous incisions for access to the temporal bone.*

The **external ligaments of the auricle** connect the ear to the side of the head. The internal ligaments connect the various parts of the auricular cartilage. The external auricular muscles connect the outer ear to the skull and scalp and move it in one piece; these muscles are less well developed in humans than in other territorial mammals. The external carotid artery, the posterior auricular artery, the anterior auricular branch of the superficial temporal artery, and a small branch from the occipital artery bring blood to the auricle. The venous return roughly parallels the arterial circulation and flows into the internal jugular system. The nerves to the outer ear are the great auricular nerve, derived from C2; the auricular branch of the vagus; the auriculotemporal branch of the mandibular nerve; and the lesser occipital nerve, a branch of C2.

➠ *Trauma to the auricle. Because it protrudes from the side of the scalp, the auricle is vulnerable to contusions, lacerations, and, on occasion, traumatic amputation. The auricle has an excellent blood supply and heals rapidly following meticulous approximation of its lacerated or incised surfaces. This rule of rapid auricular healing also holds good for reposition of all or part of the ear after traumatic amputation. ''Cauliflower ear'' is the result of subperichondrial hemorrhage and hematoma. Hematomas must be evacuated and pressure dressings applied to prevent necrosis of the auricular cartilage.*

➠ *Keratotic lesions of the auricle. Prolonged exposure of the auricle to sun and wind can lead to chronic irritation, keratotic lesions, and perhaps to squamous or basal cell carcinoma.*

The **external acoustic meatus** extends from the bottom of the concha to the outer surface of the tympanic membrane; it is usually about 2.5 cm long. The short meatal passage is cylindric in shape and has a cartilaginous and a bony portion.

The cartilaginous segment of the meatus, 6–8 mm long, is a continuation of the outer ear cartilage and is anchored to the rim of the auditory process of the temporal bone. The osseous segment of the meatus is about 15–17 mm long; it narrows toward the tympanic membrane and turns obliquely so that its anterior wall projects 3–5 mm beyond its posterior wall. The tympanic membrane, which is the termination of the auditory canal, is also slanted obliquely, making the anterior wall of the canal longer than the posterior wall. The osseous segment of the meatus lies within the tympanic portion of the temporal bone. The epithelium of the meatus is thin and firmly attached to both the cartilaginous and osseous walls.

The blood supply to the auricle is the posterior auricular from the external carotid and the anterior

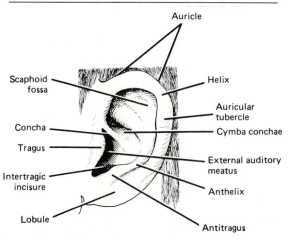

Auricle

Scaphoid fossa

Helix

Auricular tubercle

Concha

Cymba conchae

Tragus

Intertragic incisure

External auditory meatus

Anthelix

Lobule

Antitragus

Figure 4–2. The external ear.

auricular from the superficial temporal; veins accompany the arteries. Nerves are the great auricular and lesser occipital from the cervical plexus, the auricular branch of the vagus, the auriculotemporal branch, and the mandibular. These also supply the auditory canal.

⟶ ***Otitis externa.*** *Otitis externa is bacterial or fungal infection of the external auditory canal. It is relatively common and usually results from skin irritation due to scratching or the presence of foreign bodies (or water) in the external acoustic meatus.*

⟶ ***Atresia of the external acoustic meatus.*** *Atresia of the external acoustic meatus is most often congenital, but it can occur following chronic infection or trauma. Severe atresia can lead to conductive hearing loss.*

MIDDLE EAR
(Tympanum)
(Figs 4–3, 4–4, and 4–5)

The middle ear is an irregularly shaped, air-filled space in the temporal bone. It is connected via the **auditory (eustachian) tube** with the nasopharynx. Crossing from its lateral to its medial wall, a string of 3 small movable bones (ossicles) transmits vibrations from the tympanic membrane (eardrum) to the

inner ear. The tympanic cavity consists of the area immediately behind the eardrum (mesotympanum) and the tympanic attic (epitympanum), which lies just superior to the tympanic membrane. The tympanic attic contains the superior segment of the malleus and most of the incus. It extends from the tympanic membrane laterally to the lateral wall of the inner ear medially. Posteriorly, the cavity joins the tympanic antrum, which relates it to the mastoid air cells. Anteriorly, the tympanic cavity is related to the auditory tube.

The **eardrum,** or **tympanic membrane,** separates the inferior segment of the external auditory meatus from the tympanic cavity. The membrane is ovoid, thin, and almost transparent and is attached to the temporal bone by a thick fibrocartilaginous ring. The membrane is slanted obliquely, so that the anteroinferior quadrant is medial to the posterosuperior quadrant. The triangular anteriosuperior segment of the membrane (pars flaccida) is lax, while its lower, larger segment (pars tensa) is taut. The handle (manubrium) of the malleus is firmly attached to the center of the pars tensa. The central depressed area of the tympanic membrane is called the umbo.

⟶ ***Otitis media.*** *When fluid is present in the tympanic cavity, the tympanic membrane usually bulges outward. As the infection that causes the fluid clears, the drum returns to normal. The ideal way to drain the fluid is by free incision (myringotomy) into the drum through the*

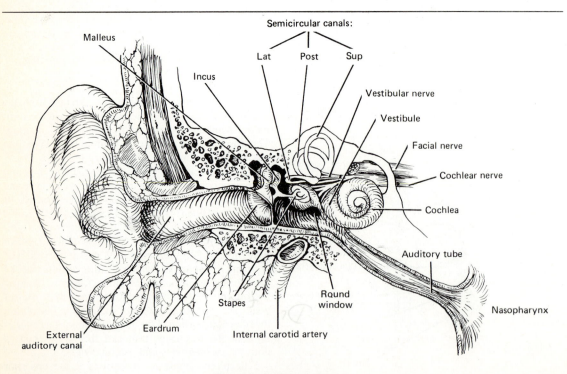

Figure 4–3. The middle ear.

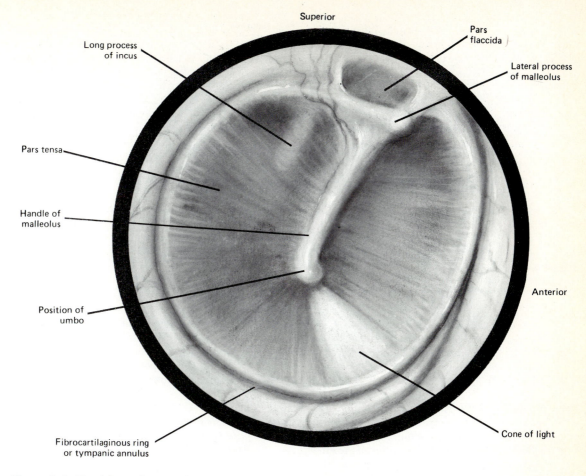

Figure 4–4. The right eardrum as viewed through an otoscope showing the location of landmarks and common sites of perforation.

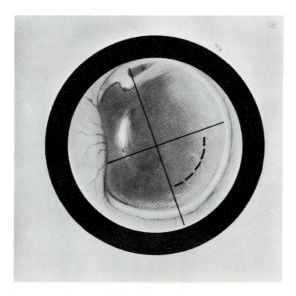

Figure 4–5. Bulging eardrum showing location of myringotomy incision.

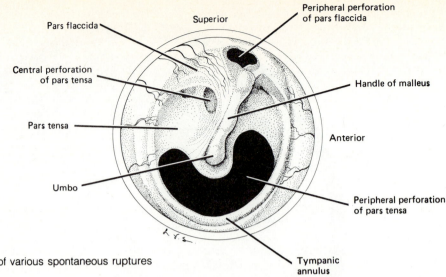

Figure 4–6. Locations of various spontaneous ruptures of eardrum.

posteroinferior or anteroinferior quadrants of the membrane well below the level of the umbo. The incision should be made in a posterior to anterior direction, keeping the knife head away from the auditory ossicles.

➧ ***Rupture of the tympanic membrane.*** *(Fig 4–6.) A sudden increase in air pressure in the external ear, such as follows a slap on the side of the head or instrumentation of the external ear canal, may rupture the tympanic membrane. Rupture may follow skull fracture; bloody discharge from the ear after head injury always suggests basal skull fracture. Acute otitis media is the most common cause of tympanic membrane perforation. Perforation of the membrane can be surgically repaired using temporalis fascia graft.*

The 4 walls of the middle ear are (1) the vertical (medial, labyrinthic) wall, made up of the fenestra vestibuli (oval window), which leads from the tympanic cavity into the inner ear, plus the promontory of the cochlea, the fenestra cochlea (round window), and the prominence of the facial canal; (2) the posterior (mastoid) wall, which contains the facial recess and nerve, the pyramidal eminence, and the fossa for the incus; (3) the anterior carotid wall, which separates the middle ear from the internal carotid artery by a thin bony diaphragm, which is pierced by the caroticotympanic nerve and the tympanic branch of the internal carotid artery; and (4) the lateral wall, formed mainly by the tympanic membrane. The roof is a thin plate of bone, the tegmen tympani, upon which rests the temporal lobe of the brain. The floor of the tympanic cavity is formed by a thin plate of bone below which is the superior bulb of the internal jugular vein.

The epitympanum (attic) and the subjacent mastoid air cells are actually an extension of the air-filled tympanic cavity and the auditory tube. Mastoid air cells of varying size and position are present throughout the mastoid prominence of the temporal bone.

➧ ***Cholesteatoma.*** *Rupture or invagination of the pars flaccida of the tympanic membrane may lead to entrapment of keratinizing squamous epithelium in the middle ear and the mastoid area. As keratin accumulates, it becomes erosive. This tumorlike mass, known as a cholesteatoma, may erode bone, producing vertigo and deafness as it approaches the membranous labyrinth. Cholesteatomas can be effectively treated only by tympanomastoid surgery.*

➧ ***Acute suppurative mastoiditis.*** *The mucoperiosteum of the air cells of the mastoid process is frequently involved secondary to acute suppurative otitis media. With formation of an abscess cavity in the mastoid process, otitis media may develop into an acute mastoiditis requiring surgical drainage. Acute mastoiditis is now rare, and the same is true of extension of mastoid inflammation into the sigmoid sinus followed by septic thrombosis in the internal jugular vein.*

The **auditory tube,** 3–4 cm long, connects the tympanum with the nasopharynx. Its walls are partly osseous and partly fibrocartilaginous. The osseous segment starts in the anterior (carotid) wall of the tympanum and gradually narrows as it approaches the junction of the squamous and petrous portions of the temporal bone. The longer cartilaginous segment is encased in a fibrocartilaginous plate that terminates at an ostium in the lateral wall of the nasopharynx, bounded posteriorly by the torus tubarius, a protrusion of the fibrocartilaginous pharyngeal end of the tube as it lies just deep to the pharyngeal mucous membrane.

The mucous membrane of the tympanum extends through the auditory tube to the nasopharynx. The epithelium varies from a ciliated columnar type near the pharyngeal opening of the tube to a nonciliated cuboid type as the tube approaches the tympanum.

Four arteries supply the middle ear: the tympanic branch of the maxillary artery, the stylomastoid branch of the posterior auricular artery, the petrosal branch of the midmeningeal artery, and a branch of the ascending pharyngeal artery. Venous drainage terminates in the pterygoid plexus and the superior petrosal sinus. The nerve supply to the tympanum is via the tympanic plexus by a branch of the glossopharyngeal nerve (Jacobsen's nerve), the caroticotympanic nerves, and the small petrosal nerve. The mastoid air cells are devoid of significant sensory innervation.

➧ ***Obstruction of the auditory tube.*** *Auditory tube obstruction may follow acute inflammation of lymphoid tissue, which lies in a submucosal position close to the pharyngeal end of the tube. Such blockage can result in negative pressure in the tympanic cavity, as a result of oxygen absorption by the tympanic epithelium. There is subsequent conductive hearing loss. Long-term obstruction of the auditory tube is often the precursor of serous otitis media and the major cause of chronic middle ear and mastoid disease.*

The Auditory Ossicles
(Fig 4–7)

Three small movable ossicles—the malleus, the incus, and the stapes—extend across the tympanic cavity. The handle of the malleus is attached to the tympanic membrane and the base of the stapes is attached to the circumference of the fenestra ovalis (oval window), while the incus sits between the malleus and stapes. The ossicles transmit sound vibrations received by the tympanic membrane to the perilymphatic fluid in the vestibule. The head of the malleus and the body of the incus lie in the epitympanum, their long processes extending into the tympanic cavity. The malleus and stapes are held in position by ligaments and supported by the tensor tympani muscle and the stapedius muscle, respectively. The incus,

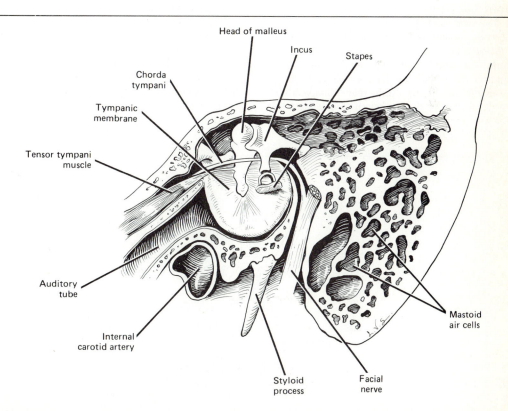

Figure 4–7. Section through mastoid air cells showing location of auditory ossicles, medial surface of tympanum, and auditory tube.

however, has only 2 suspending ligaments and no muscular attachments, making it the ossicle most susceptible to displacement secondary to trauma.

⇒ *Diseases of the ossicles. Stapedial ankylosis (otosclerosis) in young and middle-aged persons is the most common cause of progressive conductive deafness. If one or more of the ossicles are congenitally absent or are fixed, a conductive hearing defect is always present. The conductive defect can be alleviated by ossicular reconstruction or by stapedectomy.*

INNER EAR
(Labyrinth)
(Fig 4–8)

The inner ear contains the sensory organs of equilibrium and hearing and sends afferent impulses via the eighth cranial nerve to the cochlear and vestibular nuclei in the brain stem. The osseous labyrinth is part of the petrous pyramid of the temporal bone and houses the seat of hearing and balance. The sensory epithelium for hearing and balance is located in the membranous labyrinth, a group of connecting membranous fluid-filled sacs and ducts floating within the osseous labyrinth.

Osseous Labyrinth
(Figs 4–9 and 4–10)

The osseous labyrinth has 3 segments: the vestibule, the semicircular canals, and the cochlea. The **vestibule,** the middle segment, lies medial to the tympanic cavity, posterior to the cochlea, and anterior to the semicircular canals. At the rear of the vestibule are the 5 orifices of the semicircular canals, while anteriorly an oval orifice joins with the scala vestibuli

of the cochlea. On the lateral vestibular wall, the oval window is connected to the base of the stapes. The vestibule contains the utricle and the saccule, the 2 otolith organs.

The 3 **semicircular canals** (superior, posterior, and lateral) are superior and posterior to the vestibule and house the organs of the equilibrium. The **cochlea,** a spiral bone coiled about a central pillar, the modiolus, forms the anterior segment of the bony labyrinth and contains the auditory nerve. The cochlea is roughly pyramidal, with its apex pointing anterolaterally and its base forming the inferior segment of the internal acoustic meatus. Branches of the cochlear division of the acoustic nerve pass through openings in the base of the modiolus.

Membranous Labyrinth

The membranous labyrinth lies within the confines of the osseous labyrinth suspended in a fluid, the perilymph, which has an ionic concentration similar to that of extracellular fluid (high in sodium and low in potassium). It contains endolymph, a fluid of high potassium concentration (similar to intracellular fluid). It consists of 3 semicircular ducts, 2 membranous sacs (utricle and saccule), and the cochlear duct. The semicircular ducts lie within the osseous semicircular canals and are similar in form to the bony canals in which they lie. They present a dilated ampulla at one end that contains the crista ampullaris and the vestibular sensory hair cells. The ducts join the utricle through 5 openings.

The **utricle,** the larger of the otolith organs, lies in the posterosuperior segment of the vestibule. The cavity of the utricle joins posteriorly via 5 openings with the semicircular ducts. The smaller otolith organ, the **saccule,** lies near the orifice of the scala vestibuli of the cochlea and is connected with the membranous cochlear duct. Its lumen does not directly join with that of the utricle. The semicircular canals, the utricle,

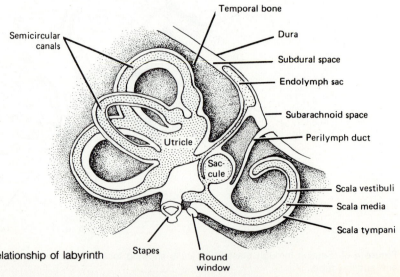

Figure 4–8. Inner ear showing relationship of labyrinth and cochlear duct.

Labels: Temporal bone, Dura, Subdural space, Endolymph sac, Subarachnoid space, Perilymph duct, Scala vestibuli, Scala media, Scala tympani, Semicircular canals, Utricle, Saccule, Stapes, Round window

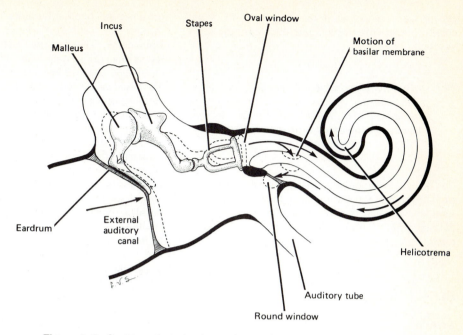

Figure 4–9. Cochlear duct showing pathway of sound.

and the saccule are suspended by several transverse fibrous bands that extend from their lateral borders to the enclosing bony walls. Additional attachment is via vestibular nerve fibers that extend through foramens in the osseous labyrinth on their way to innervate the sensory epithelium.

The cochlear duct (scala media) is a spiral-shaped sac attached to the inner osseous wall of the cochlea. It is surrounded by 2 perilymph chambers: the scala vestibuli, which communicates with the vestibule and

the oval window, and the scala tympani, which ends at the round window. The 2 perilymph chambers communicate at the helicotrema, which is located at the cochlear apex. The cochlear duct is attached at the osseous spiral lamina by the basilar membrane and to the outer wall of the cochlea by the spiral ligament. The basilar membrane supports the organ of Corti and the cochlear hair cells and separates the cochlear duct from the scala tympani. Reissner's membrane extends from the osseous modiolus to the

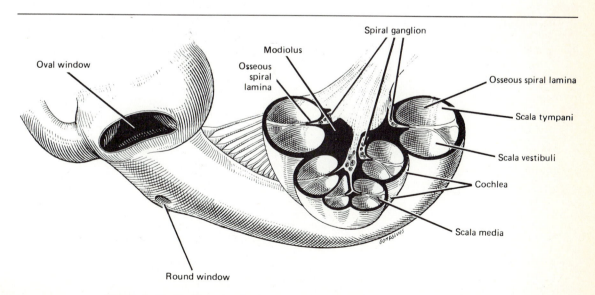

Figure 4–10. Cochlea showing scala vestibuli, scala tympani, and scala media.

end of the stria vascularis on the outer wall of the cochlea, separating the cochlear duct from the scala vestibuli.

➠ *Infectious labyrinthitis. Infection of the labyrinth, causing vertigo, may follow disease of the mastoid area, middle ear disease, or meningitis. Infection may also spread to the labyrinth from distant sites.*

The most common primary site for secondary labyrinth infection is the mastoid area; the adjacent lateral semicircular canal is also frequently involved when the labyrinth is infected or when erosive cholesteatoma is present.

BLOOD VESSELS & NERVES

Arteries

Arterial blood is supplied to the inner ear by a terminal branch of the anteroinferior cerebellar artery, a branch of the basilar artery. The vessel is also known as the labyrinthine artery and divides into cochlear and vestibular branches. The cochlear branch supplies the cochlea, saccule, and posterior ampulla; the vestibular branch supplies the lateral (horizontal) and superior ampullae and the utricle.

Veins

Venous drainage from the cochlea and ampullae is mainly via the vein of the cochlear duct. The semicircular canals are drained via the vein of the vestibular aqueduct, which reaches the sigmoid sinus, and the internal jugular venous system.

Nerves

The middle ear is supplied by special sensory fibers from the cochlea and the vestibule that connect with the eighth cranial nerve. As the eighth nerve approaches the internal auditory canal, it divides into the superior vestibular, inferior vestibular, and cochlear nerves. The superior vestibular nerve supplies the cristae of the superior and lateral semicircular canals and the saccule of the membranous labyrinth. The cochlear nerve contains the axons of the primary auditory neurons innervating the cochlea. In addition to these afferent projections from the cochlea and the vestibular system to the brain, efferent fibers project to the sensory epithelium of the inner ear. The cochlear efferents originate in the superior olivary complex (olivocochlear bundle of Rasmussen). They leave the brain stem with the inferior vestibular nerve and at the vestibulocochlear anastomosis enter the cochlea. Vestibular afferent fibers accompany the cochlear efferents in the vestibular nerve and split to innervate the slopes of the cristae and the utricle and saccule. These fibers arise from an area ventromedial to the vertical segment of the lateral vestibular nucleus.

➠ *Otosclerosis. Otosclerosis secondary to stapedial fixation causes conductive hearing loss. Stapedectomy may reestablish the function of the ossicles by replacing the stapes bone with a wire or Teflon piston prosthesis.*

➠ *Eighth nerve tumors. Tumors of the eighth (vestibulocochlear) nerve are usually benign acoustic neuroma. Other lesions that occur with some frequency in the area of the cerebellopontine angle and must be considered in the differential diagnosis of eighth nerve tumors are cysts, aneurysms, meningiomas, osteomas, and gliomas. Acoustic neuromas tend to occur within the internal acoustic meatus. Most of them arise from the superior vestibular nerve. Their removal calls for accurate anatomic knowledge of bony and membranous labyrinths, and the surgical procedure often requires the combined skills of an otologist and neurosurgeon.*

The Eye

Khalid F. Tabbara, MD

EMBRYOLOGY

The eye is formed from neural and surface ectoderm and from mesenchyme containing mesodermal and neural crest cells.

Neural ectoderm of the diencephalon gives rise to the optic cup and the optic stalk, which become the retina and the optic nerve, respectively.

The optic cup evokes a thickening of the overlying ectoderm, which sinks inward and detaches from the surface as the lens. The conjunctiva and the lacrimal and tarsal glands also arise from surface ectoderm.

From the mesenchyme are derived the choroid, the ciliary bodies, the iris, the sclera, the cornea, and the vitreous humor.

The extraocular and eyelid muscles, orbital vessels, and ciliary muscles also develop from mesenchyme, but the sphincter and dilator pupillae muscles are said to form from ectoderm.

The eyelids, composed of ectodermal and mesenchymal elements, grow toward each other and fuse near the end of the third month but separate again about 4 months later.

ANOMALIES

Congenital defects of the ocular structures fall into 2 main categories: developmental anomalies, or dysplasia of embryonal origin, and tissue reactions to intrauterine insults (due to infections or drugs). Examples of the first category are dermoid tumors, microphakia, anophthalmos, microphthalmos, and congenital glaucoma. Examples of the second category are chorioretinitis and some forms of cataract. Heredity plays a major role in the development of certain congenital deformities. Any failure of regression of primitive vascular tissue at the proper stage—or of fusion of embryonic tissue—can lead to a defect of development of iris or choroid (eg, coloboma of iris).

GROSS ANATOMY

The major structures of the external eye are shown in Fig 5–1.

OCULAR ADNEXA

1. EYEBROWS

The eyebrows are folds of thickened skin covered with hair. The folds are supported by underlying muscle fiber. The glabella is a usually hairless prominence between the eyebrows.

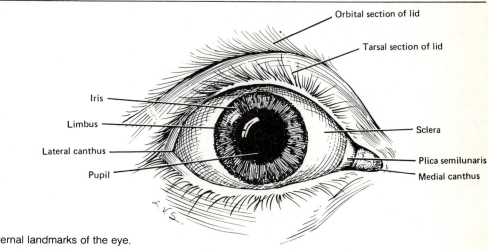

Iris

Limbus

Lateral canthus

Pupil

Orbital section of lid

Tarsal section of lid

Sclera

Plica semilunaris

Medial canthus

Figure 5–1. External landmarks of the eye.

2. EYELIDS

The upper and lower eyelids (palpebrae) are modified folds of skin that can close to protect the anterior eyeball. Blinking helps spread tear film that protects the cornea and conjunctiva from dehydration. The skin of the eyelids is thin, loose, and elastic. It possesses few hair follicles and no subcutaneous fat.

The eyelids consist of 5 principal planes of tissue (from superficial to deep): skin layer, layer of striated muscle (orbicularis oculi), areolar tissue, fibrous tissue (tarsal plates), and a layer of mucous membrane (palpebral conjunctiva).

⇒ *Ptosis. Abnormalities of the levator palpebrae superioris may cause drooping of the upper eyelid (ptosis).*

Palpebral Fissure

The palpebral fissure is the space between the open lids. The fissure terminates at the medial and lateral canthi. The lacrimal lake consists of the **caruncle,** a yellowish elevation of modified skin containing large modified sweat glands and sebaceous glands that open into follicles that contain fine hair; and the **plica semilunaris,** a vestige of the third eyelid of lower species. This is a crescentic fold lateral to the caruncle. In Orientals, the epicanthal fold (**epicanthus**) passes between the medial ends of the upper and lower lids. Epicanthal folds are present normally in infants of all races and disappear with development of the nose bridge.

Lid Margins

The free lid margin is 25–30 mm long and about 2 mm wide. It is divided by the gray line (mucocutaneous junction) into anterior and posterior margins. At the **anterior margin,** irregularly spaced **eyelashes** project from the margins of the eyelids. The **glands of Zeis** are small modified sebaceous glands that open into the hair follicles at the base of the eyelashes. The **glands of Moll** are modified sweat glands that open in a row near the base of the eyelashes.

The **posterior margin** shows the small orifices of modified sebaceous glands (**meibomian glands**). A surgical incision through the gray line can easily split the lid into anterior and posterior lamellae.

⇒ *Chalazion. A hordeolum (sty) is an acute infection of an eyelid gland (glands of Zeis, Moll, or Meibom). A chalazion is a lipogranuloma of a meibomian gland. It is characterized by nontender localized swelling without acute inflammation. Chalazion seldom subsides spontaneously.*

At the medial end of the posterior margin of each lid there is a central small opening called the **lacrimal punctum.** The puncta carry the tears down through the corresponding canaliculus to the lacrimal sac.

Structure of the Lids

The tarsal plate is the main supporting structure of the eyelids. It is a dense fibrous tissue layer with a small amount of elastic tissue. The angles of the tarsal plates are attached to the orbital margin by the lateral and medial palpebral ligaments; the upper and lower tarsal plates are also attached by a condensed, thin fascia, the orbital septum, to the upper and lower orbital margins.

⇒ *Entropion and ectropion. Entropion is inversion of the lid. The eyelashes may touch the cornea and conjunctiva (trichiasis). Senile entropion is caused by atrophic relaxation of the inferior fascial attachments to the lower eyelid, leaving a freely movable lower tarsal edge. The preseptal portion of the palpebral orbicularis muscle contracts and overrides the pretarsal portion of the muscle.*

⇒ *Cicatricial entropion. Cicatricial entropion is caused by scarring of the lid from diseases such as trachoma or membranous conjunctivitis, burns, irradiation, chemical injuries, or surgical procedures on the lids.*

The **levator palpebrae superioris muscle** arises from the apex of the orbit and passes forward to insert into the anterior surface of the superior tarsus and the overlying skin.

The lids are lined posteriorly by a layer of mucous membrane, the **palpebral conjunctiva,** which adheres firmly to the tarsus.

The **orbicularis oculi muscle** is supplied by the facial nerve; its function is to close the lids. Its muscle fibers surround the palpebral fissure in concentric fashion and spread, for a short distance, around the orbital margin. Some fibers run onto the cheek and forehead.

Blood Vessels, Lymphatics, & Nerves
(Fig 5–2)

The blood supply to the lids is derived from the facial (from the external carotid artery) and ophthalmic arteries (from the internal carotid artery) via their palpebral branches. Venous drainage from the lids empties into the ophthalmic vein and the veins that drain the forehead and temple. The veins are arranged in pre- and posttarsal plexuses.

Lymphatics from the lateral segment of the lids run into the preauricular and deep cervical lymph nodes. Lymphatics draining the medial side of the lids empty into the submandibular lymph nodes.

The sensory nerve supply to the eyelids is derived from the first and second divisions of the trigeminal (fifth) nerve. The small lacrimal, supraorbital, supra-

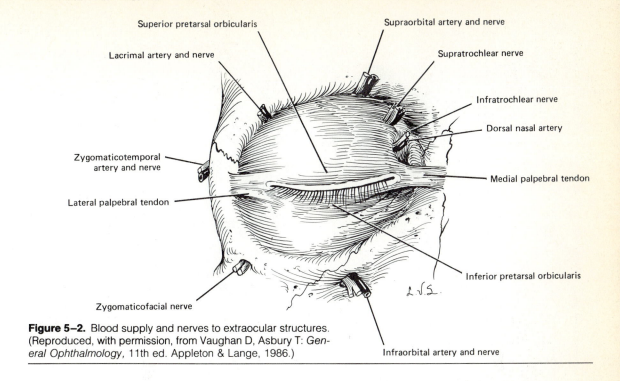

Superior pretarsal orbicularis

Lacrimal artery and nerve

Supraorbital artery and nerve

Supratrochlear nerve

Infratrochlear nerve

Dorsal nasal artery

Zygomaticotemporal
artery and nerve

Medial palpebral tendon

Lateral palpebral tendon

Zygomaticofacial nerve

Inferior pretarsal orbicularis

Infraorbital artery and nerve

Figure 5–2. Blood supply and nerves to extraocular structures. (Reproduced, with permission, from Vaughan D, Asbury T: *General Ophthalmology,* 11th ed. Appleton & Lange, 1986.)

trochlear, infratrochlear, and external nasal nerves are branches of the ophthalmic (first) division of the trigeminal nerve. The infraorbital, zygomaticofacial, and zygomaticotemporal nerves are branches of the maxillary (second) division.

➠ *Nerve VII. Denervation of the facial nerve results in paralysis of the orbicularis oculi muscle and inability to close the eyelids.*

LACRIMAL APPARATUS
(Fig 5–3)

The lacrimal apparatus consists of the lacrimal glands, the accessory lacrimal glands, the canaliculi, the lacrimal sac, and the nasolacrimal duct. The lacrimal gland consists of the almond-shaped **orbital portion** of the gland, in the lacrimal fossa in the temporal segment of the orbit; and the **palpebral portion,** smaller than the orbital portion, located just above the superior temporal conjunctival fornix. Lacrimal ducts, which open by approximately 10 fine orifices, connect the 2 portions of the lacrimal gland to the superior conjunctival fornix.

Blood Vessels, Lymphatics, & Nerves

The blood supply of the lacrimal gland is derived from the lacrimal artery; the lacrimal vein drains into the ophthalmic vein. The lymphatic drainage of the lacrimal gland joins the conjunctival lymphatics to drain into the preauricular lymph nodes.

The nerve supply to the lacrimal gland consists of (1) the lacrimal nerve (sensory), a branch of the trigeminal first division; (2) the great superficial petrosal nerve (secretory), which comes from the superior salivary nucleus via the pterygopalatine ganglion; and (3) sympathetic nerves accompanying the lacrimal artery and nerve.

Lacrimal Canaliculi

Tears secreted by the major and accessory lacrimal glands into the upper conjunctival fornix pass over the cornea and conjunctiva and drain into the lacrimal canaliculi through the lacrimal puncta. The canaliculi, about 1 mm in diameter and 8 mm long, join to form a common canaliculus just before opening into the lacrimal sac.

➠ *Acute dacryoadenitis and dacryocystitis. Dacryoadenitis is acute inflammation of the lacrimal gland. Dacryocystitis is acute or chronic infection of the lacrimal sac; it usually occurs in infants or in persons over age 40, is unilateral, and is the result of obstruction of the lacrimal duct, manifested by tearing and discharge.*

➠ *Disorders of the lacrimal gland. Benign or malignant tumors may occur in the lacrimal gland and may be manifested by dry eye syn-*

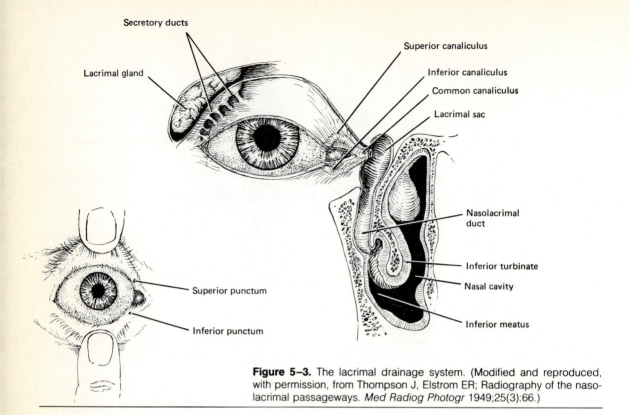

Figure 5–3. The lacrimal drainage system. (Modified and reproduced, with permission, from Thompson J, Elstrom ER; Radiography of the naso-lacrimal passageways. *Med Radiog Photogr* 1949;25(3):66.)

drome (keratoconjunctivitis sicca), which has many causes. Instillation of artificial tears is one form of therapy. The lacrimal gland may also be affected by leukemia or by systemic disorders such as sarcoidosis, amyloidosis, or Sjögren's syndrome.

The **lacrimal sac** lies in the lacrimal fossa. The nasolacrimal duct continues downward from the nasolacrimal sac in the nasolacrimal fossa and opens into the inferior meatus of the nasal cavity lateral to the inferior turbinate. Tears pass into the puncta by capillary attraction and gravity and by the constant blinking action of the eyelids.

➠ *Obstruction of nasolacrimal duct. Nasolacrimal duct obstruction with stasis predisposes to infection of the lacrimal sac (dacryocystitis). Probing of the duct can overcome congenital membranous obstruction in infants and young children. The procedure has no lasting benefits in adults.*

Related Structures

The **medial palpebral ligament** connects the upper and lower tarsal plates to the frontal process at the inner canthus anterior to the lacrimal sac.

The **angular vein and artery** lie just under the skin of the inner canthus. Skin incisions made in the course of surgical procedures on the lacrimal sac should always be placed 2–3 mm to the nasal side of the inner canthus to avoid these vessels.

THE EYEBALL
(Figs 5–4 and 5–5)

1. THE CONJUNCTIVA

The conjunctiva is a thin, transparent mucous membrane that covers the posterior surface of the lids and the anterior surface of the sclera. It is continuous with the skin at the lid margin (mucocutaneous junction) and with corneal epithelium at the limbus.

The **palpebral conjunctiva** lines the posterior surface of the lids and adheres firmly to the tarsus. At the upper and lower margins of the tarsus, the conjunctiva is reflected backward and attaches to and covers the sclera.

The **bulbar conjunctiva** is loosely attached to the orbital septum in the region of the fornices and is folded many times. This allows the eye to move freely and enlarges the conjunctival secretory surface. The ducts of the lacrimal glands open into the upper temporal aspect of the superior fornix. Except for

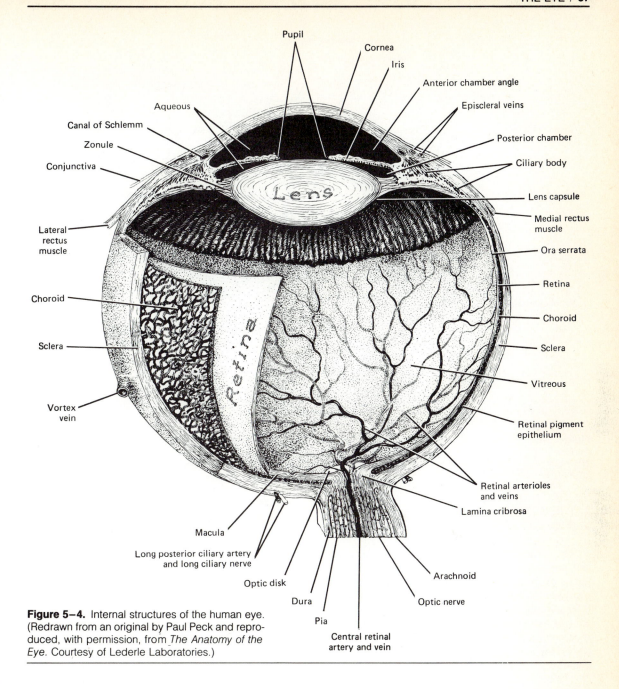

Figure 5–4. Internal structures of the human eye. (Redrawn from an original by Paul Peck and reproduced, with permission, from _The Anatomy of the Eye._ Courtesy of Lederle Laboratories.)

the limbus, the bulbar conjunctiva is loosely attached to Tenon's capsule and to the underlying sclera.

A soft, movable, thickened fold of bulbar conjunctiva at the inner canthus corresponds to the nictitating membrane of some lower animals. A small, fleshy epidermoid structure, the **caruncle,** is attached to the semilunar fold and is a transition zone containing both cutaneous and mucous membrane elements.

Blood Vessels, Lymphatics, & Nerves

The conjunctival arteries are derived from the ante-

rior ciliary and palpebral arteries. They anastomose freely with the numerous conjunctival veins to form a dense conjunctival vascular network. The conjunctival lymphatics join with the lymphatics of the eyelids to form a rich plexus. The conjunctiva receives its nerve supply from the first ophthalmic division of the trigeminal nerve. It possesses a relatively small number of pain fibers.

⇒ _**Conjunctivitis.** Inflammation of the conjunctiva is the most common eye disease._

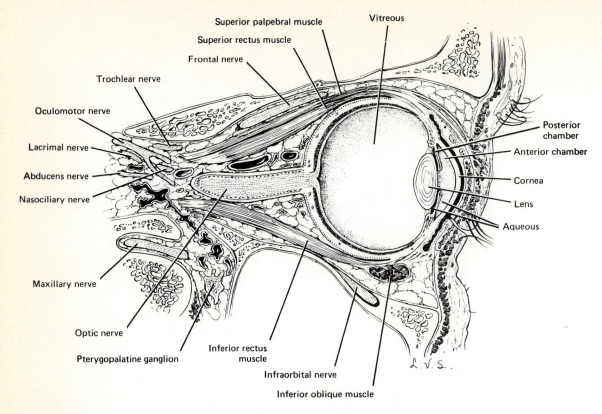

Figure 5–5. Lateral view of the eye and surrounding structures. (Reproduced, with permission, from Vaughan D, Asbury T: *General Ophthalmology,* 11th ed. Appleton & Lange, 1986.)

2. THE CORNEA
(Figs 5–4 to 5–6)

The cornea is an avascular, transparent refracting and protective membranous window through which light rays pass to the retina. Its refractive power is equivalent to +43 diopters. The adult cornea is about 0.59 mm thick at the periphery and about 0.56 mm thick at the center and is about 11.5 mm in diameter. It is composed of 5 layers: epithelium, Bowman's layer, stroma, Descemet's membrane, and endothelium.

The cornea receives nourishment from the aqueous and the tears and through the vascular limbus, through which nutrients must pass to the avascular cornea. The superficial cornea derives its oxygen from the atmosphere. The sensory nerves of the cornea are derived from the ophthalmic division of the trigeminal nerve, and there is severe pain whenever the fibers in the corneal epithelium are exposed, even by minor abrasions.

➠ *Scarring after corneal ulceration. This is a major cause of impaired vision and blindness. Ulcers may be caused by bacteria, fungi, vi-* ruses, vitamin A deficiency, exposure, or trauma.

➠ *Keratoplasty. Corneal transplantation (keratoplasty) is indicated in some cases of scarring, edema, thinning, and distortion.*

Radial keratotomy is a new surgical procedure for myopia whereby radial incisions are made to flatten the surface and decrease myopic error. Corneal incision and local excision of tissue are also occasionally performed for corneal astigmatism.

3. THE SCLERA
(Figs 5–4 to 5–6)

The sclera is the fibrous protective coating of the eye. It is white, dense, and continuous with the cornea anteriorly at the limbus and the dural sheath of the optic nerve posteriorly. It is about 0.5–1 mm thick. A few strands of modified scleral tissue pass over the optic disk (lamina cribrosa). The outer layer of the sclera is composed of thin, fine elastic tissue, the episclera, that contains the supply of blood vessels. The lamina fusca is the brownish inner continuous scleral layer. The sclera is penetrated by the long

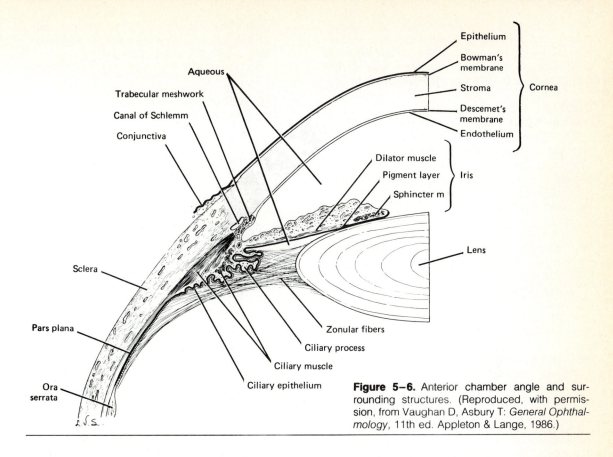

Figure 5–6. Anterior chamber angle and surrounding structures. (Reproduced, with permission, from Vaughan D, Asbury T: *General Ophthalmology*, 11th ed. Appleton & Lange, 1986.)

and short posterior ciliary arteries and the long and short ciliary nerves. About 4 mm behind the limbus, the 4 anterior ciliary arteries and veins penetrate the sclera, near the insertion of the rectus muscle. Just behind the equator of the globe, the 4 vortex veins exit the sclera, usually one in each quadrant.

⟾ *Episcleritis. Inflammation of the episclera may be caused by autoimmune diseases, granulomatous diseases, metabolic diseases, and infections. Injuries to the sclera may result from trauma or may follow irradiation or thermal or chemical burns.*

4. THE UVEAL TRACT
(Fig 5–4)

The uveal tract consists of the iris, ciliary body (ciliary process), and choroid. It is the middle vascular layer of the eye and is protected by the cornea and sclera. It contributes blood supply to the retina. The iris controls the amount of light that enters the eye by a reflex action that constricts the pupil in light and dilates it in darkness. The ciliary body forms the root of the iris and through its muscular fibers governs the thickness of the lens in accommodation.

Aqueous humor is secreted by the ciliary processes into the posterior chamber. The choroidal blood vessels nourish the outer portion of the underlying retina.

Iris
(Figs 5–4 to 5–6)

The iris is the anterior extension of the ciliary body. It presents as a flat surface with a central round hole, the pupil. It forms the posterior wall of the anterior chamber and the anterior wall of the posterior chamber. Within the stroma of the iris are the sphincter and dilator muscles of the pupil. Two heavily pigmented layers on the posterior surface of the iris represent the anterior extension of the pigment epithelium of the retina.

Ciliary Body
(Figs 5–4 and 5–6)

The ciliary body extends forward from the anterior end of the choroid to the root of the iris (about 6 mm). It consists of a corrugated anterior zone (corona ciliaris) and a flattened posterior zone (pars plana). The **ciliary muscle** is composed of longitudinal, circular, and radial fibers that contract and relax the zonular fibers (zonule). This alters the tension of the capsule of the lens, giving the lens a variable dioptic power. The blood supply to the ciliary body comes from the iris. The ciliary processes secrete **aqueous**, which circulates from the posterior chamber to the anterior chamber and drains via the angle of the anterior chamber through the trabecular meshwork and the canal of Schlemm to the venous circulation. The sensory nerve supply of the iris is through the ciliary nerves.

Choroid
(Figs 5–4 and 5–5)

The choroid is the posterior vascular segment of the uveal tract between the retina and the sclera. The deeper the vessels, the wider their lumens. The choroid is attached posteriorly to the margins of the optic nerve. Anteriorly, the choroid joins with the ciliary body.

➧ *Symptoms of uveal tract disease. Inflammation of the iris (iritis) causes pain and photophobia. Choroidal disease may be associated with visual loss. The anterior uveal tract is examined with a flashlight and loupe or with the slit lamp. The posterior uveal tract is examined with the ophthalmoscope.*

➧ *Inflammation of the uveal tract. The most common type is acute iritis, with pain, photophobia, blurred vision, and a small pupil. In such cases, it is important to rule out acute angle-closure glaucoma and then instill dilating drops to prevent posterior adhesions, referred to as posterior synechiae.*

5. THE LENS
(Figs 5–4, 5–5, and 5–6)

The lens is a biconvex, avascular, colorless, and almost completely transparent structure about 3–4 mm thick and 9 mm in diameter. It is suspended behind the iris and connected with the ciliary body by the zonules. Anterior to the lens is the aqueous; behind it, the vitreous. The zonule, or suspensory ligament, consists of fibrils that arise from the ciliary body and insert into the equator of the lens.

The sole purpose of the lens is to focus light on the retina. The physiologic interplay of ciliary muscle, zonule, and lens that focuses a nearby object on the retina is called accommodation. As the lens ages, its accommodative power is gradually reduced. There are no pain fibers, blood vessels, or nerves in the lens.

➧ *Disorders of the lens. Disorders of the lens consist of opacification (cataract formation) and dislocation. In either case, the patient complains of blurred vision without pain. Cataracts may be senile, congenital, toxic, secondary to systemic disease (hypoparathyroidism), or the result of trauma. Cataracts may cause uveitis or glaucoma. Lens dislocation may be associated with an inborn error of metabolism, may be a hereditary congenital defect, or may occur as a result of ocular trauma.*

6. THE VITREOUS
(Figs 5–4 and 5–6)

The vitreous is a clear, avascular gelatinous body that accounts for two-thirds of the volume and weight of the eye. It fills the space bounded by the lens, retina, and optic disk. It helps maintain the shape of the eye and the clarity of the visual axis. It is in contact with the posterior lens capsule, the zonular fibers, the epithelium of the pars plana, the retina, and the optic nerve head.

➧ *Rupture of the globe. Rupture of the globe may result in blindness and sometimes loss of the eyeball. Prolapse of the uvea, vitreous, and retina through a penetrating wound may lead to loss of the eye. Prompt repair of the injured eye is mandatory.*

➧ *Secondary inflammation of the vitreous. Local inflammatory lesions of the choroid and retina cause inflammation of the vitreous. There is no pain, and the external eye may appear normal; but there is blurring of vision, and the fundus may become invisible.*

7. THE AQUEOUS
(Figs 5–4, 5–5, and 5–6)

Aqueous (aqueous humor) fills the anterior and posterior chambers of the eye. It is slightly alkaline, composed mainly of water, and secreted by the ciliary process. From the posterior chamber the fluid passes through the pupil into the anterior chamber, then toward the filtering trabecular meshwork at the periphery and into the canal of Schlemm, from which arise 25–30 collector channels. The aqueous is then drained through the scleral venous plexuses and the aqueous veins into the anterior ciliary veins.

➧ *Glaucoma. Glaucoma is characterized by acute or chronic increase in intraocular pressure sufficient to cause degeneration of the optic disk and visual field defects. Therapy aims to facilitate the outflow of aqueous through existing drainage channels, using miotics or surgical procedures, and in some cases to inhibit the secretion of aqueous by drugs. In patients with acute angle-closure glaucoma, surgical iridectomy or laser iridotomy is necessary. Operative procedures, including the use of lasers, may also be indicated in chronic glaucoma.*

8. THE RETINA
(Figs 5–4, 5–5, and 5–7)

The retina is the thin, semitransparent layer of nerve tissue that forms the innermost coat of the posterior segment of the eye. It consists of 10 layers of highly organized tissue. Its outer surface is related to the choroid; its inner surface touches the vitreous. Posteriorly, the retina is continuous with the optic nerve. It extends nearly as far anteriorly as the ciliary body, ending at that point in a ragged edge (the ora serrata). In the center of the posterior segment of the retina is the macula lutea, an oval, yellowish spot whose center is depressed (fovea centralis). At this point, the retina is very thin, and one can see the dark choroid coat through it. About 3 mm medial to the macula is the optic disk, marking the position of the optic nerve. A small niche (optic cup) in the center of the disk is the point of entrance of the central artery of the retina. The disk is insensitive to light and is called the physiologic blind spot.

The 10 layers of the retina are (1) the internal limiting membrane, (2) a layer of nerve fibers, (3) a ganglion cell layer, (4) the inner plexiform layer, (5) the inner nuclear layer, (6) the outer plexiform layer, (7) the outer nuclear layer, (8) the external limiting membrane, (9) a layer of rods and cones, and (10) pigment epithelium.

The retina receives its blood supply in its outer third from the choriocapillaris. The inner two-thirds is supplied by branches from the central retinal artery, a branch of the ophthalmic artery. The central macular area is avascular.

Arteriovenous crossings are frequent in the temporal quadrants of the retina. Veins are located deep to the arteries at these crossings.

➠ **Disorders of the retina.** *Obstruction of the central retinal artery is usually unilateral and oc-* *curs in old patients. It leads to sudden loss of vision. Blockage of the central retinal vein usually results in slow, painless loss of vision. Diabetic retinopathy has become a leading cause of blindness in the Western world. Retinopathy of prematurity is a bilateral retinal disease of premature infants who receive excessive concentrations of oxygen during the first few weeks of life. The retina may be torn by mechanical force, usually vitreous traction. Since the retina is only loosely adherent to the pigment epithelium, the 2 layers may separate, allowing fluid to accumulate between them, as in cases of retinal detachment.*

EXTRAOCULAR STRUCTURES

1. TENON'S CAPSULE
(Fig 5–8)

Tenon's capsule (fascia bulbi) is a fibrous membrane that envelops the globe from the limbus to the optic nerve, touching the sclera. Its lower segment is thick and fuses with the fascia of the inferior rectus and inferior oblique muscles to form the suspensory ligament of Lockwood. The fusion forms a sling on which the globe rests. At the point where the fascia bulbi is pierced by the tendons of the extraocular muscles, it sends a tubular reflection around each of these muscles. These fascial extensions are quite tough and limit the action of the extraocular muscles ("check ligaments").

2. EXTRAOCULAR MUSCLES
(Figs 5–8 and 5–9)

There are 6 extraocular muscles: 4 recti and 2 obliques. Their blood supply is derived from the

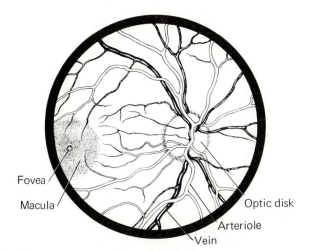
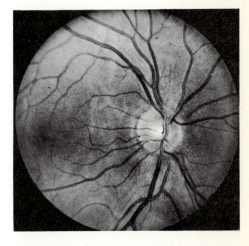

Fovea

Macula

Optic disk

Arteriole

Vein

Figure 5–7. The normal fundus. Diagram at left shows landmarks of the photograph at right. (Photo by Diane Beeston. Reproduced, with permission, from Vaughan D, Asbury T: *General Ophthalmology*, 9th ed. Lange, 1980.)

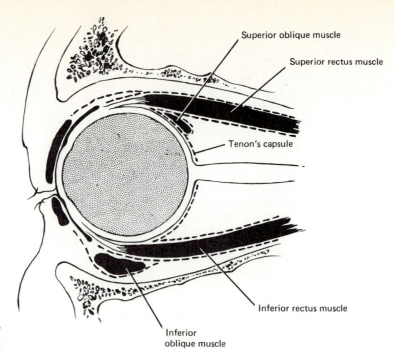

Figure 5–8. Fascia about the muscles and eyeball (Tenon's capsule). (Reproduced, with permission, from Vaughan D, Asbury T: *General Ophthalmology,* 11th ed. Appleton & Lange, 1986.)

ophthalmic artery, the lacrimal artery, and infraorbital arteries. The oculomotor nerve divides and innervates the medial, inferior, and superior rectus muscles and the inferior oblique muscle. The abducens nerve innervates the lateral rectus muscle; the trochlear nerve innervates the superior oblique muscle.

Rectus Muscles

The 4 rectus muscles originate in the tendinous ring, the annulus of Zinn, surrounding the optic nerve at the posterior apex of the orbit. The rectus muscles insert into the sclera on the surface of the eyeball anterior to its equator. They are named by site of insertion, ie, medial rectus, lateral rectus, inferior rectus, and superior rectus. The muscles are about 40 mm long and become tendinous at their insertion. The lateral rectus abducts the eye, and the medial rectus adducts the eye. The superior rectus elevates and adducts the eye and is concerned with **intorsion.** The inferior rectus depresses and adducts the eye and is concerned with **extorsion.**

➡ *Strabismus. Strabismus (*squint*) is abnormal deviation of the eye. Outward deviation is called exotropia; inward deviation is called esotropia.*

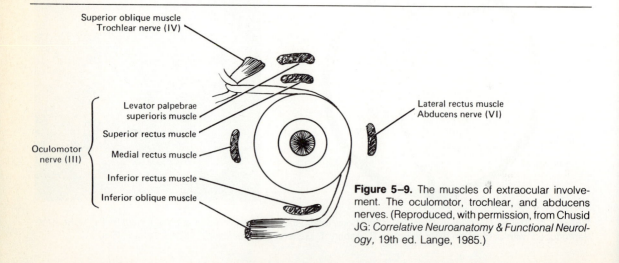

Figure 5–9. The muscles of extraocular involvement. The oculomotor, trochlear, and abducens nerves. (Reproduced, with permission, from Chusid JG: *Correlative Neuroanatomy & Functional Neurology,* 19th ed. Lange, 1985.)

Under normal conditions, the visual axes of the eyes intersect at the object of regard, the image falling on the fovea of each eye. When the eyes are positioned so that the image falls on the fovea of one eye only, the second eye is said to be deviating, and in such cases strabismus is present.

➠ ***Surgery on extraocular muscles.*** *Surgery on the extraocular muscles is indicated when nonsurgical means have failed to correct strabismus and when the cosmetic effect of the deviation is unacceptable. The objective of surgery is to place the visual axis of the deviating eye as nearly parallel to that of the contralateral eye as possible so that the eyes will be straight in all conjugate movements of gaze.*

Oblique Muscles

The **superior oblique** is the longest and thinnest of the ocular muscles. It originates above and medial to the optic foramen and passes anteriorly in the form of a tendon to its trochlea, or pulley. It then reflects backward and downward to attach to the sclera beneath the superior rectus. The superior oblique directs the eye laterally and inferiorly.

The **inferior oblique** muscle originates from the nasal side of the orbital wall just behind the inferior orbital rim. It passes beneath the inferior rectus and

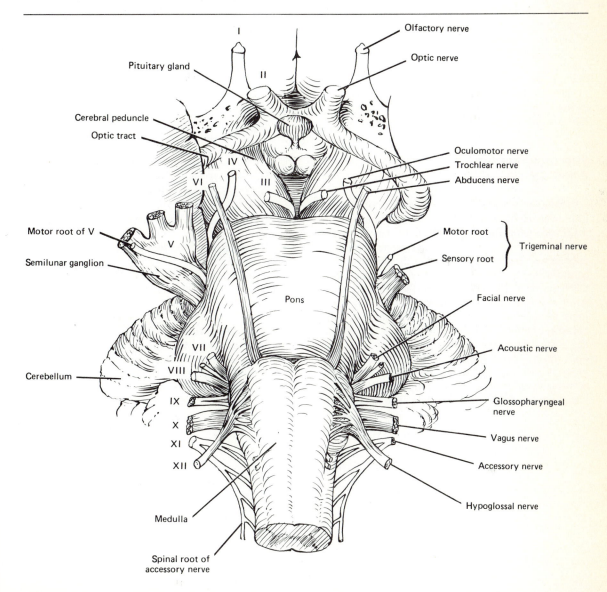

Figure 5–10. Emergence of cranial nerves from the brain. (Reproduced, with permission, from Chusid JG: *Correlative Neuroanatomy & Functional Neurology,* 19th ed. Lange, 1985.)

then under the lateral rectus to insert into the sclera with a short tendon. Its action directs the eye superiorly and laterally.

Levator Palpebrae Superioris Muscle

The levator palpebrae superioris muscle arises with a short tendon from the undersurface of the sphenoid near the optic foramen. It inserts into the skin of the eyelid and into the anterior surface of the upper tarsus. The action of the levator palpebrae superioris is to raise the upper eyelid. Part of the orbicularis oculi muscle acts as the antagonist of the levator palpebrae.

⸬➧ ***Blepharoptosis.*** *Blepharoptosis, or drooping of the upper eyelid, results from dysfunction of the levator palpebrae superioris muscle. It may be congenital or acquired and unilateral or bilateral.*

The blood supply is derived from the lateral branch of the ophthalmic artery. The levator is supplied by the superior branch of the oculomotor nerve.

THE OPTIC NERVE
(Fig 5–10)

The trunk of the optic nerve consists of about 1 million axons that arise from the ganglion cells of the retina (nerve fiber layer). The optic nerve emerges from the posterior surface of the globe through a circular opening in the sclera, near the posterior pole of the eye. The orbital segment of the nerve enters the bony optic foramen to reach the cranial cavity. After a 10- to 15-mm intracranial course, the nerve joins the opposite optic nerve and forms the **optic chiasm,** where one-half of the fibers cross, and continues posteriorly to the lateral geniculate bodies as the **optic tract.** Eighty percent of the nerve consists of visual fibers that synapse in the lateral geniculate body on neurons whose axons terminate in the primary visual cortex of the occipital lobes. The nerve fibers become myelinated on leaving the eye. Twenty percent of the fibers are pupillary and bypass the geniculate body. The ganglion cells of the retina and their axons are part of the central nervous system. They will not regenerate if severed.

The fibrous wrappings of the optic nerve are continuous with the meninges. The pia mater is closely attached to the nerve in most of its intracranial and all of its intraorbital course, but it is only loosely attached in the optic chiasm. The pia divides the optic nerve fibers into bundles by sending multiple septa into the nerve substance and continues to the sclera. The arachnoid sheathes the nerve from the intracranial end of the optic foramen to the globe, where it terminates in the sclera. The dura mater lining the inner surface of the cranial vault meets the optic nerve as it leaves the optic foramen. As the nerve enters the orbit through the optic foramen, the dura splits, one layer lining the orbital cavity and the other forming the outer covering of the optic nerve. The tough, fibrous dura becomes continuous with the outer two-thirds of the sclera.

⸬➧ ***Optic neuritis.*** *The term "optic neuritis" denotes inflammation of the optic nerve. The major symptom is loss of vision. Upon ophthalmoscopic examination, it resembles papilledema.*

In retrobulbar neuritis, the nerve is affected posteriorly, so that there are no visible ophthalmologic changes of the nerve unless optic atrophy supervenes. The most frequent cause of retrobulbar neuritis is multiple sclerosis.

⸬➧ ***Papilledema.*** *Papilledema, or choked disk, is noninflammatory congestion of the optic disk associated with increased intracranial pressure due to tumors, abscesses, bleeding, or malignant hypertension.*

⸬➧ ***Pressure of tumors on optic nerve.*** *Some pituitary tumors, craniopharyngiomas, meningiomas, and aneurysms may press on the optic nerve in the region of the optic chiasm. Loss of vision, field changes, and bony erosion of the sella are frequent findings.*

The Vertebral Column

Jack deGroot, MD, & Joseph G. Chusid, MD

6

EMBRYOLOGY

Vertebrae

The **vertebral column** originates in mesenchymal cells of the sclerotomes. Such mesenchymal cells surround the spinal cord and the notochord to form a long mesenchymal column, which retains traces of segmental origin (sclerotomic blocks) as indicated by the intersegmental arteries. The caudal portion of each sclerotome proliferates and condenses and binds to the cephalic half of the next sclerotome to form a vertebral body. Anomalies include cleft vertebrae, asymmetric fusion of adjacent vertebrae, anomalies in number (increase or decrease) of vertebrae, and fused vertebrae. Klippel-Feil syndrome consists of fused cervical vertebrae.

Intervertebral Disk

Mesenchymal cells originating from the underlying sclerotome segment fill the space between 2 precartilaginous vertebral bodies to form the intervertebral disk.

Nucleus Pulposus

The notochord persists within each intervertebral disk and undergoes mucoid degeneration to form the nucleus pulposus, which later is surrounded by the circular fibers of the annulus fibrosus.

GROSS ANATOMY
(Fig 6–1)

The vertebral (spinal) column consists of 33 vertebrae joined by ligaments and cartilage. The upper 24 vertebrae are discrete and movable; the lower 9 are fixed—5 being fused to form the sacrum and the terminal 4 fusing to form the coccyx. The normal vertebral column may be considered to have 7 cervical, 12 thoracic, 5 lumbar, 5 sacral, and 4 coccygeal vertebrae. Mobility of the vertebrae in the cervical, thoracic, and lumbar regions is relatively free compared with the mobility of the sacrum and coccyx. The spinal column in the male is 10–12 cm longer than in the female.

The vertebral column is curved in the ventrodorsal direction in several places. The cervical spine is concave posteriorly; the thoracic spine is convex; and the lumbar spine is concave, the curve ending at the lumbosacral angle. The pelvic curve is concave anteriorly from the lumbosacral angle to the tip of the coccyx.

VERTEBRAE

The typical vertebra has a body and a neural arch surrounding the vertebral canal. The **neural arch** is composed of a **pedicle** on each side supporting a **lamina** that extends posteriorly to the midline. The pedicle has a notch superiorly and inferiorly that forms the **intervertebral foramen.** The neural arch is attached to a posterior midline **spinous process,** or **spine,** and has lateral transverse processes and upper and lower articular facets.

The bodies of the vertebrae gradually increase in width from the second cervical to the first thoracic, become narrower over the next 2 to 3, and then become wider again as far down as the lumbosacral angle. The oval-shaped **intervertebral foramens** through which the spinal nerves pass are smallest in the cervical region and gradually increase in size to the lowest lumbar area. The midline spinous processes of the cervical vertebrae (C2–6) are bifid and almost horizontal; those of the thoracic vertebrae are single and slant downward; and those of the lumbar vertebrae are single and almost horizontal.

The laminae on each side of the spinous processes form shallow grooves filled by muscle layers. The **articular facets** are lateral to the laminae, while the **transverse processes** are more lateral and somewhat anterior.

Vertebrae & Spinal Nerves

Spinal nerves C1–7 (both right and left) pass over the superior aspect of their corresponding cervical vertebrae. Spinal nerve C8 passes below the body of vertebra C7. All of the remaining spinal nerves pass below the inferior margins of their corresponding vertebra.

The vertebrae **articulate** body-to-body and also by articular facets. Movement between adjacent vertebrae is slight, but the additive effect can be large. Range of motion is greatest in the cervicothoracic and thoracolumbar junctions, the 2 most common sites of vertebral injury.

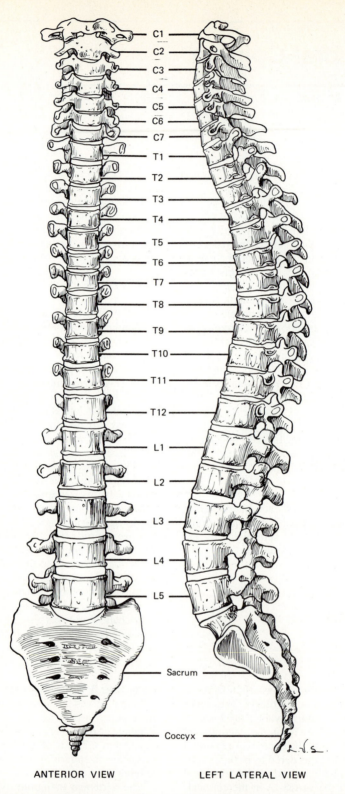

C1	C2	C3	C4	C5	C6	C7

ANTERIOR VIEW   LEFT LATERAL VIEW

Figure 6–1. The vertebral column. (Reproduced, with permission, from Chusid JG: *Correlative Neuroanatomy & Functional Neurology*, 19th ed. Lange, 1985)

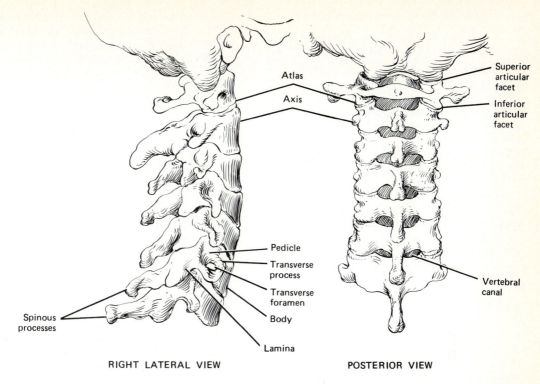

Atlas

Axis

Superior
articular
facet

Inferior
articular
facet

Pedicle

Transverse
process

Transverse
foramen

Body

Spinous
processes

Vertebral
canal

Lamina

RIGHT LATERAL VIEW

POSTERIOR VIEW

Figure 6–2. The cervical vertebrae. (Reproduced, with permission, from Chusid JG: *Correlative Neuroanatomy & Functional Neurology,* 19th ed. Lange, 1985.)

1. CERVICAL VERTEBRAE
   (Fig 6–2)

The upper cervical vertebrae are characterized by a foramen that perforates each of the transverse processes. The vertebral vessels pass through the bony canal formed by the foramens. The seventh cervical vertebra has a small foramen that is absent in about 30% of people.

C1 (Atlas)

The atlas, the first cervical vertebra, has no vertebral body or spinous process and consists mainly of 2 lateral masses and 2 arches. The anterior arch is convex ventrally and has a tubercle at its midpoint and a smooth oval facet on its posterior surface for articulation with the odontoid process of the axis (C2). The posterior arch is concave ventrally and has a tubercle at the midpoint of its posterior surface. The 2 lateral masses of the atlas have superior and inferior facets. The superior articular facets are large, oval, and concave, articulating with the condyles of the occipital bone. Small grooves for the vertebral arteries and first cervical spinal nerves are located just posterior to these facets. The inferior articular facets are circular and convex and articulate with the adjacent lower axis. The oval transverse foramen in the transverse process transmits the vertebral artery, the accompanying vertebral veins, and a sympathetic nerve.

C2 (Axis)

The axis, the second cervical vertebra, has a large **dens,** or **odontoid process,** rising perpendicularly from the superior surface of its body. An oval facet for articulation with the atlas lies on the anterior surface of the odontoid process. The spinous process of the axis is large, strong, and bifid, while the 2 transverse processes are small, terminating in a tubercle on each side.

C3–6

The third to sixth cervical vertebrae have smooth bodies, wider transversely than anteroposteriorly. The anterior surface of each body slightly overlaps the superior portion of the adjacent inferior vertebra. The pedicles arise from the lateral posterior aspect of each body, midway between its upper and lower margins.

C7

The seventh cervical vertebra has a prominent nonbifid spinous process, almost horizontal, which is usually the first readily palpable vertebral spine below the occiput.

Laminae

The vertebral laminae are narrow and thin, meeting in the midline to form a short bifid spinous process. Articular facets project laterally from the junction of the pedicle and lamina and have superior and inferior surfaces.

⇒ **Fractures and fracture-dislocations of the cervical vertebrae.** *Fractures and fracture-dislocations of the vertebrae usually result from acute hyperextension or hyperflexion of the spine due to indirect trauma. Direct trauma usually causes fracture of the spinous process and, rarely, the vertebral lamina. Penetrating or open fractures may result from gunshot wounds, stab wounds, etc.*

In vertebral column injuries, the spinal cord and its nerves are seldom injured unless bone fragments or vertebrae are displaced. Neurologic damage may occur at the time of injury or because of subsequent manipulation. In some cases, severe neurologic deficits occur with relatively minor spinal fractures.

The neurologic deficit resulting from spinal cord injury depends on the nature and level of the injury. Fractures or fracture-dislocations of cervical vertebrae may result from a blow to the head with acute flexion of the neck (as in diving). The relatively horizontal facets of the cervical vertebrae sometimes allow dislocation to occur without the facets being fractured. In anterior dislocations of the thoracolumbar area, however, the intervertebral facets are almost always fractured.

⇒ **Osteoarthritis of the cervical spine.** *Osteoarthritis is a chronic progressive arthropathy characterized by degeneration of cartilage and hypertrophy of bone along the articular margins. The disease is most frequent in men over age 50. It commonly affects the cervical and lumbar spine and the joints of the fingers, toes, hips, and knees. Articular inflammation is minimal, and there may be no deformity. X-rays usually show narrowed joint spaces, foramens, osteophytes, increased density of subchondral bone, and bone cysts.*

In severe osteoarthritis of the cervical spine, cervical radicular symptoms and cervical myelopathy may occur. Symptoms may develop from direct spinal cord or spinal root compression, angulation by the ridges on the posterior margins of the vertebral bodies, or ischemia due to compression of the anterior spinal artery and veins. Radicular symptoms include upper limb paresthesias, paresis, and dysesthesia accompanied by muscle reflex changes (depression) and atrophy. Cord involvement leads to weakness and sensory disturbances of the lower limbs, with hyperreflexia and extensor plantar responses.

⇒ **Whiplash injuries of the cervical spine.** *So-called whiplash injury is one in which the cervical spine is suddenly and unexpectedly forced in one direction and then in the opposite direction. It is often associated with rear-end automobile collisions. Symptoms usually include rapid onset of neck pain, headache, stiff neck with increased pain on motion, and radiating pains and numbness in the upper extremities.*

In severe cases, headache and neck stiffness persist for months, and the loss of normal neck motion may be striking. Forward flexion of the neck is achieved slowly and cautiously, and spasm of paravertebral neck muscles may be evident on palpation.

X-rays of the cervical spine often show straightening or reversal of its normal curvature. Analgesics, sedatives, bed rest, heat, and massage are often beneficial. Cervical traction may be necessary, and cervical collars are commonly used for neck and head support.

Blood Vessels

The vertebral artery usually enters a canal formed by foramens in the transverse processes of the cervical vertebrae through the foramen in the transverse process of C6. The foramen of the transverse process of C7 transmits only the vertebral vein and is frequently small or absent.

2. THORACIC VERTEBRAE
(Fig 6–3)

The 12 thoracic vertebrae are intermediate in size between the cervical and lumbar vertebrae and are distinguished by facets for articulation with the ribs. The bodies of the first and second thoracic vertebrae are small, like those of the cervical vertebrae, and as one proceeds from superior to inferior the bodies become larger and support more weight. The bodies of T5–8 are slightly flattened on the left by the presence of the descending thoracic aorta. The thoracic vertebral spinous processes are long and directed downward, overlapping from T5 to T8. T8 has the longest vertical spinous process.

Facets for articulation with the heads of the ribs are located on the sides of the vertebral bodies, and facets for articulation with the tubercles of the ribs are located on the transverse processes (Fig 6–3). The facets on the vertebral bodies are near the roots of the pedicles. The bodies of T2–8 have 2 facets on each side, an upper and a lower, while T9–12 have one facet. T1 is unique in having a complete facet for articulation with the head of the first rib and a demifacet for the upper half of the head of the second rib.

The articular facets on the transverse processes of T1–6 are concave and face anteriorly and laterally. In T7–10, the articular facets are flat and face superiorly, laterally, and anteriorly. This suggests that the first 6 ribs rotate at the costotransverse joints, while

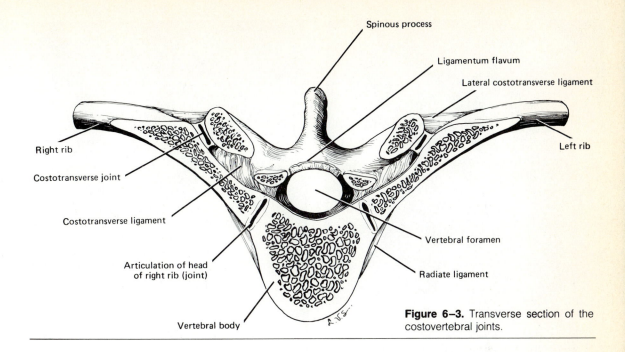

Figure 6–3. Transverse section of the costovertebral joints.

the lower 4 glide. The transverse processes of T11 and T12 have no articular facets.

The facets for articulation with the vertebrae are vertical. The superior articular facets lie at the junction of the laminae and pedicles and face dorsally and laterally, each articulating with the inferior facet of the next higher vertebra. The inferior articular facets of T12 are rotated outward, resembling those of the lumbar vertebrae.

➤ *Vertebral body osteoporosis. This very common metabolic bone disease is frequently noted on routine x-ray examinations of the vertebral column. It occurs in all of the vertebrae but more commonly in the thoracic vertebrae. It may cause backache, vertebral collapse, or spontaneous vertebral fracture, usually without spinal cord compression. Serum calcium, phosphorus, and alkaline phosphatase levels are usually normal. X-rays may show demineralization of the spine and pelvis and compression fractures of the spine. While the cause is not clear, vertebral body osteoporosis is often noted in sedentary people and in postmenopausal women. Other associated conditions include endocrine deficiencies, low calcium intake, developmental disturbances, and nutritional disorders.*

➤ *Tumors of the vertebral column. (Figs 6–4 and 6–5) Primary skeletal tumors include tumors of mesenchymal origin (bone, cartilage, connective tissue) and tumors of hematopoietic, nerve, vascular, fat cell, and notochordal origin. They are distinguished from a group of* secondary malignant tumors that extend to bone directly or by hematogenous spread.

Benign tumors of the vertebral column include osteochondromas and benign osteoblastomas. Malignant tumors include sarcomas, chordomas, and myelomas. Metastatic tumors to the spine are usually of epithelial origin.

Pain and local swelling usually occur early in the course of a vertebral tumor. Occasionally, spontaneous fracture of a vertebra occurs, accompanied by an increase in bone pain. Along with local tenderness and pain, deformity of the spine may become evident. Elevation of serum alkaline phosphatase is associated with widespread vertebral bone lesions, especially those that are osteoblastic in character. Special x-rays (laminography, angiography, CT scan, radio-isotope scan) or biopsy may be necessary for diagnosis.

Tumors of the vertebral column produce various abnormalities. Rapidly growing neoplasms may destroy bone completely, or osteoblastic changes with increased bone density may occur. Changes include erosion of the neural arches and scalloping of the posterior aspect of the vertebral bodies.

Treatment of a vertebral tumor depends on its nature and extent. Irradiation, operative resection, chemotherapy, and hormonal therapy may alleviate symptoms or help restore impaired function.

➤ *Tuberculosis of the thoracolumbar spine. About half of all cases of tuberculosis of the musculoskeletal system involve the vertebral*

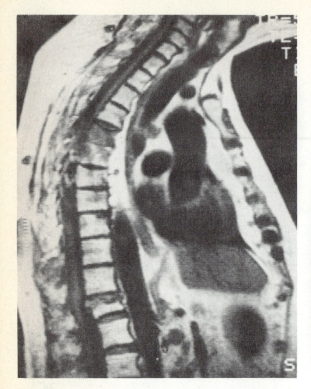

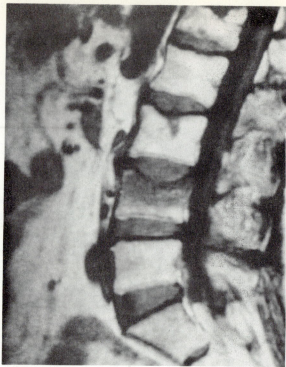

Figure 6–4. Mid-sagittal MR image through the thorax; multiple low-intensity masses in the vertebrae have led to kyphosis and compression of vertebrae (pathology: lymphoma). The patient was suffering from AIDS.

Figure 6–5. Mid-sagittal MR image through the lumbosacral spine; a low-intensity mass is present in L4 body (pathology: prostatic cancer metastases).

column, especially the thoracolumbar spine. Two or more vertebrae are usually involved, and the portion of the vertebral body adjacent to the epiphyseal plate or intervertebral disk is frequently affected early. Three-fourths of cases occur in children under 5 years of age. Paraplegia may result from epidural compression, particularly in the thoracic vertebrae. Spinal deformity and dwarfism may also occur.

➭ ***Compression fracture of the thoracolumbar spine.*** *(Fig 6–6.) Compression fractures of the vertebrae resulting from hyperflexion injury are most common in the thoracic and upper lumbar regions. If there is violent forward movement in addition to compression, a vertebra may be displaced anteriorly on the vertebra below it, with dislocation or fracture of the articular facets between the 2 vertebrae and rupture of the interspinous ligaments.*

''Seatbelt fractures''—if only a lap belt is worn—are often associated with paraparesis or worse.

3. LUMBAR VERTEBRAE
(Fig 6–7)

The 5 massive, weight-bearing lumbar vertebrae are distinguished by the absence of foramens in their transverse processes and the absence of costal articular facets on their vertebral bodies. The lumbar curve is convex anteriorly. Fibrocartilaginous disks between the vertebrae increase mobility.

The lumbar vertebrae have large, wide bodies whose superior and inferior surfaces are mildly concave and whose sides are constricted ventrally. The pedicles, which arise from the upper vertebral body, are short and strong and have superior and inferior grooves, the superior and inferior vertebral notches. The notches approximate to form foramens for egress of the spinal nerves.

➭ ***Lumbar pain.*** *Low back pain may have a variety of causes. To determine the site and cause, inspection and palpation of the painful area as well as complete pelvic and rectal examina-*

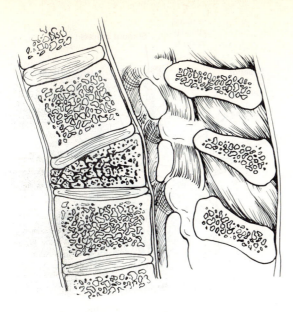

Figure 6–6. Anterior compression fracture. Note lack of neural canal involvement. (Reproduced, with permission, from Day LJ et al: Orthopedics. Chapter 44 in *Current Surgical Diagnosis & Treatment,* 7th ed. Way LW [editor]: Appleton & Lange, 1985.)

tion are necessary. *Plain x-ray films and CT scan with or without intrathecal contrast are usually very useful in determining the cause of the back pain when the lesion is in the spine.*

There may be muscle spasm and tenderness to percussion and deep pressure, particularly in association with local deformity or restriction of spinal motion. Paravertebral lumbar spasm accompanied by lumbar radiculopathy may result from several conditions, including herniated intervertebral disks, metastases to the lung (from carcinoma of the prostate or breast, lymphoma, etc), osteoarthritis, fracture of the spine, and local trauma. Lordosis, scoliosis, or list in the lumbar region may be noted when the patient stands. Psoas muscle spasm may indicate disease of the psoas muscle, the lumbar vertebrae, or soft tissues surrounding the psoas muscle, eg, epidural abscess.

Limitation of passive lumbar flexion with resulting pain often accompanies disease of the lumbar or lumbosacral articulations. Asymmetry of the articular facets is a cause of low back pain. **Spondylolysis** *— separation of the inferior articular process from the rest of the vertebrae—is an important cause of low back pain when it occurs bilaterally in L5. In such cases, the vertebra and spinal column above it may slide forward on the sacrum (***spondylolisthesis***), throwing the vertebral column out of line.*

Ankylosing spondylitis (Marie-Strümpell disease). This chronic inflammatory disease of the joints of the axial skeleton is manifested as painful and progressive stiffening of the spine. Males are most often affected, and the onset— usually in the late teens or early twenties—is gradual and marked by intermittent low back pain that may radiate into the thighs. As the disease progresses, the thoracic and cervical spine are affected and back motion becomes limited, with flattening of the normal lumbar curve and exaggeration of the thoracic curve. Atrophy of the trunk muscles and radicular symptoms may appear. In 50% of cases, transient acute arthritis of the peripheral joints occurs.

X-rays show early erosion and sclerosis of the sacroiliac joints and, late in the course of the disease, involvement of the apophyseal joints of the spine, calcification of the anterior and posterior longitudinal ligaments, and squaring and demineralization of the vertebral bodies. The late x-ray findings are sometimes called ''bamboo spine.''

The short, broad, strong laminae of the lumbar vertebrae end in a thick, broad spinous process that is almost horizontal. The articular facets lie in a sagittal plane at the base of the laminae. The superior articular facet is concave and faces medially and posteriorly, while the inferior facet faces anteriorly and laterally.

The lumbar transverse processes are comparatively slender and are anterior to the articular processes. L5 is characterized by massive transverse processes that connect with the entire lateral aspect of the pedicle and encroach on the body of the vertebra.

4. THE SACRUM
(Fig 6–8)

The large triangular wedge-shaped sacrum is formed by fusion of the 5 sacral vertebrae, which decrease in size from superior to inferior. The sacrum articulates with L5, the coccyx, and the 2 hip bones and forms the posterior wall of the bony pelvis.

The **sacral base** articulates with the inferior aspect of L5, forming the prominent **sacrovertebral angle.** Two large oval facets on either side, for articulation with L5, face dorsally and medially. Articulating with the ilium on either side of the sacrum are the lateral **auricular surfaces.** The lateral portions of the sacral base are the triangular **alae.** The **apex,** the lower extremity of the sacrum, articulates with the coccyx.

The **pelvic surface** of the sacrum is concave and grooved by 4 transverse ridges that correspond to the sites of fusion of the 5 fetal sacral bone segments. On either side of the ridges are the 4 **anterior sacral**

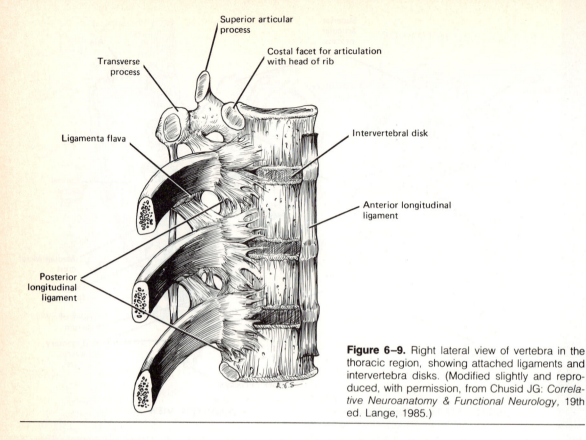

Figure 6–9. Right lateral view of vertebra in the thoracic region, showing attached ligaments and intervertebra disks. (Modified slightly and reproduced, with permission, from Chusid JG: *Correlative Neuroanatomy & Functional Neurology*, 19th ed. Lange, 1985.)

bodies to the sacrum. It is thickest in the thoracic region and intimately attached to the ventral margins of the vertebral bodies. The **posterior longitudinal ligament** runs within the vertebral canal along the middorsal surfaces of the vertebral bodies, down the entire length close to the vertebral margins. It extends from the posterior surface of the body of the axis to the sacrum. The ligament fans out at the intervertebral margins, reinforcing the intervertebral areas, and is thinnest in the cervical and lumbar regions.

Intervertebral disks are composed of fibrocartilage and lie between contiguous vertebral surfaces from the axis to the upper sacral border. In general, they conform to the vertebral surfaces where they lie and may vary considerably in size, shape, and thickness. The intervertebral disks make up about one-fourth of the length of the vertebral column. They are thicker in the cervical and lumbar areas than in the thoracic region, a characteristic permitting greater mobility in these areas. The disks help absorb stress and strain transmitted to the vertebral column. Each disk is enveloped by a thick capsule around the **annulus fibrosus** (which contains the **nucleus pulposus**). The intervertebral disks are thicker anteriorly and are intimately attached to the hyaline cartilage that covers the superior and inferior surfaces of the bodies of the vertebrae. They are reinforced laterally by the interarticular ligaments.

Herniation of an intervertebral disk. Rupture or herniation of an intervertebral disk may be caused by trauma or degeneration. The nucleus pulposus protrudes posteriorly into the vertebral canal through the defective annulus fibrosus and impinges on nerve roots. In over 90% of cases, rupture of the disk occurs at the L4–5 and L5–S1 interspaces. Usually only a single nerve root is compressed, but several may be involved (eg, cauda equina by the disk at the L5–S1 interspace). Large disk protrusions in the thoracic regions, though very rare, may even compress the spinal cord.

In lumbosacral disk herniations there may be back and radicular pain, straightening of the normal lumbar curve, scoliosis toward the contralateral side, impaired straight leg raising, tenderness to palpation along the sciatic nerve, depressed ankle or knee reflexes, and impaired perception of pain and touch in dermatomal distribution to the calf or ankle.

In about 5–10% of cases, herniation of the disk occurs in the cervical region, usually at C5–6 and C6–7 interspaces. Paresthesias, pain, and weakness occur in the upper extremities in the affected cervical root distribution (C6 or C7), with diminution of the appropriate tendon reflexes. Mobility of the neck is re-

stricted, with accentuation of radicular and neck pains by neck motion, coughing, sneezing, or straining. Long tract signs (extensor plantar response, sensory or motor impairment in lower limbs and trunk, etc) occasionally occur, indicating compression of the spinal cord by the disk.

Narrowing of the affected disk space is often seen in x-rays of the spinal column, and characteristic defects can usually be demonstrated by myelography, CT scan, or MRI.

Cervical disk disease may be helped by bed rest with a cervical collar, local heat, and analgesics. Lumbosacral disk disease is benefited by rest on a firm surface, heat, and analgesics. Traction may be helpful, and surgery may be necessary in some cases.

2. LIGAMENTS OF ARTICULATION BETWEEN VERTEBRAL ARCHES

The joints between the laminae and the spinous and transverse processes have several ligaments. The **ligamenta flava** join the laminae of adjacent vertebrae. They lie on either side of the spinous processes and extend laterally as far as the articular facets. Each ligament attaches to the dorsal margins of the lamina below and to the undersurface of the lamina above. The ligamenta flava are thinnest in the cervical region and grow thicker in extending inferiorly to the lumbar vertebrae.

The **supraspinous ligament** joins the tips of the spinous processes from C7 to the sacrum. It is dense and fibrous, fuses with the interspinal ligaments, and increases in width and thickness as it descends to the lumbar region. The ligament continues upward as the ligamentum nuchae of the cervical region.

The **interspinal ligaments** connect adjacent spinous processes, running from the tip to the root of each process. The ligaments fuse with the supraspinous ligaments dorsally and with the ligamenta flava ventrally. They are widest and densest in the lumbar region.

3. CRANIOCERVICAL LIGAMENTS

These ligaments connect the cervical vertebrae with the cranium and provide great mobility and protection for the head and neck. In side-to-side head movement, the joint between the atlas and axis is involved, since the atlas moves with the occipital bone. In nodding movements, the atlanto-occipital joints on each side are involved.

External Ligaments

The ligamentum nuchae is the superior extension of the supraspinous ligament. It is fan-shaped and strong and extends from the external occipital protuberance to the spine of C7. Its anterior border attaches to the cervical spinous processes, while its free posterior border blends with the investing layer of the deep cervical fascia. The ligament forms a septum in the midline by joining the spinous processes of the cervical vertebrae from roots to apexes. It gives origin to the splenius capitis, rhomboid, and trapezius muscles.

The anterior atlanto-occipital membrane is a broad ligament that extends from the anterior margin of the foramen magnum to the upper border of the anterior arch of the atlas (C1). It blends on each side with the atlanto-occipital capsule. The posterior atlanto-occipital membrane is a thin broad ligament that connects the margins of the foramen magnum with the superior margin of the posterior arch of the atlas. The vertebral artery and first cervical nerve pierce the inferior lateral portion of this membrane. The atlantoaxial ligament is a strong ligament that runs from the anterior arch of the atlas to the front of the body of the axis.

Internal Ligaments

The tectorial membrane is the superior extension of the posterior logitudinal ligament of the vertebral column. It extends downward from the occipital bone, covering the posterior surface of the body of the atlas and attaching to the odontoid process of the axis. Its superior vertical segment extends from the tip of the odontoid process to the midpoint of the anterior edge of the foramen magnum. The thick transverse portion forms a sling across the posterior surface of the odontoid process and is attached at both ends to the arch of the atlas. In fractures of the odontoid process, the cruciate ligament, by virtue of its position, helps prevent compression of the upper cervical spinal cord and the medulla.

The alar ligaments are 2 light, strong fibrous cords that reach from the medial sides of the occipital condyles to either side of the odontoid process. They limit rotation and flexion of the head.

BLOOD VESSELS

Arteries

A. Cervical Vertebrae: The cervical vertebrae are supplied by spinal branches that leave the cervical course of the vertebral artery. These cervical spinal arteries enter the vertebral column through the intervertebral foramens, and each divides into 2 vessels: The first supplies the spinal cord and its covering membranes; the second branches into ascending and descending divisions that join with the segmental spinal arteries above and below, on the dorsal surfaces of the vertebral bodies near the pedicle attachments. Small branches run to the vertebral bodies and their periosteum.

B. Thoracic Vertebrae: The thoracic vertebrae are supplied by the dorsal rami of the posterior intercostal arteries. The dorsal intercostal ramus gives off a spinal branch that reaches the vertebral canal

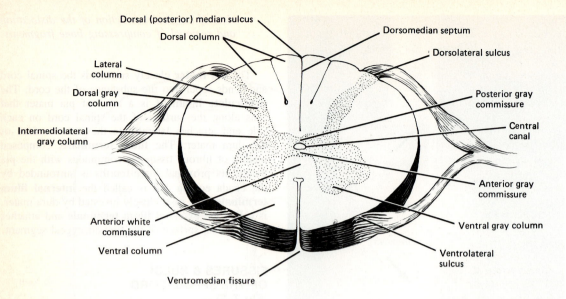

Figure 7–3. Anatomy of the spinal cord. (Reproduced, with permission, from Chusid JG: *Correlative Neuroanatomy & Functional Neurology,* 19th ed. Lange, 1985.)

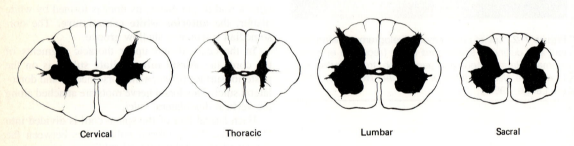

Cervical   Thoracic   Lumbar   Sacral

Figure 7–4. Transverse segments of the spinal cord at various levels. (Reproduced, with permission, from Chusid JG: *Correlative Neuroanatomy & Functional Neurology,* 19th ed. Lange, 1985.)

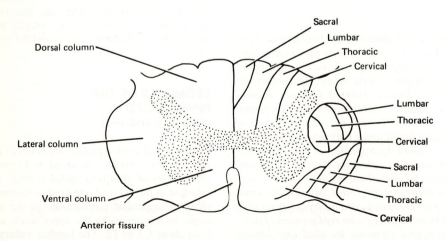

Figure 7–5. Segmental arrangement in the spinal cord. (Modified after Walker.) (Reproduced, with permission, from Chusid JG: *Correlative Neuroanatomy & Functional Neurology,* 19th ed. Lange, 1985.)

origin to the nerves of the brachial plexus; the lumbar enlargement, which is less extensive, corresponds to the area of origin of the nerves of the lumbosacral plexus. The thoracic and sacral cord segments are small, as no extremities are served.

Because of the different growth rates of the spinal cord and the vertebral column, the cord segments are higher than their corresponding vertebrae, the discrepancy becoming greater as one passes caudally along the cord. Thus, the lower the nerve root, the greater the distance between its origin in the cord and its point of exit from the spinal canal.

⟱ *Relationship between cord segments and vertebrae. (Table 7–1.) The relationship between the cord segments, vertebral bodies, and spinous processes is of clinical importance in locating the level of a cord lesion or the site for surgical approach.*

1. INTERNAL STRUCTURE OF THE SPINAL CORD (Fig 7–6)

Gray Matter of the Spinal Cord

In transverse section, the cord is seen to contain an H-shaped internal mass of gray substance surrounded by white matter. The gray matter is made up of 2 symmetric halves joined across the midline by a transverse connection (commissure) of gray substance through which runs the very small **central canal,** which extends the length of the spinal cord. The central canal is lined with ependymal cells and filled with cerebrospinal fluid and is continuous superiorly with the fourth ventricle in the medulla oblongata.

The **anterior ventral gray column** (anterior horn) is ventral to the central canal. It contains the cells of origin of the fibers of the ventral roots. The **lateral column** (lateral horn) is a triangular projection of gray matter that is prominent in the upper cervical, thoracic, and midsacral regions. It contains preganglionic cells for the autonomic nervous system. The **posterior dorsal gray column** (posterior horn) is a long, slender column that reaches almost to the dorsolateral sulcus. It is capped by a crescentic mass of translucent tissue containing nerve cells called the

substantia gelatinosa (of Rolando). The **reticular formation** is a network of processes extending into the lateral column between the anterior and posterior columns. The central canal divides the transverse commissure into anterior and posterior gray commissures.

The form, quantity, and appearance of the gray substance of the cord varies at different levels. The greatest proportion of gray to white matter is in the lumbar and sacral segments. In the cervical region, the posterior gray column is comparatively narrow and the anterior column is broad and expansive. In the thoracic region, the posterior and anterior columns are narrow and a lateral column is evident. In the lumbar region, both the posterior and anterior columns are broad and expanded.

⟱ *Syringomyelia. Syringomyelia, a disease of the spinal cord of unknown cause, is marked by cavitation and gliosis. It is characterized clinically by muscular wasting and weakness, sensory defects, long tract signs, and trophic disturbances. The cervical cord segments are usually affected, but the disease is sometimes seen in the lumbar cord and the brain stem (syringobulbia). Developmental defects are frequently associated with it, such as "pigeon breast," scoliosis, hydrocephalus, and Arnold-Chiari malformation.*

The symptoms of syringomyelia usually commence in the second or third decade of life and are characterized by early loss of pain and temperature sense in the lower cervical and thoracic dermatomes with preservation of touch and deep pressure sense. The loss of pain and temperature sensation is often in a shawllike distribution (Fig 7–7). Presenting symptoms include wasting of small muscles of the hand and painless burns of the fingers or forearm. Weakness and atrophy of the shoulder girdle muscles are associated with the disease, as are Horner's syndrome, Charcot joints, nystagmus, and vasomotor and trophic disturbances of the upper extremities. Tendon reflexes of the upper extremities may be absent. Long tract spinal cord damage may result in pyramidal deficits and ataxia of the lower extremities and impaired bladder function.

⟱ *Posterolateral sclerosis. Posterolateral sclerosis (subacute combined degeneration) is characterized by progressive degeneration of the posterior and lateral columns of the spinal cord, sometimes with mental changes and peripheral neuropathy. It is often a complication of pernicious anemia but also occurs with nutritional deficiency states. Degeneration of the spinal cord may develop before other clinical manifestations of pernicious anemia.*

Table 7–1. Anatomic relationships of spinal cord and bony spine in adults

Cord Segments	Vertebral Bodies	Spinous Processes
C8	Lower C6, upper C7	C6
T6	Lower T3, upper T4	T3
T12	T9	T8
L5	T11	T10
S	T12, L1	T12, L1

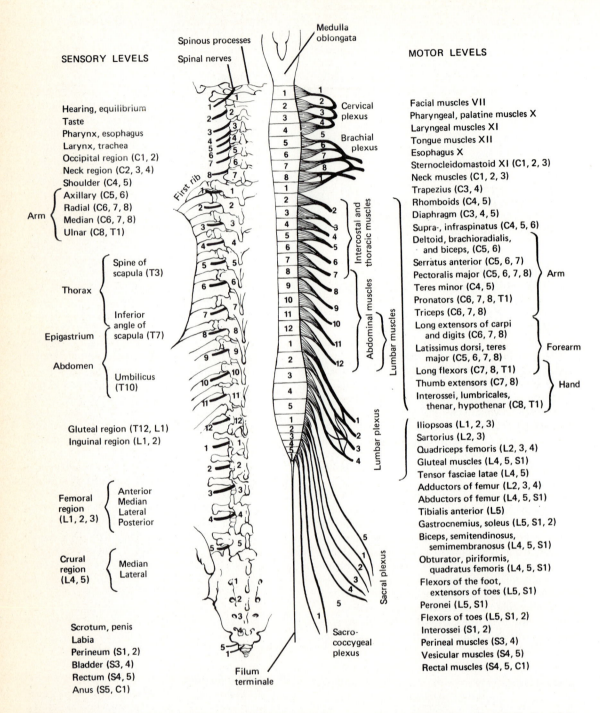

SENSORY LEVELS

Spinous processes
Spinal nerves
Medulla oblongata

MOTOR LEVELS

Hearing, equilibrium
Taste
Pharynx, esophagus
Larynx, trachea
Occipital region (C1, 2)
Neck region (C2, 3, 4)
Shoulder (C4, 5)
Arm {
Axillary (C5, 6)
Radial (C6, 7, 8)
Median (C6, 7, 8)
Ulnar (C8, T1)

Thorax {
Spine of scapula (T3)
Inferior angle of scapula (T7)
Epigastrium
Abdomen {
Umbilicus (T10)

Gluteal region (T12, L1)
Inguinal region (L1, 2)

Femoral region (L1, 2, 3) {
Anterior
Median
Lateral
Posterior

Crural region (L4, 5) {
Median
Lateral

Scrotum, penis
Labia
Perineum (S1, 2)
Bladder (S3, 4)
Rectum (S4, 5)
Anus (S5, C1)

First rib
Filum terminale

Cervical plexus
Brachial plexus
Intercostal and thoracic muscles
Abdominal muscles
Lumbar muscles
Lumbar plexus
Sacral plexus
Sacro-coccygeal plexus

Facial muscles VII
Pharyngeal, palatine muscles X
Laryngeal muscles XI
Tongue muscles XII
Esophagus X
Sternocleidomastoid XI (C1, 2, 3)
Neck muscles (C1, 2, 3)
Trapezius (C3, 4)
Rhomboids (C4, 5)
Diaphragm (C3, 4, 5)
Supra-, infraspinatus (C4, 5, 6)
Deltoid, brachioradialis, and biceps, (C5, 6)
Serratus anterior (C5, 6, 7)
Pectoralis major (C5, 6, 7, 8) } Arm
Teres minor (C4, 5)
Pronators (C6, 7, 8, T1)
Triceps (C6, 7, 8)
Long extensors of carpi and digits (C6, 7, 8)
Latissimus dorsi, teres major (C5, 6, 7, 8) } Forearm
Long flexors (C7, 8, T1)
Thumb extensors (C7, 8) } Hand
Interossei, lumbricales, thenar, hypothenar (C8, T1)

Iliopsoas (L1, 2, 3)
Sartorius (L2, 3)
Quadriceps femoris (L2, 3, 4)
Gluteal muscles (L4, 5, S1)
Tensor fasciae latae (L4, 5)
Adductors of femur (L2, 3, 4)
Abductors of femur (L4, 5, S1)
Tibialis anterior (L5)
Gastrocnemius, soleus (L5, S1, 2)
Biceps, semitendinosus, semimembranosus (L4, 5, S1)
Obturator, piriformis, quadratus femoris (L4, 5, S1)
Flexors of the foot, extensors of toes (L5, S1)
Peronei (L5, S1)
Flexors of toes (L5, S1, 2)
Interossei (S1, 2)
Perineal muscles (S3, 4)
Vesicular muscles (S4, 5)
Rectal muscles (S4, 5, C1)

Figure 7–6. Relation of spinal cord to vertebral column. (Reproduced, with permission, from Chusid JG: *Correlative Neuroanatomy & Functional Neurology*, 19th ed. Lange, 1985.)

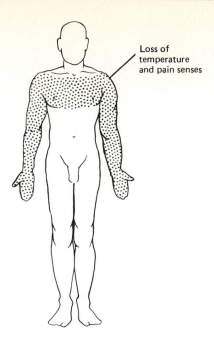

Figure 7–7. Syringomyelia. (Reproduced, with permission, from Chusid JG: *Correlative Neuroanatomy & Functional Neurology*, 19th ed. Lange, 1985.)

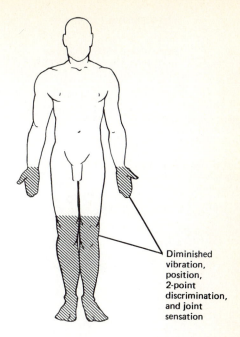

Figure 7–8. Posterolateral sclerosis. (Reproduced, with permission, from Chusid JG: *Correlative Neuroanatomy & Functional Neurology*, 19th ed. Lange, 1985.)

The onset is characterized by tingling, numbness, and "pins-and-needles" sensations, first in the toes and feet and later in the fingers. Mental symptoms may occur, including hallucinations, disorientation, memory defects, and personality changes. With pronounced peripheral nerve involvement, there may also be tenderness of the calf and sole muscles, stocking distribution of impaired touch sensibility up to the level of the knees (Fig 7–8), distal weakness of the lower extremities, and depressed or absent knee and ankle jerks.

Posterior column disease may be evidenced by loss of position sense in the extremities, a positive Romberg test, an ataxic, broad-based gait, impaired 2-point discrimination, and loss of vibratory sensation. Lateral column disease leads to pyramidal weakness, spasticity, and hyperreflexia, with extensor plantar responses.

Vitamin B_{12} therapy is specific, and neurologic symptoms are reversible if of relatively short duration.

2. WHITE MATTER OF THE SPINAL CORD

The white matter of the spinal cord consists of myelinated and unmyelinated nerve fibers (Fig 7–9) in a network of neuroglia. These nerve fibers link the various segments of the spinal cord and connect the spinal cord with the brain. The white matter of

the spinal cord is divided into 3 columns: ventral, lateral, and dorsal.

Anterior White Column

The anterior white column lies between the ventrolateral sulcus and the ventromedian fissure.

A. Descending Tracts: The **ventral corticospinal tract** (direct pyramidal tract, anterior cerebrospinal tract) lies close to the anteromedian fissure and ends in the midthoracic region. Its cells of origin are in the large pyramidal cells of the ipsilateral pre-Rolandic motor cortex. The **vestibulospinal tract** is located in the marginal portion and extends from the vestibular nerve nuclei to the sacral segments. The **tectospinal tract** lies immediately posterior to the vestibulospinal tract and takes its origin from the contralateral superior colliculus of the midbrain, crossing in the fountain decussation of Meynert in the midbrain. The **reticulospinal tract** in the sulcomarginal zone comes from the reticular substance of the medulla and midbrain.

B. Ascending Tracts: The **ventral spinothalamic tract** is located in the marginal portion of the anterior column and is derived from cells of the opposite posterior gray column. The **spino-olivary tract** is located in the anterior marginal zone and contains fibers going to the inferior olivary nucleus of the medulla oblongata.

Lateral White Column

The lateral white column extends between the ven-

DESCENDING PATHWAYS

ASCENDING PATHWAYS

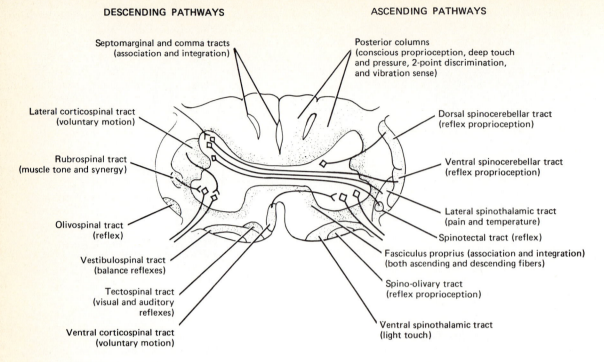

Figure 7–9. Pathways in spinal cord (lower cervical region). (Reproduced, with permission, from Chusid JG: *Correlative Neuroanatomy & Functional Neurology*, 19th ed. Lange, 1985.)

trolateral and dorsolateral sulci, the line of origin of the anterior nerve roots.

A. Descending Tracts: The **lateral corticospinal tract** (crossed pyramidal tract, lateral cerebrospinal tract) extends the entire length of the spinal cord between the dorsal spinocerebellar tract and the fasciculus proprius. Its fibers arise from pyramidal cells of the contralateral precentral motor cortex and are so arranged that the fibers of the upper extremity are situated medially and those of the lower extremity peripherally. The **rubrospinal tract** is situated just anterior to the lateral corticospinal tract. Its fibers originate in the red nucleus of the midbrain, cross the median plane, and then descend in the spinal cord. The **olivospinal tract** lies close to the most lateral of the anterior nerve roots in the cervical cord region and originates in the medulla oblongata in the vicinity of the inferior olivary nucleus.

B. Ascending Tracts: The **dorsal spinocerebellar tract** lies at the periphery of the posterior part of the lateral column just ventral to the posterior lateral sulcus. Its fibers arise from cells of the ipsilateral dorsal nucleus and proceed to the cerebellum via the inferior cerebellar peduncle. The **ventral spinocerebellar tract** is located at the periphery of the lateral column anterior to the dorsal spinocerebellar tract. Its fibers arise from cells of the posterior gray column and intermediate gray substance of both sides and enter the cerebellum via the superior cerebellar

peduncle. The **lateral spinothalamic tract** lies on the medial and anterior side of the ventral spinocerebellar tract. Its fibers arise from cells of the opposite posterior gray column and cross via the anterior white commissure shortly after their origin to end in the thalamus. The **spinotectal tract** passes ventrally to the lateral spinothalamic tract; its fibers arise from the opposite posterior gray column to end in the tectum of the midbrain.

Posterior White Column

The posterior white column lies between the dorsolateral and dorsomedian sulci.

A. Descending Tracts: The **fasciculus interfascicularis** is situated between the fasciculus gracilis and the fasciculus cuneatus. Its fibers are of intraspinal and dorsal root origin. The septomarginal fasciculus is located near the dorsomedian sulcus.

B. Ascending Tracts: The **fasciculus gracilis** is located next to the dorsomedian sulcus, beginning in the lowest portion of the spinal cord and increasing in size as one proceeds anteriorly. It receives fibers from the medial group of nerve fibers of the posterior roots and terminates in the nucleus of the funiculus gracilis in the medulla. The **fasciculus cuneatus** lies between the fasciculus gracilis and the posterior gray column and is similarly derived from the posterior nerve roots of the thoracocervical region. It terminates in the nucleus of the funiculus cuneatus in the medulla.

3. FASCICULUS PROPRIUS

The dorsal fasciculus proprius, located immediately adjacent to the gray matter, is composed of a mixture of fiber pathways: (1) short fibers running in both directions and serving to integrate the functions of the cord through intersegmental and intrasegmental association connections; (2) fibers of the **medial longitudinal fasciculus,** descending from the medulla in the anterior portion of the dorsal fasciculus proprius and conveying impulses from the vestibular, oculomotor, trochlear, and abducens nuclei concerned with equilibratory reflexes; and (3) fibers of the reticulospinal tract, conveying part of the extrapyramidal flow for the regulation of muscle tone.

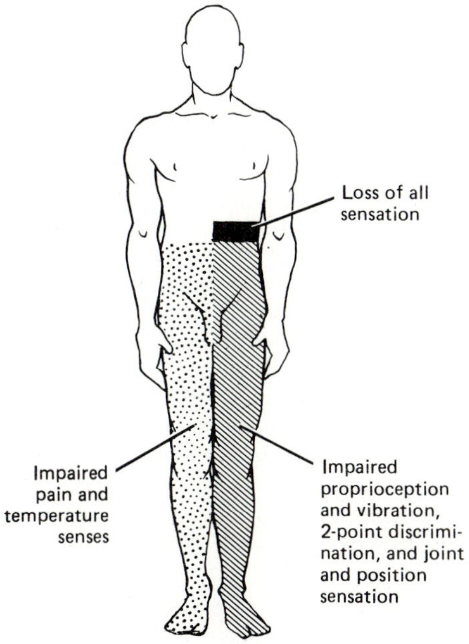

➡ ***Brown-Séquard syndrome.*** *This condition is caused by hemisection of the spinal cord, regardless of cause. It usually consists of (1) ipsilateral lower motor neuron paralysis at the level of the lesion; (2) ipsilateral upper motor neuron paralysis below the level of the lesion; (3) ipsilateral loss of proprioceptive, vibratory, and 2-point discrimination sense below the level of the lesion; (4) contralateral loss of pain and temperature sense below the lesion; and (5) loss of all sensation at the level of the lesion (Fig 7–10).*

Loss of all sensation

Impaired pain and temperature senses

Impaired proprioception and vibration, 2-point discrimination, and joint and position sensation

Figure 7–10. Brown-Séquard syndrome, with lesion at left tenth thoracic level. (Reproduced, with permission, from Chusid JG: *Correlative Neuroanatomy & Functional Neurology,* 19th ed. Lange, 1985.)

4. SPINAL ROOTS & NERVES (Fig 7–11)

Thirty-one pairs of spinal nerves arise from the spinal cord. Each nerve has an anterior, or ventral, root and a posterior, or dorsal, root. The **spinal ganglion,** or **dorsal root ganglion,** is a swelling containing cells in the dorsal root of each nerve. Each root contains bundles of nerve fibers. The groups of spinal nerves are divided into 8 cervical, 12 thoracic, 5 lumbar, 5 sacral, and one coccygeal nerve. The nerve roots become increasingly oblique as one proceeds down the spinal cord. In the lumbosacral region, the

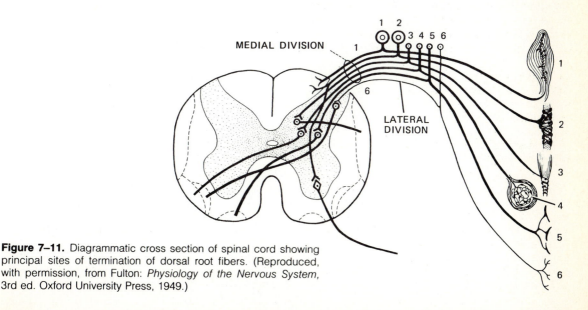

Figure 7–11. Diagrammatic cross section of spinal cord showing principal sites of termination of dorsal root fibers. (Reproduced, with permission, from Fulton: *Physiology of the Nervous System,* 3rd ed. Oxford University Press, 1949.)

roots descend almost vertically to exit from the bony vertebral canal. Because of their length and appearance, the collection of lumbosacral nerve roots is referred to as the **cauda equina** (''horse's tail'').

The **anterior nerve root** consists of efferent fibers originating in the ventral and lateral gray columns. These become medullated shortly after their origin and emerge from the spinal cord in 2 or 3 irregular rows over an area about 3 mm wide. The **posterior nerve root,** made up of 6–8 rootlets attached in the dorsolateral sulcus in a linear series, contains afferent fibers from the nerve cells in the spinal ganglion. In general, the most medial fibers pass to the fasciculus cuneatus; most of the remaining fibers terminate in the substantia gelatinosa and the dorsal gray column.

SPINAL CORD CIRCULATION

Arteries

The **anterior spinal artery,** formed by the midline union of paired branches of the vertebral arteries, descends along the ventral surface of the cervical spinal cord, narrowing somewhat near the fourth thoracic segment.

The **posterolateral spinal arteries** arise from the vertebral arteries and course downward to the lower cervical and upper thoracic segments.

The **anterior medial spinal artery** is the prolongation of the anterior spinal artery below the fourth thoracic cord segment.

Some but not all intercostal arteries from the aorta supply **segmental or radicular branches** to the spinal cord to the level of the first lumbar cord segment; the largest of these branches, the great ventral radicular artery, enters the spinal cord between the eighth thoracic and fourth lumbar cord segments. This artery, also known as the **arteria radicularis magna** (artery of Adamkiewicz), usually arises on the left and is responsible for most of the arterial blood supply of the lower half of the spinal cord in most people.

Occlusion of this artery is rare; when it does occur, occlusion results in major neurologic deficits (paraplegia, loss of sensation in the legs, urinary incontinence, and more).

In the lumbosacral area, some **radicular arteries** are present, derived from the lumbar, iliolumbar, and lateral sacral arteries. The largest such vessel appears to enter the intervertebral foramen at the second lumbar vertebra to form the lowermost portion of the anterior spinal artery—called the **terminal artery**—which runs along the filum terminale.

The paired **posterior spinal arteries** are much smaller than the single large anterior spinal artery; they branch to form the posterolateral arterial plexus at various levels. The posterior spinal arteries supply the dorsal white columns and the more posterior part of the dorsal gray columns.

Segmentally, the branches of radicular arteries that enter the intervertebral foramens accompany the dorsal and ventral nerve roots, respectively. These branches unite directly with the posterior and anterior spinal arteries to form an irregular ring of arteries, an arterial corona, with vertical connections. One branch of these coronal arteries, occurring at most levels, is a sulcal artery. **Anterior sulcal arteries** arise at various levels along the cervical and thoracic cord within the ventral sulcus and supply the ventral and lateral columns on either side of the spinal cord. At any given cord segment, only one side of the cord is supplied by this vessel; the other side receives blood from the coronal arteries.

Veins

An irregular **external venous plexus** lies in the epidural space; it communicates with segmental veins, basivertebral veins from the vertebral column, the basilar plexus in the head, and—by way of the pedicular veins—with a smaller **internal venous plexus** that lies in the subarachnoid space. All venous drainage is ultimately into the venae cavae. Both plexuses extend the length of the cord.

Neck Region 8

EMBRYOLOGY
(Figs 8–1, 8–2, and 8–3)

The outline of embryology presented here applies also to structures discussed in the following 4 chapters.

Many of the structures of the neck originate from the branchial arches or the pouches or clefts between them. Initially there are 6 pairs of arches, but the fifth is transient and soon becomes unrecognizable. The clefts are external structures, and the pouches are internal structures.

Arches

The first branchial arch (responsible for much of the development of the face) is called the **mandibular arch** and is supplied by the mandibular branch of cranial nerve V. From it evolve the maxillary process dorsally and the mandibular process ventrally. Within the latter lies Meckel's cartilage, whose membrane will eventually ossify and form the body of the mandible. Within the maxillary and mandibular processes evolve a number of structures: the incus, the malleus, the maxilla, the zygoma, the mandible, the spheno-mandibular ligament, the anterior ligament of the malleus, the muscles of mastication, the anterior belly of the digastric muscle, and the mylohyoid, tensor tympani, and tensor palatini muscles. Anomalies include those of the eyelids, the ears, the mandible, the palate, and certain features of syndromes such as Treacher Collins (mandibular facial dysostosis) and Pierre Robin (cleft palate and hypoplasia of the mandible).

The second branchial arch is called the **hyoid arch** and is supplied by cranial nerve VII. It grows laterally and inferiorly to partly cover the third and fourth arches, forming a transient cervical sinus in the process. From the hyoid arch are derived the stapes, the styloid process of the temporal bone, the stylohyoid ligament, the lesser horn and superior part of the body of the hyoid bone, the muscles of facial expression, the stapedius and stylohyoid muscles, and the posterior bellies of the digastric muscles. Anomalies include remnants of the cervical sinus, such as branchial fistulas, and cervical or branchial cysts.

The third branchial arch (**glossopharyngeal arch**) is supplied by cranial nerve IX. It is covered in part by the second branchial arch (see above) as it grows inferiorly. From the glossopharyngeal arch are derived the lower part of the body and the greater horn of the hyoid bone and the stylopharyngeus muscle.

The fourth and sixth branchial arches form the thyroid, cricoid, and small laryngeal cartilages. The fourth arch is supplied by the superior laryngeal branch of the vagus, which innervates the cricothyroid muscle. The intrinsic muscles of the larynx are supplied by the nerve of the sixth arch, the recurrent laryngeal branch of the vagus. The levator veli palatini and the 3 pharyngeal constrictors, supplied by the pharyngeal plexuses, probably arise from fourth and sixth arch elements.

The fifth branchial arch is rudimentary and either disappears or merges with the fourth and sixth arches.

Pouches

The first pharyngeal pouch develops into the tubotympanic recess, which surrounds the developing ossicles of the middle ear. Its distal portion forms the mastoid antrum, while its central part becomes the primitive middle ear cavity and contributes to the tympanic membrane. The junction of the proximal part of the recess with the pharynx forms the auditory tube.

The second pharyngeal pouch is largely obliterated as the palatine tonsil develops. A portion of it, however, remains as the intratonsillar cleft. The endoderm of the pouch forms the surface epithelium of the tonsil and lines the tonsillar crypts.

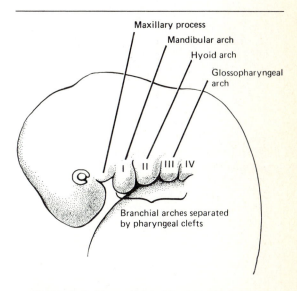

Figure 8–1. Topography of the branchial region.

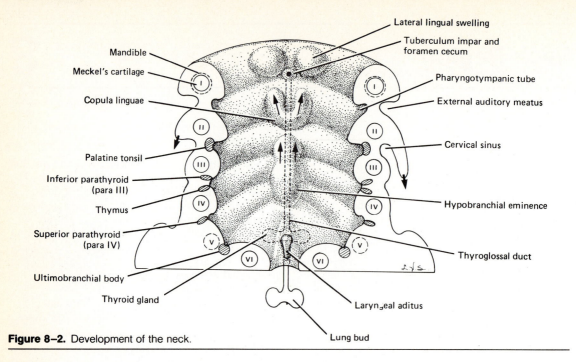

Figure 8–2. Development of the neck.

Each third pharyngeal pouch develops dorsal and ventral wings of epithelial cells, and its pharyngeal connection is obliterated. The cells of the dorsal wings form the inferior parathyroid glands, while those of the ventral wings migrate medially and inferiorly and fuse to form the thymus. The inferior parathyroid glands may vary in position (at the lower pole of the thyroid, or within the thymus). Thymic fragments also may be found high in the lateral neck or within the thyroid gland. Anomalies include congenital thymic aplasia and absence of the parathyroid glands (DiGeorge's syndrome).

Each fourth pharyngeal pouch also develops ventral and dorsal wings. The epithelium of the dorsal wing develops into the superior parathyroid gland, which also may be anomalously found in the lateral

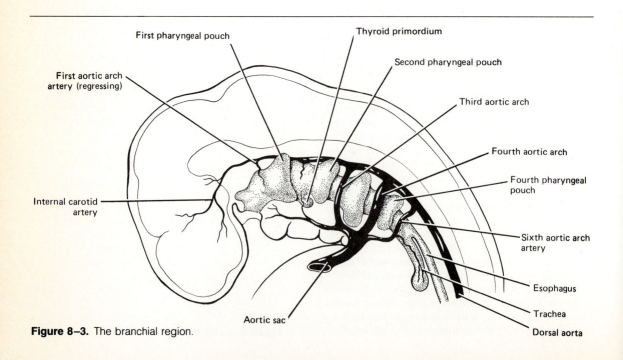

Figure 8–3. The branchial region.

neck somewhere along its path of descent. The fate of the ventral pouch is uncertain, but it may contribute to the thymus.

The fifth pharyngeal pouch usually becomes part of the fourth pouch, and the epithelium associated with it gives rise to the ultimobranchial body, whose cells become the C-cells (calcitonin-producing) of the thyroid gland.

Clefts

The first pharyngeal cleft is present during the fourth and fifth fetal weeks and separates the first and second branchial arches externally. Its dorsal extremity persists as the external acoustic (auditory) meatus.

The third and fourth pharyngeal clefts disappear. The lateral and inferior growth of the second branchial arch creates the cervical sinus, which normally disappears completely.

Branchial Anomalies (Figs 8–4 and 8–5)

Anomalies of the branchial system are relatively uncommon. When present, they are mostly due to the persistence of structures that normally disappear during fetal development. They include the following: congenital auricular cysts and sinuses; branchial or

lateral cervical sinuses; branchial fistulas; branchial or lateral cysts; branchial vestiges (cartilaginous or bony); and ectopic, absent, or supernumerary parathyroids.

GROSS ANATOMY

The neck is bounded superiorly by the mandibular symphysis and by the body of the mandible. A line drawn from the angle of the mandible to the styloid process of the temporal bone marks the course of the stylomandibular ligament and the inferior border of the retromandibular fossa. The posterosuperior border runs from the styloid process around the external auditory meatus on to the mastoid process of the temporal bone. It then continues along the superior nuchal line of the occipital bone to the external occipital protuberance in the midline.

Inferiorly and anteriorly, the neck is bounded by the notch and the superior border of the manubrium and by the sternoclavicular joint. The clavicle, the acromioclavicular joint, and a line drawn from the

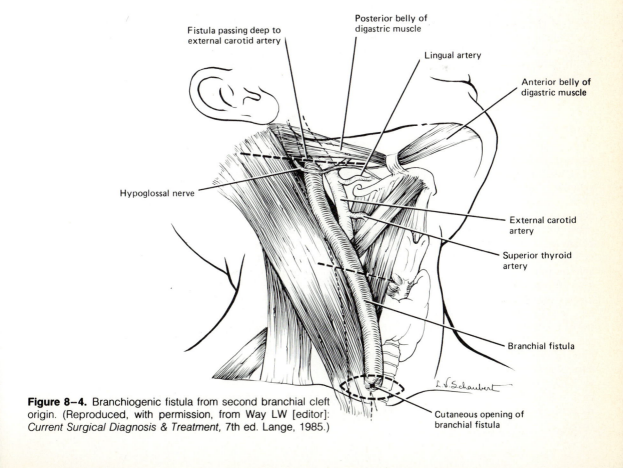

Figure 8–4. Branchiogenic fistula from second branchial cleft origin. (Reproduced, with permission, from Way LW [editor]: *Current Surgical Diagnosis & Treatment,* 7th ed. Lange, 1985.)

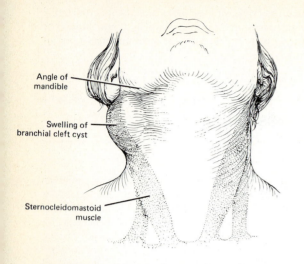

Angle of mandible

Swelling of branchial cleft cyst

Sternocleidomastoid muscle

Figure 8–5. Branchial cleft cyst. Cyst lies posterior to the angle of the mandible, partially hidden by the sternocleidomastoid muscle.

acromioclavicular joint to the spinous process of C7 complete the lateral and posteroinferior borders of the neck.

The external appearance of the neck differs with age, sex, and habitus. Women and children usually have smoother, more rounded necks than men, because of the greater amount of adipose tissue and the smaller size of the visible bones, muscles, and cartilages. Surface landmarks of the cervical region are therefore harder to distinguish in women and children than in men. As people age, much of the cervical subcutaneous adipose tissue is lost.

SURFACE LANDMARKS

Bony Landmarks

Bony landmarks of the neck include mandibular symphysis (symphysis menti); the transverse ramus of the mandible to its termination at the mandibular angle; the mastoid process of the temporal bone; the manubrium (manubrium sterni), with its midline notch; the 2 clavicles; the elongated spinous process of C7; the hyoid bone at the level of C3; and the anterior tubercle of the transverse process of the C6. The C6 transverse process anterior tubercle is at the level of the cricoid cartilage and thus marks the lower border of the larynx and the beginning of the cervical trachea. C6 is at the level of the downward bend of the inferior thyroid artery. The middle cervical ganglion lies just ventral to the latter. The vertebral artery enters the foramen in the vertebral transverse process at C6. The common carotid artery may be compressed against the transverse process of C6 as an emergency measure to control severe upper neck or facial hemorrhage.

Cartilaginous Landmarks

The cartilaginous landmarks of the neck are the thyroid cartilage, with the notch on its mid upper border at the level of C4, which helps to mark the anterior midline of the neck; the cricoid cartilage at the level of C6; and the cartilaginous tracheal rings, which normally are midline neck structures.

⏩ *Clinical importance of midline surface anatomy. Deviation of the larynx or tracheal rings from the midline of the neck suggests pressure or traction upon these structures. A mass (tumor, collection of fluid or air) can push the air passage to the contralateral side. The passage may be pulled to the ipsilateral side by the presence of a sclerosing cancer or by fibrosis in malignant or infected lymph nodes. Deviations from the midline may also be due to changes in pressure within the pleural cavities. Diminished pressure, as in atelectasis, can draw the trachea toward the affected side, whereas increased pressure from pneumothorax, hemothorax, pneumohemothorax, or pyothorax can push the trachea to the opposite side of both the mediastinum and the neck.*

Cervical Muscular Landmarks (Fig 8–6)

The cervical muscular landmarks are the massive **sternocleidomastoid** muscle, the **omohyoid** muscle as it obliquely crosses the neck, the **trapezius** muscle, the **sternohyoid** muscles (visible), and the **digastric** muscles (visible and palpable).

FASCIAE & SPACES OF THE NECK (Fig 8–7)

Superficial Cervical Fascia & Platysma Muscle

The superficial fascia of the neck lies between the skin and subcutaneous tissue and the deep cervical fascia. It is usually quite thin. Over the ventrolateral area, it encloses the platysma muscle. This muscle arises from the fascia covering the pectoralis major and from the fascia covering the deltoid muscle. The platysma crosses the clavicles and the upper sternum and inserts into the mandible and subcutaneous tissues of the lower face, where it interlocks with the inferior facial muscles. The platysma may reach up to the lower border of the orbit. The platysma is the muscle of expression in the neck. It is innervated by the descending cervical branch of the facial nerve.

⏩ *Platysma muscle in neck surgery. Meticulous closure of the platysma during the final stages of neck surgery will prevent adhesion of cervical*

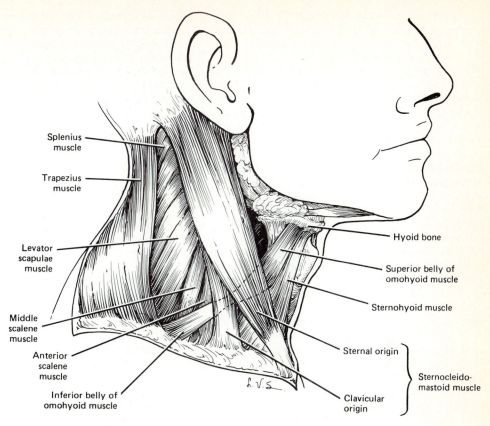

Splenius muscle

Trapezius muscle

Levator scapulae muscle

Middle scalene muscle

Anterior scalene muscle

Inferior belly of omohyoid muscle

Hyoid bone

Superior belly of omohyoid muscle

Sternohyoid muscle

Sternal origin

Clavicular origin

Sternocleido-mastoid muscle

Figure 8–6. Lateral view of the neck muscles.

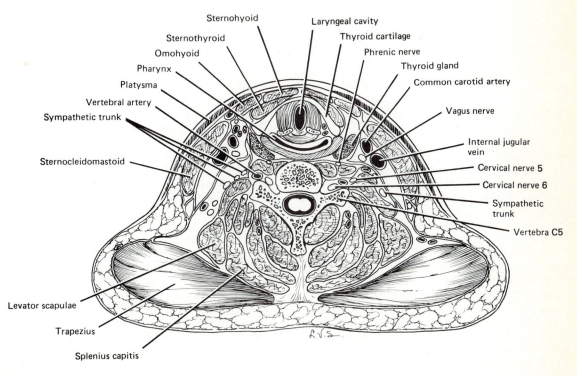

Sternohyoid

Sternothyroid

Omohyoid

Pharynx

Platysma

Vertebral artery

Sympathetic trunk

Sternocleidomastoid

Levator scapulae

Trapezius

Splenius capitis

Laryngeal cavity

Thyroid cartilage

Phrenic nerve

Thyroid gland

Common carotid artery

Vagus nerve

Internal jugular vein

Cervical nerve 5

Cervical nerve 6

Sympathetic trunk

Vertebra C5

Figure 8–7. Cross section of the neck at C5, showing arteries, veins, nerves, muscles, adipose tissue, and investing fascia.

skin and subcutaneous tissues to the deeper neck muscles, which move as they contract and relax. Such adhesions lead to cosmetically unacceptable movable scars.

Subplatysmal Space

Deep to the superficial fascia and the platysma muscle but superficial to the deep cervical fascia are a group of structures of great clinical interest.

A. Branches of the Facial Nerve: The **mandibular branch** descends into the neck from the level of the stylomandibular ligament, at first lying posterior to the angle of the jaw and then about 0.75 cm below the lower border of the transverse ramus of the mandible. It then runs forward, paralleling the lateral third of the mandible, before turning superiorly to cross the mandible (just medial to the masseter) and run to the angle of the mouth, where it supplies the muscles of the lower lip and chin.

➠ *Injury to the mandibular branch of the facial nerve. A transverse incision just below the mandible must be made with care so that the physician may locate and retract the mandibular branch of the facial nerve. Injury to the nerve results in a disfiguring ipsilateral mouth droop. Excessive pressure on the middle section of the transverse ramus of the mandible may result in temporary palsy of this nerve.*

The **descending cervical branch** is the nerve to the platysma. It lies between the superficial and deep neck fasciae as it runs inferiorly, posterior to the mandibular branch of the facial nerve. As it descends to the mid neck, it arches medially to supply the platysma muscle. It is seldom exposed in routine neck incisions. It is usually transected in radical neck dissections in which the platysma muscle is removed.

➠ *Sparing of the descending cervical branch. The cervical branch of the facial nerve is usually the last branch of the nerve to be involved in facial palsy, and it is usually the first branch to recover. When it is cut, the neck on the affected side becomes flat, flaccid, and expressionless.*

B. Branches of the Cervical Plexus: The terminal segments of 3 superficial branches of the cervical plexus, which arise from the anterior primary divisions of C2, C3, and C4, lie within the subplatysmal space. The nerves are the smaller occipital, the great auricular, and the cutaneous nerve of the neck. The 3 supraclavicular nerves—anterior, middle, and posterior—are derived from the cervical plexus. They lie in the subplatysmal space and eventually supply

cutaneous sensation to the shawl area of the shoulder. These nerves have an important junctional relay with the phrenic nerve, which arises from C3, C4, and C5 within the cervical plexus. The cervical plexus relay produces anterolateral shoulder area pain secondary to phrenic nerve irritation as a result of sub- or supradiaphragmatic irritative pathologic processes.

➠ *Shoulder pain secondary to diaphragmatic irritation. Pain in the shawl area of the shoulder may be due to basilar pulmonary pneumonia with a pleuritic component, cancer of the lower lobe of the lung with pleuritic spread, and pericarditis. It may also result from irritation of the inferior surface of the diaphragm by air, blood, serum, or pus.*

C. Arteries: The submental artery, a branch of the facial artery, runs medially and dips beneath the arterial belly of the digastric muscle to supply the submental area.

D. Venous Drainage: A plexus of veins occupies the space between the superficial and deep fasciae in the submental area. From this plexus, at the level of the hyoid bone, arise the 2 anterior jugular veins that run inferiorly in the subplatysmal space to the level of the thyroid cartilage, where they pierce the deep cervical fascia.

➠ *Submental hematoma. Trauma to the submental area may result in swelling in the suprahyoid area. The cause is rupture of the superficial submental veins, and trapping of blood between the platysma and the deep cervical fascia.*

Deep Cervical Fascia

The deep cervical fascia invests all of the neck structures lying deep to its own superficial layer, the investing fascia. It has 4 main divisions: the investing fascia (enveloping fascia, superficial layer of deep cervical fascia), the middle cervical fascia, the pretracheal (visceral) fascia, and the prevertebral fascia.

A. Cervical Investing Fascia: The cervical investing fascia (the superficial layer of the deep cervical fascia) begins along the spines of the cervical vertebrae. It ensheathes the trapezius and the dorsal paravertebral muscles. At the anterior border of the trapezius muscle, it gives off the prevertebral fascia. Farther forward, it covers the triangular area of the neck between the trapezius and the sternocleidomastoid muscle. At the lateral border of the sternocleidomastoid, the investing fascia splits to enclose the muscle. From the anterior border of the muscle, it is again a single layer of fascia. It then covers the most ventral portion of the neck and joins the contralateral sheath of investing fascia in the midline.

Ventrally and superiorly, the fascia is attached

to the mandibular symphysis and to the transverse ramus of the mandible to the angle of the jaw. There, it splits and proceeds superiorly as 2 layers that ensheathe the parotid gland. At the superior margin of the parotid gland, the fascial layers fuse with the zygomatic arch. Between the angle of the jaw and the styloid process of the temporal bone, the investing fascia forms the stylomandibular ligament. Farther laterally, the fascia attaches to the bony external auditory meatus. The superior attachment of the fascia then follows the insertion of the sternocleidomastoid muscle to the mastoid process, nuchal line of the occiput, and the external occipital protuberance.

Between the hyoid bone and the mandible, the investing fascia covers the submental and submandibular triangles. It fuses with the superficial surfaces of the anterior and posterior bellies of the digastric muscles. Collections of fluid (blood, pus) lying deep to the investing fascia will thus be confined to the suprahyoid area and will not ordinarily spread to other neck regions. In the submandibular area, the investing fascia forms a sheath for the submandibular salivary gland.

The investing fascia fuses to the hyoid bone. In the midline, below the hyoid bone, the investing fascia is a single sheet to the level of the thyroid cartilage. There, it splits into a ventral and a dorsal layer to ensheathe the sternocleidomastoid muscle. Inferiorly, the 2 layers are attached to the manubrium and to the clavicles. In the midline, just above the sternum, the split layers of the investing fascia enclose a small suprasternal space. This space (space of Burns) contains the sternal head of the sternocleidomastoid muscle, the anterior jugular veins and their connecting midline transverse venous arch, areolar tissue, and a few lymph nodes. At the level of the thyroid cartilage, the anterior jugular veins pierce the ventral layer of the split investing fascia. They then run inferiorly between the 2 layers to terminate in the anterior jugular arch, about 1.5 cm superior to the sternum. Venous blood then empties into the external jugular vein, on the surface of the sternocleidomastoid muscle.

B. Middle Cervical Fascia: The middle cervical fascia ensheathes both the superficial and deep layers of the infrahyoid muscles and thus possesses superficial, mid, and deep septa. Superiorly, each septum attaches to the hyoid bone. Inferiorly, all 3 fascial divisions attach to the sternum. Laterally, the fascia is attached to the clavicle. Just superior to the clavicular attachment, the fascia forms the pulley for the intermediate tendon of the omohyoid muscle. The lateral border of the middle cervical fascia is attached to the carotid sheath.

C. Visceral Fascia: The visceral (pretracheal) fascia lies deep to both the middle cervical and investing fasciae. It encloses the hypopharynx, the esophagus, the larynx, and the trachea. It also forms the carotid sheath, which encloses the internal jugular vein, the common carotid artery, and the vagus nerves. The carotid sheath is thick and strong where it envelops the common and internal carotid arteries; it is quite thin where it envelops the internal jugular vein.

The visceral fascia, after enveloping the thyroid gland and forming its false capsule, runs ventral to the trachea and the carotid sheath, to reach the root of the neck and enter the mediastinum. Here it ultimately blends with the superior portion of the fibrous pericardium.

A fascial cleft surrounds the visceral fascia and separates it from the middle cervical fascia ventrally and from the prevertebral fascia dorsally. This allows the esophagus, the trachea, and the thyroid gland to move freely up and down during swallowing.

D. Prevertebral Fascia: The prevertebral fascia lies just ventral to the prevertebral muscles and forms the fascial floor of the posterior triangle of the neck (Fig 8–6). It is derived from the investing fascia at the anterior border of the trapezius muscle. The prevertebral fascia is extremely strong and fibrous as it runs transversely across the neck, joining its fellow from the contralateral side just ventral to the vertebral bodies. It lies ventral to the scalene muscles and the levator scapulae, longus colli, longus capitis, and rectus capitis muscles. In the midline, it lies just ventral to the anterior longitudinal ligament of the vertebral column. It is dorsal to the carotid sheath and the esophagus, to which it is attached by multiple fibrous septa. It lies on the ventral surface of the longus capitis muscle and can be traced superiorly to the occipital bone. Inferiorly, the prevertebral fascia continues into the thorax, blending with the anterior longitudinal ligament covering the ventral surface of the upper thoracic vertebrae and with the endothoracic fascia.

➠ *Posterior esophageal fibrous septa. The fibrous septa running from the posterior esophageal wall to the adjacent prevertebral fascia funnel material that may leak from the posterior surface of the pharynx or esophagus directly into the posterosuperior mediastinum, with resulting mediastinitis.*

The prevertebral fascia is attached to the transverse processes and to the spinous processes of the cervical vertebrae, thus firmly enclosing the paravertebral compartment of the neck.

Lateral and deep to the sternocleidomastoid muscle, the prevertebral fascia is tightly adherent to the more anterior investing fascia. Fat separates the 2 fasciae as they reach the clavicle. The retropharyngeal cleft or space divides the anterior surface of the prevertebral fascia from the posterior surface of the visceral fascia.

➠ *Migration of pus from cervical vertebral infections. Collections of pus dorsal to the prevertebral fascia resulting from cervical vertebral infection may travel along the axillary and brachial arteries down to the mid arm. This is made possible by prolongation of prevertebral fascia inferiorly and laterally as the axillary and brachial arterial sheaths. Such purulent collections, however, usually point in the posterior triangle of the neck. In such cases, they are deep to both the prevertebral fascia and the investing fasciae of the neck, which are adherent.*

The anterior primary rami of the cervical nerves lie dorsal to the prevertebral fascia, as do the deep loops of the cervical plexus. As the phrenic nerve and accessory phrenic nerve descend, they lie dorsal to the prevertebral fascia on the ventral surface of the scalenus anterior muscle. The long thoracic nerve, the suprascapular nerve, the nerve to the rhomboid (dorsal scapular), and the nerve to the subclavius lie dorsal to the prevertebral fascia as they arise from the brachial plexus. The cervical sympathetic chain and its 3 ganglia lie just ventral to the prevertebral fascia.

Anterior Neck

9

THE SUPRAHYOID AREA OF THE NECK

The suprahyoid area is the most superior segment of the anterolateral neck. Superiorly, it is bounded in the midline by the **mandibular symphysis** (symphysis menti); laterally, by the body of the mandible up to the mandibular angle and by the **stylomandibular ligament.** Inferiorly, the area is bounded by the body of the hyoid bone, the posterior belly of the digastric muscle, and the stylohyoid muscle. The suprahyoid area is composed of 2 lateral submandibular areas and a central submental area.

THE SUBMENTAL REGION

The submental area is bounded superiorly by the mandibular symphysis and the mandible; laterally by the anterior bellies of the digastric muscles; and caudally by the body and the lesser cornu of the hyoid bone. The area is roughly triangular and is roofed by the investing layer of the deep cervical fascia, which is attached to the mandible superiorly, the hyoid bone inferiorly, and the anterior bellies of the digastrics laterally. The floor of the submental triangle is formed by the 2 mylohyoid muscles, which meet the midline in a central fibrous raphe. Enclosed within the submental area are lymphatics, the submental lymph glands, and some areolar tissue. Deep to the mylohyoid floor of the submental area are the 2 midline, thin geniohyoid muscles and areolar tissue that separates the submental area from the mucous membrane of the floor of the mouth near the lower anterior incisor teeth, the frenulum of the tongue, and the openings of the 2 submandibular salivary ducts.

⟹ *Investing fascial attachments. The investing fascia of the neck covers the suprahyoid region and seals off collections of blood, pus, or serum within the area. Seldom do such collections spill over into the infrahyoid or carotid areas of the neck; instead, they cause the investing fascia covering the suprahyoid area to bulge outward.*

⟹ *Connections between the floor of the mouth and the submandibular region. Cellulitis of the floor of the mouth, if not treated early, may lead to formation of a woody phlegmon of the submandibular area (Ludwig's angina). This is due to (1) the thin muscular barrier between the floor of the mouth and the submandibular area; (2) the presence of the mylohyoid cleft, which connects the neck and the oral cavity; and (3) the profuse network of lymphatic channels between the floor of the mouth and the submandibular area.*

Muscles of the Submental Area (Fig 9–1)

The **mylohyoid muscles** arise from the mylohyoid line on the inner surface of the mandible. The more posterior fibers of the muscle insert into the body of the hyoid bone. The central and anterior fibers insert into the submental central fibrous raphe. The muscle serves to elevate both the hyoid bone and the tongue. It is supplied by the inferior alveolar nerve, a branch of the mandibular division of the trigeminal nerve.

The **geniohyoid muscle** is thin and lies just superior to the mylohyoid central raphe and just deep to the mylohyoid muscle. It arises from the inferior mental spine on the mandibular symphysis and inserts into the hyoid bone. It abuts the contralateral geniohyoid muscle tightly. It pulls the tongue and hyoid bone anteriorly and is supplied by C1 through the hypoglossal nerve.

⟹ *Approach to the floor of the mouth. Incisions through the skin and investing fascia in the submental area should be made in a transverse direction. If it is necessary to explore the area deep to the mylohyoid muscle, the incision should be a vertical one through the median raphe of the mylohyoid and between the 2 geniohyoid muscles.*

Lymph Glands

The 6–8 submental lymph glands lie on the floor of the submental area on either side of its central raphe. The glands drain the central cutaneous area

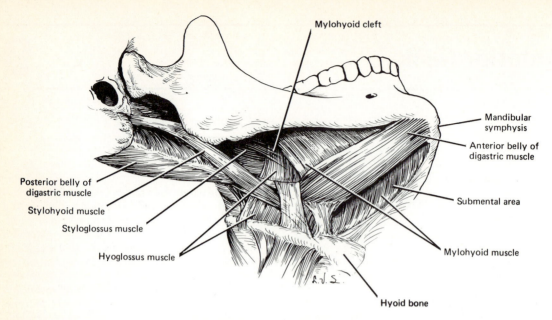

Figure 9–1. The submandibular muscles.

of the chin, a frequent site of furuncles and acne vulgaris; the central portion of the lower lip, a frequent site of lip cancer and ulceration; the anterior area of the floor of the mouth; the lower central incisor teeth and their adjacent gingiva; the oral openings of the ducts of the submandibular salivary glands; and occasionally the tip of the tongue. All of these areas may drain directly into the submandibular lymph nodes, bypassing the submental nodes; or drainage may occur into both groups of nodes. Efferents from the submental nodes pass to the submandibular nodes. There is some lymph drainage across the midline and into the contralateral nodes.

Venous Drainage

The anterior jugular veins begin in a venous plexus that lies superficial to the investing layer of the deep cervical fascia. This plexus makes approaches to the area quite vascular.

⫸ *Lymphatic drainage in the submental area. In planning a dissection for cancer of the upper neck, oropharynx, face, or scalp, the surgeon must be aware of cross-midline lymphatic drainage in the submental region, which always calls for a* bilateral *suprahyoid area dissection.*

Remnant Tissues

Remnants of the thyroglossal duct may occasionally appear in the submental area as cysts, abscesses, fistulas, or ectopic thyroid tissue. They appear as midline structures, since the thyroglossal duct always occupies a midline position.

THE SUBMANDIBULAR (DIGASTRIC) TRIANGLES OF THE NECK

The 2 submandibular areas extend from the anterior bellies of the digastric muscles to the sternocleidomastoid muscle and from the floor of the mouth to the posterior bellies of the digastric and stylohyoid muscles. The submandibular triangle is bounded superiorly by the transverse ramus of the mandible to the mandibular angle and the **stylomandibular ligament.** Inferiorly, the area is bounded by the posterior belly of the digastric muscle and the stylohyoid muscle. The submandibular area is roofed by the investing layer of the deep fascia of the neck, which is firmly attached inferiorly to the bellies of both digastric muscles and superiorly to the body of the mandible and the stylomandibular ligament.

Muscles of the Submandibular Area
(Fig 9–1)

The **digastric muscle** is composed of 2 muscle bellies united by a central fibrous tendon. The muscle runs from the mastoid process to the mandibular symphysis. Its central tendon holds the muscle to the greater cornu of the hyoid bone. The digastric muscle helps to open the jaws; the anterior belly pulls the hyoid bone anteriorly, and the posterior belly pulls it posteriorly. The anterior belly of the muscle is supplied by the mylohyoid nerve, a branch of the mandibular nerve. The posterior belly is supplied by a branch of the facial nerve.

The **stylohyoid muscle** lies superficial and superior to the posterior belly of the digastric. It arises from the styloid process of the temporal bone and inserts into the hyoid bone. Close to its insertion, it is perforated by the central digastric tendon. The muscle moves the hyoid bone superiorly and laterally and is supplied by a branch of the facial nerve.

The floor of the submandibular area is made up of 3 muscles whose fibers run in different directions. Anteriorly, it is formed by the posterior fibers of the **mylohyoid muscle.**

The **hyoglossus muscle,** which forms the mid portion of the floor, arises from the greater cornu of the hyoid bone. The hyoglossus is thicker than the mylohoid. It inserts between the styloglossus and the inferior longitudinal muscle of the tongue. The hyoglossus depresses the tongue. It is supplied by the hypoglossal nerve.

Because the hyoglossus lies on a more dorsal plane than the mylohoid, a cleft is present between the two. This **mylohyoid cleft** (submandibular cleft) leads from the upper neck into the floor of the mouth and connects the suprahyoid region and the floor to the mouth. Through this cleft extends the posterior segment of the submandibular salivary gland, the excretory duct of the submandibular gland, a branch of the facial artery which is to supply the floor of the mouth, the lingual and hypoglossal nerves, and numerous small veins and lymphatics.

The most posterior portion of the floor of the submandibular area is formed by the **middle constrictor of the pharynx,** which lies deeper than the hyoglossus. The muscle arises from the greater and lesser cornua of the hyoid bone and the stylohyoid ligament. It inserts into the posteromedian fibrous raphe of the hypopharynx. It is supplied by branches from the pharyngeal plexus of nerves. It helps move boluses of food inferiorly into the esophagus.

➠ ***Branchial cleft cysts.*** *Branchial cleft cysts appear in the most posterior segment of the submandibular area, usually deep to the sternocleidomastoid muscle, and lie upon the fibers of the middle contrictor of the pharynx.*

Superficial Contents of the Submandibular Region

Three structures lie just superficial to the investing fascia, roofing the submandibular area.

Posteriorly lies the cervical branch of the facial nerve as it descends to the mid neck to innervate the platysma muscle.

About 2 cm anterior to the descending cervical nerve, the mandibular branch of the facial nerve runs anteriorly, paralleling the body of the mandible while lying about 2 cm caudal of it. The nerve then arches superiorly to cross the transverse ramus of the mandible and run to the lateral commissure of the mouth.

The descending anterior facial vein crosses the transverse ramus of the mandible obliquely, to enter the submandibular area. At first it lies superficial to the investing fascia; later it pierces the fascia to occupy the submandibular space.

Structures Enclosed Within the Submandibular Space (Fig 9–2)

The most superficial of these structures is a plexus of veins that lies just deep to the investing fascia. The veins lie mainly upon the surface of the mandibular salivary gland. The venous plexus is formed when the posterior and the anterior facial veins combine to form the common facial trunk. The common facial trunk is joined from below by the ascending thyrocervical trunk, which drains the upper pole of the thyroid gland and the tissues of the upper central neck. This venous junction drains into the **common facial vein,** which joins the internal jugular vein deep to the sternocleidomastoid muscle.

The **submandibular salivary gland** lies at the center of each submandibular area under the transverse ramus of the mandible and directly on the hyoglossus muscle. From the deep surface of the gland the submandibular salivary duct (Wharton's duct), surrounded by a prolongation of submandibular gland tissue, extends superiorly and medially through the mylohyoid cleft to reach the oral cavity. The duct is joined in the floor of the mouth by excretory ducts from the sublingual salivary gland. The joined ducts then terminate in the floor of the mouth on the apex of a papilla just lateral to the frenulum of the tongue.

➠ ***Relationship of submandibular gland tissue to the sublingual gland.*** *Within the oral cavity, the submandibular salivary duct and its covering glandular tissue come into direct contact with sublingual glandular tissue, which lies just lateral to them. This close contact explains in part the rapid spread of infection from the floor of the mouth into the submandibular region of the neck and the frequency with which these salivary glands are involved in the same infectious and malignant processes.*

The submandibular salivary gland is normally about 3.5 × 2 × 2 cm in size. The gland is innervated by sympathetic nerves from the carotid plexus and by parasympathetic fibers from the facial and glossopharyngeal nerves. It is a compound racemose gland and a multilobular structure, each lobule draining into a major branch of its major excretory duct. Its alveoli secrete fluid of alkaline pH. An extension of the investing fascia of the neck encases the gland, lying just superficial to the actual gland capsule. This fascial covering must be incised before the gland can be inspected.

➠ ***Ranula.*** *Submandibular salivary gland tissue is a frequent site of acute infection, often fol-*

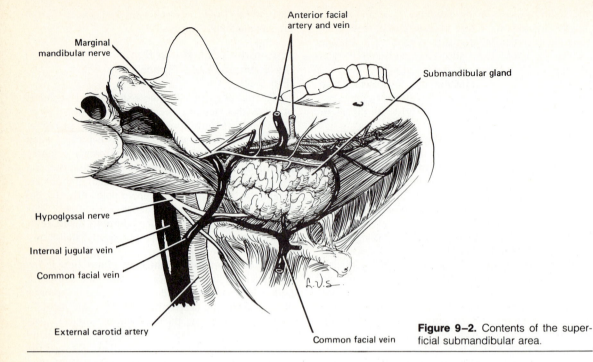

Marginal
mandibular nerve

Anterior facial
artery and vein

Submandibular gland

Hypoglossal nerve

Internal jugular vein

Common facial vein

External carotid artery

Common facial vein

Figure 9–2. Contents of the superficial submandibular area.

lowed by chronic infection and fibrosis of the gland. The fibrosis may lead to blockage of the excretory ducts, with subsequent stone formation and cystic degeneration of the gland. A ranula is a swelling of a blocked submandibular or sublingual duct.

Lymph Glands, Arteries, & Nerves (Fig 9–3)

The 8–16 **submandibular lymph nodes** are arranged in 3 main groupings (Fig 9–3): (1) a group superficial and lateral (but unrelated) to the submandibular salivary gland; (2) a group lying beneath the capsule of the submandibular gland; and (3) lymph nodes within the substance of the salivary gland. The 3 groups of submandibular nodes receive lymph drainage (1) from the submental glands; (2) by direct flow of lymph from all areas draining into the submental glands; (3) from the entire floor of the mouth; (4) from all of the lower teeth and adjacent gingiva and the corresponding buccal mucosa; (5) from the angle of the mouth; (6) from the lymph nodes lying superficial to the parotid gland; (7) from the lateral portions of the upper and lower lips; (8) from the cheek; and (9) from the tip of the tongue. The efferents from the submandibular lymph glands drain into the superior deep cervical nodes, which lie just deep to the sternocleidomastoid muscle.

➠ *Relationship of the submandibular lymph nodes to the submandibular salivary gland.*

The close relationship of these structures makes removal of the salivary gland mandatory in lymph node dissection for cancer metastatic to or primary in the submandibular area.

➠ *Tumors in the submandibular area. Both primary and metastatic tumors are common in the submandibular area. The submandibular lymph nodes lie along the route of spread of cancer cells and bacterial pathogens from the face, the oropharynx, the thyroid gland, the scalp, and the upper neck.*

The **external maxillary or facial artery,** the third anterior branch of the external carotid artery, is the principal artery of the submandibular area. It runs obliquely across the area, pursuing a tortuous course deep to the submandibular salivary gland. It is so closely applied to the deep surface of the gland that it grooves the gland. The artery runs beneath the posterior belly of the digastric muscle. It crosses the mandible at the anterioinferior border of the masseter muscle and runs to the angle of the mouth. It gives off muscular and glandular branches within the submandibular area. A large branch of the artery accompanies the duct of the submandibular salivary gland through the mylohyoid cleft to become the major artery of the lateral portion of the floor of the mouth. The facial artery also gives off branches to the palatine tonsil and the soft palate. A branch of the facial artery, the submental artery, dips beneath the anterior belly of the digastric and supplies the submental area.

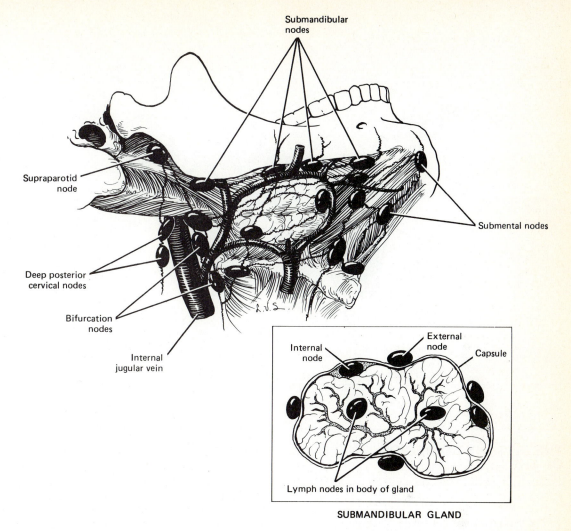

Figure 9–3. Lymphatics of the submandibular area.

Nerves related to the submandibular area are as follows:

The **mandibular branch of the facial nerve** lies superficial to the submandibular area, external to the investing layer of the deep cervical fascia.

The **hypoglossal nerve** (Fig 9–4) descends vertically from deep in the retromandibular fossa to reach the level of the angle of the mandible. It gives off the **ansa cervicalis** (hypoglossi), multiple small branches that innervate all of the ribbon muscles with the exception of the thyrohyoid, which is innervated by the main hypoglossal trunk. The hypoglossal nerve continues anteriorly until it lies inferior to the posterior belly of the digastric muscle. It then enters the submandibular area by passing deep to the posterior belly of the digastric and stylohyoid muscles. It lies on the surface of the hyoglossus muscle for only 0.75 cm, then enters the mylohyoid cleft to continue into the floor of the mouth, where it serves as the motor nerve to the tongue. It lies deep to the anteroinferior border of the submandibular gland and must always be located and isolated during operations upon the gland and its excretory duct.

The **lingual nerve,** a branch of the mandibular division of the trigeminal nerve, runs across the submandibular area under cover of the transverse ramus of the mandible and upon the surface of the hyoglossus muscle. It then enters the mylohyoid cleft, where it crosses both the submandibular salivary duct and the hypoglossal nerve from medial to lateral. It then runs forward into the floor of the mouth, where it lies lateral to the hypoglossal nerve and the submandibular salivary duct. It supplies the sublingual salivary gland and the mucous membrane of the floor of the mouth and lower gums. It also supplies tactile sensation to the anterior two-thirds of the tongue.

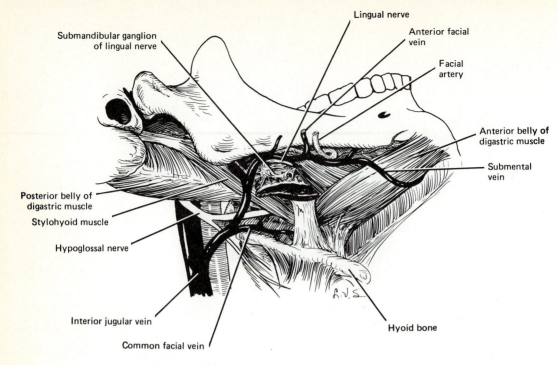

Figure 9–4. Deep dissection of the submandibular area.

THE INFRAHYOID REGION OF THE NECK

The infrahyoid region of the neck occupies the midline area, inferior to the hyoid bone and superior to the upper border of the sternum, the sternoclavicular joints, and the medial segments of the clavicles. Laterally, the area is bounded by the posterior belly of the digastric muscle and the sternocleidomastoid muscle. The area contains the infrahyoid muscles, the thyroid gland, the laryngotracheal tube, the lower hypopharynx, the cervical esophagus, and the anterior cervical lymph nodes. The anterior jugular veins are the most superficial structures in the area.

LINEA ALBA

The linea alba of the neck is a vertical fibrous structure formed by a coalescence in the midline of the investing fascia, the sheaths of the infrahyoid muscles, and the false capsule of the thyroid gland. It reaches from the hyoid bone to the sternum. It represents a relatively avascular surgical pathway to the anterior surface of the thyroid gland and to structures of the visceral compartment of the neck if the infrahyoid muscles are retracted laterally.

THE INFRAHYOID MUSCLES (Figs 9–5 and 9–6)

These paired muscles are divided into superficial (sternohyoid, omohyoid) and deep (sternothyroid, thyrohyoid) groups.

The **sternohyoid** muscle arises from the medial end of the clavicle, the sternoclavicular joint, and the posterosuperior surface of the sternum. It inserts into the body of the hyoid bone. It is supplied by branches from the ansa cervicalis (C1–3).

The **omohyoid** muscle is made up of 2 muscular bellies, superior and inferior, joined by a flat central tendon. The muscle arises from the superior border of the scapula and runs obliquely to insert into the body of the hyoid bone lateral to the sternohyoid insertion. The muscle passes deep to the sternocleidomastoid muscle, dividing that muscle into supra- and inframomohyoid segments. The omohyoid draws the hyoid bone caudally. It is supplied by the ansa cervicalis (C1–3).

The **sternothyroid** muscle arises from the manubrium and from the first rib cartilage. It inserts into the oblique line on the anterolateral surface of the thyroid cartilage. It draws the thyroid cartilage caudally. It is supplied by the ansa cervicalis (C1–3).

The **thyrohyoid** muscle arises from the oblique line of the thyroid cartilage and inserts into the inferior margin of the greater cornu of the hyoid bone. It draws the hyoid bone inferiorly and the thyroid cartilage superiorly. It is supplied by fibers from C1 via the hypoglossal nerve.

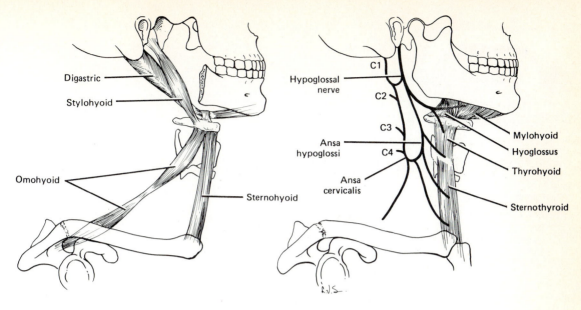

Figure 9–5. The suprahyoid and infrahyoid muscles.

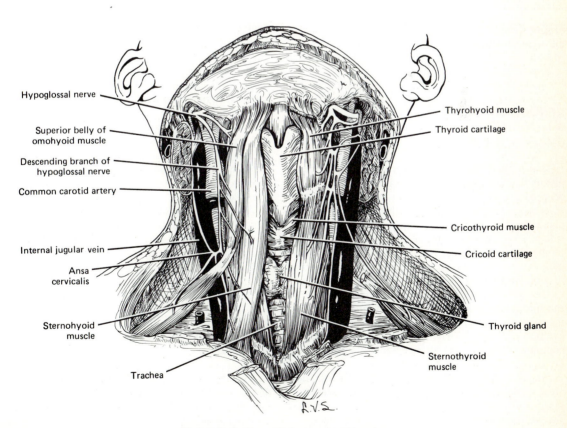

Figure 9–6. The anterior cervical triangle.

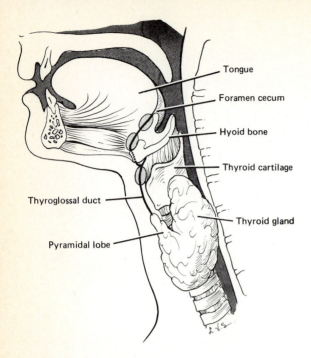

Figure 9–7. The course of the thyroglossal duct, showing sites of possible aberrant glands.

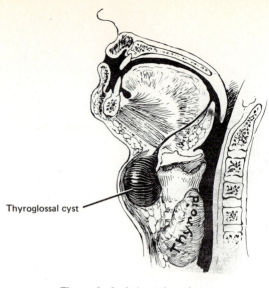

Figure 9–8. A thyroglossal cyst.

During swallowing, all infrahyoid muscles move the hyoid bone and the thyroid cartilage inferiorly. In addition, the omohyoid moves the hyoid bone dorsally and slightly laterally.

VENOUS DRAINAGE & LYMPHATICS (Figs 9–7 and 9–8)

The **anterior jugular** veins arise from a venous plexus that occupies the submental area of the neck deep to the platysma muscle but superficial to the investing fascia. At the level of the hyoid bone, the plexus forms 2 veins that run inferiorly, one on each side of the anterior midline of the neck. At the level of the thyroid cartilage, each anterior jugular vein pierces the superficial layer of the split investing fascia of the lower anterior neck. Between the split layers of the investing fascia, the 2 anterior jugular veins run a short distance and about 2.5 cm superior to the sternum; they arch laterally to join the ipsilateral external jugular vein. The 2 anterior jugulars usually communicate across the midline about 2.5 cm above the sternum (jugular venous arch).

Three or 4 inconstant anterior cervical nodes lie close to the midline of the neck, deep to the investing fascia and superficial to the trachea and the larynx. They receive lymph from the inferior half of the thyroid, the trachea, and the larynx.

THE THYROID GLAND

EMBRYOLOGY OF THE THYROID GLAND

Epithelium proliferates from the floor of the pharyngeal gut between the tuberculum impar and the copula (location indicated in adult life by the foramen cecum of the tongue) to form the thyroglossal duct. The thyroid develops as an outgrowth of that duct, which grows ventrally between the first and the second arches. At the level of the hyoid bone it changes direction and grows inferiorly to the level of the second tracheal ring, at which point the lateral thyroid lobes develop.

Anomalies. (Figs 9–7 and 9–8.) Anomalies of the thyroid include persistence of the thyroglossal duct as a cyst or sinus; aberrant thyroid tissue—always near the midline between the tongue and the mediastinum (tongue, floor of mouth, high neck, mediastinum); persistence of a pyramidal lobe; and abnormal position (too high or too low; substernal thyroid).

GROSS ANATOMY (Fig 9–9)

The thyroid gland is made up of 2 lateral lobes and a connecting central isthmus. The isthmus usually lies at the level of the upper 3 tracheal rings, rarely rising to the level of the cricoid cartilage or the cricotracheal membrane. The lateral lobes of the gland

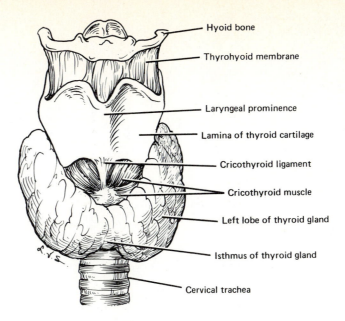

Figure 9–9. Relationships of the thyroid to the larynx.

usually cover the lateral aspects of the thyroid cartilage and are firmly attached to the cartilage by the suspensory ligament of the thyroid gland. The ligament results from thickening of the visceral fascia which ensheathes the thyroid gland as its false capsule. The lateral thyroid lobes lie in close approximation to the surfaces of the trachea, being connected by fascial condensations and by small blood vessels (Fig 9–9).

The **isthmus** of the thyroid varies markedly in extent and thickness. On occasion it is composed only of connective tissue; at other times it may cover the trachea with thyroid tissue up to 2.5 cm thick. The isthmus is usually less vascular than the lateral lobes. The isthmus often extends superiorly as a triangular prolongation on the ventral surface of the trachea and larynx, the pyramidal lobe.

The thyroid gland lies deep to the infrahyoid muscles, separated from them by its false capsule, derived from the visceral fascia. The true capsule of the thyroid is tightly applied to the external surface of the gland. From the true capsule, multiple fibrous prolongations run into the deep structure of the gland, dividing it into multiple small lobules.

Between the true and false capsules of the thyroid are placed the large surface veins that drain the gland.

⮕ *Size of thyroid. The thyroid normally weighs 30–40 g. This weight may triple or quadruple in hyperthyroidism, and the gland may weigh as little as 10–20 g in some cases of thyroid hypofunction. The gland is normally a vascular organ, the supplying vessels entering along fibrous prolongations of the true glandular cap-*

sule. The vascularity increases in toxic hyperplasia and decreases in colloid goiter disease and in Riedel's struma (chronic fibrous thyroiditis).

Relationships of the Thyroid (Figs 9–10 and 9–11)

Ventrally, the thyroid is closely related to its false capsule and to the sternothyroid and sternohyoid muscles. Superiorly and laterally, each thyroid lobe is related to the thyroid cartilage just superior to its cricothyroid articulation. Posterolaterally, the thyroid is related to the common carotid artery, the internal jugular vein, and the vagus nerve, all encased in the carotid sheath. In the midline posteriorly, the gland may be related to the cricothyroid membrane and the cricoid cartilage and is always related to the upper tracheal rings. The thyroid gland is closely related posteriorly on the left side of the neck to the esophagus. On the right side of the neck, a deep tracheoesophageal groove is present.

⮕ *Hyperthyroidism. Hyperthyroidism is usually associated with a diffusely hyperplastic thyroid gland. It may also be secondary to one or more toxic thyroid nodules. Treatment may be with antithyroid drugs or radioactive iodine or by subtotal thyroidectomy. If the patient is operated on, a small remnant of tissue is usually left on either side, with care for preservation of the parathyroids and the fibers of the superior and recurrent laryngeal nerves.*

Figure 9–10. Relationships of the anterior neck muscles and the thyroid and larynx.

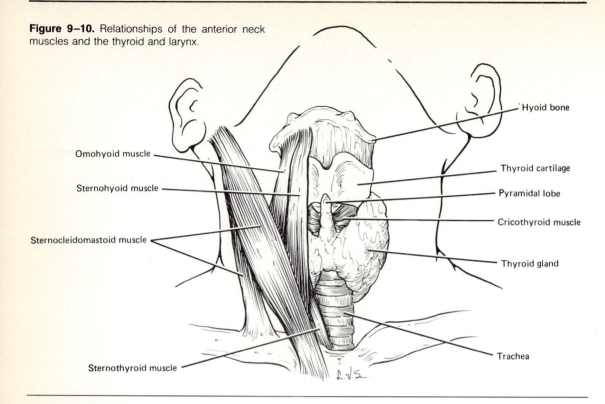

Hyoid bone

Thyroid cartilage

Pyramidal lobe

Cricothyroid muscle

Thyroid gland

Trachea

Omohyoid muscle

Sternohyoid muscle

Sternocleidomastoid muscle

Sternothyroid muscle

➠ ***Nodular thyroid.*** *Thyroid nodules, single or multiple, are removed surgically for the alleviation of pressure symptoms, to rule out cancer, to prevent extension into the mediastinum, as treatment for hyperthyroidism, and for cosmetic reasons. Needle biopsy or a radioactive iodine scan can help in assessing malignant change and in locating the exact position of deep glandular nodules. Ultrasound helps to determine whether a nodule is solid or cystic.*

➠ ***Thyroiditis.*** *Inflammation of the thyroid gland may be acute, subacute, or chronic and suppurative or nonsuppurative. Late or prolonged thyroiditis may result in Hashimoto's disease or Riedel's struma. Surgery is rarely indicated in Hashimoto's disease. In Riedel's thyroiditis, surgery is usually limited to removal of that portion of the gland that overlies the trachea and is the cause of tracheal compression symptoms. Needle biopsy is of help in confirming the diagnosis.*

➠ ***Thyroid cancer.*** *Thyroid cancer is classified as follows: (1) papillary adenocarcinoma, (2) follicular adenocarcinoma, (3) medullary carcinoma, (4) undifferentiated carcinoma, (5) lymphoma, (6) sarcoma, and (7) metastases from distant primary tumors. Methods of surgical treatment include removal of the single malignant nodule and removal of the involved lobe and thyroid isthmus. Carcinoma is usually*

treated by total thyroidectomy with ipsilateral partial or complete neck dissection. Lymphoma and sarcoma may require treatment by external radiation following thyroidectomy. The metastases of papillary and follicular carcinoma occasionally may be treated with radioactive iodine after thyroid removal by surgery.

BLOOD VESSELS, LYMPHATICS, & NERVES

Arteries
(Figs 9–12 and 9–13)

The superior thyroid arteries normally supply 15–18% of blood to the gland, the inferior thyroid arteries 76–78%, the inconstant thyroid ima 2%, and branches running from the sternothyroid muscle or from the trachea to the gland, 1%.

The **superior thyroid artery** may arise as the first anterior branch of the external carotid artery or directly from the common carotid artery just proximal to its bifurcation. The artery varies in length from 2.5 cm to 6 cm depending upon the level of the superior pole of the thyroid gland. The superior thyroid artery runs caudally, lying just lateral to the thyroid cartilage. Just before it reaches the thyroid, it divides into ventral and dorsal terminal descending branches. The ventral branch sends a sizable twig toward the midline and a small branch to the suspensory ligament of the gland. The dorsal branch runs along the dorsolateral border of the gland to join

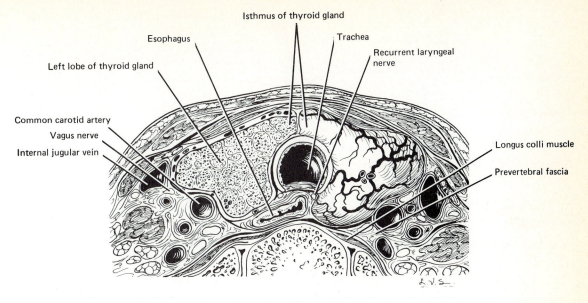

Figure 9–11. Cross section of the neck at the level of T1, showing thyroid relationships.

with the ascending dorsal branch of the inferior thyroid artery. About 1.5 cm after the superior thyroid artery it gives off the superior laryngeal artery, which enters the larynx along with the internal branch of the superior laryngeal nerve by piercing the thyrohyoid membrane.

The **inferior thyroid artery** is the continuation of the thyrocervical trunk, which arises from the first portion of the subclavian artery. The inferior thyroid artery runs across the vertebral triangle. It lies on a plane just ventral to the vertebral artery, the longus colli muscle, and the prevertebral fascia. It ascends as high as the cricoid cartilage, then loops inferiorly and comes to lie in a plane dorsal to the carotid sheath and the cervical sympathetic chain. It runs inferiorly, and just before it reaches the lower pole

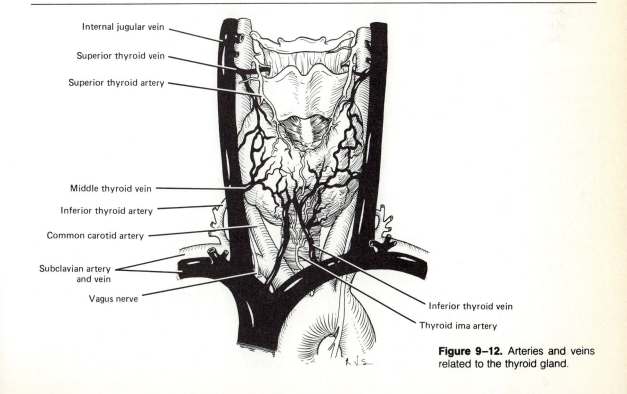

Figure 9–12. Arteries and veins related to the thyroid gland.

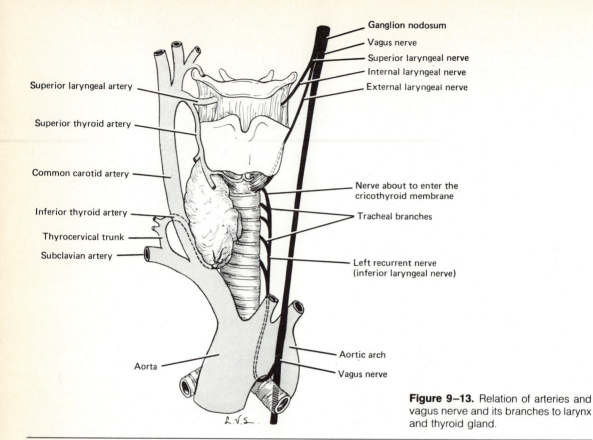

Figure 9–13. Relation of arteries and vagus nerve and its branches to larynx and thyroid gland.

of the gland, it divides into 2 branches that supply the dorsal and ventral surfaces of the inferior half of each thyroid lobe. The 2 ascending terminal branches of the artery anastomose with the descending branches of the ipsilateral superior thyroid artery and with the branches of the contralateral inferior thyroid artery. Just inferior to the lower thyroid pole, the inferior thyroid artery becomes closely related to the recurrent laryngeal nerve. At the level of its medial and inferior bend, the inferior thyroid artery lies just dorsal to the middle cervical ganglion of the cervical sympathetic chain. At this level, the artery picks up the autonomic nerve fibers it carries to the thyroid gland.

➡ *Ligation of the inferior thyroid artery. In order to avoid injury to the current laryngeal nerve and not deprive the parathyroids of arterial blood, the sites of election for ligation of the inferior thyroid artery are (1) at the level of C6, just distal to the point where the artery makes its inferior bend; (2) within the tissue of the lower pole of the thyroid; or (3) just proximal to where the vessel bifurcates before reaching the inferior pole of the gland. Site (1) is dangerous because it may interrupt the arterial supply to the parathyroid glands. Sites (2) and (3) are most commonly used.*

The **thyroid ima artery** is a branch of either the superior surface of the arch of the aorta or of the brachiocephalic artery. It runs superiorly on the ventral surface of the tracheal rings to reach the thyroid isthmus.

➡ *Bleeding from the thyroid ima artery during tracheostomy. The thyroid ima artery should be searched for, isolated, and ligated in performing elective tracheostomy. If this is not done, it is liable to bleed into the opened trachea during the procedure.*

Small arterial branches from the vessels supplying the sternothyroid muscle penetrate the superior lateral surface of the false capsule of the thyroid and supply a small amount of arterial blood to the gland.

Small tracheal arterial vessels enter the posterior and lateral surfaces of the thyroid gland.

➡ *Bleeding from tracheal arterial branches during thyroidectomy. During the late stages of total thyroid lobectomy or total thyroidectomy, tracheal arterial branches may bleed. This occurs during the stage of elevation of the gland from the underlying trachea.*

Veins
(Fig 9–12)

Venus return from the thyroid gland begins with some large veins that coalesce on the glandular surface within the true capsule. The veins then pierce the true capsule and lie just deep to its false capsule. Venous return from these large surface veins is via one of the following 3 routes.

The superior pole of the thyroid is drained by the **superior thyroid vein,** which runs alongside the superior thyroid artery to empty into the common facial vein and into the common facial venous trunk. It receives multiple muscular branches from the superior reaches of the neck.

The lateral surfaces of the thyroid gland are drained by 2–6 lateral thyroid veins that empty into the **internal jugular vein.** The lateral thyroid veins are 1–1.5 cm long and usually hypertrophy greatly in disease of the gland. They must be ligated and retracted laterally in order to properly mobilize the lateral and dorsal surfaces of the thyroid gland.

Issuing from the inferior pole of each lobe of the thyroid is a venous plexus of **inferior thyroid veins.** The veins run caudally on tracheal surfaces to empty into the right and left brachiocephalic veins.

Lymphatics

Lymphatic drainage from the thyroid gland pursues 2 major directions.

Ascending lymphatic drainage from the superior half of the thyroid proceeds via 2 pathways: (1) A medial group of lymphatics collect lymph from the isthmus and the medial superior portion of the lateral lobes; this lymph drains into the nodes lying on the cricothyroid membrane (prelaryngeal nodes). (2) A lateral pathway runs from the superior pole of the thyroid lobe and from the isthmus into lymphatics that follow the superior thyroid artery. These lymphatics empty into deep cervical nodes above the level where that chain crosses the omohyoid muscle.

Descending lymphatic drainage from the thyroid also takes 2 pathways: (1) Lymph from the isthmus and from the medial inferior portions of the lateral lobes runs to lymph glands situated on the ventral surface of the trachea (pretracheal glands). (2) Lateral inferior lymphatic drainage from the thyroid occurs along the inferior laryngeal nerves. This lymph empties into the deep cervical nodal chain below the crossing of the omohyoid muscle. There is also some inferior drainage via lymphatics that parallel the lateral thyroid veins. This lymph runs to the paraesophageal nodes that lie in the tracheoesophageal groove.

▸ *Paraesophageal lymph nodes during thyroid surgery. The paraeosophageal lymph nodes must be identified and biopsied in suspected thyroid carcinoma. If the nodes contain carcinoma, the nodes in the deep cervical chain must be located. The question of whether the lateral thyroid lobes drain lymph across the midline into the contralateral lobe is still unanswered.*

Nerves Related to the Thyroid Gland
(Figs 9–13 and 9–14)

The **superior laryngeal nerve** arises from the inferior vagal ganglion in the retromandibular region and descends along the lateral wall of the pharynx deep to the internal carotid artery. At the level of the greater cornu of the hyoid bone, it lies just superior to the superior thyroid artery. It follows the descending course of the superior thyroid artery for about 0.5 cm and then bifurcates into internal and external branches.

The **internal branch** of the superior laryngeal nerve runs medially to reach the thin thyrohyoid membrane. It is accompanied by the superior laryngeal branch of the superior thyroid artery. Both the nerve and the artery perforate the lateral portion of the thyrohyoid membrane and together enter the larynx. The internal division of the superior laryngeal nerve is purely sensory and supplies sensation to the larynx above the vocal cords. It also sends small branches to the base of the tongue and the aryepiglottic folds. The **external branch** of the superior laryngeal nerve descends close to the external surface of the larynx and supplies the cricothyroid muscle. The external branch of the nerve leaves the superior thyroid artery to innervate the muscle about 1.5 cm superior to the upper pole of the gland.

The **recurrent (inferior) laryngeal nerve** runs a different course on the right and left sides of the body. The **right recurrent laryngeal nerve** arises from the descending vagus nerve just after it has crossed the first portion of the subclavian artery. The right recurrent nerve moves superiorly on a plane dorsal to the subclavian artery and then runs across the vertebral triangle, deep to the common carotid artery and ventral to the inferior thyroid artery. After reaching the inferior pole of the thyroid, the nerve continues superiorly in the tracheoesophageal groove close to the posterior capsule of the thyroid gland and to both the inferior and superior parathyroid glands. It passes beneath the inferior pharyngeal constrictor muscle and enters the larynx through the cricothyroid membrane. The right recurrent nerve is a motor nerve and supplies all of the right-sided intrinsic laryngeal muscles except the cricothyroid. It is also sensory to the larynx below the vocal cords.

The **left recurrent laryngeal nerve** arises from the vagus nerve after the vagus has crossed the subclavian artery, just to the left of the termination of the aortic arch. The left vagus lies anterior to the left surface of the descending aorta. The left recurrent nerve at first runs superiorly and medially and becomes closely related to the ligamentum arteriosum and the pulmonary artery. The nerve continues its superior course, closely related to the dorsal surface of the aortic arch. It reaches the left lateral surface

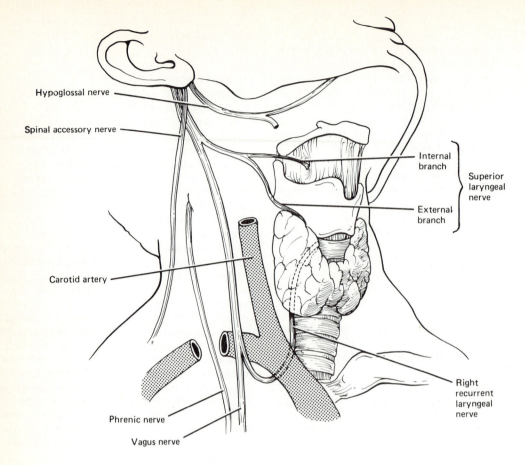

Figure 9–14. Nerves related to the thyroid.

of the thoracic trachea, which it accompanies superiorly. The left recurrent laryngeal nerve is related to the upper medial surface of the left lobe of the lung, to the thoracic duct, and to the esophagus.

⟾ *Injury to left inferior laryngeal nerve. The left recurrent laryngeal nerve is more vulnerable to trauma and disease than the right. Lying in the shallow left tracheoesophageal groove makes it more vulnerable to iatrogenic injury. The close association of the left nerve to both the arch and the descending aorta makes it susceptible to inclusion in pathologic processes such as aneurysm, aortitis, and aortic coarctation. Operative vascular procedures performed on the aorta may injure the nerve. The close relationship of the left recurrent nerve to a patent ductus arteriosus makes it vulnerable to injury during surgery. The long thoracic course of the left recurrent nerve makes it vulnerable to injury in cases of thoracic trauma. The nerve may also become involved in late*

cases of carcinoma of the upper lobe of the left lung (Pancoast's syndrome). Such involvement is a signal that operative lung removal will not effect a cure.

Extralaryngeal branching of the recurrent laryngeal nerve (Fig 9–14) occurs frequently. Branching may start near the takeoff of the nerve from the vagus, but generally it begins close to the inferior pole of the thyroid gland and becomes more frequent as the nerve approaches the cricothyroid membrane and the interior of the larynx. The extralaryngeal branchings of the inferior laryngeal nerve may vary from one to 6 and may cause confusion during thyroid surgery.

Innervation of the thyroid gland per se is via the middle and inferior cervical ganglia of the autonomic system. It is thought that this innervation has mainly a vasomotor function. There is a network of sympathetic fibers terminating in the basement membrane of the follicular cells, supporting the belief that neurogenic stimuli can influence thyroid function directly.

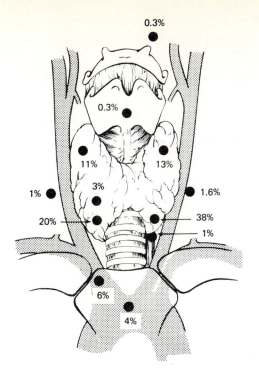

Figure 9–15. Sites of aberrant parathyroid tissue. (Reproduced, with permission, from Way LW [editor]: *Current Surgical Diagnosis & Treatment,* 7th ed. Lange, 1985.)

THE PARATHYROID GLANDS

GROSS ANATOMY
(Figs 9–15 and 9–16)

The parathyroid glands appear as small reddish-orange bodies about 4 mm wide and 6–7 mm long. It may be difficult to distinguish them from small fatty lobules. There are 1–8 glands, but 4 is the usual number. There are usually 2 superior and 2 inferior parathyroids. Collectively, the glands weigh about 120–140 mg. Parathyroid glands or remnants of parathyroid tissue may be found in ectopic position (1) anywhere in the visceral compartment of the neck along the course of their embryonic migration; (2) within the substance of the thyroid gland; or (3) in the superior mediastinum. Normally, the superior parathyroids lie high on the dorsal surface of the thyroid gland, between the false capsule of the thyroid and the intrinsic glandular capsule. The inferior parathyroids lie on the dorsal surface, close to the lower pole of the thyroid. On occasion they may lie dorsal to the false capsule of the thyroid, so that they cannot be seen at surgery unless this capsule has been incised. Occasionally, the inferior parathyroids may be found either in the lower neck or the mediastinum, where they may abut the trachea or esophagus or be related to the left brachiocephalic vein and the remnants of the thymus.

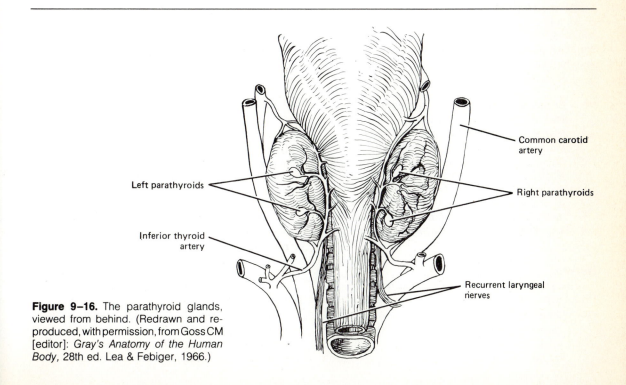

Figure 9–16. The parathyroid glands, viewed from behind. (Redrawn and reproduced, with permission, from Goss CM [editor]: *Gray's Anatomy of the Human Body,* 28th ed. Lea & Febiger, 1966.)

➠ *Position of superior parathyroids. Since the superior parathyroids lie ventral to the false capsule of the thyroid gland, they are more easily injured during thyroidectomy than are the inferior parathyroids, which frequently lie dorsal to the false capsule of the gland. The left parathyroids lie in a more narrow tracheoesophageal groove and are more often injured at surgery than the right-sided glands.*

BLOOD VESSELS, LYMPHATICS, & NERVES

Arteries

Both the superior and the inferior parathyroids are served by small branches from the inferior thyroid arteries and by thyroid arterial anastomoses. The tiny parathyroid artery enters hilumlike areas which distinguishes the gland from a lobule of fat.

One must take care to ligate the inferior thyroid artery distal to the point of takeoff of the parathyroid vessels, ie, well below the level of the arterial bend at C6.

➠ *Identification of the parathyroid gland by isolation of its arterial supply. The surgeon is frequently able to trace the small arterial branch that runs from the inferior thyroid artery to the individual parathyroid. Great care must be taken not to injure this extremely vulnerable vessel.*

Veins & Lymphatics

Venous return and lymphatic drainage from the parathyroid gland is into channels that empty into the veins and lymphatics which primarily drain the thyroid gland.

➠ *Location of parathyroids containing adenomas or hyperplastic tissue. The localization of a parathyroid that contains tumor or hyperplastic tissue can be assisted by selective arteriography, CT scan, and ultrasonography. Knowledge of the pathways of embryologic descent of the parathyroids is helpful. Almost 90% of ectopic parathyroid tissue lies within the neck. Only after the neck has been thoroughly searched should the mediastinum be explored.*

Nerves

The parathyroid glands receive their nerve supply from the middle and inferior cervical ganglia of the autonomic system.

THE LARYNGOTRACHEAL TUBE

The laryngotracheal tube, composed of the larynx and the cervical trachea, normally occupies the midline of the neck. In most males and in a small number of females it projects forward beyond the ventral plane of the neck.

THE LARYNX
(Fig 9–17)

The larynx begins at the base of the tongue at the level of vertebra C4. In infants (6–12 months), the superior laryngeal border is at the level of the disk between C2 and C3. Until the onset of puberty, the larynx is about the same size in males and females. When girls reach puberty, there is only a slight increase in the size of the larynx; in boys at puberty, all of the laryngeal cartilages become enlarged. The thyroid cartilage becomes particularly prominent, and the anteroposterior diameter of the rima glottidis almost doubles its prepubescent measurement.

1. GROSS ANATOMY

The larynx is composed of bone, cartilage, and connecting membranes. The larynx regulates tension of the vocal cords and thus increases or decreases the size of the air space at the level of the rima glottidis. Widening or narrowing of the air space at the rima is of importance in phonation and respiration and in protection of the tracheobronchial tree from foreign bodies or noxious vapors. The space closes completely as an aid to certain physiologic functions, eg, urination, defecation, and parturition (Valsalva's maneuver).

Relations of the Larynx

Laterally, the larynx is close to the major neurovascular bundle of the neck. The narrowing hypopharynx lies immediately dorsal to the larynx. The lowest part of the cricoid cartilage forms the posterior laryngeal wall at the level of the beginning of the esophagus (C6). Ventrally, the lower segment of the larynx is on occasion related to the isthmus of a high-lying thyroid gland or to a pyramidal thyroid lobe. In the adult, the laryngeal length is at the levels of C4–6.

➠ *Injuries to the ventral projection of the larynx. The larynx may be injured by a direct blow to its ventral surface (as in automobile and airplane injuries). The laryngeal cartilages, particularly the protruding thyroid cartilage,*

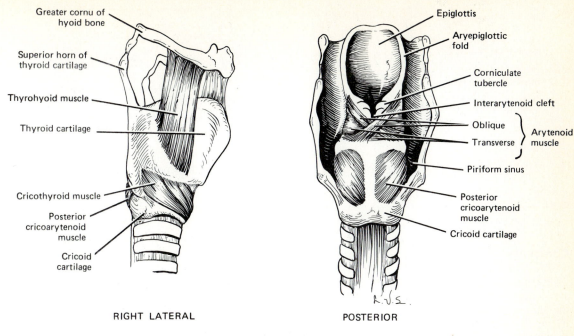

Figure 9–17. The larynx.

may be fractured or displaced, and edema of the submucosa quickly ensues. With such injuries, it is mandatory to perform an immediate tracheostomy so that the displacement or the edema will not block the central air passage. Because of the ossification within the laryngeal cartilages—particularly the thyroid cartilage—that appear in later life, the larynx is more easily fractured in the elderly.

Low-lying thyroglossal cysts or sinus tracts may be ventral to the larynx. The sternothyroid and thyrohyoid muscles lie just ventral to the larynx. Both the larynx and the trachea are ensheathed by fibrous septa from the visceral fascia of the neck. The descending arm of the inferior thyroid artery lies lateral to the inferior half of the larynx.

➡ ***Direct and indirect laryngoscopy.*** *The larynx may be examined by indirect or direct laryngoscopy. Indirect laryngoscopy can be performed only upon adults, since children cannot tolerate placement of a mirror against the soft palate. In cooperative patients, using indirect laryngoscopy, most laryngeal structures can be inspected. Direct laryngoscopy (Fig 9–18) calls for introduction of an endoscope directly into the larynx. This gives a much better view. Laryngeal endoscopy can be employed to remove foreign bodies and tumors and for laryngeal biopsy and other minor surgical procedures.*

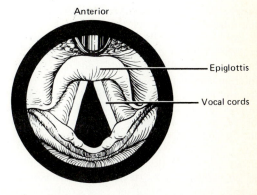

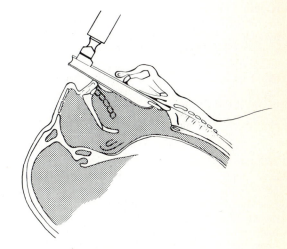

Figure 9–18. Direct laryngoscopy with view of glottis.

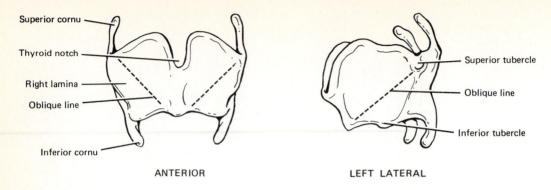

Figure 9–19. Thyroid cartilage.

Components of the Larynx

The **hyoid bone** is the single bony component of the larynx. It is roughly horseshoe-shaped and suspended from the tips of the styloid processes of the temporal bones by the stylohyoid ligaments and by the stylohyoid muscle and the posterior belly of the digastric muscle. It is made up of a body, 2 lesser cornua (horns), and 2 greater cornua. Superiorly, the hyoid bone is attached to the mandible by the mylohyoid, geniohyoid, and anterior digastric muscles; to the temporal bone of the skull by the posterior digastric and stylohyoid muscles; and to the tongue by the genioglossus, chondroglossus, and hyoglossus muscles. Caudally, the hyoid is attached to the thyroid cartilage by the thyrohyoid membrane and thyrohyoid muscle; to the sternum by the sternohyoid muscle; and to the scapula by the omohyoid muscle. Dorsally, the hyoid is attached to the epiglottis by the hyoepiglottic ligament. The hyoid bone acts as the superior anchor of the central air passage of the neck.

The **thyroid cartilage** (Fig 9–19) is composed of 2 quadrilateral plates of cartilage that meet at an acute angle (facing ventrally) in the midline of the neck. In the later decades of life, the thyroid cartilage tends to ossify wholly or in part, and as a consequence during later life fractures of the semi-bony cartilage may occur as a result of direct trauma. In the midline, where the 2 cartilaginous plates join, is the **thyroid notch.** The notch is an excellent landmark for delineating the midline of the neck at the laryngeal level. Two slender hornlike projections called the **superior cornua** extend upward. To these are attached the lateral thyrohyoid ligaments. The shorter inferior cornua join with the lateral borders of the anterior ring of the cricoid cartilage. An oblique line is present on the ventral surface of the mid portion of the thyroid cartilage. The line gives insertion to the sternothyroid muscle and origin to the thyrohyoid and inferior pharyngeal constrictor muscles. On the dorsal surface of the thyroid cartilage are the sites of attachment for the thyroepiglottic ligament, the anterior terminations of the false cords (ventricular folds), and the anterior terminations of the true cords

(vocal folds). The thyroepiglottic ligament, from which the epiglottis arises, is a midline structure at the mid posterior surface of the cartilage. The inner surface of the thyroid cartilage is covered by the mucous membrane of the laryngeal cavity. The sites of attachment of the false and true cords are just lateral to the midline, one above the other, slightly lower than the attachment of the thyroepiglottic ligament.

The **cricoid cartilage** (Fig 9–20) lies just inferior to the thyroid cartilage. It is shaped like a signet ring, the signet portion facing dorsally. The ventral projection of the cartilage lies at C6. The cricoid ring is slightly thicker, broader, and more easily palpable than the subjacent tracheal rings. Most of the signet (dorsal) portion of the cartilage extends above the level of C6, almost to the mid portion of the thyroid cartilage. The signet portion of the cricoid is strong and thick, and its superior lateral borders are notched for its articulation with the arytenoid cartilages. The mid posteroinferior surface of the cricoid signet presents a small ridge, the site of origin of the longitudinal muscles of the esophagus. Ventrally, the narrow cricoid arch is attached to the lower border of the thyroid cartilage by the cricothyroid ligament and to the first tracheal ring by the cricotracheal ligament. On the posterior cricoid body is a facet for articulation of the cricoid with the inferior cornu of the thyroid cartilage.

The **arytenoids** are small paired, roughly pyramidal cartilages that articulate at their bases with the cricoid cartilage via a diarthrodial joint. From this joint the 2 arytenoid cartilages rise, so that their apexes project farther posteriorly than do their bases. At the lateral inferior angle of each arytenoid (muscular process) insert the lateral and posterior cricoarytenoid muscles. Its anteroinferior angle (vocal process) is pointed and holds the posterior end of the true vocal cord. Just superior to the vocal process is the posterior attachment of the false cords. The medial surface of each arytenoid is lined with mucous membrane. The vocal ligaments are tensed, loosened, approximated, or separated by the gliding and rotating action of the arytenoids upon the cricoid lamina.

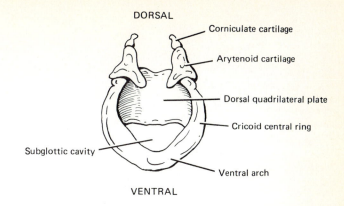

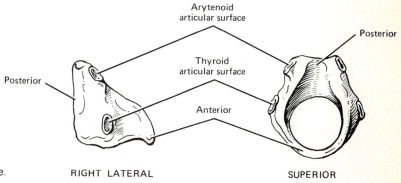

Figure 9–20. The cricoid cartilage. Right lateral and superior views.

The **corniculates** are small paired conical cartilages that sit atop the apexes of the arytenoids. They serve to lengthen and bring closer together the apexes of the arytenoid cartilages and are the dorsal inferior attachments of the aryepiglottic folds.

The **cuneiform cartilages** lie within the free border of the aryepiglottic folds, near the arytenoid apical insertions of the folds. They are small cigar-shaped cartilages that tend to strengthen the dorsal ends of the folds. They appear grossly as pearly white ridges lying just deep to the mucous membrane that covers the surface of the folds.

The **epiglottis** (Fig 9–21) is a yellowish single cartilage that lies just dorsal to the thyroid cartilage, the thyrohyoid membrane, the hyoid bone, and the root of the tongue. It guards the superior opening of the larynx. The cartilage is racket-shaped, composed of a handle and a body. The body faces convexly forward and has a dorsal concavity. The long thin handle of the epiglottis is attached by the thyroepiglottic ligament to the midline of the dorsum of the thyroid cartilage just superior and medial to the attachments of the ventricular folds. The epiglottis is attached to the base of the tongue and the lateral pharyngeal walls by 3 loose folds of mucous membrane, a central glossoepiglottic fold, and 2 lateral pharyngoepiglottic folds which are attached loosely to the side walls of the pharynx. The depressions on either side of the central fold are called the valleculae. Ventrally, the epiglottis is separated from the thyrohyoid membrane and the hyoid bone by a fat pad. It is connected to the body of the hyoid bone by the hyoepiglottic ligament. The supraglossal half of its anterior surface and the entire posterior surface of the epiglottis are covered with mucous membrane. The smooth dorsal concave surface of the cartilage presents at its base a midline tubercle that marks the level of the laryngeal opening. There are small pits in the cartilage, the sites of mucous glands that serve to lubricate the true vocal cords. During deglutition, the epiglottis falls dorsally in valvelike fashion over the laryngeal opening and then rapidly regains its upright position. The convex ventral surface of the epiglottis serves to deflect the ingested bolus of food or liquid to either side of the pharynx.

Ligaments of the Larynx

The laryngeal ligaments, which serve to bind the individual laryngeal structures together, are extrinsic or intrinsic. The extrinsic ligaments connect the laryngeal structures to extralaryngeal structures. The intrinsic ligaments connect the several cartilages of the larynx one to another.

A. Extrinsic Ligaments: The **thyrohyoid membrane** extends from the superior border of the thyroid cartilage to the margins of the body and lesser cornua

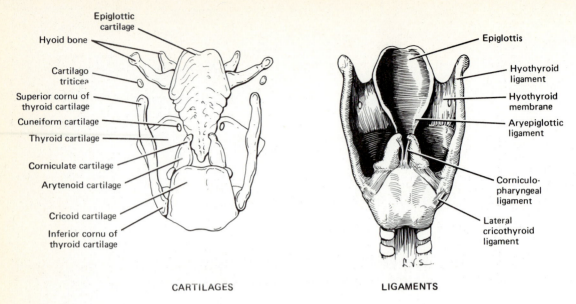

Figure 9–21. Posterior view of the larynx and epiglottis.

of the hyoid bone. The ligament is separated from the dorsal surface of the body of the hyoid bone by a mucous bursa that facilitates smooth motion of the larynx during deglutition. The lateral superior portions of the ligament thicken into short cords, the lateral thyrohyoid pillars, which secure the tips of the 2 long superior cornua of the thyroid cartilage to the hyoid bone. The lateral thin portion of the thyrohyoid ligament is pierced by the superior laryngeal vessels and lymphatics and by the internal branch of the superior laryngeal nerve.

The **hyoepiglottic ligament** connects the handle of the epiglottis to the hyoid bone. The **cricotracheal ligament** connects the anterior portion of the cricoid cartilage to the highest cervical tracheal ring.

B. Intrinsic Ligaments: The **thyroepiglottic ligament** binds the handle of the epiglottis to the dorsal surface of the thyroid cartilage. Deep to the mucous membrane of the larynx is a sheet of fibrous tissue, the **elastic membrane** of the larynx. The superior portion of the membrane is poorly defined and extends from the arytenoids to the mid epiglottis. The inferior portion of the membrane is very thick and well marked and connects the thyroid, cricoid, and arytenoid cartilages to one another.

The **cricothyroid membrane** (Fig 9–22) (conus elasticus) is made up of an anterior segment and 2 lateral segments. The anterior segment connects the thyroid cartilage to the anterior cricoid ring and is covered by the cricothyroid muscle. It is pierced laterally by the recurrent laryngeal nerves and by branches of the inferior thyroid artery. The central portion of the ligament is much thicker than its lateral segments. The lateral portions of the ligament reach from the upper limits of the cricoid cartilage to the caudal limits of the vocal cords with which they blend.

Interior of the Larynx (Fig 9–23)

The cavity of the larynx extends from the level of the epiglottic tubercle superiorly to the first tracheal cartilage inferiorly. The interior of the larynx is divided into the vestibule, the rima glottidis, and the infraglottic compartment.

The **vestibule** is triangular, with the base of the triangle facing ventrally. It is bounded ventrally by the posteroinferior surface of the epiglottis; dorsally by the apexes of the arytenoids, capped by the corniculates; and laterally on either side by the aryepiglottic folds. These folds enclose the mucous membrane, ligamentous and smooth muscle fibers that proceed from the margins of the epiglottis to the apexes of the arytenoids. Within each fold is the cuneiform cartilage, which serves to strengthen the fold just before it attaches to the arytenoid.

The piriform sinuses are narrow troughs that lie lateral to each aryepiglottic fold. They are pharyngeal pouch remnants. They are bounded medially by the aryepiglottic fold and laterally by the thyroid cartilage and by the thyrohyoid membrane.

The **ventricular folds (false vocal cords)** are 2 thick folds of mucous membrane that enclose a thin strip of fibrous tissue (the ventricular ligaments). The folds are attached ventrally to the thyroid cartilage next to the epiglottic attachment. They are attached dorsally to the base of the arytenoids next to the vocal process of these cartilages. The inferior borders form a free crescentic margin that spans the cavity. The ventricular folds do not extend as far medially into the laryngeal canal as do the true vocal cords. Consequently one may see both the ventricular folds and the vocal folds as one looks down into the cavity of the larynx.

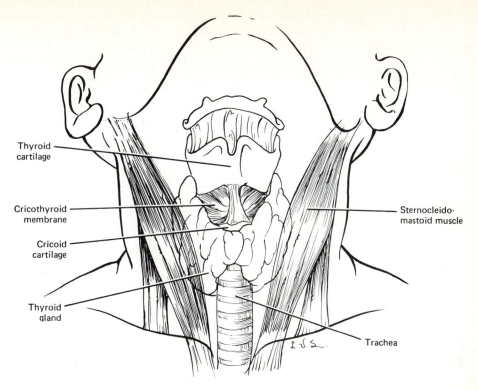

Figure 9–22. Anterior view of the larynx showing the cricothyroid membrane. (Reproduced, with permission, from Dunphy JE, Way LW [editors]: *Current Surgical Diagnosis & Treatment,* 5th ed. Lange, 1981.)

The **vocal folds (true vocal cords)** are 2 extremely strong ligamentous bands (vocal ligaments) covered by a thin, tightly attached mucous membrane. They are attached ventrally to the dorsal surface of the thyroid cartilage just inferior to the attachments of the ventricular folds. Dorsally they are attached to the vocal processes of the arytenoids.

The **ventricle of the larynx** is a fusiform fossa lying inferior to the ventricular folds and superior to the vocal folds. It extends almost the entire antero-posterior diameter of the larynx. Laterally, it is bounded on either side by the mucous membrane covering the thyroarytenoid muscle. The most anterior portion of each ventricle leads via a small aperture

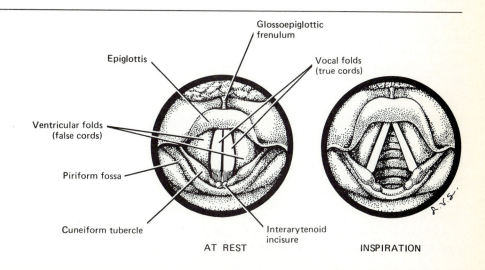

Figure 9–23. Interior of the larynx.

into a pouch of mucous membrane called the appendix.

The **appendix of the ventricle** is a membranous sac occupying the space between the ventricle of the larynx and the thyroid cartilage. It runs superiorly as a blind sac, almost as high as the superior border of the thyroid cartilage. It contains 50–80 mucus-secreting glands. When the surrounding muscular and cartilaginous structures compress the sac, a mucoid secretion is expressed from the glands that serves to lubricate the vocal folds.

The **rima glottidis** is the aperture of the larynx at the level of the true vocal cords. Ventrally, the aperture lies between the vocal cords; dorsally, it lies between the bases and the vocal processes of the arytenoid cartilages. The dorsal boundary of the rima is the mucous membrane running between the 2 arytenoid cartilages. The rima is the narrowest portion of the larynx and the level at which most aspirated foreign bodies lodge. The average ventrodorsal width of the larynx at the rima level is 23 mm in men, 18 mm in women, and 8–15 mm in children. The shape of the aperture of the rima varies from a narrow elliptical central slit to a lozenge-shaped opening.

The **mucous membrane of the larynx** is continuous with the mucous membrane of the oropharynx and with the tracheobronchial mucous membrane. It covers the superior half of the anterior surface of the epiglottis and all of its dorsal surface. The mucous membrane is prolonged to form the epiglottic folds. The mucous membrane covers the ventricular folds, continues into the appendix of the ventricle, and is reflected onto the vocal ligaments. The upper halves of the anterior dorsal surfaces of the epiglottis, the ventral half of the aryepiglottic folds, and the vocal folds are covered with stratified squamous epithelium. The remaining laryngeal mucous membrane is of the columnar ciliated epithelium type.

Muscles of the Larynx

The muscles of the larynx perform 2 major functions: opening and closing of the glottis and regulation of the tension of the vocal cords. The laryngeal muscles are extrinsic and intrinsic.

A. Extrinsic Muscles: The extrinsic muscles of the larynx are (1) the sternothyroid, which runs from the manubrium to the oblique line of the thyroid cartilage; (2) the thyrohyoid, which runs from the oblique line of the thyroid cartilage to the hyoid bone; and (3) the constrictor pharyngis inferior, which runs from the thyroid and cricoid cartilages to the central raphe on the posterior surface of the pharynx.

B. Intrinsic Muscles: The paired **cricothyroid muscles** arise from the cricoid cartilage and run to the thyroid cartilage. Their function is to tighten and elongate the vocal folds. By tilting the thyroid cartilage anteriorly, they tighten the folds; and by tilting it ventrally they loosen the posterior one-fourth of the folds.

The paired **posterior cricoarytenoid muscles** arise from the posterior surface of the cricoid cartilage

and insert into the muscular process of the arytenoid cartilage. The 2 muscles separate the vocal cords by rotating the arytenoid cartilages laterally at the cricoarytenoid joints. This movement opens the glottis.

The paired **lateral cricoarytenoid muscles** arise from the arch of the cricoid cartilage and insert into the muscular process of the arytenoid cartilage. These muscles rotate the arytenoids medially, closing the glottis.

The **arytenoid** is a single muscle that fills the space between the medial surfaces of the arytenoid cartilages. It arises posteriorly and laterally on one arytenoid and runs to the posterolateral surface of the contralateral one. It approximates the 2 arytenoids and thus is important in closing the posterior portion of the glottis.

The **thyroarytenoids** are paired muscles that parallel the vocal folds while lying just lateral to them. They arise from the angle of the thyroid cartilage and insert into the base of the arytenoid. Their major action is to pull the arytenoids ventrally toward the thyroid cartilage, with consequent shortening and relaxation of the vocal folds. This action is aided by relaxation of the cricoarytenoids.

Infraglottic Compartment

The infraglottic compartment is a short segment of the laryngeal cavity that extends from the rima glottidis to the first tracheal ring inferiorly. It is limited anteriorly by the cricothyroid ligament and the ring of the cricoid cartilage. If the vocal cords are approximated, the compartment becomes dome-shaped, the roof of the dome being formed by the mucosa-covered conus elasticus.

⇒ *Operations on the larynx. Median thyrotomy (laryngofissure) is a procedure in which a midline incision is made through the thyroid cartilage and the thyrohyoid membrane. It is used for removal of laryngeal tumors that do not necessitate total laryngectomy and for removal of foreign bodies lodged in the larynx that cannot be removed by endoscopy.*

Laryngotomy is performed when severe edema or an impacted foreign body calls for rapid admission of air into the lower larynx and trachea. A transverse cutaneous incision is made in the midline of the neck at the level of the upper border of the cricoid cartilage. The incision is continued through the cricothyroid membrane into the laryngeal cavity, and a laryngotomy tube is inserted. This is not a good procedure to use in children, since their vocal cords lie very close to the cricothyroid membrane. Tracheostomy is generally preferable.

Total laryngectomy is indicated for advanced or widespread malignant laryngeal tumor in cases where more conservative measures such as irradiation and local excision would be futile or have been tried without success. Total laryngectomy is usually indicated also for removal of tumors contiguous to the larynx, such as cancers of the cervical esophagus and hypopharynx. Total laryngectomy is usually accompanied by radical lymphatic nodal dissection on the side of dominance of the tumor in the larynx.

2. BLOOD VESSELS, LYMPHATICS, & NERVES

Arteries

The major arterial supply to the larynx is via branches of the superior and inferior thyroid artery. The superior laryngeal artery, a branch of the descending superior thyroid artery, perforates the lateral portion of the thyrohyoid membrane along with the internal branch of the superior laryngeal nerve and supplies blood to the upper half of the larynx. The inferior laryngeal artery, a branch of the inferior thyroid artery, enters the larynx through the cricothyroid membrane and supplies blood to the inferior half of the larynx. Small amounts of blood come via arteries that supply the pharynx and esophagus. Entrance of these vessels into the larynx from the closely applied pharyngeal and esophageal walls tend to bind the larynx closely to them.

Veins

The laryngeal veins accompany the laryngeal arteries. Superior laryngeal venous flow is into the superior thyroid veins and then into the internal jugular vein. the inferior laryngeal veins empty mainly into the inferior thyroid veins. Further flow is then into the internal jugular or brachiocephalic venous systems.

Lymphatics

The superior lymphatics accompany the superior laryngeal veins. They pierce the thyrohyoid membrane and run to the superior, vertical lymph nodes near the bifurcation of the common carotid artery. The inferior lymphatics pass out from the larynx via the cricothyroid membrane and run to deep vertical cervical nodes just inferior to the crossing of the deep vertical lymph chain by the omohyoid muscle. Some laryngeal lymphatic channels pass directly forward through the cricothyroid ligament and drain into nodes that lie on the upper tracheal rings. When these superficial nodes are palpable, they must always suggest laryngeal infection or cancer.

Nerves

The nerve supply to the larynx has been discussed in the section on the thyroid. The internal branch of the superior laryngeal nerve supplies sensation to the interior of the larynx above the vocal cords and a few motor filaments to the arytenoid muscle. The external branch of the superior laryngeal nerve supplies the cricothyroid muscle. The inferior (recurrent) laryngeal nerve supplies all of the other intrinsic muscles of the larynx. There is also a rich sympathetic nerve supply to the larynx, mainly via its major supplying arteries.

⟸ *Injuries to the superior laryngeal nerve. Injury to the main trunk of the superior laryngeal nerve causes only transient weakness of phonation as a result of loss of the action of the cricothyroid muscle. It does, however, decrease the sensory acuity of the laryngeal mucous membrane on the ipsilateral side. Transient weakness of phonation is accompanied by hoarseness, often mistakenly attributed to the passing of the endoscope during induction of anesthesia. Actually, the hoarseness is due to paralysis of the dorsal one-fifth of the vocal cord secondary to inability of the cricothyroid muscle to maintain tension on the posterior segment of the cord. The main trunk of the superior laryngeal nerve is vulnerable during procedures to correct internal carotid arteriosclerotic stenosis. The external branch of the superior laryngeal nerve comes quite close to the termination of the superior pole vessels supplying the upper lobe of the thyroid gland. The nerve must be searched for during ligation of these vessels and retracted from the operative field.*

Injury to the external branch of the superior laryngeal nerve causes paresis of the cricothyroid muscle, whose action is responsible for tonus of the posterior segment of the true vocal cord. The injury results in minor vocal changes. In such cases, examination of the larynx shows the posterior one-fourth of the involved cord to be quite lax. Such an injury can occur in surgical procedures upon the lower segment of the internal carotid artery (endarterectomy) and in procedures for mobilization of the upper pole of a high-lying thyroid gland.

THE CERVICAL TRACHEA
(Fig 9–24)

The cervical trachea is composed of 4 or 5 cartilaginous rings plus their connecting membranes. It extends in the midline of the neck, from the lower border of the larynx at C6 to the level of the upper border of the sternum (T2). The highest tracheal ring is attached to the cricoid cartilage by the cricotracheal membrane. Tracheal diameter is greater in men than in women and is quite small in early childhood. This is of importance in selecting a tracheostomy tube

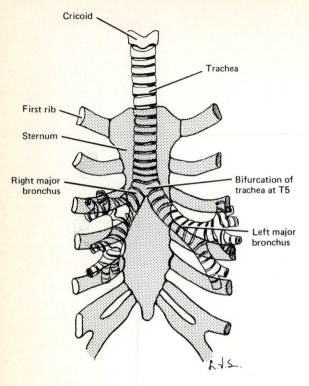

Cricoid

Trachea

First rib

Sternum

Right major
bronchus

Bifurcation of
trachea at T5

Left major
bronchus

Figure 9–24. The laryngotracheal tube.

with the proper curvature so that it will not injure the posterior wall of the trachea.

The cervical trachea is related ventrally to the thyroid isthmus superiorly and the inferior thyroid veins and thyroid ima artery inferiorly. The trachea is covered ventrally by the sternothyroid and sternohyoid muscles and by the investing fascia of the neck. Dorsally, the cervical esophagus is tightly attached to the trachea, protruding from behind the left side of the cervical trachea. Lateral to the trachea lie the lateral lobes of the thyroid gland, the inferior thyroid arteries, and the neurovascular bundle. The inferior laryngeal nerves lie in the tracheoesophageal groove.

Each tracheal cartilage forms an imperfect ring that is deficient posteriorly, smooth muscle fibers and fibrous tissue making up the dorsal arch. The lining mucous membrane of the trachea is of the stratified ciliated type.

The cervical trachea is supplied by the inferior thyroid artery, is drained mainly by the inferior thyroid veins, and is innervated by the vagus nerve, the recurrent laryngeal nerves, and the cervical autonomic nervous system. Lymphatic drainage from the cervical trachea is into the inferior (infraomohyoid) deep cervical nodes. A few small nodes occasionally lie on

the surface, draining both the trachea and the inferior larynx.

➡ *Position of cervical trachea. Movement of the cervical trachea from the midline suggests force exerted on the trachea by either cervical or superior thoracic structures. Increases or decreases in intrathoracic pressure may also be reflected in changes in cervical tracheal position.*

➡ *Trauma to the trachea. Tracheal trauma often affects the tightly adherent adjacent esophagus. Marked edema follows tracheal injury, and in cases of severe anterior neck injuries tracheal intubation from above (or tracheostomy) should be performed as low in the neck as possible, so that posttraumatic edema will not block the tracheal air passage. Since the trachea does not project as far ventrally in the neck as does the larynx, it is less often injured as a result of direct trauma.*

➡ *Tracheostomy. Tracheostomy is performed as a concurrent procedure in total laryngectomy and following extensive operative procedures upon the neck in which the possibility of postoperative laryngeal edema exists. It is performed as a surgical emergency when there is sudden obstruction of the upper segment of the cervical central air passage owing to foreign body aspiration; when there is blockage of the air passage due to infections or edema of the pharynx or larynx; and when vocal cord palsy with laryngeal stridor has occurred.*

Tracheostomy may be performed either above or below the level of the thyroid isthmus. The low tracheostomy is preferable. The neck is opened through either a vertical or a transverse skin incision. The midline arch connecting the lower anterior jugular veins may have to be divided, and the ribbon muscles are then opened via an incision into the linea alba of the neck. The ribbon muscles are retracted laterally. The thyroid isthmus is either divided or retracted superiorly. The second and third tracheal rings are hooked ventrally and opened vertically, and a tracheostomy tube is inserted. Care must be used in the selection of tracheostomy tube size so that the posterior projection of the tube will not cause pressure necrosis of posterior tracheal wall. This is particularly important when the procedure is performed on infants and young children, who have narrow tracheas and whose thin posterior tracheal walls easily become necrotic.

The Sternocleidomastoid (Carotid) Region of the Neck

10

THE STERNOCLEIDOMASTOID MUSCLE
(Fig 10–1)

The large sternocleidomastoid muscle is the major anatomic feature of the sternomastoid (carotid) region of the neck. It arises from 2 heads—a medial sternal head and a lateral clavicular head—separated from each other by a triangular space whose apex points superiorly. The space is usually filled by a thin layer of muscle fibers but often is covered only by a fibrous membrane.

➠ *Sympathetic ganglion injections. The interval between the 2 sternocleidomastoid heads may be used as a site of needle insertion for injections into the inferior cervical ganglion or the most superior thoracic ganglion of the sympathetic chain.*

In vasospastic disease of the upper extremity (eg, Raynaud's disease), injection of a local anesthetic into and around the stellate ganglion may relieve the spasm. In vascular disease of the intracranial area, stellate ganglion injection may relieve the vascular spasm that is secondary to hemorrhage or thrombosis of an intracranial artery. The procedure is now seldom used since the advent of more efficient vascular procedures (carotid endarterectomy, etc).

The sternocleidomastoid muscle inserts into the mastoid process of the temporal bone. As the muscle runs from origin to insertion, it covers the mid portion of the anterior neck. The muscle draws the vertebral column to the ipsilateral side and the head to the ipsilateral shoulder. In addition, it rotates the head superiorly and to the contralateral side. When both muscles work in unison, they flex the neck anteriorly.

The **sternocleidomastoid sulcus** lies alongside the medial border of the muscle. The sulcus is used as an incisional landmark in the anterior approach to the retrosternomastoid region. The muscle is divided into 2 segments by the omohyoid muscle as it crosses

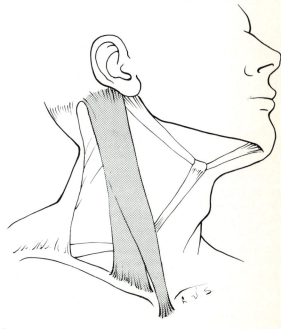

Figure 10–1. The sternocleidomastoid muscle.

deep to the sternocleidomastoid. This results in a long supraomohyoid segment and a short infraomohyoid segment. The transverse cervical and suprascapular arteries also lie deep to the inferior fourth of the muscle as they run laterally after branching from the thyrocervical trunk.

The sternocleidomastoid sheath is derived from the investing fascia of the neck. Above the level of the omohyoid crossing, the sheath of the muscle is quite thick, while below the omohyoid crossing the sheath is much thinner. Because various septa of the visceral fascia actually arise from its deep sheath, the lower half of the muscle is always more difficult to mobilize. The muscle is primarily supplied by the accessory nerve, which crosses it in oblique fashion from anterior to posterior. The muscle is also supplied to some extent by branches from the second and third cervical nerves.

➠ *Sternocleidomastoid "tumor" and congenital torticollis. Just deep to the anterior sheath and lying within the body of the muscle is a thick plexus of veins. During parturition, as a result of movements of the fetal head, these veins may rupture and bleed either into the muscle belly or just under the anterior sheath. The bleeding usually results in eventual formation of a fibrosed hematoma in the lower one-fifth of the muscle ("sternocleidomastoid tumor"); in infants, this mass must be distinguished from fibrous lymphatic tumors. If bleeding within the muscle belly is not minor and is untreated, a fibrous contracture of one or both of the inferior heads of the muscle may occur, with resultant shortening of these heads. Severe shortening results in torticollis (wryneck), which causes the head to be pulled toward the side of the injury. This differs from torticollis of neurologic origin, in which the muscle heads appear normal. Neurologic torticollis may also follow parturition as a result of traumatic stretching or avulsion of the accessory nerve, which supplies both the sternocleidomastoid and the trapezius muscles.*

STRUCTURES DEEP TO THE STERNOCLEIDOMASTOID MUSCLE

Deep to the sternocleidomastoid muscle—and shielded by it—are important cervical structures: (1) the carotid sheath, containing the carotid arterial system, the internal jugular vein, and the vagus nerve; (2) the vertical deep chain of cervical lymph nodes; (3) the spinal accessory nerve; (4) the omohyoid muscle; (5) the prevertebral fascia, which separates the deep surface of the sternocleidomastoid muscle from the anterior and middle scalene muscles; (6) the cervical plexus of nerves; (7) the cervical sympathetic chain and ganglia; and (8) the vertebral triangle of

the neck, containing the first portion of the subclavian artery with its branches, the thoracic duct (on the left side only), the stellate ganglion, the phrenic nerve, and the inferior laryngeal nerve.

THE CAROTID ARTERIAL SYSTEM (Fig 10–2)

The major vessel lying deep to the sternocleidomastoid muscle is the common carotid artery, whose site of origin differs on the right and left.

The right common carotid artery begins dorsal to the right sternoclavicular joint as the continuation of the brachiocephalic (innominate) artery. The left common carotid artery arises from the most superior portion of the aortic arch, to the left of the brachiocephalic artery. The left common carotid artery ascends from its origin on the aortic arch and passes through the superior mediastinum until it reaches the left sternoclavicular joint. Lying ventral to the left common carotid are the manubrium, the sternal origins of the strap muscles, the anterior portions of the left pleura and lung, the long left brachiocephalic vein, and the remnants of the thymus gland. When present, a substernal thyroid also lies ventral to the artery. Lying dorsal to the vessel are the trachea, the esophagus, the left recurrent laryngeal nerve, and the major (left) thoracic duct.

➠ *Disorders involving the common carotid artery. As a result of its superior thoracic course, the left common carotid artery may be injured by penetrating or crushing wounds of the superior chest. It may be eroded by an enlarging tumor of the upper left lung or of the superior portion of the thoracic esophagus. Aneurysms of the aortic arch can alter the course of the left common carotid artery and may obliterate the vessel.*

At their points of origin, the right and left common carotid arteries are fairly close together, separated only by the lower tracheal rings. Each artery ascends from the level of the sternoclavicular joint, lying just anterior to the transverse processes of the lower cervical vertebrae and deep to the body of the sternocleidomastoid muscle as it bears obliquely laterally and eventually reaches to the level of the greater cornu of the hyoid bone. As a result, the vessels are farther apart at their site of bifurcation than at their site of cervical origin.

➠ *Carotid compression hemostasis. At the level of the anterior ring of the cricoid cartilage (C6), the common carotid artery may be compressed against the transverse process of C6. This procedure is occasionally useful in emer-*

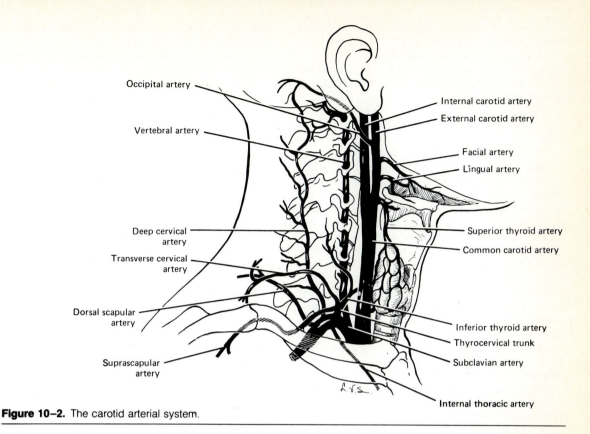

Figure 10–2. The carotid arterial system.

gency situations as a means of stopping hemorrhage from the vessel.

At the level of the superior border of the thyroid cartilage, the common carotid artery divides into the **internal and external carotid arteries.** Normally, there are no branches of the common carotid artery proximal to its bifurcation. Occasionally, the common carotid may give off the **superior thyroid artery** and rarely the lingual artery. As the common carotid arteries ascend, they are contained within the carotid sheath. Also within this sheath are the internal jugular vein, which lies lateral to the artery, and the vagus nerve, which lies deep to the artery. The omohyoid muscle crosses anterior to the common carotid from medial to lateral, about 4.5 cm below the level of its bifurcation.

The **carotid body** (one on each side) is a reddish brown oval structure 3–6 mm long that lies behind the angle of bifurcation of the common carotid artery. It has an outer fibrous capsule and is made up of epithelioid cells and multiple nerve fibers. The carotid body plays a role in the control of blood pressure, circulation, and respiration. It is firmly attached to the bifurcation of the common carotid artery and to the most proximal segments of the internal and external carotid arteries.

➡ ***Tumors of the carotid body.*** *Carotid body tumors are usually benign but occasionally may infiltrate the adjacent arteries, and total tumor removal calls for major vascular surgery. The tumors are rarely palpable and are usually diagnosed on the basis of vasomotor symptoms aided by the use of carotid arteriography. A "vascular blush" at the carotid bifurcation and widening of the arms of the bifurcation by the mass are of help in diagnosis.*

The internal carotid artery ascends superiorly in approximately the same line as did the common carotid artery. At its origin, the internal carotid is relatively superficial, lying just dorsal and lateral to the external carotid artery.

As the **internal carotid artery** ascends to the level of the angle of the mandible, it lies in the retromandibular fossa deep to the parotid gland and just ventral to the transverse processes of the upper 3 cervical vertebrae. At the level of the angle of the jaw, the internal carotid artery lies deep to the external carotid artery, which now lies in the inferior segment of the retromandibular fossa, with the internal jugular vein lateral to the internal carotid artery and the vagus nerve deep to it. The internal carotid artery enters the skull via the carotid foramen in the petrous portion of the temporal bone and, in the middle cranial fossa, divides into the anterior and middle cerebral arteries. There are no extracranial branches of the internal carotid artery, but some branches of the artery which are given off within the bony cranium terminate in an extracranial position. Because of the deep position of the internal carotid in the retromandibular space, this segment of the vessel is seldom injured by external trauma.

The **external carotid artery** supplies the anterior portion of the superior segment of the neck, including the upper half of the larynx and the thyroid gland, structures in the retromandibular fossa, the face, the scalp, and the oropharynx. The vessel arises from the common carotid artery at the level of the superior border of the thyroid cartilage and at first passes anteriorly and superiorly. It then turns rather sharply posteriorly to enter the retromandibular fossa at the level of the angle of the jaw. It ascends in the retromandibular fossa to about the midpoint of the overlying parotid gland and enters the deep cotyledon of the gland, to break up into its terminal branches. As it passes superiorly, the external carotid rapidly diminishes in size as a result of the many relatively large branchings.

Branches of the Carotid Artery

There are 4 major sets of branchings from the external carotid artery: anterior, posterior, ascending, and terminal.

A. Anterior Group: The **superior thyroid artery** is given off from the external carotid soon after the common carotid artery has bifurcated. It is a 5-cm trunk running from the hyoid bone to the upper pole of the thyroid gland. The vessel first arches superiorly, then turns inferiorly under the infrahyoid muscles to descend just lateral to the thyroid cartilage. It finally reaches the superior pole of the thyroid gland. The artery is closely associated with the main trunk and later with the external division of the superior laryngeal nerve. The superior thyroid artery supplies the upper half of the thyroid gland, the infrahyoid muscles of the neck, the hyoid bone, the superior half of the larynx, a portion of the sternocleidomastoid muscle, and the cricothyroid muscle.

➧ *Ligation of the superior thyroid artery. In ligating the superior thyroid artery just superior to the upper pole of a high-lying thyroid gland, care must be taken to identify and avoid the external (motor) branch of the superior laryngeal nerve.*

The **lingual artery** arises from the external carotid about 0.5 cm superior to the origin of the superior thyroid artery. Its immediate course is toward the greater cornu of the hyoid bone. It then curves inferiorly and anteriorly, forming a loop that is always crossed by the hypoglossal nerve before it passes

under the posterior belly of the digastric muscle to enter the submandibular space.

➧ *Relationship of the lingual artery and the hypoglossal nerve. The loop of the lingual artery is important in locating the hypoglossal nerve during radical neck dissection. The lingual artery is best ligated at the level of the greater cornu of the hyoid bone just prior to the formation of its loop in order to avoid injury to the hypoglossal nerve.*

After being crossed by the hypoglossal nerve, the lingual artery ascends deep to the posterior belly of the digastric and the stylohyoid muscles, lying upon the middle constrictor of the pharynx in the submandibular area. It then runs horizontally forward deep to the hypoglossus and genioglossus muscles. Terminally, it ascends into the floor of the mouth, where it turns forward to run on the inferior surface of the tongue to its tip (the profunda linguae). The lingual artery gives off suprahyoid, dorsal lingual, sublingual, and deep lingual branches.

The **facial (external maxillary) artery** arises from the external carotid within the carotid triangle. Its origin is slightly superior to the takeoff of the lingual artery sheltered by the transverse ramus of the mandible. It ascends in an obliquely superior and anterior direction deep to the posterior belly of the digastric and stylohyoid muscles. In the suprahyoid area, it lies superficial to the hyoglossus in a tortuous oblique course across the muscle, grooving the deep surface of the submandibular salivary gland. It gives branches to the deep surface of the submandibular salivary gland and to its duct, to the muscles of the suprahyoid area, and to the floor of the mouth via a branch that travels through the mylohyoid cleft along with the submandibular salivary duct. The facial artery finally climbs superiorly over the transverse ramus of the mandible at the anteroinferior border of the masseter muscle.

➧ *Relationship of the facial artery to the gland of Stahr. As it crosses the mandible, the facial artery is closely related to the lymph gland of Stahr, which is often palpable in children with scalp or face infections. The gland must be removed along with the deep lymph chain of the neck in radical neck dissection performed for tongue cancer. It is frequently the site of recurrence.*

The facial artery continues toward the lateral commissure of the mouth, then to the medial palpebral fissure. The artery sends off ascending palatine, tonsillar, glandular, submental, inferior and superior labial, lateral nasal, angular, and muscular branches.

B. Posterior Group: The **occipital artery** arises from the external carotid, opposite the anterior takeoff of the facial artery. Its origin is near the posterior belly of the digastric muscle where it crosses the hypoglossal nerve. The occipital artery runs toward the posteroinferior area of the scalp close to the occipital group of lymph nodes. It is accompanied in its terminal portion by the greater occipital nerve. It gives off muscular, sternocleidomastoid, auricular, meningeal, descending, and terminal branches.

The **posterior auricular artery** arises from the external carotid artery superior to the level of the posterior belly of the digastric, opposite the tip of the styloid process of the temporal bone. It ascends to the groove between the cartilage of the ear and the mastoid process, where it divides into its terminal auricular and occipital branches. It also gives off a small stylomastoid branch.

C. Ascending Group: The **ascending pharyngeal artery** is a long slender vessel situated deeply in the neck. It arises from the external carotid just superior to the point of bifurcation of the common carotid artery. It ascends almost vertically, between the internal carotid artery and the lateral wall of the pharynx, to the base of the skull and gives off palatine, pharyngeal, prevertebral, meningeal, and tympanic branches.

D. Terminal Group: As the **external carotid artery** passes superiorly, it enters the retromandibular fossa and comes into contact with the deep surface of the inferior pole of the parotid gland at the level of the angle of the jaw. The artery continues in the retromandibular fossa, deep to the parotid gland; then it enters the substance of the gland. Within the parotid, it lies deep to both the facial nerve and the posterior facial vein and divides into its 2 terminal branches. The **maxillary artery** arises behind the neck of the mandible and passes forward between the ascending ramus of the mandible and the sphenomandibular ligament. It gives off multiple branches to the face and the deep facial fossae. It also gives off the middle meningeal branch, which terminates intracranially. The **superficial temporal artery,** the smaller terminal branch of the external carotid, is a continuation of the vessel. It begins behind the neck of the mandible within the substance of the parotid gland, ascends, and leaves the parotid gland by crossing the posterior root of the zygomatic process. About 2 cm above the zygoma it divides into frontal and parietal branches whose divisions supply the temporal and parietal areas of the scalp.

➠ *Collateral circulation following ligation of the carotid arteries. Following ligation of the common carotid artery, excellent collateral circulation is maintained via the free communication between the external and internal carotids, both intra- and extracranially. The chief extracranial communications are via the superior and inferior thyroid arteries, between the deep cervical artery and the descending arm of the occipital artery. The intracranial source of collateral circulation is via the vertebral branch of the subclavian artery. Ligation of the common carotid artery is usually feasible in younger people, but in older people it is best to check the adequacy of the collaterals by temporary occlusion of the vessel before permanent ligation.*

*When the **external carotid artery** is ligated, fairly good collateral circulation develops between those intracranial branches of the internal carotid that terminate extracranially and the facial and scalp branches of the external carotid. Intracranial branches of the internal carotid, which supply collateral circulation, terminate in the orbit and in the upper pharynx. There is also anastomosis between the external carotid branches of the contralateral sides. If possible, the external carotid should be ligated as far proximally as possible, usually just above the takeoff of the superior thyroid artery, care being taken to secure the dorsal branching ascending pharyngeal artery so that it will not bleed following carotid transection.*

*When the **internal carotid artery** is ligated, collateral circulation is supplied via the intracranial circle of Willis, with the vertebral artery supplying blood from both the ipsilateral and contralateral sides. Small amounts of blood come also from anastomosis of the extracranial endings of intracranial branches of the internal carotid with facial branches of the external carotid artery.*

VEINS OF THE STERNOCLEIDOMASTOID REGION (Fig 10–3)

The **internal jugular vein** collects blood from the cranial cavity, the scalp, the face, and the neck. The vessel begins at the jugular foramen of the skull as a continuation of the sigmoid sinus. At its origin, it is dilated into a bulblike swelling. The vein runs inferiorly, deeply placed in the retromandibular fossa. It lies at first lateral to the internal carotid artery, then ventral to the artery. At the root of the neck, it joins the subclavian vein to form the **brachiocephalic vein.** In the subclavian region, the right internal jugular vein lies away from the right common carotid artery as it crosses ventral to the subclavian artery. The left internal jugular vein usually overlaps the left common carotid artery in the lower neck and is usually smaller than the vein on the right. The internal jugular vein receives cervical blood from the inferior petrosal sinus, the thyrocervical facial trunk, the lingual veins, the pharyngeal veins, the lateral thyroid veins, and occasionally the occipital vein.

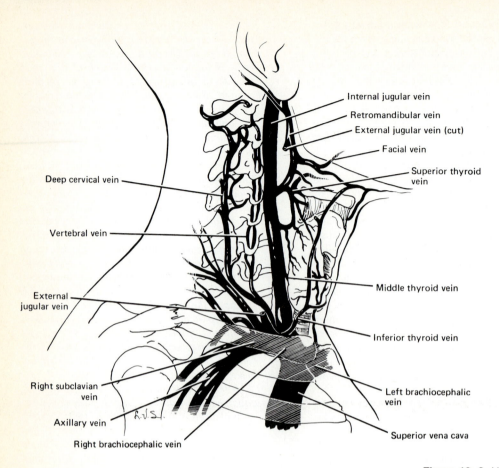

Figure 10–3. Veins of the neck.

Transverse sinus thrombophlebitis. The intracranial transverse sinus may become involved with a septic thrombophlebitis secondary to a middle ear or mastoid air cell infection. The process in the transverse sinus process may extend into the internal jugular vein. Although antibiotics usually will control the infection, the internal jugular vein may require ligation in the neck distal to the inferior margin of the thrombophlebitis to prevent its extension and the propagation of infected emboli.

The **vertebral veins** pass from the foramen magnum of the skull just superior to the posterior arch of the axis and are joined by venous branches from the deep cervical muscles. As a result, several venous trunks of fair size are formed that run to C6, alongside the vertebral artery in the foramens in the transverse processes of the cervical vertebrae. The veins form a thick venous plexus about the vertebral artery. The veins empty into the brachiocephalic veins. The vertebral veins play an important role in maintenance of intracranial venous flow following ligation of the internal jugular vein.

The **external jugular vein** (Fig 10–4) collects blood from the exterior of the cranium (scalp) and the deep parts of the face. It is formed by the junction of the posterior facial vein (retromandibular vein) with the posterior auricular vein. It begins at the lower edge of the parotid gland and runs obliquely and inferiorly on the external surface of the sternocleidomastoid muscle.

Just superior to the clavicle, the external jugular vein perforates the investing layer of the deep cervical fascia and terminates in the subclavian vein lateral to the anterior scalene muscle. It receives venous blood from the occipital, posterior external jugular (if present), transverse cervical, suprascapular, and anterior jugular veins.

LYMPHATICS OF THE HEAD & NECK (Figs 10–5 to 10–7)

The lymphatic tissues of the head and neck present a complex system of lymphatic pickup, relay, and dispersal. The lymphatic tissues are divided into 3

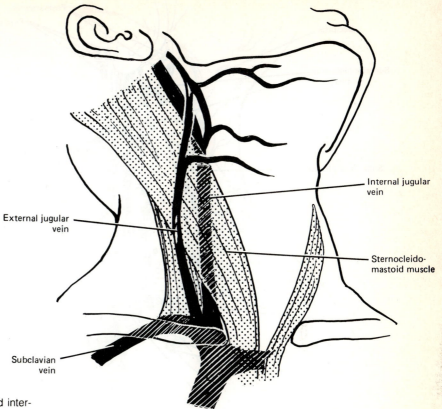

Figure 10–4. External and internal jugular veins.

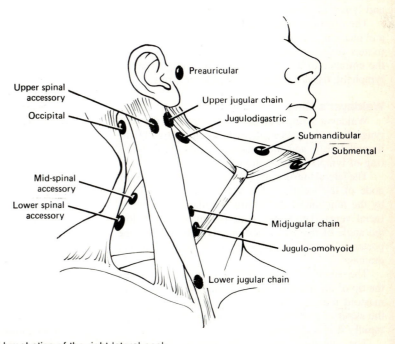

Figure 10–5. Schematic illustration of lymphatics of the right lateral neck.

meatus. They are frequently enlarged in infectious mononucleosis.

The **preauricular (anterior auricular) lymph nodes** are situated just anterior to the tragus. This positioning is so constant that a swelling not exactly in this position is not due to involvement of a lymph node. The nodes lie superficial to the external capsule of the parotid gland. They drain the skin covering the pinna and a segment of the temporal region of the scalp. They also drain the conjunctiva and enlarge in viral conjunctivitis. They are on occasion mistaken for a tumor mass within the superficial lobe of the parotid gland.

The **parotid group of lymph nodes** is situated both within the substance of the parotid gland and just external to its deep capsule, where the nodes lie between the deep surface of the gland and the lateral pharyngeal wall. The deep group of parotid lymph nodes drains the nasopharynx and the mucous membrane lining of the nose. The superficial or intra-parotid nodes receive lymph from the eyelids, the anterior and temporal segments of the scalp, and the external auditory meatus.

The **facial lymph nodes** are divided into superficial and deep groups. The **superficial group** consists of (1) the infraorbital lymph nodes just inferior to the orbit; (2) the buccal lymph nodes, which lie on the buccinator muscle just lateral to the lateral commissure of the mouth; and (3) the mandibular lymph nodes, which lie on the mandible just anterior to the masseter muscle, in close proximity to the anterior facial artery and vein as those vessels cross the mandible. The superficial group of facial lymph nodes receives lymph from the conjunctiva, the eyelids, the nose, and the cutaneous surface of the cheek.

The **deep group of facial lymph nodes** lies close to the internal maxillary vessels and to the internal pterygoid muscle. The nodes drain the temporal fossa, the infratemporal fossa, the deep structures of the nose, and portions of the pharynx.

The **lingual nodes** lie on the posterior third of the tongue deep to the genioglossus muscle. Lymph from the tongue flows to these glands.

The **retropharyngeal nodes** lie dorsal to the superior segment of the pharynx, just anterior to the arch of the atlas (C1). They lie within the buccopharyngeal fascia and drain the nasal cavity, the nasopharynx, and the auditory tube.

The **submental lymph nodes** lie in the submental area on the medial segment of the mylohyoid muscle. They drain the central portion of the lower lip, the anterior portion of the floor of the mouth, the anterior hairy portion of the chin, the lower incisor teeth and their adjacent gingiva, and the tip of the tongue. The submental nodes drain into the submandibular nodes and across the midline to the contralateral submental group of nodes.

The **submandibular lymph nodes** lie in the submandibular area superficial to the hyoglossus and medial pharyngeal constrictor muscles. The nodes lie deep to the investing fascia of the neck and either close to or actually within the submandibular salivary gland.

➠ *Removal of submandibular salivary gland in suprahyoid lymphatic dissection. In radical neck dissection for cancer, the submandibular salivary gland must be removed along with the adjacent submandibular lymph nodes, since involved nodes frequently lie within the gland substance. Additionally, since there is cross-midline drainage in the submental area, both suprahyoid areas must be cleaned out in a unilateral lymphatic neck dissection.*

The submandibular lymph nodes drain the side of the nose, the inner canthus of the eye, the cheek, the angle of the mouth, the whole of the upper lip, the outer portion of the lower lip, the gingiva, the lateral surfaces of the tongue, and the submental lymph nodes. In addition, many of the nodes of the superficial chain drain into the submandibular nodes before they finally drain into the deep cervical chain.

The **superficial cervical lymph nodes** lie on the external surface of the sternocleidomastoid muscle just inferior to the parotid gland and close to the external jugular vein. They drain the parotid area and the lobe of the ear. Their efferents empty into the deep cervical chain.

The **anterior cervical nodes and the superficial cervical nodes** (Fig 10–8) lie near the midline of the neck ventral to the larynx and the trachea. They consist of a superficial and a deep set of nodes. The superficial set lies along the course of the anterior jugular veins and drains only the skin of the neck. The deep set consists of the infrahyoid lymph nodes, which lie on the thyrohyoid membrane and drain the superior half of the larynx; and the prelaryngeal lymph nodes, which lie on the cricothyroid membrane and drain the inferior half of the larynx. The afferent channels to these glands pass through small foramens in the cricothyroid membrane. The prelaryngeal lymph nodes are often the first to become enlarged in cancer of the larynx, and if they are palpable that diagnosis should be suspected. The prelaryngeal lymph nodes also drain the inferior segment of the thyroid gland. The pretracheal lymph nodes lie alongside the inferior thyroid veins on the ventral surface of the trachea and drain lymph from the lower half of the thyroid and larynx, and from the trachea. The efferents from the anterior cervical nodes drain into the deep cervical nodes.

B. Deep Cervical Chain: The deep chain of cervical lymph nodes consists of a large number of lymph nodes that lie deep to the sternocleidomastoid muscle and in close relationship to the internal jugular vein within the carotid sheath. Some of the most inferior nodes project laterally beyond the sternocleidomastoid muscle, thus occupying the posterior triangle of the neck. These lymph nodes lie adjacent to the inferior

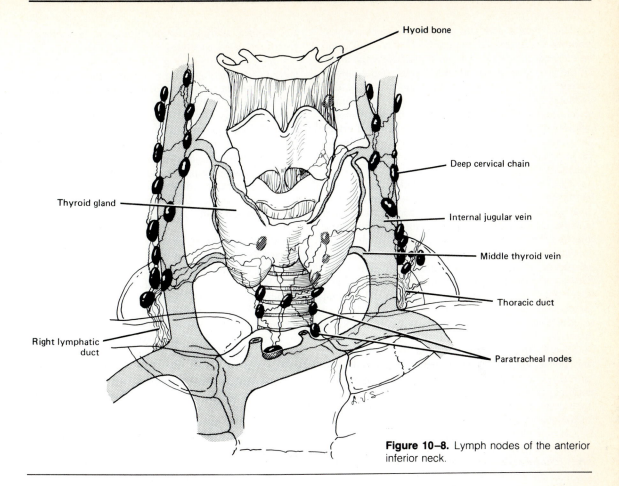

Figure 10–8. Lymph nodes of the anterior inferior neck.

trunk of the brachial plexus, the subclavian artery and vein, the dome of the pleura, and the highest nodes of the axilla. Some of the highest deep cervical lymph nodes project forward into the submandibular area. They thus become related to some superficial cervical nodes in the submandibular area. Several of the deep cervical nodes lie in the groove between the trachea and the esophagus close to the ascending recurrent laryngeal nerve and the parathyroid glands. These are called the paratracheal or tracheoesophageal lymph nodes. The thyroid and parathyroid lymph nodes drain into the paratracheal nodes, and on occasion these glands contain the first malignant metastases from the thyroid and parathyroid glands.

➠ ***Deep cervical radical neck dissection.*** *Removal of the entire deep cervical chain of lymphatics and lymph nodes as well as the overlying sternocleidomastoid muscle and the adjacent internal jugular vein is part of radical neck dissection. The close proximity of the chain to the deep surface of the sternocleidomastoid muscle and the internal jugular vein may cause these structures to become adherent to the deep vertical lymph chain. The procedure accompanies or*

follows removal of the primary focus of cancer of the head or neck. In recent years, "berry picking" of the involved cervical nodes has been used in the treatment of papillary and follicular carcinoma of the thyroid with cervical metastases. This procedure calls for the removal only of grossly involved nodes and then careful observation and reoperation if further nodal involvement occurs. Care must be taken not to injure the inferior laryngeal, hypoglossal, vagus, and accessory nerves, which are in close proximity to the tissues removed in radical neck dissection.

➠ ***The dome of the pleura.*** *In performing radical neck dissection, the surgeon must not injure the dome of the pleura while attempting to remove the nodes in the inferior lateral segment of the subclavian area.*

➠ ***Virchow's node.*** *The presence of Virchow's node, palpable just superior to the middle third of the left clavicle and close to the termination of the major thoracic duct, suggests a tumor below the level of the diaphragm, particularly a tumor of the stomach or lower esophagus.*

Three lymph nodes of the deep vertical cervical group deserve special mention: (1) the main node of the palatine tonsil, which lies just below the angle of the jaw between the internal jugular and common facial veins; (2) the main node of the tongue, which is situated at the level of the bifurcation of the common carotid artery; and (3) the supraomohyoid lymph node, which lies superficial to the common carotid artery just above its omohyoid crossing. This node plays an important role in lymph drainage from the tongue, especially from its apex.

The deep cervical nodes eventually receive—directly or indirectly—all of the lymph from the entire head and neck. Lymph from the deep cervical chain is collected finally into a single major lymphatic trunk that lies low in the neck: the jugular lymph trunk. On the right side, this trunk drains into the junction of the right subclavian and internal jugular veins. On the left side, the trunk enters the thoracic duct just before it empties into the subclavian and internal jugular venous junction.

Under normal circumstances, with no abnormal blockage of lymph channels, there is little or no cross-midline lymphatic drainage in the neck. However, this rule is violated in the submental area and quite probably within the thyroid gland as it straddles the midline of the neck. Midline areas of the tongue may drain to the deep chain of nodes on either side of the neck.

➠ *Thoracic duct trauma. Following deep wounds of the left lower neck or extensive surgery in that area, a lymphatic fistula may develop secondary to transection of the cervical portion of the thoracic duct. A right thoracic duct is rarely transected. The left thoracic duct fistula complicates wound healing and is a postoperative nuisance. Severe limitation of the diet with carefully controlled intravenous feedings usually results in spontaneous closure of the fistula.*

THE VAGUS NERVE

The vagus nerve runs the entire length of the neck after leaving the jugular foramen of the skull. Just after its exit via the jugular foramen of the skull, along with the accessory nerve, it presents 2 ganglia, the superior and inferior vagal ganglia, which are the sensory ganglia of the organs supplied by the nerve. The superior ganglion is quite small and actu-

ally is placed within the jugular foramen. The inferior ganglion (ganglion nodosum), which lies about 1.5 cm distal to the superior ganglion, is spindle-shaped and must be distinguished from the superior cervical ganglion of the autonomic chain that lies nearby at the level of C2–3. The vagus is contained within the carotid sheath as it descends in the neck. It is joined by the cranial segment of the accessory nerve just caudad to the inferior vagal ganglion. Within the carotid sheath, the vagus lies deep to both the internal jugular vein and the internal and common carotid arteries. In the root of the neck, the vagus lies ventral to the subclavian artery and dorsal to the subclavian vein.

Cervical Branches of the Vagus Nerve

In the **jugular fossa,** the vagus gives off a meningeal branch to the dura of the posterior fossa and an auricular branch to both the skin of the posterior ear and to the posterior segment of the external acoustic meatus.

In the **neck,** the vagus gives off (1) pharyngeal branches that participate in formation of the pharyngeal plexus, branches of which run to the pharynx and the soft palate; (2) nerves to the carotid body from the pharyngeal plexus and the superior laryngeal nerve; (3) the superior laryngeal nerve, which provides sensation to the mucous membrane of the larynx and motor power to the cricothyroid muscle; (4) the 2 superior cardiac branches, one emerging from the vagus high in the neck and the other at the level of the first rib; (5) the right inferior laryngeal nerve, providing motor power to the muscles of the right side of the larynx (see Chapter 8); and (6) tracheal and pharyngeal branches to the mucous membranes and muscle coats of the trachea and the pharynx.

➠ *Injury to the vagus nerve and its superior laryngeal branch. Because of its relatively deep position in the neck, lying under the sternocleidomastoid muscle and protected by the carotid sheath, the vagus nerve is seldom transected as a result of cervical trauma. However, its superior laryngeal branch is occasionally injured in vascular procedures performed near the bifurcation of the common carotid artery, and the external motor branch to the cricothyroid muscle is on occasion injured during mobilization of the superior pole of a high-lying thyroid gland.*

Paravertebral, Posterior, & Subclavian Regions of the Neck

11

PARAVERTEBRAL REGION

The paravertebral region of the neck lies between the cervical vertebrae and the prevertebral fascia. It should be studied in relationship to the adjacent visceral compartment of the neck, which contains the pharynx and the cervical esophagus, the cervical sympathetic chain and its ganglia, the inferior thyroid artery, the vertebral artery, and the recurrent laryngeal nerves. All of these structures lie ventral to the prevertebral fascia.

➠ *Protective role of prevertebral fascia. Because of the toughness of the prevertebral fascia, inflammatory processes arising dorsal to it seldom spread into the visceral compartment of the neck. However, on occasion they may spread laterally and inferiorly within the sheath of the subclavian artery and the axillary artery. The subclavian arterial sheath is derived from the prevertebral fascia and surrounds the vessel as it passes laterally and inferiorly from behind the anterior scalene muscle. A subsheath abscess may point either in the inferior portion of the posterior triangle of the neck or in the axilla or near the midpoint of the arm where the arterial sheath fuses tightly with the adventitia of the brachial artery.*

MUSCLES OF THE PARAVERTEBRAL AREA OF THE NECK
(Fig 11–1)

The muscular floor of the paravertebral area is composed of the following muscles: medially, the longus colli and longus capitis muscles; and laterally, the anterior, middle, and posterior scalene muscles. The latter 2 muscles are frequently described as being part of the subclavian area.

The 2 **longus colli muscles** lie just anterior to the anterior longitudinal ligament of the vertebral column. The entire muscle stretches from C1 to T3. Each muscle is divided into 3 segments. The superior oblique segment arises from the transverse processes of C3–5 and inserts into the anterior arch of C1 (the atlas). The inferior oblique segment arises from the bodies of C1–3 and inserts into the anterior tubercles of C5 and C6. The vertical segment arises from the bodies of C5–7 and T1–3 and inserts into the bodies of C2–4. The longus colli muscles flex the head and neck and rotate the cervical vertebral column; they are supplied by spinal nerves C2 to T1.

The **longus capitis muscle** arises from the transverse processes of vertebrae C3–6. It runs medially and superiorly to insert into the undersurface of the occipital bone. It also is a flexor of the head and neck. It is supplied by spinal nerves C1–3.

The **anterior scalene muscle,** the closest to the vertebral column of the 3 scalenes, arises from the transverse processes of C3–6 and descends obliquely. It inserts by a narrow flat tendon into the scalene tubercle on the first rib. The muscle is deeply situated in the neck under the cover of the sternocleidomastoid muscle and just dorsal to the prevertebral fascia.

The **middle scalene muscle** arises from the transverse processes of the lower 6 cervical vertebrae and descends obliquely. It is lateral and dorsal to the anterior scalene muscle. It inserts via a broad attachment into the first rib, lateral to the scalene tubercle. The insertion is just lateral to the groove made by the subclavian artery as it passes from the neck into the axilla. Since the anterior scalene muscle arises from the anterior tubercles of the transverse processes of the lower cervical vertebrae and the middle scalene muscle arises from the posterior processes, a cleft exists between the anterior and middle scalene muscles. Projecting inferiorly and laterally through this cleft are the 3 trunks of the brachial plexus and the subclavian artery.

The smaller **posterior scalene muscle** has a tendinous origin from the transverse processes of the lower 2 or 3 cervical vertebrae and inserts by a thin tendon into the second rib.

The 3 scalene muscles can elevate the first and second ribs, raising the upper chest wall and acting as accessory muscles of respiration. When acting from below and unilaterally, the scalenes flex the neck to the ipsilateral side. When both sides act together from below, they flex the cervical vertebrae forward upon the thoracic cage. They are supplied by branches from the ventral rami of the lower 3 cervical nerves.

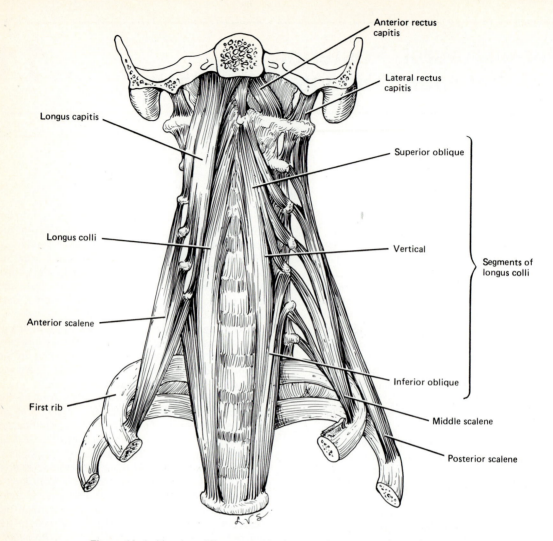

Figure 11–1. Muscles of the prevertebral or anterior vertebral area of the neck.

THE CERVICAL PORTION OF THE SYMPATHETIC CHAIN (Fig 11–2)

The cervical segment of the sympathetic trunk consists of 3 ganglia and their intervening chain. It lies just ventral to the prevertebral fascia and just medial to the transverse processes of the cervical vertebrae. The chain and ganglia lie immediately dorsal to the thick carotid sheath, almost embedded in it. The trunk is a continuation of the thoracic sympathetic chain.

The **superior cervical ganglion** (the largest of the three) is reddish and fusiform and lies at the level of C2 and C3. It is believed to arise from coalescence of the 4 ganglia corresponding to the upper 4 cervical nerves. It lies dorsal to the internal carotid artery and the internal jugular vein and just ventral to the prevertebral fascia covering the longus capitis

muscle. The ganglion must be distinguished from the nearby ganglion nodosum of the vagus nerve. The superior cardiac nerve branches from the superior cervical ganglion, and as it descends it sends gray rami communicantes to spinal nerves C1–4. The superior ganglion also gives off the internal carotid nerve, branches to the second, third, and fourth spinal nerves, pharyngeal branches, branches to the external carotid artery, and branches to the internal carotid plexus.

The **middle cervical ganglion** is about 3 mm in diameter and the smallest of the three. On occasion it may be absent. It is located at the level of C6, the level of the cricoid cartilage. It lies just ventral to the bend of the inferior thyroid artery. The middle cervical ganglion gives off the middle cardiac nerve, gray rami communicantes to nerves C5–6, and sympathetics to the thyroid.

The **inferior cervical ganglion** is clinically the most important. It lies between the transverse process

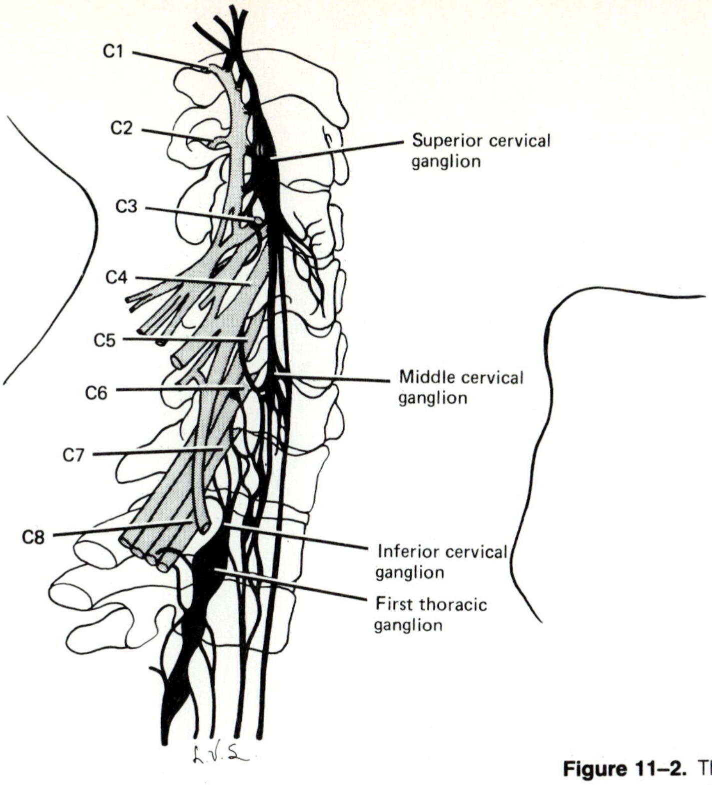

Figure 11–2. The cervical portion of the sympathetic trunk.

of C7 and the first rib and is difficult to expose via a cervical incision. It is situated just medial to the descending branch of the costocervical branch of the subclavian artery. The ganglion is irregular in shape and often fused to the first thoracic sympathetic ganglion. The inferior cervical ganglion gives off the inferior cardiac nerve and the vertebral nerve, which ascends through foramens of the transverse processes of the cervical vertebrae along with the vertebral artery. It sends gray rami to nerves C7 and C8. None of the 3 cervical ganglia receive white rami from the cervical nerves.

The entire cervical sympathetic system gives off branches to the great vessels supplying the head, the neck, the intracranial area, and the upper extremities. The nerves help to maintain tone in these vessels.

➡ ***Horner's syndrome.*** *Horner's syndrome is evidenced by a constricted pupil, ptosis of the upper eyelid, enophthalmos, and flushing and dryness of the face ipsilaterally. It results from disruption of the autonomic supply to the eye and lateral face. The syndrome follows injuries to or pressure upon the cervical sympathetic chain in the mid and lower neck. The syndrome may be secondary to trauma, tumor, or degenerative neurologic disease. It may follow gunshot or stab wounds to the lower neck.*

➡ ***Removal of ganglia of the upper extremity.*** *In treating vasospastic disease of the upper extremity (Raynaud's disease), the inferior cervical and upper thoracic ganglia are on occasion removed to alleviate severe arm or hand pain. The descending branch of the costocervical artery, lying close to the superior thoracic ganglion, is often ligated to facilitate stellate ganglion removal. A low cervical or axillary approach to the ganglion is used.*

THE PHRENIC NERVE (Fig 11–3)

The phrenic nerve is 2 parts motor to one part sensory fibers. It arises in the cervical plexus from spinal nerves C3–5 and runs obliquely from lateral to medial across the anterior surface of the anterior scalene muscle. It lies deep to the sternocleidomastoid muscle, the lateral belly of the omohyoid muscle, the transverse cervical and suprascapular vessels, and the prevertebral fascia. As it descends into the mediastinum, it passes ventral to the subclavian vein. It crosses the internal mammary artery at the thoracic inlet—a constant anatomic relationship. Within the thorax, the phrenic nerve descends almost vertically, lying ventral to the root of the lung and between the pericardium and the mediastinal pleura. Upon

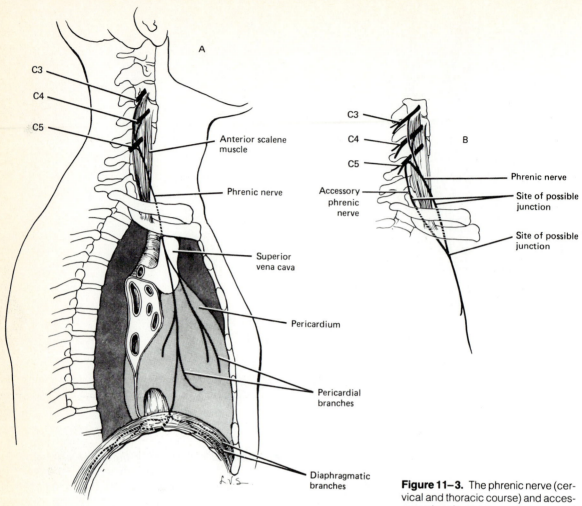

Figure 11–3. The phrenic nerve (cervical and thoracic course) and accessory phrenic nerve.

reaching the diaphragm, the nerve divides into motor branches for the ventrolateral diaphragmatic musculature and sensory branches for both surfaces of the diaphragm.

The phrenic nerve is longer on the left side than on the right, since the left diaphragm is lower than the right. In the neck, the left phrenic nerve is closely related to the thoracic duct, which must be searched for and dissected free in procedures to section the phrenic nerve for the purpose of paralyzing the diaphragm.

ACCESSORY PHRENIC NERVE

In 10–15% of persons, an accessory phrenic nerve is found. It may be a thin filament originating from C5 that joins the major phrenic nerve trunk in the lower neck; it may originate from C5, pass into the thorax, and innervate the diaphragm independently; or it may be a branch of C3 joining the phrenic nerve trunk high in the thorax.

The presence of an accessory phrenic nerve helps to explain residual diaphragmatic movement after the major trunk has been pinched or sectioned. Alternatively, such continued movement may be attibutable to diaphragmatic innervation from lower intercostal and upper lumbar segmental nerves.

THE POSTERIOR CERVICAL TRIANGLE
(Fig 11–4)

The posterior triangle of the neck is bounded anteriorly by the posterior border of the sternocleidomastoid muscle, posteriorly by the anterior border of the trapezius muscle, inferiorly by the clavicle, and superiorly by the converging trapezius and sternocleidomastoid muscles. The omohyoid muscle divides the posterior cervical triangle into a large superior and a smaller inferior segment. The superior segment is clinically unimportant. The infraomohyoid segment constitutes

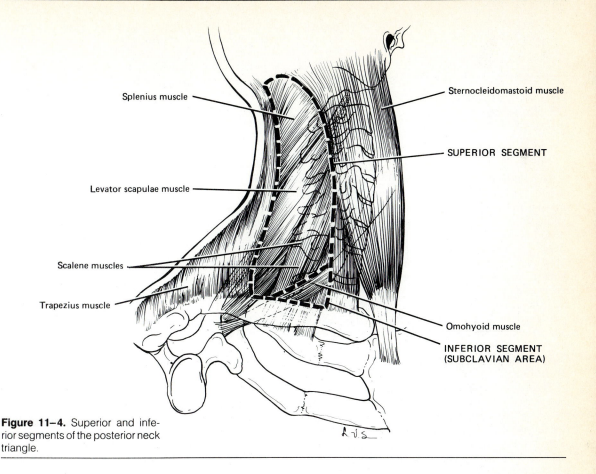

Figure 11–4. Superior and inferior segments of the posterior neck triangle.

the supraclavicular area of the neck and is of great clinical importance.

From medial to lateral, the floor of the posterior triangle of the neck is formed by the anterior, middle, and posterior scalene muscles and the levator scapulae. The splenius capitis and semispinalis muscles contribute to the floor of the triangle.

The **levator scapulae** arises from the transverse processes of C1–4 and inserts along the vertebral border of the scapula. It forms the dorsolateral floor of the posterior triangle of the neck. It elevates and aids in lateral rotation of the scapula. It is supplied by branches of C3 and C4 via the cervical plexus and by a branch of C5.

The **splenius muscle** of the head arises from the nuchal ligament and from the spinous processes of C7–T3. Its fibers run superiorly to insert into the mastoid process of the temporal bone and into the superior nuchal line of the occiput. The muscle pulls the head and neck in a dorsal and lateral direction. Both muscles acting together aid in extending the head and neck. The splenius muscle is supplied by lower cervical nerves.

The **semispinalis muscle** of the head arises by tendinous slips from the transverse processes of C7–T7 and from the articular processes of C4–6. It passes superiorly to insert on the occiput. The semispinalis

usually lies deep to the splenius capitis. It rotates the head to the contralateral side and aids in extension of the head. The muscle is supplied by cervical nerves.

BLOOD VESSELS & NERVES
(Figs 10–2 and 10–4)

The superior four-fifths of the posterior cervical triangle contains some major arteries and veins, parts of the cervical plexus derived from C1–4, and a segment of the accessory nerve.

The **accessory nerve** crosses the posterior triangle, appearing at the posterior border of the sternocleidomastoid muscle. As it crosses the area obliquely, it receives some branches from spinal nerve C2. It then passes beneath the trapezius muscle, which it supplies, and sends branches to the sternocleidomastoid muscle.

➥ *Trauma to accessory nerve. The accessory nerve lies in a relatively superficial position lateral to the sternocleidomastoid muscle and is often injured. Injury can occur during radical neck dissection or deep lymph node biopsy or during removal of tumor masses in the postero-superior neck. If the trapezius loses its acces-*

sory nerve supply, the arm cannot be completely abducted.

THE CERVICAL PLEXUS OF NERVES
(Figs 11–5 and 11–6)

The cervical plexus is made up of the anterior divisions of spinal nerves C1–4. Nerves C2–4 divide into superior and inferior branches, the branches reuniting to form 3 loops. The accompanying sympathetic rami may join either the primary nerve or the loops. The plexus is situated at the level of vertebrae C1–4 and covered by the upper half of the sternocleidomastoid muscle and by the prevertebral fascia. It receives fibers from cranial nerves X, XI, and XII and is joined by sympathetic rami. The major nerves that leave the cervical plexus may be classified as cutaneous (superficial) or muscular (deep) branches.

Cutaneous (Superficial) Branches

The **lesser occipital nerve** supplies the skin behind the external ear. The **great auricular nerve** supplies the skin of the face over the parotid gland. The posterior division of the great auricular nerve supplies the skin over the mastoid process of the temporal bone and the lobe of the ear. The **anterior cutaneous nerve** of the neck supplies the skin of the anterior and lateral portions of the neck. The 3 **supraclavicular nerves** (medial, intermediate, and lateral) supply sensation to the shawl area of the shoulder.

Muscular (Deep) Branches

Branches extend to the rectus capitis anterior and lateralis, to the longus colli and longus capitis, and to the musculature that attaches to the hyoid bone. The C1 branches to the geniohyoid and thyrohyoid and to the superior belly of the omohyoid reach these muscles via the hypoglossal nerve. The ansa cervicalis consists of fibers from the cervical plexus (C1, C2, and C3). C1 fibers travel on the hypoglossal nerve and then loop inferiorly into the neck to supply the omohyoid, sternohyoid, and sternothyroid muscles. They lie superficial to the carotid sheath.

The phrenic nerve is illustrated and described in Fig 11–3 and its accompanying text.

Deep muscular branches of the cervical plexus run to the sternocleidomastoid, trapezius, levator scapulae, and middle scalene muscles.

THE SUPRACLAVICULAR AREA
(See also Chapter 10.)

The inferior segment of the posterior cervical triangle, above the clavicle, is called the supraclavicular area. From medial to lateral, the floor of the area is formed by the longus colli muscle, the 3 scalene muscles, and the levator scapulae. These muscles all lie deep to the prevertebral fascia.

The medial segment of the supraclavicular area is the vertebral triangle, formed by the longus colli medially, the anterior scalene anterolaterally, and the clavicle inferiorly. The entire vertebral triangle is covered by the sternocleidomastoid muscle.

The lateral aspect of the supraclavicular area is more superficial and is bounded by the clavicle inferiorly, the sternocleidomastoid medially, and the omohyoid superiorly.

The major structures in the supraclavicular area include the subclavian artery and vein and their branches, the vagus and phrenic nerves, the lower segment of the cervical sympathetic chain, the internal jugular vein, and the left and right thoracic ducts. The subclavian artery dominates the supraclavicular region of the neck.

BLOOD VESSELS, LYMPHATICS, & NERVES

Arteries
(Fig 11–6)

The cervical portion of the **subclavian artery** is divided into 3 portions by the anterior scalene muscle. The first portion of the artery lies medial, the second portion deep, and the third portion lateral to the muscle. The origins and primary courses of the subclavian artery differ on the right and left sides of the body.

A. First Portion of the Subclavian Artery: The **right subclavian artery** originates from the innominate artery high in the mediastinum behind the right sternoclavicular joint. Together with the common carotid artery, the right subclavian artery enters the visceral compartment of the neck. It first crosses the inferior segment of the vertebral triangle, lying deep to the sternocleidomastoid muscle and separated from it by the subclavian and internal jugular veins. In the medial segment of the vertebral triangle, it is more superficial and related ventrally to the phrenic and vagus nerves, the loop of the cervical sympathetic chain, and the internal jugular and vertebral veins.

As the right subclavian artery crosses the vagus nerve, the recurrent laryngeal nerve branches off and runs dorsal to the artery. The phrenic nerve crosses the artery ventrally near the border of the scalene muscle. Just inferior to the first portion of the right subclavian artery is the dome of the right pleura, which separates the artery from the apex of the lung, which may be grooved by the vessel. Dorsal to the first part of the subclavian artery are parts of the cervical sympathetic trunk, the longus colli muscle, and the first thoracic vertebra.

The right subclavian artery ascends only slightly higher than the superior border of the clavicle, the height varying with the position of the arm. This is important in positioning the arm for surgery on the lower neck. If the arm is raised above the horizontal,

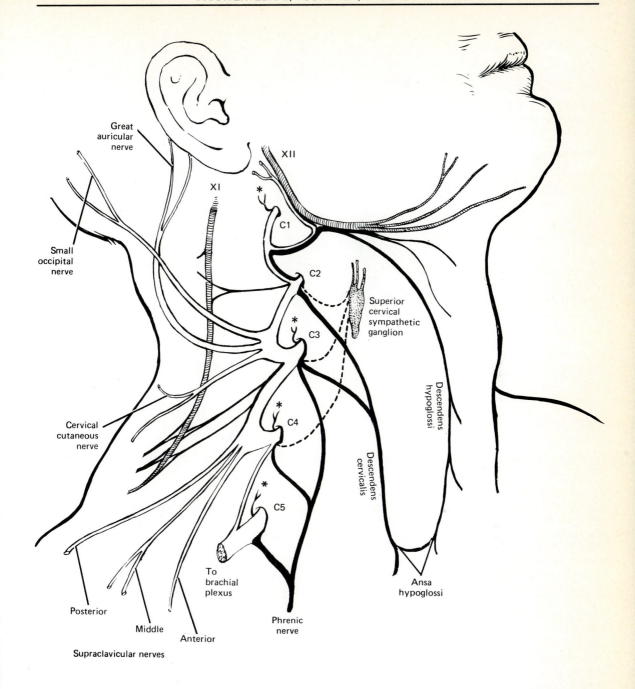

Figure 11–5. The cervical plexus. (Modified and reproduced, with permission, from Chusid JG: *Correlative Neuroanatomy & Functional Neurology,* 19th ed. Lange, 1985.)

the artery disappears behind the clavicle. If the arm hangs down alongside the body, the vessel becomes a true lower neck structure.

The right lymphatic duct (when present) lies ventral to the right subclavian artery just before the duct empties into the right internal jugular vein.

The **left subclavian artery** arises from the arch of the thoracic aorta at the level of T4, on planes

dorsal and lateral to the takeoff of the left common carotid artery. It rises to just below the left sternoclavicular joint. Because of its level of origin, the left subclavian artery has a superior mediastinal as well as a cervical course. In the superior mediastinum, the left vagus and phrenic nerves are ventral to the artery. The left common carotid artery lies medial to the left subclavian artery. In the lower left neck,

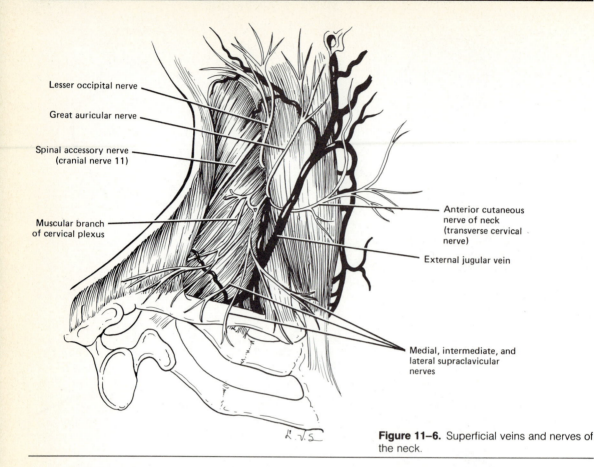

Figure 11–6. Superficial veins and nerves of the neck.

the left internal jugular, vertebral, and brachiocephalic veins all lie ventral to the left subclavian artery. In the mediastinum, the left subclavian artery is related dorsally to the esophagus, the left recurrent laryngeal nerve, the inferior cervical ganglion of the sympathetic chain, and the longus colli muscle. The thoracic duct crosses ventral to the artery as it passes laterally to enter the junction of the internal jugular and subclavian veins. The left apical pleura and the apex of the left lung lie behind the artery. The course of the left subclavian artery is almost twice as long as that of the right subclavian vessel, and as a consequence the left subclavian artery is correspondingly more vulnerable to injury. As the left subclavian artery reaches its highest thoracic level, it lies under the origins of the sternocleidomastoid, sternohyoid, and sternothyroid muscles.

The 4 or 5 major branches of each of the subclavian arteries arise from the first (or sometimes the second) portion of the vessel.

The **vertebral artery** arises from the posterosuperior aspect of the subclavian artery near the medial border of the base of the vertebral triangle. It ascends in the vertebral triangle between the longus colli medially and the anterior scalene laterally. It is surrounded at its origin by a plexus of nerve fibers derived from the inferior cervical ganglion of the cervical sympa-

thetic trunk. The internal jugular vein and the vertebral veins lie ventral to the vertebral artery. The inferior thyroid artery and the left thoracic duct cross the artery from lateral to medial as they lie ventral to it. Lying dorsal to the origin of the vertebral artery is the transverse process of C7, the cervical sympathetic chain, and the inferior cervical ganglion. The vertebral artery at its origin lies ventral to the prevertebral fascia, but during its ascent in the vertebral triangle to the level of vertebra C6 it pierces the fascia to reach the transverse process of vertebra C6. The vertebral artery then ascends through foramens in the transverse processes of vertebrae C6–C1. It enters the vertebral canal in the base of the skull and joins with the vertebral artery of the contralateral side to form the basilar artery. The vertebral artery and vein play important roles in maintenance of intracranial arterial and venous circulation following ligation or occlusion of the internal carotid artery or the internal jugular vein.

➡ *Ligation of the vertebral artery. The vertebral artery can be ligated in the space between its point of origin and where it enters the foramen of the transverse process of C6. In this segment, it lies dorsal to the prevertebral fascia and is surrounded by a plexus of autonomic nerves. Injection of the vertebral artery with opaque medium may aid in localization of an intracranial aneurysm or tumor.*

The **internal mammary** or **internal thoracic artery** arises from the inferior surface of the subclavian artery, opposite the origin of the thyrocervical trunk. It descends through the thorax, lying dorsal to the costal cartilages of the upper 6 ribs just lateral to their junction with the sternum. Just above the superior surface of the diaphragm, it terminates by dividing into the musculophrenic and superior epigastric arteries. At the point where the internal thoracic artery enters the chest cavity, it is crossed from lateral to medial by the phrenic nerve.

The **thyrocervical trunk** is a short artery that arises from the superior surface of the subclavian artery close to the medial border of the anterior scalene muscle. Almost immediately after its takeoff, it divides into 3 branches. The **suprascapular (transverse) artery** runs laterally dorsal to the clavicle. It crosses ventral to the anterior scalene muscle, the phrenic nerve, the subclavian artery, and the inferior trunk of the brachial plexus. The artery runs deep to the inferior belly of the omohyoid muscle, then enters the supraspinous fossa of the scapula and descends dorsally to the neck of the scapula through the greater scapular notch. It finally reaches the infraspinous fossa, where it anastomoses with the circumflex scapular artery, the descending branch of the transverse cervical artery, and the thoracoacromial trunk of the axillary artery, thus providing collateral circulation around the shoulder joint.

The **transverse cervical artery** also passes transversely across the lower neck from medial to lateral. It lies dorsal to the posterior belly of the omohyoid muscle but ventral to the phrenic nerve and the scalene muscles. It lies ventral to or entwined among the 2 lower trunks of the brachial plexus. When it reaches the trapezius muscle, it divides into superficial and deep branches. The superficial branch distributes branches to the trapezius and neighboring muscles and lymph nodes. The deep branch passes beneath the levator scapulae muscle to the superior angle of the scapula. It then descends deep to the rhomboid muscles along the vertebral border of the scapula to its inferior angle.

The **inferior thyroid artery,** the terminal branch of the thyrocervical trunk, ascends in the vertebral triangle, just ventral to the prevertebral fascia. It rises toward the mid portion of the lateral lobe of the thyroid gland, then bends medially to run to the lower pole of the thyroid gland. The arterial bend is at the level of vertebra C6 and the cricoid cartilage. The vessel lies deep to the carotid sheath and the cervical autonomic chain but ventral to the vertebral artery and the longus colli muscle. While ascending, the artery gives off anterior laryngeal, tracheal, esophageal, ascending cervical, and **muscular branches.**

➠ *Ligation of the inferior thyroid artery. The preferred site for ligation of the inferior thyroid artery is either well distal to its bend at C6, after it has entered the substance of the lower pole of the thyroid gland, or just lateral to its point of entry into the gland. At these locations, there is less risk of damage to the inferior laryngeal nerve, which is close to the artery in the lower pole of the thyroid gland. Care must be taken to ligate the vessel distal to the takeoff of its parathyroid branches to avoid parathyroid infarction.*

The **costocervical trunk** arises from the subclavian artery just dorsal and medial to the medial border of the anterior scalene muscle. It passes initially in a dorsal direction and gives off its ascending branch, then turns abruptly toward the thorax and descends dorsally to the pleural cavity. At this point, the artery is called the highest intercostal artery. It continues to descend just ventral to the necks of the first and second ribs and just lateral to the junction of these 2 ribs with the upper 2 thoracic vertebrae. Near the necks of the first and second ribs, the vessel lies lateral to the stellate ganglion of the sympathetic chain, and in the operative approach to the ganglion it must be located and ligated. The highest intercostal artery supplies the first and second dorsal thoracic interspaces and lies medial to the anterior division of the first thoracic nerve.

B. Second Portion of the Subclavian Artery:
The second portion of the artery lies deep to the anterior scalene muscle and forms the apex of the superior arch of the vessel. It gives off no branches except occasionally the right costocervical trunk. In order to pass dorsally from the visceral compartment of the neck, the subclavian artery pierces the prevertebral fascia and picks up an external sheath from this fascia.

C. Third Portion of the Subclavian Artery:
The third portion of the subclavian artery runs inferiorly from the lateral margin of the anterior scalene muscle toward the first rib, where it enters the axilla proper as the axillary artery. There are usually no branches from the third segment of the subclavian artery, but the descending scapular (transverse cervical) artery may arise from it rather than as a branch of the thyrocervical trunk.

In the inferior lateral portion of the supraclavicular area of the neck, the subclavian artery is covered only by the skin, platysma, investing fascia, and a condensation of the visceral fascia and the prevertebral fascia into a single fascial layer. The vessel is crossed by the descending external jugular vein. Farther laterally, the artery lies dorsal to the clavicle and the subclavius muscle. The suprascapular vessels lie ventral to the artery. The most inferior trunk of the brachial plexus is placed between the artery and the middle scalene muscle. Superior and lateral to the artery are the superior and middle trunks of the bra-

12 The Pharynx & Cervical Esophagus

THE PHARYNX
(Figs 12–1, 12–2, & 12–3)

EMBRYOLOGY

A tubelike endodermal diverticulum derived from the roof of the yolk sac develops dorsal to the pericardial cavity and the septum transversum as the foregut. Its cranial portion becomes separated from the stomodeum by the buccopharyngeal membrane. The pharyngeal gut, or pharynx, extends from the buccopharyngeal membrane to the tracheobronchial diverticulum. At the end of the fourth fetal week, the buccopharyngeal membrane ruptures.

GROSS ANATOMY

The pharynx is the inferior continuation of the oral and nasal cavities. It begins at the superior epiglottic tip, just above the level of the hyoid bone, and ends at the level of vertebra C6 at the lower border of the cricoid cartilage, where it becomes the cervical esophagus. The pharynx lies just ventral to the vertebral column, separated from it only by the anterior longitudinal ligament, the longus colli muscles, and the alar and prevertebral fasciae. Just anterior to the superior segment of the pharynx is the laryngeal orifice, formed by the epiglottis and the aryepiglottic folds. Farther inferiorly, the larynx pushes dorsally into the pharynx and creates 2 pharyngeal fossae, one on each side of the laryngeal cavity. These are called the piriform fossae, or sinuses.

➠ *Foreign bodies in the piriform sinuses. Foreign bodies often find their way into the piriform sinuses of the larynx. Fish bones and chicken bones frequently lodge at these sites, causing pain and pharyngeal irritation. They are usually removed by direct laryngoscopy.*

The pharynx is lined with stratified squamous epithelium and possesses a thick fibrous submucosa. External to it are the pharyngeal muscles: the superior, middle, and inferior pharyngeal constrictors (Fig 12–

2). External to the muscular layer is a thin sheath of areolar tissue. There is no serous outer layer. The pharynx is wide at its inception; however, it narrows rapidly, and at the level of C6 it is only half as wide as at its beginning.

The musculature of the pharynx is composed of the 3 pharyngeal constrictor muscles, which are related to the dorsolateral surface of the organ. The quadrilateral **superior constrictor of the pharynx** is the thinnest. It arises from the inferior one-third of the medial pterygoid plate, the alveolar ridge of the mandible, and the side of the tongue. The fibers insert into the most superior segment of the central constrictor raphe and onto the pharyngeal spine of the occipital bone. The **middle constrictor of the pharynx** is a fan-shaped muscle that arises from the hyoid bone and the stylohyoid ligament. The fibers fan out posteriorly to insert into the median fibrous raphe of the pharynx, joining along that line with the contralateral median constrictor muscle. The **infe-**

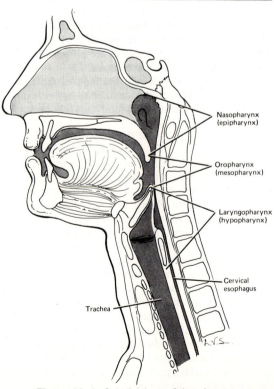

Nasopharynx (epipharynx)

Oropharynx (mesopharynx)

Laryngopharynx (hypopharynx)

Cervical esophagus

Trachea

Figure 12–1. Subdivisions of the pharynx.

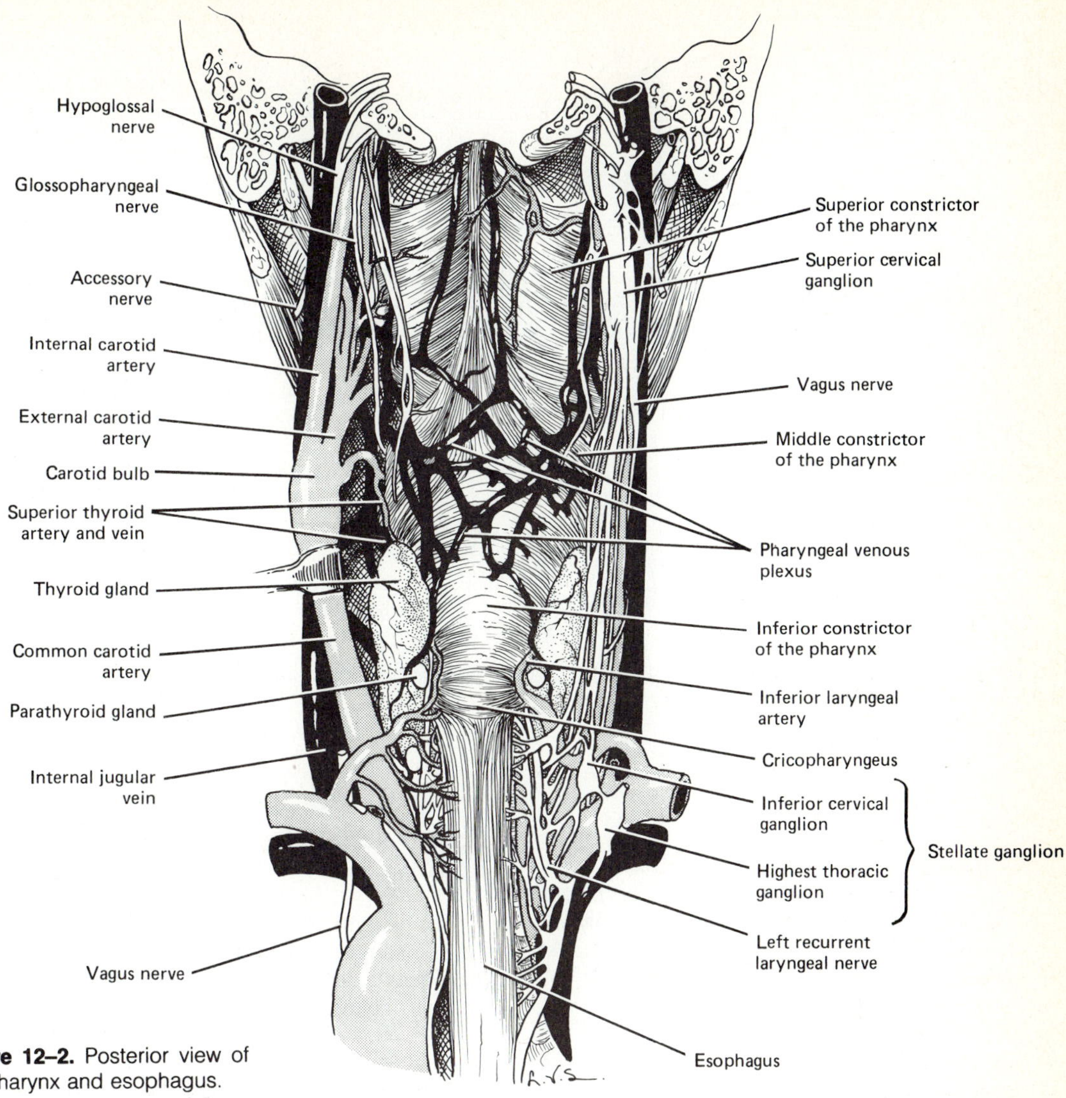
Hypoglossal nerve
Glossopharyngeal nerve
Accessory nerve
Internal carotid artery
External carotid artery
Carotid bulb
Superior thyroid artery and vein
Thyroid gland
Common carotid artery
Parathyroid gland
Internal jugular vein
Vagus nerve
Superior constrictor of the pharynx
Superior cervical ganglion
Vagus nerve
Middle constrictor of the pharynx
Pharyngeal venous plexus
Inferior constrictor of the pharynx
Inferior laryngeal artery
Cricopharyngeus
Inferior cervical ganglion
Highest thoracic ganglion
Stellate ganglion
Left recurrent laryngeal nerve
Esophagus

Figure 12–2. Posterior view of the pharynx and esophagus.

rior constrictor of the pharynx is the thickest. It arises from the cricoid cartilage, from the superior surface of the thyroid cartilage, and from the inferior cornu of that cartilage. Its fibers run posteromedially to insert into the central fibrous raphe of the pharynx. Its superior fibers run obliquely upward, while its most inferior fibers are transverse (cricopharyngeus muscle) and are continuous with esophageal sphincters.

➠ ***Traction and pulsion diverticula of the lower pharynx and upper esophagus.*** *Traction on the pharynx or esophagus by adjacent inflamed or cancerous tissues may cause* ***traction diverticula,*** *usually ventral or ventrolateral in position, which are composed of cell casts of the pharyngeal wall and are seldom large enough to cause symptoms.*

Pulsion diverticula *most commonly occur in the midline of the dorsal wall of the lower pharynx about 1 cm above the superior margin of the cervical esophagus. They usually originate at the point where the inferior oblique fibers of the inferior constrictor of the pharynx meet the transverse fibers of the cricopharyngeus segment of that muscle. There is normally a slight midline gap called "Killian's dehiscence" between these 2 sets of muscle fibers. Excessive enlargement of this midline dimple results in formation of a* ***Zenker's diverticulum,*** *the most common of the food-channel diverticula in the neck. The pharyngeal mucous membrane is gradually forced dorsally, forming a pouch just below the level of the oblique fibers of the inferior constrictor of the pharynx. The walls of the diverticulum consist of mucous membrane, submucosa, and an outer fibrous*

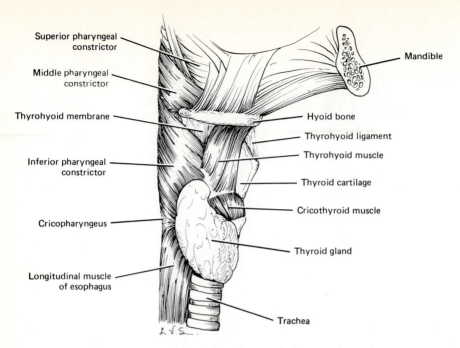

Figure 12–3. Right lateral view of external pharyngeal muscles.

layer derived from the external aponeurosis of the pharynx. As the left border of the esophagus protrudes from beneath the left border of the overlying trachea, the diverticulum, which is pulled inferiorly by the weight of the contents of the sac, nearly always descends in the left tracheoesophageal groove.

Symptoms of pharyngeal diverticula are (1) progressive difficulty in swallowing; (2) late regurgitation of ingested food or fluid into the oropharynx; and (3) late in the disease, symptoms suggesting esophagitis and upper esophageal stricture. Aspiration pneumonitis is common.

➡ ***Surgical repair of a pulsion pharyngeal diverticulum.*** *The surgical approach for repair of large pulsion diverticulum of the pharynx is usually a left-sided one, along the medial border of the sternocleidomastoid muscle, which is retracted laterally. The ribbon muscles, the thyroid gland, and the trachea are retracted medially, opening up the left tracheoesophageal groove. The left recurrent laryngeal nerve must be identified and retracted medially. The sac is dissected free from the surrounding tissues, dissected superiorly to its neck, ligated, and removed, and the pharynx is repaired. For small symptomatic sacs, the transverse fibers of the cricopharyngeus muscle are isolated, and sphincterotomy is performed.*

BLOOD VESSELS, LYMPHATICS, & NERVES

The pharynx receives its major blood supply from the ascending pharyngeal artery—a dorsal branch of the external carotid—and from the superior and inferior thyroid arteries. Venous return is into the internal jugular vein via a plexus of veins that lies in the external areolar sheath of the pharynx.

Lymphatic drainage from the pharynx is either into the retropharyngeal group of nodes or directly into the deep cervical chain above the level of the omohyoid crossing.

The pharyngeal branches of nerves IX and X give motor and sensory supply to the pharynx.

THE CERVICAL ESOPHAGUS

The cervical esophagus begins at the lower border of the pharynx at the level of C6 and the lower border of the cricoid cartilage and terminates at the top of the posterior mediastinum, where it becomes the thoracic esophagus. It descends along the ventral surface of the vertebral column, separated from the column by the prevertebral fascia, the alar fascia, the longus colli muscle, and the anterior longitudinal ligament of the vertebral column.

The esophagus presents 2 curvatures in the cervical region: (1) a lateral curvature, with its convexity facing to the left; and (2) an anteroposterior curvature, with a ventral convexity that conforms to the cervical spine. The lateral curvature is not corrected until the esophagus has reached the level of the fifth thoracic vertebra in the superior mediastinum. A knowledge of these curvatures makes passage of the esophageal endoscope easier for the physician and more comfortable for the patient.

At rest, the cervical esophagus presents merely as a longitudinal tube that is flattened in the anteroposterior plane. Both the pharynx and the cervical esophagus are loosely attached dorsally to the prevertebral fascia by loose sagittal septa which tend to funnel retropharyngeal and retroesophageal collections of fluid into the superior posterior mediastinum.

➠ ***Posterior septal attachments.*** *The posterior septal attachments of the esophagus permit considerable anterior and lateral mobility of the digestive tube at the cervical level and are of importance in cervical esophageal mobilization and anastomosis. They also tend to funnel esophageal contents toward the mediastinum following superior esophageal or inferior pharyngeal perforation.*

➠ ***Stenosis, atresia, and valve formation in the esophagus.*** *(Fig 12–4.) Failure of recanalization of all or a portion of the esophageal tube, failure of development of nutrient arteries to the esophagus, or pressure by an aberrant band upon a nutrient artery leading to the primitive esophagus may lead to esophageal stenosis, atresia, or valve formation. It is often accompanied by stenosis, atresia, and valve formation in the duodenum, by imperforate anus, and by agenesis of one or both of the lung buds. Early vomiting and marked salivation immediately after delivery are the first signs noted with anomalies of the esophageal lumen. The condition must be differentiated from tracheoesophageal fistula, annular pancreas, stenosis, atresia, or valve formation of the duodenum. The progress of an orogastric tube will be obstructed proximal to the stomach, and an x-ray with contrast medium verifies the presence of the obstruction and demonstrates its level.*

➠ ***Congenital tracheoesophageal fistulas.*** *(Fig 12–4.) Tracheoesophageal fistula is a congenital anomaly in which a fistula forms between the thoracic trachea or a major stem bronchus and the subjacent esophagus. The proximal segment of esophagus above the level of the fistula is usually connected to the distal esophagus by an area of atretic or stenotic esophagus.*

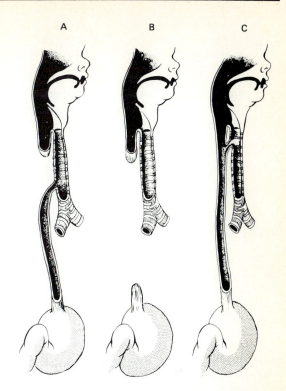

Figure 12–4. Congenital esophageal anomalies. The most common is esophageal atresia, with a tracheoesophageal fistula to the distal segment (**A**). The second most common is esophageal atresia without a tracheoesophageal fistula (**B**). Tracheoesophageal fistula without esophageal atresia (**C**) is the third most common anomaly.

However, there may be actual separation of the proximal and distal esophageal segments. Although there are multiple combinations of the congenital tracheoesophageal fistula, by far the most commonly encountered fistula presents with a short, blind superior esophageal pouch and a connection between the distal segment of the esophagus and the dorsal surface of the inferior segment of the trachea.

➠ ***Symptoms of congenital tracheoesophageal fistula.*** *Infants with congenital tracheoesophageal fistulas have dyspnea, marked salivation, cyanosis, and the presence of air in the proximal gastrointestinal tract despite failure of passage of an esophagogastric tube. Regurgitation of acid gastric juice into the pulmonary tree eventually results in pneumonia, which is life-threatening if early surgical repair is not done.*

➠ ***Surgical repair of tracheoesophageal fistula.*** *Surgical repair of a congenital tracheoesophageal fistula depends for success upon (1) early diagnosis; (2) correction of fluid, electrolyte, and blood imbalance in the infant; (3) use of antibiotics; and (4) the efficacy of positive pres-*

sure anesthesia. The operative procedure calls for closing of the fistulous opening into the trachea and construction of an anastomosis between the upper and lower esophageal segments. The operative procedure is performed through the right chest, preferably in an extrapleural fashion. In order to secure proper exposure, the azygos vein is ligated as it enters the superior vena cava. If such an anastomosis cannot be constructed, the proximal portion of the esophagus is made to empty as a cutaneous fistula in the lower left neck, and life is maintained by a feeding gastrostomy. The feeding gastrostomy is maintained for several weeks following the second attempt at anastomotic surgery, which is performed at about age 6–12 months.

➠ ***Enteric cysts of the esophagus.*** *A reduplication or enteric cyst of the esophagus may be found, usually in relationship to the distal thoracic esophagus but on rare occasions in the cervical region. Because such cysts are usually located 0.5–5 cm from the wall of the esophagus, they may complicate thoracic tumor diagnosis. Ultimate diagnosis may rest upon the finding of esophageal muscle fibers in the cyst wall.*

ANATOMIC FEATURES OF THE CERVICAL ESOPHAGUS (Fig 12–5)

Relations

Ventrally, the cervical esophagus is closely attached by loose areolar tissue to the trachea and to multiple small blood vessels. Since the cervical esophagus curves gently to the left of the midline of the neck, it is also related ventrally to the dorsal surface of the left lobe of the thyroid gland, the left recurrent laryngeal nerve, the left parathyroid glands, and the left inferior thyroid artery. Laterally, the esophagus is related to the neurovascular bundle (particularly on the left side), the recurrent laryngeal nerves, the cervical sympathetic chain, and the descending arm of the inferior thyroid artery. Low in the neck, it is adjacent to the thoracic duct. Dorsally, the esophagus is related to the alar and prevertebral fasciae.

➠ ***Pressure of thyroid and parathyroid tumors upon the esophagus.*** *Large adenomas of the left lobe of the thyroid and left-sided parathyroid adenomas may occasionally indent and compress the ventral surface of the esophagus. On occasion, this may be demonstrated by x-ray following a thick barium swallow.*

➠ ***Close attachment of the ventral surface of the esophagus to the trachea.*** *Since the ventral*

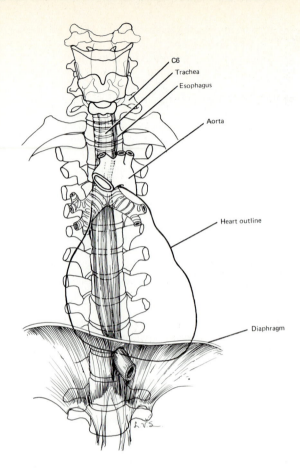

Figure 12–5. The esophagus and its intrathoracic relationships.

surface of the cervical esophagus and the dorsal surface of the trachea and lower larynx are so close, the ventral esophageal surface must be removed in the course of total laryngectomy for cancer; conversely, the larynx must usually be removed in resection of advanced cancer of the lower pharynx and upper esophagus.

Course of the Esophagus (Fig 12–5)

From its midline cervical origin at the termination of the pharynx, the esophagus curves gently to the left as far as the level of the thoracic inlet. From this level to the level of T5, the esophagus gradually regains its midline position. At the T5 level, it once again moves to the left to finally pierce the diaphragm to the left of the midline at T10. Since in the cervical region the esophagus is not completely covered ventrally by the trachea, a left-sided cervical incision offers good surgical access to the esophageal tube in the neck.

The cervical esophagus is capable of marked superior, ventral, and lateral displacement, both because of its intrinsic elasticity and because of its relatively loose connection to both the trachea and the prevertebral fascia.

The esophagus is anatomically constricted at 3 levels: (1) at its orifice in the neck at C6, the level of the cricopharyngeal segment of the inferior constrictor of the pharynx; (2) at the level of the bifurcation of the trachea (T5); and (3) at the level of the esophageal hiatus in the diaphragm (T10). Between these 3 constrictions are 2 compensatory dilatations. These constrictions and dilatations are easily seen in barium swallow x-ray examination of the organ.

➠ *Esophageal burns at the level of C6. The physiologic narrowing of the cervical esophagus at C6 is frequently the site of caustic burns with subsequent mucosal sloughing and luminal stricture. This is a common complication of swallowing of caustic substances by children.*

➠ *Perforations of the esophagus at C6. The esophagus is occasionally perforated secondary to ingestion of sharp objects or instrumentation. The physiologic narrowing at C6 makes this one of the more common sites of traumatic perforation.*

Layers of the Esophagus (Fig 12–6)

The esophagus is composed of 4 layers: (1) an external thin fibrous coat, (2) a muscular layer, (3) a layer of submucosa, and (4) an inner mucosal layer.

A. Fibrous Coat: The esophagus is enclosed in a thin fibrous (adventitial) coat in which run the vessels and nerves supplying the organ. The esophagus has no outer serosal covering, making esophageal anastomoses more prone to leakage.

B. Muscular Layer: The muscular layer of the esophagus consists of an outer layer of longitudinal muscle and an inner layer of circular muscle. The longitudinal musculature is grouped into 3 fasciculi: a ventral fascicular bundle arising from the cricoid cartilage by the cricopharyngeal tendon and 2 lateral bundles that are continuous with the musculature of the inferior constrictors of the pharynx. The 3 fasciculi blend together and invest the entire esophagus except for the dorsal surface of the tube just distal to the transverse fibers of the cricopharyngeus. This leaves a triangular area of the superior dorsal esophagus with no covering of longitudinal muscle. Deep to the longitudinal muscle, the esophagus is completely invested by a layer of circular muscle that is continuous superiorly with the musculature of the inferior constrictor of the pharynx. In the cervical region, the esophageal muscle fibers are reddish and chiefly striated; as the esophagus descends into the thorax, the musculature assumes the characteristics of involuntary smooth muscle and is quite pale.

➠ *True esophageal pulsion diverticula below the level of the cricopharyngeus. Since the longitudinal muscle does not cover the extreme superior dorsal wall of the esophageal tube, this*

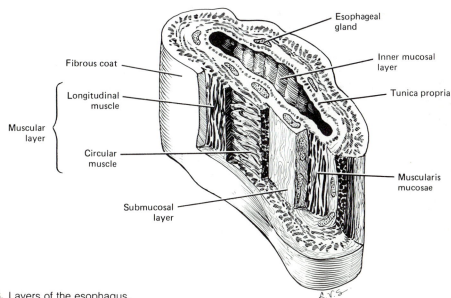

Figure 12–6. Layers of the esophagus.

area is a potentially weak one. It lies just inferior to the cricopharyngeus muscle, and although it is partially reinforced by the most inferior fibers of the cricopharyngeus, it remains quite weak. Herniation through this area (accounting for 5–7% of total pharyngeal-esophageal herniations) constitutes a true esophageal diverticulum. It causes symptoms similar to those of pharyngeal diverticulum, and the procedure for its exposure and repair is similar to that carried out for cure of a more superior pharyngeal diverticulum.

C. Submucosal Layer: The esophageal submucosal coat lies between the mucous membrane and the deepest of the circular smooth muscle fibers. Lodged in this coat are the esophageal mucous glands, which empty on the surface of the mucosal layer via a long-necked excretory duct. The submucosal coat also contains plexuses of blood vessels, lymphatics, and nerves.

D. Inner Mucosal Layer: The thick mucosal coat is arranged into longitudinal columns that tend to smooth out when the esophagus is distended. The mucosal lining is of the stratified squamous type save for the segment just proximal to the esophagogastric junction. At this point, there is frequently some metaplasia of the esophageal mucosal lining, tending toward the columnar gastric type of cellular pattern. On occasion, this makes it difficult to determine whether a tumor at the gastroesophageal junction is a primary gastric or esophageal lesion.

BLOOD VESSELS, LYMPHATICS, & NERVES

Arteries
The cervical esophagus receives its blood supply from branches of the inferior thyroid artery and from the ascending pharyngeal artery (first dorsal branch of the external carotid artery).

Veins
The cervical esophagus is drained mainly by the inferior thyroid veins, which receive blood from the plexus of veins that lies in the outer fibrous coat of the organ. The inferior thyroid veins empty into the brachiocephalic veins. The venous flow may also empty directly into the internal jugular vein or into the lateral thyroid veins.

Lymphatics
Lymphatic drainage from the cervical esophagus is mainly into the small paratracheal nodes, in the esophagotracheal groove close to the recurrent laryngeal nerves. These nodes usually drain directly into the inferior deep cervical nodes, lying below the level of the crossing of the omohyoid muscle.

Nerves
The cervical esophagus is supplied by the pharyngeal plexus of nerves. The plexus is formed by the junction of fibers from the vagus and glossopharyngeal nerves. Additional fibers from the cervical autonomic chain also supply the cervical esophagus.

The Thoracic Cage

13

EMBRYOLOGY

Ribs

The **ribs** originate in the mesenchymal costal processes of the thoracic vertebrae. They are cartilaginous during fetal life and early childhood, when final ossification occurs.

Anomalies. Accessory ribs (cervical or lumbar) are caused by retention and lateral development of a costal process on a cervical or lumbar vertebra. Fused ribs may be associated with the anomaly known as hemivertebra.

Sternum

The precise site of mesenchymal origin of the **sternum** is uncertain. The adult sternum develops from fusion of 2 sternal bands in the midline of the thorax to form the entire sternum. Sternal ossification begins before birth.

Anomalies. Cleft sternum consists of varying degrees of separation of the 2 sternal components. Totally cleft sternum may be accompanied by ectopia cordis. Pectus excavatum (funnel chest) is probably due to traction on the dorsal inferior surface of the sternum.

Vertebrae

Mesenchymal cells of the sclerotomes give rise to the **thoracic vertebrae** (see Chapter 7).

GROSS ANATOMY
(Fig 13–1)

The thoracic cage is composed of osseous, cartilaginous, fibrous, and muscular structures which together form a specialized type of ''armor plate'' that provides both rigidity and pliability and serves to house and protect the major respiratory and circulatory organs.

The thorax is roughly conical. Its short anterior bony wall is made up of the sternum, the ventral portions of the superior 10 ribs, and their attached costal cartilages. Laterally, its wall is formed by the rib cage, the ribs slanting obliquely, caudally, and ventrally. Dorsally, it is formed by the 12 thoracic vertebrae and by the attached dorsal segments of the 12 thoracic ribs as they run laterally and inferiorly to their angles. In adults, the thoracic cavity is roughly oval; in infants and young children, it is more circular.

Thoracic Inlet

The kidney-shaped thoracic inlet is the narrowest of any segment of the thoracic cage—about 6.5 cm in anteroposterior diameter and about 12.5 cm in transverse diameter. The thoracic inlet rises to a higher level dorsally than ventrally, the first thoracic vertebra—its dorsal landmark—being situated higher than the manubrium, whose superior rim, the ventral landmark, is at the level of T2. This difference in ventral and dorsal inlet height allows the apical portion of the lung and the dome of its pleura to rise above the level of the manubrium but still to be contained within the thorax dorsally, where the lungs rise to the level of the neck of the first rib.

Thoracic Outlet

The thoracic outlet is much more spacious than the thoracic inlet. The inferior boundary of the thorax is the musculotendinous diaphragm, which separates the abdominal cavity from the thoracic cavity. The thoracic outlet is bounded dorsally by the 12th thoracic vertebra. Passing anteriorly, the boundary moves ventrally and is delineated by the 12th, 11th, and tenth ribs from lateral to medial and farther anteriorly by the joined costal cartilages of the tenth, ninth, eighth, and seventh ribs. In the midline anteriorly, it is bounded by the joint between the body and the xiphoid process of the sternum.

Vertebral Column

The ventrodorsal inclination of the vertebral column accounts for the amount of space present in the various segments of the thoracic cavity. Normally, the vertebral column has a forward curve in the upper thoracic area, and as a consequence there is a narrowing of the anteroposterior thoracic diameter at the level of T2–4. The distance between the posterior surface of the manubrium and the ventral surface of the vertebral bodies is only 5–6 cm at the level of the thoracic inlet. Into this narrow inlet area are crowded the great vessels of the thorax, the trachea and esophagus, many major nerves, the thoracic duct, remnants of the thymus, and occasionally some retrosternal thyroid tissue. Conversely, in the mid thorax the vertebral column shows a ventral concavity; consequently, at this level (T5–9), the distance between the dorsal surface of the sternum and the vertebral bodies increases markedly. The inferior 3 thoracic vertebrae project ventrally, and so the thorax narrows somewhat as the thoracic outlet is approached.

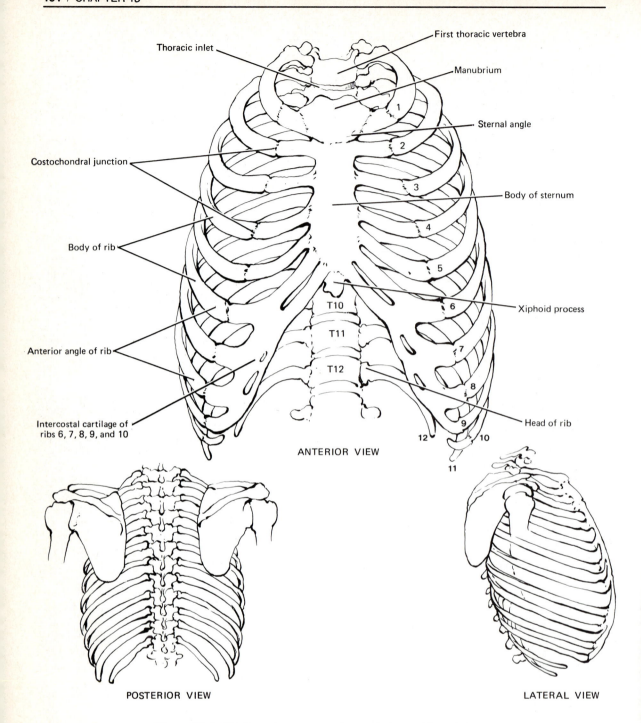

First thoracic vertebra

Thoracic inlet

Manubrium

Sternal angle

Costochondral junction

Body of sternum

Body of rib

Xiphoid process

T10

T11

Anterior angle of rib

T12

Head of rib

Intercostal cartilage of ribs 6, 7, 8, 9, and 10

ANTERIOR VIEW

POSTERIOR VIEW

LATERAL VIEW

Figure 13–1. The thoracic cage: anterior, posterior, and lateral views.

⇒ **Abnormalities of the thoracic cage.** *Variations in the size and shape of the thoracic cage may occur as congenital anomalies, or they may be due to a variety of pathologic conditions. Functional scoliosis of the thoracic vertebral spine may occur. Kyphosis of the thoracic vertebrae may occur as a result of demineralization* (*osteoporosis*), *with subsequent vertebral collapse. One or more thoracic vertebrae may collapse as a result of metastatic spread from a malignant breast or prostatic tumor. Collapse of a thoracic vertebra may occur if severe trauma results in the compression of one or more vertebrae. Poliomyelitis may cause unilat-*

eral atrophy of the thoracic musculature, with resultant thoracic vertebral scoliosis. Osteomyelitis of the dorsal spine may cause collapse of one or more thoracic vertebrae and kyphosis of the dorsal spine.

"Lines" of the Thorax
(Table 13–1; Fig 13–2)

For purposes of exact anatomic and clinical description, the external surface of the thoracic cage is delineated by a series of vertical lines that run parallel with the long axis of the body.

THE STERNUM
(Fig 13–3)

Divisions of the Sternum

The sternum forms the central anterior segment of the bony thoracic cage and is composed of 3 major divisions.

A. Manubrium Sterni: The manubrium, the most superior segment of the bone, is roughly quadrilateral, with a slightly roughened ventral surface and a smooth dorsal surface. A midline superior notch called the suprasternal or jugular notch lies at the level of T2. The superior lateral margins of the manubrium are notched for reception of the clavicular heads. The manubrium joins the body of the sternum at the level of T5. The costal cartilage of the first rib joins the midlateral surface of the manubrium via a synchondrosis. The manubrium articulates with the body of the sternum via a strip of fibrocartilage strengthened ventrally by fibrous tissue derived from the pectoralis fascia. The second costal cartilage joins the manubrium at the level of its junction with the sternal body.

B. Body: The body of the sternum lies just inferior to the manubrium and is about 10–14 cm in length. It is multiply faceted laterally on each side for junction with the costal cartilages of ribs 2–7. The costosternal articulations, with the exception of the most superior one, are of the gliding type. The sternal body joins with the xiphoid process via a cartilaginous synchondrosis at the level of T10. The manubrium and the sternal body join at an acute angle, with a ventral convexity (sternal angle) (Fig 13–4). The sternal angle is often visible and is easily palpable in most individuals. It serves as a convenient starting point for counting the ribs, since the costal cartilage of rib 2 always articulates with the sternum at this level; due to the overhanging clavicle, rib 1 is almost impossible to palpate.

⇒ *Sternal fractures and sternal trauma. Despite its extremely vulnerable location, fractures of the sternum are not common; when they do occur, displacement of the fragments is rare. This is because the sternum is protected ventrally by the midline decussations of the dense investing fascia of the 2 pectoralis major muscles. Dorsally, the sternum is well supported by the endothoracic fascia. The most common site of sternal fracture is at the sternal angle. Even when displacement of sternal fragments occurs, there is seldom any injury to the underlying mediastinal structures. In every case of fracture of the sternum, however, the physician should be alert to the possibility of traumatic diaphragmatic laceration with herniation of abdominal contents (immediately or later) into the thoracic cavity. Sternal trauma should also arouse a suspicion of trauma to the heart. This possibility should be checked by electrocardiographic tracings, and a close clinical watch should be kept for the onset of a bloody pericardial effusion, which may lead to cardiac tamponade.*

Table 13–1. "Lines" of the thorax.

Midsternal line (MSL)	Divides the sternum into halves and serves as a guide to the position of the midline of the dorsal surface of the thorax when scoliosis is not present.
Midclavicular line (MCL)	A line dropped vertically from the mid clavicle. It usually passes just medial to the nipple in a breast with normal posture.
Parasternal line (PSL)	Halfway between the midclavicular and midsternal lines.
Anterior axillary line (AAL)	Runs inferiorly from the anterior axillary fold, formed by the inferior border of the pectoralis major muscle as it leaves the chest to run to its humeral insertion.
Posterior axillary line (PAL)	Passes inferiorly from the posterior axillary fold formed by the lateral border of the latissimus dorsi muscle as it leaves the posterior thoracic wall to run to its insertion on the humerus.
Midaxillary line (MAL)	Runs inferiorly from the center of the axilla.
Midscapular line (MSL)	Runs vertically through the inferior angle of the scapula.
Paravertebral line (PVL)	Just lateral to the vertebral bodies. As it descends, it passes through the tips of the vertebral transverse processes.

domastoid, and the sternohyoid, sternothyroid, and transverse thoracic muscles. The muscular fibers of the anterior mid segment of the diaphragm, the linea alba, and the rectus abdominis muscle also have sternal attachments.

The Sternoclavicular Joint
(Fig 13–4)

This is a double synovial joint of the gliding type, the 2 halves of the joint being separated by a fibrocartilaginous articular disk. The disk absorbs much of the shock delivered to the joint in trauma to the upper extremity or shoulder girdle. This joint arrangement permits movement in all directions but is quite limited. The centrally placed articular disk divides the joint into a pair of cavities, each with its separate synovial membrane. There are 3 supporting joint ligaments: (1) Superiorly, the transverse sternal or interclavicular ligament runs from the medial end of one clavicle, across the superior margin of the sternum, to the medial end of the contralateral clavicle. It is bound down tightly to the superior surface of the manubrium as it runs transversely. (2) The anterior and posterior collateral ligaments strengthen the joint ventrally and dorsally and prevent abnormal anteroposterior joint movement. (3) The costoclavicular ligament is a short trapezoid-shaped ligament running from the cartilage of the first rib to the undersurface of the most medial portion of the clavicle.

⇒ *Dislocation of the sternoclavicular joint. The sternoclavicular joint is rarely dislocated, since the clavicle usually breaks instead. About 90% of the dislocations that do occur are in a ventral direction, and injury to the important retroclavicular vessels and nerves is thus avoided.*

THE CLAVICLE
(Collarbone) (Fig 13–5)

The clavicle is a gently curved bone that transversely overlies the superior ventral segment of the thorax. It lies just superior to the first rib and makes up the anterior unit of the shoulder girdle. The bone presents 2 curvatures: a lateral curvature with a dorsal convexity and a medial curvature with a ventral convexity. The clavicle articulates medially with the manubrium and laterally with the acromial process of the scapula. The bone lies in a very superficial position, just deep to the skin, subcutaneous tissues, and platysma muscle, and can easily be palpated along its entire course. It acts as a fulcrum that enables the muscles of the shoulder girdle to give lateral movement to the arm. It is usually well developed in animals with prehensile digits and usually absent in animals who use their forequarters only for progression. The bone is covered ventrally by the platysma muscle, which runs across it from the anterosuperior chest wall onto the neck and lower face.

The clavicle gives attachments to the following muscles: the deltoid, the trapezius, the pectoralis major, the clavicular head of the sternocleidomastoid, and the subclavius. Attached also to the clavicle are the coracoclavicular ligament, with its conoid and trapezoid components, and the costoclavicular ligament.

The divisions of the brachial plexus, the subclavian artery, and the subclavian vein all pass dorsal to the clavicle en route from the lower neck to the axilla.

⇒ *Trauma to the clavicle. (Fig 13–6.) The clavicle is the most frequently fractured bone in the body. The most common site is at the junc-*

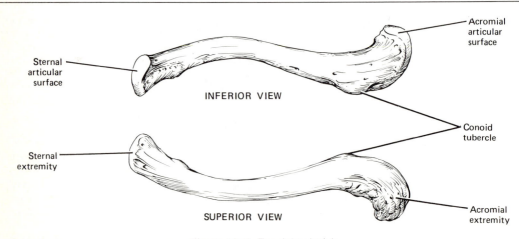

Sternal articular surface

Acromial articular surface

INFERIOR VIEW

Conoid tubercle

Sternal extremity

SUPERIOR VIEW

Acromial extremity

Figure 13–5. The right clavicle.

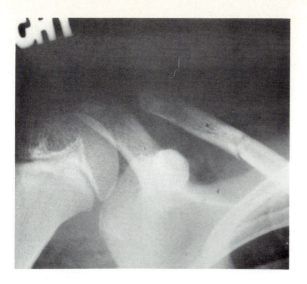

Figure 13–6. Fracture of the clavicle.

tion of the mid and lateral thirds. Owing to the superior pull of the sternocleidomastoid and trapezius muscles, the medial clavicular fragment tilts superiorly. The lateral fragment is pulled inferiorly by the weight of the arm and the combined action of the pectoralis major and teres major muscles and medially by the adductors of the shoulder. Dorsal displacement of the clavicular fragments following trauma, with resultant injuries to the vascular and nervous structures at the base of the neck, is rare.

➠ **Metastases to the clavicle.** Malignant diseases that tend to metastasize to bone frequently involve the clavicle. The breast and prostate are common primary sites. The clavicle does not possess a medullary cavity.

THE SCAPULA
(Shoulder Blade) (Fig 13–7)

Borders of the Scapula

The scapula is a flattened triangular bone that covers the superior dorsolateral portion of the chest wall, reaching from the second rib superiorly to the eighth

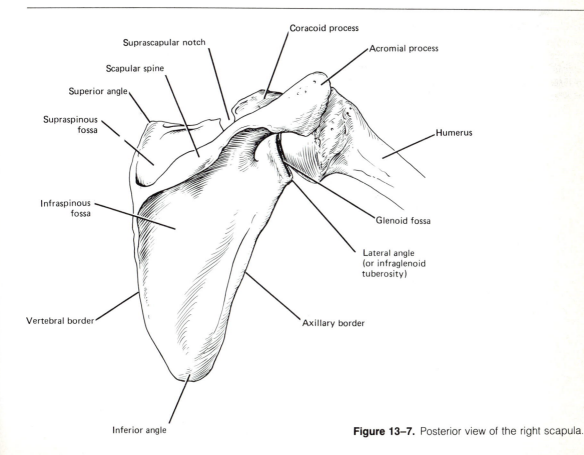

Figure 13–7. Posterior view of the right scapula.

rib inferiorly. Its short superior border runs laterally and presents the suprascapular notch through which the suprascapular nerve passes on its way to innervate both the supra- and infraspinous muscles. The superior border of the scapula is quite thin and gives attachment only to the posterior belly of the omohyoid muscle. The medial (vertebral) border of the scapula is its longest and is thicker than the superior border. It gives attachment to the levator scapulae and the major and minor rhomboid and serratus anterior muscles. The lateral (axillary) border of the scapula runs from the inferior scapular angle to the inferior border of the glenoid fossa. The superior end of the lateral border of the scapula is the triangular area from which the long head of the triceps muscle arises.

Angles of the Scapula

The scapula presents 3 angles: (1) The superior angle lies between the superior and medial borders. It is masked by the trapezius muscle and is difficult to palpate. (2) The inferior angle is easy to visualize and palpate. Its tip is usually at the level of the seventh intercostal interspace when the arm is held in full adduction at the side of the body. (3) The lateral angle of the scapula is formed by the shallow glenoid cavity, which permits articulation of the head of the humerus with the scapula.

Surfaces of the Scapula

The dorsal (external) surface of the scapula is divided by the scapular spine into a small supraspinous and a large infraspinous fossa. The 2 fossae are filled in by the supraspinous and infraspinous muscles, respectively. The deep costal or ventral surface of the scapula is moderately concave. Its concavity is filled in by the subscapularis and serratus anterior muscles.

Bony Processes of the Scapula

The scapula possesses 2 bony processes: coracoid and acromion. The proximal segment of the **coracoid process** projects ventrally from a wide base on the superior border of the scapula near its neck. The lateral concave surface allows for passage of the subscapularis tendon. The distal segment of the coracoid process makes a right-angle turn in the direction of the humeral head and lies in a transverse position. The coracoid process is usually palpable about 2.5 cm inferior to the lateral third of the clavicle despite the fact that it is covered by the relatively thick deltoid muscle. The short head of the biceps brachii and the coracobrachialis muscles arise from the tip of the coracoid process, whereas the pectoralis minor muscle inserts into the medial and superior borders of the process. The coracoacromial ligament, which arches over the shoulder joint, and the coracoclavicular ligament, which binds the clavicle to the coracoid process, both attach to the coracoid process of the scapula.

The **acromial process** of the scapula (acromion) represents the terminal lateral projection of the scapular spine. The acromion at first projects laterally and

then makes a right-angle turn in a ventral direction (acromial angle). The ventral terminal portion of the acromial process is subcutaneous and gives rise to the coracoacromial ligament and to fibers of the deltoid muscle. Its concave medial border presents a spherical surface centrally for its articulation with the clavicle.

➡ *Fractures of the scapula. Fracture of the scapula with posttraumatic subscapular hematoma is fairly frequent. After healing of the fracture and fibrous organization of the hematoma, the usually smooth motion of the scapula on the posterolateral chest wall may be markedly impeded. Consequently, it is important to encourage early scapulothoracic motion following such fractures.*

➡ *Sprengel's deformity. Congenital elevation of the scapula (Sprengel's deformity) is a rare, usually unilateral anomaly associated with some degree of scoliosis of the dorsal spine. The affected shoulder is carried high, and the involved side is shortened and thickened. The trapezius muscle is thickened ipsilaterally, and the superior border of the involved scapula becomes prominent.*

Ligaments & Movement of the Scapula

Under normal conditions the scapula moves freely on the underlying chest wall, sometimes referred to as movement of the "scapulothoracic joint," although obviously no such joint exists in the true sense. The **acromioclavicular joint** fixes the lateral extremity of the spine of the scapula to the lateral end of the clavicle. The articular surfaces of the joint are oval and flattened and occasionally separated by an interarticular cartilage. The joint has a weak capsular structure but is strengthened by the superior and anterior acromioclavicular ligaments. A slight forward and backward sliding motion occurs in the joint, and when the shoulder is thrust ventrally it creates a small angle between the clavicle and the acromion. Strength is added to the acromioclavicular joint by the coracoclavicular ligament, which fixes the superior edge of the coracoid process to the undersurface of the lateral end of the clavicle, thus helping to retain the clavicle in contact with the acromion. The coracoclavicular ligament is divided into 2 segments: conoid and trapezoid. The trapezoid (ventrolateral) segment of the ligament runs from the coracoid process to the lateral inferior surface of the clavicle. The conoid (dorsomedial) segment is conical, with its apex attached to the base of the coracoid process. The coracoclavicular ligament is attached by its base to the undersurface of the clavicle. Lying ventral to the ligament are the deltoid and subclavius muscles; dorsal to it is the trapezius muscle. The coracoacromial ligament forms a strong arch superior to the shoulder joint, helping to prevent superior dislocation of the shoulder.

➡ ***Dislocations of the acromioclavicular joint.*** *Inferior dislocations of the acromioclavicular joint seldom occur, but superior dislocations are a common athletic injury. The superior dislocation is easy to reduce but difficult to hold in reduction, as the conoid and trapezoid ligaments that keep the joint in apposition are usually torn by the trauma. Permanent, stable reduction is achieved by placement of a nail through the joint line, occasionally combined with repair of the 2 segments of the coracoclavicular ligament.*

THE RIBS
(Fig 13–1)

1. THE RIB CAGE

The rib cage is made up of 12 bony and cartilaginous arches on either side of the midline of the thoracic cavity. The composite rib arches form the greater part of the thoracic cage. Occasionally, a cervical or lumbar rib may increase the number of ribs on one or both sides to 13. Rarely, there are only 11. The first 7 ribs (the "true" or vertebrosternal ribs) articulate posteriorly with the vertebral column and anteriorly via their individual costal cartilages with the sternum. The lower 5 ribs (the "false" ribs) also articulate posteriorly with the vertebral column. However, anteriorly, ribs 8, 9, and 10 have their costal cartilages attached to the costal cartilage of the rib above (vertebrochondral ribs) while ribs 11 and 12 have no articulation anteriorly ("floating ribs").

Between the ribs are the intercostal spaces. They are wider anteriorly than posteriorly, and the upper intercostal spaces are usually wider than the lower ones.

The first 7 ribs increase gradually in length from rib 1 to rib 7, and the lower 5 ribs diminish progressively in length. The upper ribs are the widest, with the greatest width at the sternal extremities. It is usually possible to palpate all of the ribs except the first, which lies under the clavicle. The 11th and 12th ribs may be difficult to palpate in a heavily muscled or obese person. The second rib articulates with the sternum at the sternal angle and is often called the "indicator rib," since it is used as the starting point for counting ribs.

Typical Rib
(Figs 13–8 and 13–9)

A typical rib (2–9) consists of a head with 2 facets that articulate with the facets of the same-numbered vertebra and with the vertebra just above. Lateral to the rib head, the rib neck is moderately constricted

and positioned anterior to the transverse process of the more inferior of the 2 vertebrae with which the rib articulates. An articular tubercle lies just dorsal to the junction of the neck and the rib body. It has a smooth facet for articulation with the periphery of the transverse process of the inferior vertebra. The typical rib shows a dorsal shaft and an angle where the dorsal rib curves ventrally, continuing as the anterior shaft. The typical rib possesses a sternal extremity for junction with a costal cartilage. The external surfaces of the ribs are smooth and covered with muscle; their smooth internal surfaces are covered with endothoracic fascia and parietal pleura. The superior surface of each rib is smooth and rounded, whereas the inferior surface is notched or grooved, with an external bony overhang. Protected by the overhang lie the intercostal vessels and nerves.

First Rib

The first rib is special: It is the highest, widest, strongest, flattest, shortest, and most curved of all of the ribs. Its surfaces face superiorly and inferiorly rather than ventrally and dorsally. It articulates with only one vertebra—its own—rather than with 2, as do most of the other ribs. Its anterosuperior surface has a scalene tubercle for insertion of the anterior scalene muscle. Medial to it, the rib is grooved for passage of the subclavian vein; lateral to it is a groove for passage of the subclavian artery. The outer border of the first rib marks the beginning of the apex of the axilla. The first rib lies almost completely beneath the clavicle and is attached to its undersurface by the subclavius muscle and the costoclavicular ligament. It is attached to the coracoid process of the scapula by the costoclavicular ligament.

Costal Groove

The costal groove is located on the inner surface of a sharp external overhang on the inferior border of a typical rib. From above downward, the overhang protects the intercostal vein, artery, and the intercostal nerve as they are related to the inferior dorsal surface of the anterior ribs. Dorsal to the angle of the ribs, the intercostal nerve lies midway between the ribs, unprotected by the costal groove, and in this position it is relatively accessible to local anesthesia. Posterior to the rib angle, the costal groove is related to the inferior surface of the rib rather than to its dorsal inferior segment. Consequently, there is no protective overhang.

2. PERIOSTEUM

Unlike the periosteum of the sternum, which strips with difficulty, the rib periosteum strips quite easily, and this makes subperiosteal resection of a rib possible. The ribs—along with the sternum, the vertebrae, and the diploë of the skull—are the great reservoirs of red blood cell-producing marrow. Rib marrow

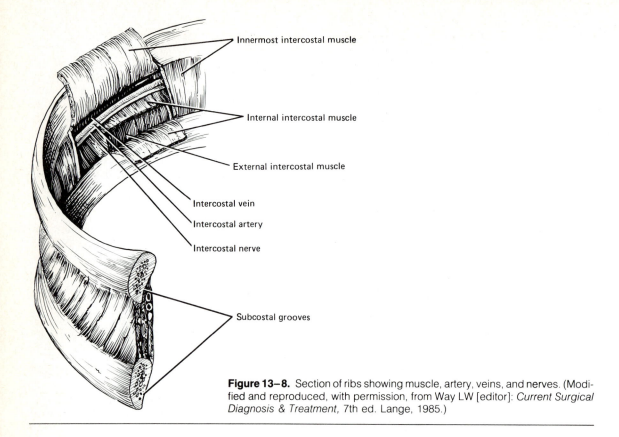

Figure 13–8. Section of ribs showing muscle, artery, veins, and nerves. (Modified and reproduced, with permission, from Way LW [editor]: *Current Surgical Diagnosis & Treatment,* 7th ed. Lange, 1985.)

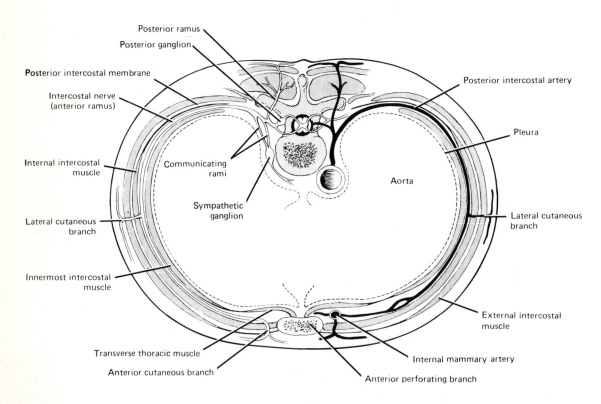

Figure 13–9. Cross section of chest. (Reproduced, with permission, from Way LW [editor]: *Current Surgical Diagnosis & Treatment,* 7th ed. Lange, 1985.)

biopsy is easy to perform in suspected blood or malignant neoplastic disease.

⇒ **Metastases to the ribs.** *The ribs are a frequent site of metastases from primaries in the breast or prostate. Rib pain with subsequent x-ray demonstration of a metastasis may be the first symptom of cancer of these organs.*

⇒ **Rib fractures.** *Because of their exposed position and relative thinness, fractures of the rib are common sequelae of trauma to the thoracic cage. The thoracic cage is much more elastic in infants and children than in adults, and as a consequence rib fractures are less common among younger people. Rib fractures may be single or multiple, bilateral or unilateral, and may be accompanied by fractures of the sternum and the thoracic vertebrae.*

⇒ **First rib fractures.** *Because of its protected position, the first rib is rarely fractured. When the first rib is fractured, it may signal the presence of severe trauma and multiple injuries to the mediastinum and lower neck.*

⇒ **Complications of rib fracture.** *Rib fractures may cause pleural lacerations and pneumothorax with or without mediastinal shift, subcutaneous emphysema, or hemothorax secondary to lung laceration or tear of an intercostal vessel. Pericardial lacerations or contusions may occur in severe cases. Lower rib fractures may be associated with tears of the diaphragm and* a subsequent diaphragmatic hernia. Fractures of the right lower rib cage may lacerate the liver; fractures of the left lower rib cage—particularly those related to the inferior midaxillary area—should suggest possible damage to the spleen.

⇒ **Flail chest.** *Severe bilateral multiple fractures of the ribs may lead to flail chest, with resultant paradoxic respiration. In other words, the floating section (flail segment) moves inward during inspiration and outward during expiration. This makes breathing difficult, decreases the tidal air flow, and calls for prompt mechanical stabilization of the chest or use of a respirator with controlled pressure respiration.*

3. COSTAL ARTICULATIONS (Figs 13–10 and 13–11)

Costovertebral Articulations

The costovertebral articulations fall into 2 categories: (1) articulations of the rib heads with one or 2 vertebral bodies, and (2) the articulation of the rib necks and tubercles with the vertebral transverse processes.

The typical rib head forms a sliding joint with the articular facets on the dorsolateral margins of the 2 adjacent vertebrae. The rib heads also articulate with the intervertebral disk, which lies between the 2 vertebral bodies with which a typical rib articulates. The heads of the first, tenth, 11th, and 12th ribs articulate with only a single vertebra, while the remaining rib heads articulate via sliding joints with their own vertebra and with the vertebra just above.

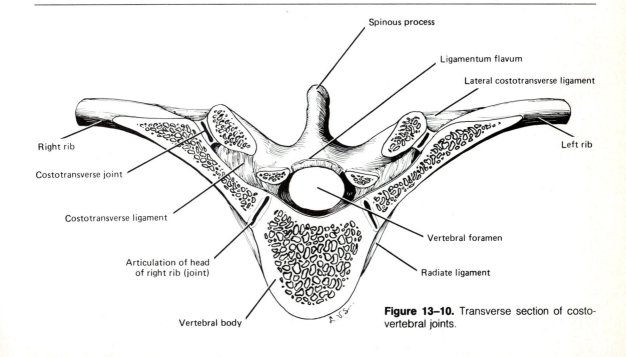

Figure 13–10. Transverse section of costovertebral joints.

Spinous process

Ligamentum flavum

Lateral costotransverse ligament

Left rib

Right rib

Costotransverse joint

Costotransverse ligament

Articulation of head of right rib (joint)

Vertebral foramen

Radiate ligament

Vertebral body

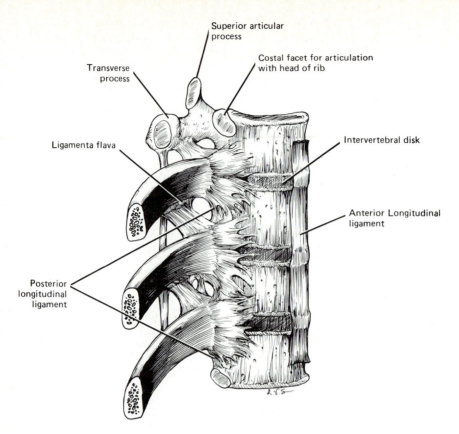

Figure 13–11. Right lateral view of intervertebral disks in thoracic region showing attached ligaments. (Reproduced, with permission, from Chusid JG: *Correlative Neuroanatomy & Functional Neurology,* 19th ed. Lange, 1985.)

Costotransverse Process Articulations
(Fig 13–9)

There are sliding joints between the articular surface of the tubercles of the ribs and the neighboring transverse processes. Costotransverse process articulations are present on ribs 1–10; ribs 11 and 12 do not have this type of articulation.

Other Articulations

Articulations between the sternum and the costal cartilages of the true ribs—with the exception of rib 1—are sliding joints. The first rib unites with the sternum via a synchondrosis. The lateral margin of each costal cartilage fits into a depression on the sternal end of the rib. The costal cartilage and the bone of the rib are tightly joined by the covering periosteum. The costal cartilages are joined to the sternum by an articular capsule, a radiate sternocostal ligament, and an intra-articular sternocostal ligament. The sternal ends of costal cartilages 8–10 have a pointed apex which is joined to the costal cartilage just superior.

4. INTERCOSTAL SPACES

The intercostal spaces are 11 in number. The first 9 are closed anteriorly, whereas the 2 lowest spaces remain open anteriorly. The spaces are wider anteriorly than posteriorly and wider on inspiration than on expiration except when there is a fixed chest, as in severe emphysema. One can increase the width of an intercostal space by flexing the thoracic cage toward the contralateral side. The intercostal spaces are filled in by the 2 sets of intercostal muscles and by intercostal membranes, which are present either anteriorly or posteriorly; and the spaces are bounded deeply by the transverse thoracic muscle and the endothoracic fascia.

➠ *Intercostal space incisions. The fifth, sixth, and seventh interspaces laterally and posteriorly are important sites for thoracotomy incisions. If the ipsilateral arm is elevated and placed behind the patient's head, the inferior angle of the scapula rises, leaving the dorso-*

lateral segments of the fourth and fifth interspaces cleared for surgical incisions.

5. INTERCOSTAL MUSCLES

External Intercostal Muscles
(Fig 13–8)

The 11 external intercostal muscles make up the most superficial layer of the intercostal space. The external intercostal muscle fibers do not reach as far anteriorly as the sternum but become membranous (anterior intercostal membrane) as they reach the lateral margins of the costal cartilages. The external intercostal muscle fibers arise from the inferior margin of the rib above to insert into the superior surface of the rib below. The external intercostal muscles are twice as thick as the internal intercostal muscles.

Internal Intercostal Muscles
(Fig 13–8)

Through the thin anterior intercostal membrane, the surgeon can perceive the deeper fibers of the internal intercostal muscles, which—unlike those of the external intercostal muscles—run to the lateral border of the sternum. Their fibers run in an oblique direction, perpendicular to those of the exterior intercostals, which tends to strengthen the intercostal spaces. The internal intercostal muscles arise from the inferior surface of the rib above and insert into the superior surface of the rib below. The internal intercostals are thinner than the external ones. The internal intercostals that reach the sternum anteriorly extend only as far as the angles of the ribs posteriorly. There they are replaced by the posterior intercostal membrane (Fig 13–10). The combined action of the 2 intercostal muscles is to pull adjacent ribs together. The muscles are supplied by the intercostal nerves.

Deepest Intercostal Muscles
(Fig 13–8)

The deepest intercostal muscle layer consists of the subcostal muscles and the transverse thoracic muscles. The neurovascular bundle lies in the plane between the internal intercostal and the deepest layer of intercostal muscles. The transverse thoracic muscle radiates laterally in fanlike fashion from its origin on the sternum to attach to the inner surfaces of the ventral segments of the second to sixth ribs. It draws anterior ribs inferiorly. It is served by the segmental intercostal nerves. The subcostal muscles are present only in the inferior thorax, where they reinforce the internal intercostals. Their fibers run from the rib near its angle to a rib 2 or 3 spaces below. They are supplied by the adjacent intercostal nerves and pull the lower ribs close together.

The deep surface of these muscles is covered by the endothoracic fascia, the lining fascia of the thoracic cavity. Deep to the endothoracic fascia is the thin subserous fascia, which lies between the parietal pleura and the lining fascia of the thoracic cavity.

In making an interspace surgical approach to the pleural cavity, the surgeon usually opens the internal intercostal muscle, the deepest intercostal muscles, the endothoracic fascia, the subserous fascia, and the parietal pleura all as a single layer, since they are bound closely together.

BLOOD VESSELS, LYMPHATICS, & NERVES

Arteries

The **posterior intercostal arteries** are segmental branches from the thoracic aorta. Each of the segmental thoracic aortic branches divides into a ventral and a dorsal branch. The dorsal branch supplies the dorsal thoracic musculature, the spinal cord, and the skin of the back. The ventral branch runs obliquely across the posterior intercostal space toward the inferior surface of the rib just superior to it. It then runs laterally and ventrally in the subcostal groove. The posterior intercostal artery lies at first between the pleura and the posterior intercostal membrane. It then passes through the membrane and continues ventrally between the internal and deepest intercostal muscles. It finally anastomoses anteriorly with the intercostal branch of either the internal thoracic or the musculophrenic arteries. Posterior interspaces 1 and 2 are supplied with arterial blood by the descending thoracic branch of the costocervical trunk, the fourth branch of the subclavian artery.

▱▶ *Coarctation of the aorta. Nearby intercostal arteries hypertrophy markedly in congenital coarctation of the aorta because they provide the collateral circulation around the coarctation. As they run in the subcostal groove of the anterior ribs, the enlarged arteries erode the lower borders of the ribs, giving them a characteristic notched appearance on chest x-rays.*

The first through sixth anterior interspaces are supplied by the **anterior intercostal arteries,** branches of the internal thoracic artery. The remainder of the anterior intercostal spaces are supplied by intercostal branches of the musculophrenic artery, one of the 2 terminal branches of the internal thoracic artery. The anterior intercostal arteries run laterally, close to the inferior surface of the rib above, to finally merge with the posterior intercostal vessels. The anterior intercostals supply the anterior chest wall muscles and the muscles of the anterior intercostal spaces and lie between the internal and deepest intercostal muscles.

The **perforating branches of the internal thoracic artery** are given off close to the lateral border of the sternum. They pierce the musculature and membranes of the ventral chest wall in the upper 6 interspaces. The perforating branches in the second, third, and fourth interspaces are quite large, particularly in women, and especially during pregnancy. They come to the surgeon's attention when the pectoralis major muscle is removed from the sternum as part of radical mastectomy.

Veins

The upper 3 posterior intercostal spaces are drained by the **highest intercostal vein.** On the right side, this vein descends to end in the azygos vein. On the left side, the highest intercostal vein passes obliquely across the aortic arch and the proximal portion of the left common carotid and subclavian arteries to empty into the left brachiocephalic vein. The lower right posterior intercostal veins usually empty into the azygos vein, whereas the lower left posterior intercostal veins empty into the hemiazygos vein. Each posterior intercostal vein has (1) a dorsal tributary that reaches it from the muscles and skin of the posterior thorax, and (2) a spinal tributary that links up with the venous plexus surrounding the spinal cord and vertebral column. Venous return via the anterior intercostal veins reaches the internal thoracic veins that accompany the internal thoracic artery. The internal thoracic veins empty into the superior vena cava via the right and left brachiocephalic veins.

The azygos, hemiazygos, and accessory hemiazygos veins are the collecting veins of the posterior thoracic parietes. (See Chapter 17.)

The **azygos vein** begins in the retroperitoneal tissues of the superoposterior abdomen at the level of L2 as the ascending right lumbar vein. It is formed by the junction of superior branches from the first and second lumbar veins. Once formed, the azygos vein enters the thorax through the aortic hiatus of the diaphragm and runs superiorly along the right side of the vertebral column as high as vertebra T4. At T4 it passes ventrally across the root of the right lung to terminate in the superior vena cava just prior to the entrance of that vein into the pericardial sac. The tributaries of the azygos vein are the right subcostal and posterior intercostal veins, the right superior intercostal vein, the hemiazygos vein, the accessory hemiazygos vein, and a few small branches that reach it from the thoracic viscera.

The **hemiazygos vein** is the superior continuation of the ascending left lumbar vein that reaches the thorax by passing through the left crus of the diaphragm and runs superiorly along the left side of the vertebral column as high as vertebra T9. At this level, the hemiazygos vein then passes horizontally to the right, between the vertebral column and the thoracic aorta, esophagus, and thoracic duct to finally terminate in the medial side of the azygos vein. The tributaries of the hemiazygos vein are the lower 5 left posterior intercostal veins, the left subcostal vein, and occasionally the accessory hemiazygos vein and a few small esophageal and mediastinal veins.

The **accessory hemiazygos vein** is a small vessel that runs inferiorly on the left side of the vertebral column as far as vertebra T8, at which level it either crosses to the right side of the thorax to join the azygos vein or terminates by joining the hemiazygos vein. There is an excellent venous anastomosis between the azygos and hemiazygos veins that connects with both the superior and inferior venae cavae. The azygos and hemiazygos veins also join up with the common iliac veins via the ascending lumbar veins and multiple small branches of the inferior vena cava. This anastomosis is of clinical importance in both superior and inferior caval blocks.

Lymph Drainage

The lymph nodes of the thoracic wall are divided into internal mammary (or sternal), intercostal, and diaphragmatic groups. The intercostal nodes lie deep within the intercostal spaces, closely related to the intercostal vessels. They drain variably into the cisterna chyli, the thoracic duct, or the right lymphatic duct. The diaphragmatic nodes lie on the superior aspect of the diaphragm. They drain into the sternal nodes or the posterior mediastinal nodes.

Both the number and the position of these lymph nodes and their connecting lymph chains are quite variable. They are most apt to lie in relation to the second, third, and fourth interspaces just deep to the area of junction of the costal cartilages with the sternum, close to the internal thoracic vessels. They are usually larger in women than in men and in younger people.

➡ *Carcinoma in sternal lymph nodes. The internal mammary or sternal lymph nodes are occasionally involved in carcinoma of the breast when the tumor is in the medial half of the breast or when the axillary nodes are blocked with metastatic tumor and lymph flow is diverted medially.*

Nerves

Intercostal nerves 2, 3, 4, 5, and 6 run in the intercostal space deep to the internal intercostal muscle. They are separated from the endothoracic fascia and the parietal pleura by the deepest intercostal muscles. In their course, the intercostal nerves give off muscular branches that supply the muscles of the intercostal spaces. The nerves also give off the lateral and anterior cutaneous branches.

The nerves and blood vessels running in the intercostal spaces have a variable relationship to the ribs. Dorsally, the posterior intercostal artery lies in the central portion of the intercostal space with the intercostal nerve superior to it and the intercostal vein superior to the intercostal nerve. Farther anteriorly, beyond the rib angle, the 3 structures change relationships. At the midaxillary line, they become closely associated with the inferior surface of the rib above. In the anterior interspaces, the intercostal vein lies superior to the artery and the intercostal nerve inferior to the artery. All 3 structures then continue forward in this relationship under the overhang of the lower border of the rib.

⟫ *Injections of intercostal nerves. The intercostal nerves may be injected with procaine or alcohol or subjected to surgical ablation for the relief of severe intractable residual chest wall pain associated with herpes zoster or old chest wall injuries. In the performance of a thoracic paracentesis through the anterolateral interspaces, the entering needle should be placed in the mid portion of the interspace rather than close to the upper or lower border of a rib. In this way the needle will avoid the neurovascular bundle. In contrast, nerve block anesthesia of an intercostal nerve in the anterolateral chest wall area should be delivered close to the inferior border of the rib that lies superior to the interspace in question.*

MUSCLES OF THE THORACIC WALL

1. MUSCLES OF THE VENTROLATERAL THORACIC WALL (FIG 13–12)

Pectoralis Major Muscle

The pectoralis major is a bulky, fan-shaped muscle that covers the anterosuperior chest wall. From its insertion on the upper humerus it fans out. It has a continuous origin from the sternal half of the clavicle; from the lateral anterior surface of the sternum from the manubrium to the seventh rib; from the cartilages of all the true ribs; and from the aponeurosis covering the superior portion of the external oblique muscle. From this wide arc of origin, there is a convergence of the pectoralis fibers toward their humeral insertion, all fibers finally joining to form a flat thick tendon 4–6 cm wide. The tendon inserts at the intertubercular sulcus of the humerus. The clavicular fibers tend to be separated from the remainder of the fibers of the muscle by a narrow but easily dissectable and recognizable cleft.

⟫ *Pectoralis major infraclavicular cleft. This cleft is of clinical interest in radical breast surgery. The clavicular fibers are usually spared so that the upper chest wall will have a better cosmetic appearance. It is easy to separate the clavicular fibers from the more inferior pectoral fibers, since no important nerves or vessels cross the cleft.*

The great bulk of the pectoralis major muscle gives shape to the anterior chest wall. The muscle flexes,

adducts, and internally rotates the arm. It has a multiple nerve supply from the medial and lateral anterior thoracic nerves (pectoral nerves), from the medial and lateral cords, respectively, that contain fibers derived from the brachial plexus (C5 through T1).

Pectoralis Minor Muscle

The pectoralis minor is thinner and much smaller than the pectoralis major, beneath which it lies. It is triangular, originating from the third, fourth, and fifth ribs, close to their respective costal cartilages. The pectoralis minor also arises from the intervening aponeurosis of the external intercostal muscles. The pectoralis minor fibers converge into an apical flat tendon that inserts into the coracoid process of the scapula. The apex of the muscle overlies the central structures of the axilla. The muscle draws the scapula ventrally and inferiorly. In forced respiration, it becomes an accessory muscle of respiration by raising the third, fourth, and fifth ribs with the scapula in fixed position. It is supplied by the medial pectoral nerve, a branch of the brachial plexus with fibers from C6–8.

Subclavius Muscle

The subclavius muscle is a short, rounded muscle that lies deep to the clavicle, between it and the external surface of the first rib. It arises from the first rib at its junction with the first costal cartilage and inserts onto the undersurface of the clavicle close to the conoid portion of the coracoclavicular ligament. It lies in the same plane on the anterior thoracic wall as does the pectoralis minor muscle. It is an accessory muscle of respiration, since in forced respiration it raises the first rib. It is supplied from the superior trunk of the brachial plexus with fibers from C5–6.

Serratus Anterior Muscle

The serratus anterior muscle is a thin, broad muscular sheet that arises from the external surfaces of the first 8 ribs and their intervening fibrous aponeuroses. From its origin, it sweeps laterally on the anterolateral chest wall as a series of fleshy digitations. It lies finally between the external surfaces of the upper posterior ribs and the deep surface of the scapula. It inserts along the inner surface of the vertebral border of the scapula. It is one of the accessory muscles of respiration. The serratus anterior is supplied by the long thoracic nerve with fibers from C5–7. The long thoracic nerve is formed in the neck and thus must pursue both a cervical and a thoracic course. The serratus anterior muscle raises the point of the shoulder during full flexion and abduction of the arm, and in addition it causes scapular rotation and draws the scapula forward, as in the act of pushing forward.

⟫ *Injuries to the long thoracic nerve. If the long thoracic nerve (of Bell), which supplies the serratus anterior muscle, is injured during breast or chest wall surgery or at the time of*

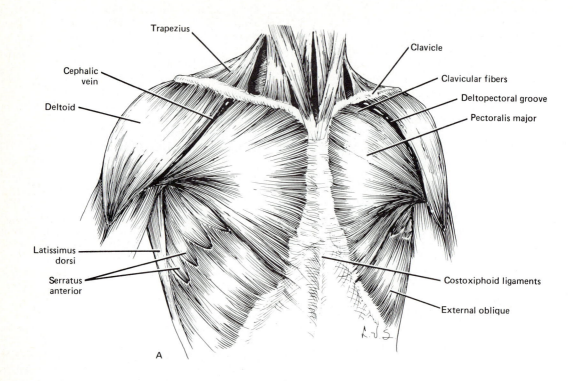

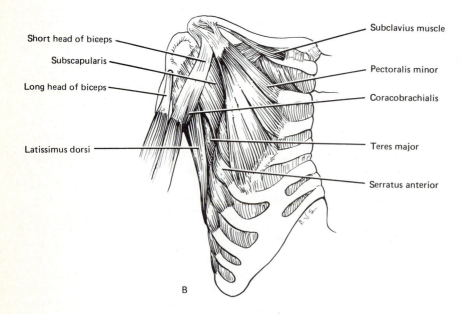

Figure 13–12. Anterior chest wall muscles. *A:* superficial; *B:* deep.

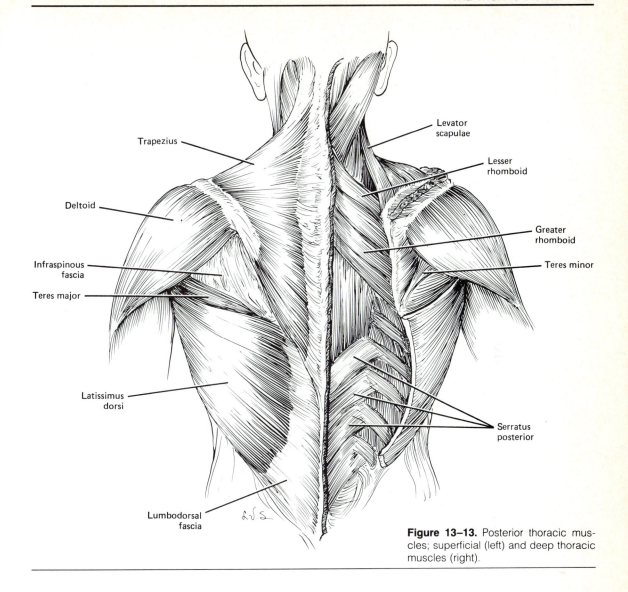

Levator scapulae

Lesser rhomboid

Greater rhomboid

Teres minor

Serratus posterior

Trapezius

Deltoid

Infraspinous fascia

Teres major

Latissimus dorsi

Lumbodorsal fascia

Figure 13–13. Posterior thoracic muscles; superficial (left) and deep thoracic muscles (right).

passage of a fetus through the birth canal, a scapular deformity results. Both the vertebral and inferior borders of the scapula lose their contact with the chest wall, and the scapula projects like a wing. The deformity is accentuated if the patient presses against a wall with arms fully extended at shoulder level.

Latissimus Dorsi Muscle

The latissimus dorsi muscle forms the posterior axillary fold. It is a large muscle, roughly triangular. It arises from the deep sheet of the thoracolumbar fascia, the spinous processes of the lower 6 thoracic vertebrae, the spinous processes of all of the lumbar and sacral vertebrae, the crest of the ilium, and fleshy slips from the lower 4 posterior ribs. It covers about seven-eighths of the lumbar region of the back and the inferolateral portion of the dorsal thorax. Its fibers

converge superiorly and end in a quadrilateral tendon that passes anterior to the teres major and inserts into the intertubercular groove of the humerus. It adducts, extends, and medially rotates the arm. It is supplied by the thoracodorsal nerve, which arises from the posterior cord of the brachial plexus with fibers coming from C6–8.

2. MUSCLES OF THE POSTERIOR THORACIC WALL (Fig 13–13; Table 13–2)

Trapezius Muscle

The trapezius is a large, thin triangular muscle that covers the neck and upper thorax. It is the most superficial of the dorsal thoracic muscles and arises from the external occipital protuberance, from the

Table 13–2. Muscles connecting the upper limbs to the vertebral column.

Muscle and Origin	Insertion	Innervation	Function
Trapezius From the external occipital protuberance and the medial third of the superior nuchal line of the occipital bone; the ligamentum nuchae; the spinous processes of C7 and of all the thoracic vertebrae; and from the supraspinal ligament dorsal to the above-mentioned vertebrae.	Into the posterior border of the lateral third of the clavicle, the medial margin of the acromion, the superior lip of the posterior border of the spine of the scapula, and the tubercle on the triangular surface of the medial end of the spine of the scapula.	Spinal accessory nerve (cranial nerve XI); branches from the anterior rami of C3 and C4 (sensory).	Entire muscle acting in unison rotates the scapula, raising the point of the shoulder; adducts the scapula; upper portion draws scapula upward, lower part draws it downward; both sides draw the head backward; the upper part draws the head to the same side and turns the face to the opposite side.
Latissimus dorsi From the broad lumbar aponeurosis, which is attached to the lower 6 thoracic and all of the lumbar and sacral vertebrae; the supraspinal ligament and the posterior iliac crest; by muscular fasciculi from the external lip of the iliac crest; by fleshy digitations from the lower 4 ribs; and by the muscular fasciculi from the inferior angle of the scapula.	Into the bottom of the intertubercular groove of the humerus via a broad tendon.	Thoracodorsal nerve (C6–8).	Extends, adducts, and rotates the arm medially; draws the shoulder downward and backward.
Rhomboideus major By the tendinous fibers from the spinous processes of T2–5 and the supraspinal ligament connecting their spines.	Into a narrow tendinous arch attached superiorly to the lower part of the triangular surface at the root of the spine of the scapula and inferiorly to the inferior angle of the scapula.	Dorsal scapular nerve (C5).	Adducts the scapula; rotates the scapula to depress its lateral angle.
Rhomboideus minor From the lower portion of the ligamentum nuchae and from the spinous process of C7–T1.	Into the base of the triangular surface at the root of the spine of the scapula.	Dorsal scapular nerve (C5).	Adducts the scapula; rotates the scapula to depress its lateral angle.
Levator scapulae From the transverse processes of C1 and C2 and from the posterior tubercles of the transverse processes of C3 and C4.	Into the vertebral border of the scapula between the superior angle and the root of its spine.	C3 and C4 via the cervical plexus.	Raises the scapula; moves the neck laterally if the scapula is fixed.

superior nuchal line of the occipital bone, from the nuchal ligament, from the spinous process of C7, and from all of the spinous processes from T1 to T12 and the intervening supraspinal ligaments. Its superior fibers insert into the lateral third of the clavicle. Its middle fibers insert into the acromion and the spine of the scapula. Its inferior fibers end in a fascial sheet that covers the medial end of the scapular spine and then inserts into the apex of the medial end of that spine. The muscle rotates the scapula and raises the point of the shoulder when the arm is flexed and in full abduction. It also adducts the scapula, draws the head to the ipsilateral side, and turns the face toward the contralateral side. It is supplied by the spinal accessory nerve and branches from C3 and C4.

Greater & Lesser Rhomboid Muscles

The greater rhomboid muscle arises from the spinous process of T2–5 and from the intervening supraspinal ligaments. It inserts into a narrow fibrous strip that runs from the root of the spine of the scapula superiorly to the inferior angle of the scapula caudally.

The lesser rhomboid muscle arises from the spinous processes of C7 and T1 and from the inferior segment of the nuchal ligament. It inserts into the root of the spine of the scapula.

The 2 rhomboid muscles draw the scapula toward the vertebral column on a plane deep to the trapezius muscle. The muscles are supplied by the dorsal scapular nerve, a branch of the brachial plexus, with fibers from C4 and C5.

The Breast

14

The breasts (mammae) are auxiliary reproductive glands of ectodermal modified sweat gland origin. Each breast lies on the superior mid surface of the chest wall. In women, the breasts are the organs of lactation; in men, the breasts are normally functionless and undeveloped.

LOBULAR STRUCTURE OF BREAST

The adult female breast contains glandular and ductal tissue, a stroma of fibrous tissue that binds the individual lobes together, and fatty tissue within and between the lobes.

Each breast consists of 12–20 conical lobes. The base of each lobe is close to the ribs; the apex, which contains the major secretory duct of the lobe, is situated close to the areola and nipple. Each lobe consists of a group of lobules, and the many lactiferous ducts in each lobule unite to form a major duct that drains a lobe as it converges toward the areola. Each of the major ducts widens to form an ampulla as it reaches the areola and then narrows for its individual opening on the nipple. The lobules are held in place by a meshwork of fatty areolar tissue. The fatty tissue increases toward the periphery of the lobule and gives the breast its bulk and its hemispheric shape.

About 80–85% of the normal breast is fat. The breast tissues are joined to the overlying skin and subcutaneous tissue by fibrous strands.

In the nonpregnant, nonlactating breast, the alveoli are small and tightly packed. During pregnancy, the alveoli enlarge and their lining cells increase in number. During lactation, the alveolar cells secrete milk proteins and lipids.

The deep surface of the breast lies on the fascia that covers the chest muscles. The fascial stroma, derived from the superficial fascia of the chest wall, is condensed into multiple fascial bands that run from the breast into the subcutaneous tissues and the corium of the skin overlying the breast. The fascial bands—Cooper's suspensory ligaments—support the breast in its upright position on the chest wall. When the ligaments are stretched, as may occur during pregnancy, or become flaccid, as occurs with old age or debilitating disease, the breast loses its good "pos-

ture" and tends to sag inferiorly on the chest wall and occasionally onto the upper abdomen.

➠ *Suspensory ligaments (of Cooper). In advanced cancer of the breast, an "orange-peel" appearance of the skin usually indicates the presence of infiltrating cancer which is ascending toward the cutaneous area along Cooper's ligaments—though the same picture may be due to fibrosis that pulls upon Cooper's ligaments during the course of healing of fat necrosis secondary to trauma. Mammograms, ultrasound, aspiration biopsy, and open biopsy are useful in distinguishing between the 2 entities.*

CHANGES IN LOBULAR STRUCTURE IN THE FEMALE BREAST DURING THE LIFE SPAN

During puberty, in response to multiglandular stimulation, the female breast begins to enlarge and eventually assumes its conical or spherical shape. Growth is due to increase in acinar tissue, ductal size and branching, and deposits of fat. Also during puberty, the nipple and areola enlarge. Smooth muscle fibers surround the base of the nipple, and the nipple becomes more sensitive to touch.

Once menses are established, the breast undergoes a periodic **premenstrual phase** during which the acinar cells increase in number and size, the ductal lumens widen, and breast size and turgor increase slightly. Many women have breast tenderness during this phase of the cycle. Menstrual bleeding is followed by a **postmenstrual phase** characterized by decrease in size and turgor, reduction in the number and size of the breast acini, and decrease in diameter of the lactiferous ducts. Individual response of the breast to cyclic hormonal influences is variable, including the degree of hypertrophic and regressive changes. Many feel that recurrent breast engorgement and regression during the reproductive years may cause cystic disease and ductal ectasia and may even play a part in neoplasia.

During pregnancy, in response to progesterone, breast size and turgidity increase markedly. These changes are accompanied by deepening nipple and areolar pigmentation, nipple enlargement, areolar widening, and an increase in the number and size of the lubricating glands in the areola. The breast ductal system branches markedly, and the individual ducts widen. The acini increase in number and size. In late pregnancy, the fatty tissues of the breasts are almost completely replaced by cellular breast parenchyma. After delivery, the breasts, now fully mature, start to secrete milk. With cessation of nursing or administration of estrogens to inhibit lactation, the gland rapidly returns to its prepregnancy state, with marked diminution of cellular elements and an increase in fat deposits.

Between the fifth and sixth decades of life, when menses cease, the breast gradually involutes. There is a decrease in the number and size of acinar and ductal elements, and adipose tissue may or may not atrophy. Consequently, the postmenopausal breast may still be well-shaped and filled with fat but contains few glandular elements.

GROSS ANATOMY
(Fig 14–1)

The adult female breast usually forms an almost hemispheric protrusion on each side of the chest wall, usually extending from just below the level of the second rib and extending to the sixth or seventh rib. The gland is usually situated between the lateral sternal border and the anterior axillary fold. The superior surface of the breast emerges gradually from the chest wall, whereas the lateral and inferior borders are quite well defined. The major portion of the breast, lying atop the pectoralis major muscle, projects ventrally; smaller portions lie atop the serratus anterior and external oblique muscles. A triangular tongue-shaped tail of breast tissue (the axillary tail) extends toward the axilla, perforates the deep axillary fascia, and terminates in close apposition to the axillary lymph vessels and nodes and the axillary blood vessels and nerves.

⤵ **Breast trauma.** *The breast is often subjected to external trauma, and some women with breast tumors relate the appearance of the mass to an episode of trauma. However, no connection has been established between breast trauma and breast cancer. Breast trauma occasionally results in fat necrosis or deep hematoma formation. Fat necrosis heals with marked fibrosis; in some cases, fat necrosis can only be distinguished from breast cancer by biopsy.*

⤵ **Axillary tail of the breast.** *The axillary tail of the breast is frequently the site of painful fibrocystic disease and less commonly the site of breast cancer. Its cyclic premenstrual swellings and postmenstrual regressions often cause anxiety. Occasionally, the swelling must be distinguished from that due to acute axillary lymphadenitis.*

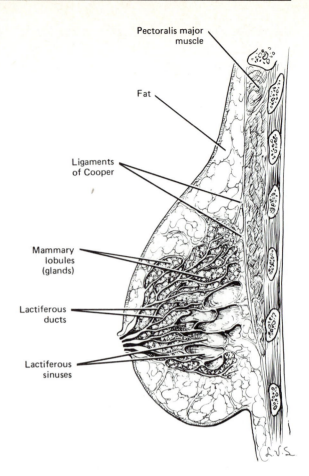

Figure 14–1. Sagittal section of the breast.

Labels: Pectoralis major muscle; Fat; Ligaments of Cooper; Mammary lobules (glands); Lactiferous ducts; Lactiferous sinuses

The skin over the breast is usually thinner than the skin of the adjacent chest wall and axilla; it is not unusual for veins in the subcutaneous tissue to be visible through the skin of the breast.

THE NIPPLE & AREOLA

The areola is a circular pigmented zone 2–6 cm in diameter at the tip of the breast. Its color varies from pale pink to deep brown depending upon age, parity, and skin pigmentation. The skin of the areola contains multiple small elevated nodules beneath which lie the sebaceous glands (glands of Montgomery). The glands are responsible for lubrication of the nipple and help prevent nipple and areolar cracks and fissures. During the third trimester of pregnancy, the sebaceous glands hypertrophy markedly.

⤵ **Diseases of the areola.** *The areola is frequently the site of fissures, chronic eczema, and small subcutaneous abscesses, the latter usually sec-*

ondary to infection of the lubricating glands of Montgomery.

➡ ***Paget's disease of the breast.*** *Paget's disease of the breast appears as a chronic eczematous condition that affects both the nipple and the areola. It always signifies carcinoma within the breast parenchyma. Paget cells can usually be recovered from the nipple or areola by smear or tissue biopsy. Paget cells resemble enlarged ductal lining cells, and the malignant neoplasm associated with the central cutaneous eczema is of the ductal type.*

The nipple is an elevated mound of tissue in the center of the areola. In the nulliparous, well-supported breast, the nipple is usually at the level of the fourth intercostal space. In multiparous women or when the ligaments of Cooper are relaxed or stretched, this position varies considerably.

A circular smooth muscle band surrounds the base of the nipple. Longitudinal smooth muscle fibers branch out from the ring of circular smooth muscle to encircle the lactiferous ducts as they converge toward the nipple. The many small punctate openings situated at the top of the nipple are the terminals of the major lactiferous ducts. The ampullae of the lactiferous ducts lie just deep to the nipple and the areola.

➡ ***Gynecomastia.*** *Gynecomastia is unilateral or bilateral enlargement of all or a portion of the male breast. It usually appears during pubescence but can occur at any time. A firm, tender discoid lump is often present just deep to the areola. Diffuse fibrous, usually painful breast enlargement is common in men kept on severely restricted diets for long periods ("prison camp disease"). Gynecomastia is often associated with cirrhosis of the liver, hyperthyroidism, some types of testicular and adrenocortical neoplasms, and administration of certain drugs (eg, thiazides). Treatment is usually expectant except when cancer is suspected or when the cosmetic deformity is a psychologic problem.*

BLOOD VESSELS, LYMPHATICS, & NERVES

Arteries
(Fig 14–2)

The breast has a multiple arterial supply. Perforating branches from the internal thoracic artery that appear in interspaces 2, 3, and 4 supply blood to the medial quadrants of the breast. These arteries perforate the intercostal muscles and the anterior intercostal membrane to supply both the breast and the

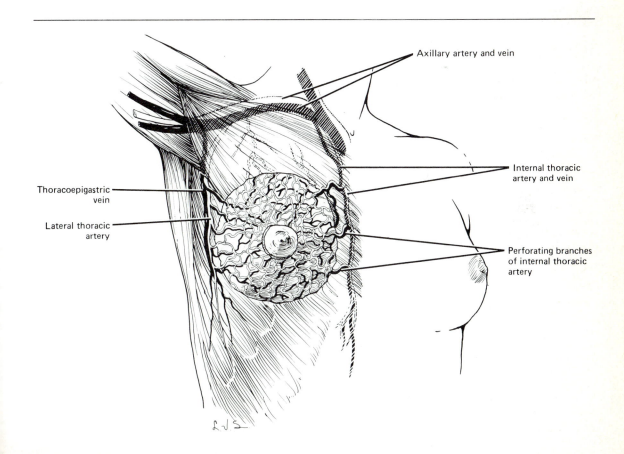

Axillary artery and vein

Internal thoracic artery and vein

Thoracoepigastric vein

Lateral thoracic artery

Perforating branches of internal thoracic artery

pectoralis major and minor muscles. During pregnancy and in advanced breast disease, the intercostal perforators generally enlarge. The breast is also supplied medially by small branches from the anterior intercostal arteries. It is nourished laterally by the pectoral branch of the thoracoacromial branch of the axillary artery and by the external mammary branch of the lateral thoracic artery, which also is a branch of the axillary artery. The external mammary artery passes along the lateral free border of the pectoralis major muscle to reach the lateral half of the breast, the artery usually lying medial to the long thoracic nerve.

The medial and lateral arteries arborize mainly in the supra-areolar area; consequently, the arterial supply to the upper half of the breast is almost twice that of the lower half.

Veins
(Fig 14–2)

Venous return from the breast closely follows the arterial supply. Blood returns to the superior vena cava via the axillary and internal thoracic veins. It also returns via the vertebral venous plexuses, which are fed by the intercostal and azygos veins. There is a rich subareolar anastomotic plexus of superficial breast veins. In thin-skinned individuals, these veins are normally visible. They always become visible during pregnancy. Their presence makes for marked vascularity of sub- and para-areolar incisions. There is a greater amount of venous flow in the superior quadrants than in the inferior quadrants of the breast.

➠ *Placement of surgical incisions. Because the inferior quadrants of the breast are less vascular than the superior quadrants, incisions should be placed when possible in the inferior half of the gland, preferably in the inferior cutaneous crease.*

Because the inferior half of the breast usually overhangs the chest wall, an incision just below the inferior margin of the gland in the inferior cutaneous crease will frequently be obscured by the droop of the breast. Incisions in the nipple and areolar areas are usually placed radially or in gently curved fashion lateral or medial to the areola.

➠ *Venous spread of breast cancer. The malignant cells of breast cancer frequently enter tributaries of the axillary and internal thoracic veins, initiating dissemination of cancer cells via venous routes to the lungs, brain, liver, and bones.*

Lymphatics
(Figs 14–3 and 14–4)

Modern surgical concepts of management of breast cancer are based to a large extent on an understanding of the pattern of lymphatic drainage from the breast.

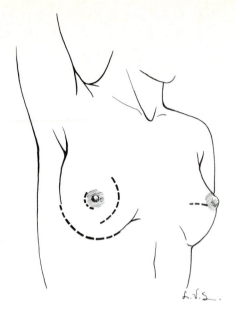

Figure 14–3. Types of breast incisions.

Lymphatic drainage from the breast may be divided into 2 main categories: superficial (including cutaneous) drainage and deep parenchymatous drainage.

A. Superficial Drainage: A large lymphatic plexus lies in the subcutaneous tissues of the breast just beneath the areola and the nipple. This plexus drains the areola and nipple areas and the cutaneous and subcutaneous tissues adjacent to the areola. It also drains the deep central parenchymatous region of the breast, the lymph rising from these areas to pool in the superficial plexus.

B. Deep Parenchymatous Drainage: The deep parenchymatous lymph channels drain most of the breast. Small periductal and periacinal lymph channels collect parenchymal lymph and deliver it to the larger interlobar lymphatics. Lymph from the cutaneous and areolar areas may drain either directly into the subareolar plexus or deeply into the parenchymatous lymph channels and is secondarily delivered to the subareolar plexus for efferent transport.

From both the retroareolar and the deep interlobar lymphatics, most breast lymph passes via 2 major trunks to the ipsilateral axillary group of lymph nodes. One major trunk drains the supra-areolar half of the breast and the other the infra-areolar half. There are no predetermined pathways by which breast lymph reaches the highest axillary node or nodes. Most breast lymph usually goes first to the anterior axillary or subpectoral group of nodes that lie just beneath the lateral border of the pectoralis major muscle, close to the lateral thoracic artery. From these nodes, lymph usually passes to nodes lying close to the mid portion of the axillary vein. The lymph then passes superiorly, via the axillary chain of lymph vessels and nodes, to nodes lying alongside the superior half of the axil-

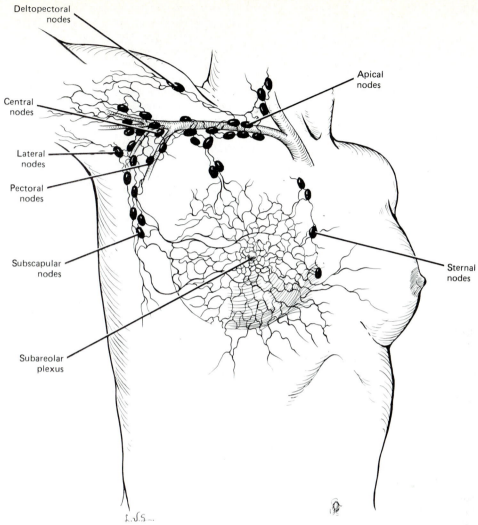

Deltopectoral nodes

Apical nodes

Central nodes

Lateral nodes

Pectoral nodes

Subscapular nodes

Sternal nodes

Subareolar plexus

L.J.S.

Figure 14–4. Lymphatics of the breast and surrounding areas.

lary vein. The lymph eventually reaches the highest nodes of the axilla. Although this is the so-called normal pattern of drainage, other paths of drainage are fairly common, particularly when the lateral and superiorly directed channels are obstructed by tumor masses.

Alternate Pathways for Lymphatic Flow

1. From the breast directly to the highest axillary node, completely bypassing all other axillary nodal tissue. This frequently occurs with superior quadrant breast tumors.

2. From the breast to the midaxillary group of nodes that lie deep to the pectoralis minor tendon, bypassing the subpectoral group of nodes.

3. From the breast directly to the subscapular group of axillary nodes, subsequently progressing through channels lying close to the axillary vein.

4. From the breast directly to the most inferior group of supraclavicular cervical nodes. Supraclavicular nodes are more commonly involved via direct extension from the apical axillary nodes.

5. From the breast across the sternal midline to the lymphatics of the contralateral breast.

6. From the breast directly to the contralateral axilla.

7. From the breast to the internal mammary group of nodes when the primary breast tumor is in the medial quadrant (as is usually the case also in 5 and 6, above).

8. From the breast to lymphatics closely related to the sheaths of the superior segments of the rectus abdominis and external oblique muscles and thence inferiorly toward the upper abdominal wall, the diaphragm, and the intra-abdominal viscera (especially the liver).

Nerves Related to the Breast Area

The lateral and anterior cutaneous branches of T4–6 supply the cutaneous tissues covering the breasts. The following nerves lie close to the breast area and assume importance in major breast surgery:

(1) The **thoracodorsal nerve,** a branch of the posterior cord of the brachial plexus (C5–7), runs along with the subscapular artery close to the posterior axillary wall and the ventral surface of the subscapular muscle. The nerve innervates the superior half of the latissimus dorsi muscle and is usually surrounded by a large venous plexus that drains into the subscapular veins.

(2) The **long thoracic nerve** (external respiratory nerve of Bell) arises from the anterior primary divisions of C5–7 at the level of the lower half of the anterior scalene muscle. In the neck, the nerve descends dorsal to the trunks of the brachial plexus on the middle scalene muscle, then dorsal to the clavicle and the axillary vessels. On the lateral thoracic wall, it descends on the external surface of the serratus anterior muscle along the anterior axillary line. The line of the lateral thoracic artery is a guide to the long thoracic nerve, the nerve usually lying just posterior to this vessel. The long thoracic nerve supplies filaments to the serratus anterior muscle. Care must be taken not to injure the nerve during operative procedures upon the medial axillary wall.

(3) The **intercostal brachial nerves** are 3 relatively minor cutaneous nerves that supply the skin of the medial surface of the upper arm. They cross transversely from the lateral chest wall to the upper inner surface of the arm, passing across the base of the axilla. It is usually not feasible to preserve these nerves in radical breast surgery, although their interruption may be followed by minor brachial areas of hyperesthesia.

(4) The **medial and lateral pectoral nerves** that supply the 2 pectoral muscles pass from the axilla to the lateral chest wall, reaching it by piercing the costocoracoid membrane. The medial pectoral nerve arises from the medial cord of the brachial plexus; the lateral pectoral nerve arises from the lateral cord of the plexus.

➠ *Preservation of medial and lateral pectoral nerves. The medial and lateral pectoral nerves must be isolated and preserved in the performance of modified radical mastectomy in order to preserve the pectoralis major and minor muscles. If these nerves are damaged, atrophy of the pectoralis major and minor muscles and fibrosis of their tendons will prevent full arm abduction and will impair internal rotation and adduction of the arm.*

➠ *Breast abscesses. Breast abscesses are most common in the puerperium but may occur at any time. Location of the abscess will determine*

the best position of incision. Drainage of these abscesses may be through a radial incision in the subareolar quadrants of the breast. Breast abscesses may also be drained by an incision through the submammary fold. Submammary fold incisions give better drainage and are usually less vascular, and the resulting scar is frequently less visible.

➠ *Benign breast tumors. Benign tumors of the breast include fibroadenoma, periductal fibromas, intraductal papillomas, retention cysts, lipomas, myxomas, chronic cystic mastitis, and fat necrosis. They occur most frequently during and just following the reproductive period of life and rarely early or late in life. It is often difficult to distinguish between benign and malignant tumors of the breast, and a persistent breast mass, particularly if it increases in size or has associated lymphadenopathy, calls for incision and biopsy to rule out cancer. Mammograms, ultrasound, thermography, Papanicolaou staining of nipple discharge, and aspiration of cystic masses may aid in diagnosis.*

➠ *Malignant breast tumors. Malignant breast tumors are carcinomas of various types and, rarely, sarcoma. Paget's disease of the nipple is always accompanied by underlying parenchymatous carcinoma of the ductal type. Management for cure or palliation depends upon the patient's age and clinical status, the type and size of the tumor, the degree of local tumor spread, the estrogen relationship of the tumor, and the presence or absence of distant metastases. Five procedures are in common use today:*

(1) Radical mastectomy. This involves removal of the breast and the pectoralis major and minor muscles and complete axillary nodal dissection. The procedure may be preceded or followed by x-ray therapy, depending largely on the presence or absence of axillary metastases.

(2) Modified radical mastectomy. This consists of removal of the entire breast and the axillary lymph glands, with preservation of the pectoralis major and minor muscles. The tendon of the pectoralis minor muscle is occasionally severed or retracted near its insertion into the coracoid process to aid in axillary visualization and lymphatic clean-out. The procedure is often followed by x-ray therapy.

(3) Simple mastectomy with or without x-ray therapy.

(4) Segmental mastectomy, for early small lesions, with or without x-ray therapy.

(5) X-ray therapy alone.

➠ *Treatment of late cancer of the breast. Late neighboring or distant malignant breast metas-*

tases may be treated by bilateral oophorectomy, adrenalectomy, pituitary ablation, androgen or estrogen therapy, chemotherapy, or any combination of these forms of treatment. The choice of late therapy will be influenced by the patient's age and clinical status, the site of metastases (visceral or bony), information gained from estrogen receptor assay, and the number of years since menopause. Late metastases respond on occasion to x-ray therapy, particularly bony and cutaneous metastatic lesions.

Aspiration of breast cysts. (*Fig. 14–5.*) Breast cysts and suspected breast cysts are being aspirated with increasing frequency. This procedure saves the patient the expense and loss of time which exploratory surgery and hospital entry entail. Aspiration frequently helps to distinguish between benign and malignant breast lesions.

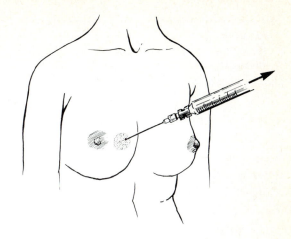

Figure 14–5. Aspiration of breast tumors.

15 — Axilla

GROSS ANATOMY
(Figs 15–1 and 15–2)

The axilla (armpit) is a pyramid-shaped compartment situated between the lateral chest wall and the medial surface of the arm. It consists of 4 walls, an apex, and a base. The axillary compartment contains blood vessels, nerves, lymphatic channels, lymph nodes, and varying amounts of adipose tissue.

BOUNDARIES OF THE AXILLA

The **anterior wall** of the axilla is composed of 2 layers of muscle: superficial and deep. The superficial layer consists of the pectoralis major muscle and its investing fascia; the deep layer is formed by the pectoralis minor and subclavius muscles with their investing fascia and by the clavipectoral fascia that runs inferiorly from the clavicle to the axillary base.

The **posterior (scapular) wall** of the axilla is formed mainly by the subscapularis muscle as it covers the ventral surface of the scapula. The inferior segment of the posterior wall of the axilla is formed by the teres major and latissimus dorsi muscles.

The **medial (thoracic) wall** of the axilla is formed

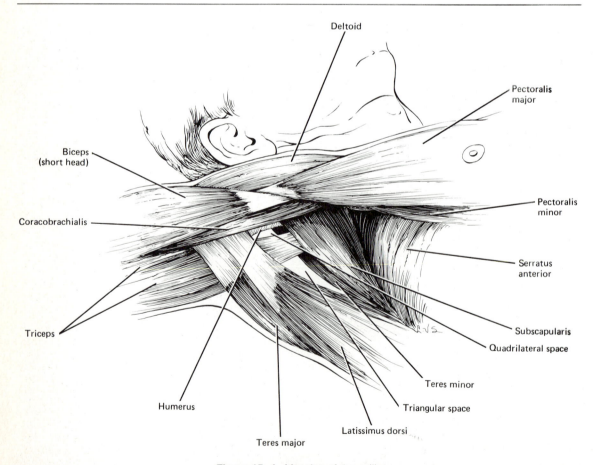

Figure 15–1. Muscles of the axilla.

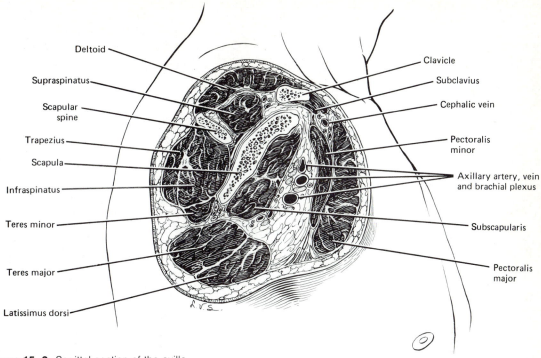

Figure 15–2. Sagittal section of the axilla.

by ribs 2–6, along with their intervening intercostal muscles, which are covered in part by the serratus anterior muscles.

The **lateral (humeral) wall** of the axilla is formed by the bicipital groove of the humerus, which contains the tendon of the long head of the biceps. The 2 lips of the bicipital groove are the sites of attachment of the muscles that constitute the major portions of the anterior and posterior axillary walls. The short head of the biceps and the coracobrachialis muscle also participate in the lateral axillary wall.

The **stubby apex** of the axilla—the superior limit of the compartment—terminates at the outer border of the first rib. The axillary apex is limited anteriorly by the clavicle, posteriorly by the superior margin of the scapula, and medially by the first rib. The adipose tissue of the apex of the axilla is continuous with adipose tissue in the posteroinferior region of the neck.

The **base** of the axilla is made up of skin, subcutaneous tissue, and the axillary fascia. It extends from the lateral border of the pectoralis major muscle to the anterior border of the latissimus dorsi muscle. When the base is tented superiorly, it forms the hollow of the armpit. The deep layer of the axillary fascia, which forms the deepest layer of the axillary base, is continuous with the fasciae of the pectoral, latissimus dorsi, serratus anterior, and brachial muscles. Attached at a right angle to the axillary fascia is the inferior termination of the clavipectoral fascia, as it descends from the inferior border of the pectoralis minor muscle. Since the clavipectoral fascia attaches

to the axillary base, it is called the suspensory ligament of the axilla, and its contraction is responsible for the superior convexity of that boundary of the axilla. The subcutaneous adipose tissue lying between the superficial and deep fascia of the base of the axilla frequently pierces the deep layer of the axillary fascia to become continuous with the true axillary adipose tissue.

➠ ***Subcutaneous fat at base of axilla.*** *Since the subcutaneous fat in the base of the axilla frequently pierces the deep layer of the axillary fascia, the deep fascia does not serve as an efficient barrier to the spread into the axilla of superficial axillary infections. The axillary tail of the breast pierces the subcutaneous tissue and superficial fascia of the axillary base and comes to lie in the true axilla. Inflammation of this area of the breast will cause symptoms in the axilla.*

➠ ***Hidradenitis.*** *The base of the axilla contains numerous sweat and sebaceous glands. The glands are frequently the site of acute and chronic infections (hidradenitis) that may be difficult to eradicate and are often complicated by the presence of multiple draining sinuses. In long-standing infections, the axillary skin, subcutaneous tissue, and deep fascia may have to be completely excised and the denuded axillary base then closed primarily or skin-grafted.*

FASCIA & MEMBRANES RELATED TO THE AXILLA

Pectoral Fascia

Two major divisions of the fascial envelopes enclose the muscles of the pectoral region and are of importance in breast surgery. The **pectoral fascia proper** originates along the clavicle. It runs inferiorly, clothing the pectoralis major muscle both superficially and deeply. In the floor of the axilla, it blends with the deep axillary fascia. The pectoralis fascia is attached to the midline of the sternum, where it decussates with the pectoral fascia of the opposite side—the decussation giving strong fascial support to the ventral surface of the sternum. Inferiorly and medially, the pectoral fascia blends (1) with the fascia covering the anterior segments of the serratus anterior muscle, and (2) with the fascia of the upper portion of the external oblique muscle. Laterally, the fascia blends with the fasciae covering the muscles of the medial upper arm. Lying ventral to the pectoral fascia proper is the breast, separated from the fascia only by the thin deep capsule of the breast, which is simply a condensation of subcutaneous tissue.

⇒ *Relationship of deep breast carcinoma to the pectoral fascia. Even a deeply situated carcinoma of the breast seldom involves the underlying pectoral fascia and musculature—even though a few lymphatics run from the breast to the fasciae covering the pectoralis major. This fact has supported modified radical mastectomy without removal of the pectoralis major muscle.*

Clavipectoral Fascia

The clavipectoral fascia lies on a plane deep to the pectoralis major muscle and its investing fascia. The clavipectoral fascia begins at the clavicle, where it immediately splits to enclose the small subclavius muscle. It fuses again into a single layer at the inferior border of the subclavius and continues until it reaches the pectoralis minor muscle, which it encloses. Farther inferiorly, it attaches at right angles to the deep fascia of the base of the axilla.

The most inferior clavipectoral segment of the clavipectoral fascia is the suspensory ligament of the axilla. The lateral half of the clavipectoral fascia, between the subclavius muscle and the pectoralis minor muscle immediately inferior to the coracoid process, is called the costocoracoid membrane. The **costocoracoid membrane** runs medially as far as the first and second costal cartilages, and laterally it is attached to the coracoid process of the scapula.

Where the clavipectoral fascia overlies the subclavius muscle, it is thickened by membranous fibers that continue as the costocoracoid ligament.

The costocoracoid membrane is pierced by the cephalic vein on its way to empty into the axillary vein; by the thoracoacromial branch of the axillary artery; and by the lymph vessels carrying lymphatic drainage from the upper outer quadrant of the breast to the axillary nodes. When the costocoracoid membrane is incised and reflected inferiorly along with the previously transected pectoralis minor muscle, the axillary sheath encircling the axillary vessels and the major nerves of the brachial plexus is visualized. In obese patients, however, the axillary structures are hidden by a layer of adipose tissue that lies just deep to the costocoracoid membrane.

Axillary Sheath

The axillary sheath is an extension of the prevertebral fascia of the neck which is continued into the axilla as a covering sheath for the major axillary vessels and nerves. The subclavian artery and brachial plexus must pierce the prevertebral fascia as they descend from the neck toward the axilla. The sheath of the axillary artery and brachial artery continues down the arm to about 5 cm superior to the elbow joint, at which level the sheath terminates by fusing with the adventitia of the brachial artery.

BLOOD VESSELS, LYMPHATICS, & NERVES

Arteries
(Figs 15–3 and 15–4)

The **axillary artery,** about 12–13 cm long, is the major artery of the axilla. It starts at the first rib as a continuation of the subclavian artery; after traversing the axilla, it becomes the brachial artery at the lower border of the teres major muscle. Throughout its course, it tends to lie dorsal and slightly superior to the axillary vein and is intimately related to the cords of the brachial plexus. The tendon of the pectoralis minor muscle, ascending to the coracoid process, divides the axillary artery into 3 parts. The first part of the artery lies medial and superior to the tendon; the second part lies dorsal to the tendon; and the third part lies lateral and inferior to the tendon.

⇒ *Arteriovenous fistula. The proximity to each other of the axillary artery and vein can lead to fistula formation. Such fistulas are fairly common sequelae of penetrating injuries of the axilla.*

⇒ *Axillary aneurysms. Axillary aneurysms present as soft pulsating masses that are often palpable through the base of the armpit. A bruit may be heard at the base of the axilla. The aneurysmal mass may press upon the nerves of the brachial plexus, with resultant sensory and motor deficits of the upper extremity. If the axillary vein is compressed by the mass, it may cause upper extremity edema. Vascular surgery makes it possible to resect the aneurysm and use a vein graft to bridge the area of deficit.*

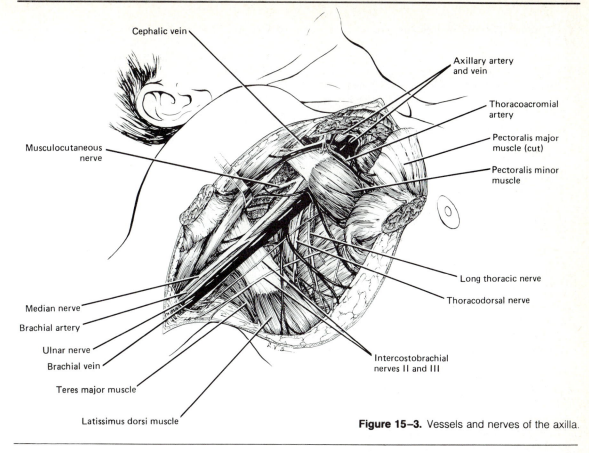

Figure 15–3. Vessels and nerves of the axilla.

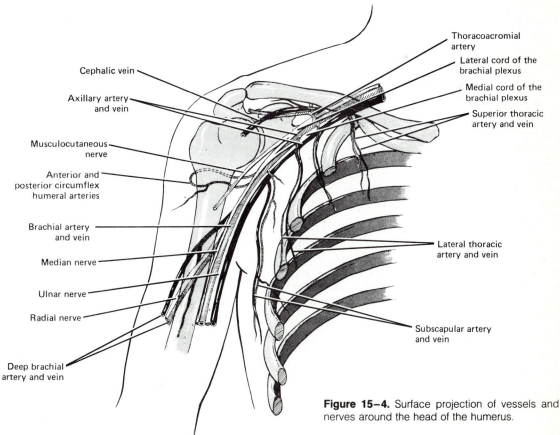

Figure 15–4. Surface projection of vessels and nerves around the head of the humerus.

➠ *Elective ligation of the axillary artery. Axillary artery ligation is usually performed near the crossing of the artery by the pectoralis minor muscle. The preferred site for ligation is usually just inferior to the muscle crossing, at a point between the subscapular and circumflex humeral branches of the vessel.*

➠ *Relationship of axillary artery to the shoulder joint. Because of the close relationship of the axillary artery to the capsule of the shoulder joint, the artery may be damaged if the joint dislocates anteriorly. The artery may be damaged during reduction of the anterior dislocation if the position of the vessel is not kept in mind.*

➠ *Axillary artery injuries with fractures of the upper humerus. Injury to the axillary artery may be secondary to fractures of both the anatomic and surgical necks of the humerus. Such injury is more common in fractures with fragment displacement.*

The **first portion** of the axillary artery lies deep to the costocoracoid membrane, superior to and on a more dorsal plane than the axillary vein. The artery lies fairly close to the anterior surface of the shoulder joint. It has one branch—the highest thoracic artery—which runs to the superior lateral chest wall, where it anastomoses with branches of the internal thoracic and anterior intercostal arteries.

The short **second portion** of the axillary artery has 2 branches: (1) the thoracoacromial trunk, which pierces the costocoracoid segment of the clavipectoral fascia and divides into pectoral, acromial, deltoid, and clavicular branches; and (2) the lateral thoracic (external mammary) artery, which runs inferiorly, lying along the lateral border of the pectoralis minor muscle. The lateral thoracic artery gives off lateral mammary and chest wall branches. Its mammary branch runs along the lateral free border of the pectoralis major muscle, medial to the long thoracic nerve, before turning medially to supply the lateral quadrants of the breast.

The **third portion** of the axillary artery lies inferior and lateral to the tendon of the pectoralis minor muscle and close to the surgical neck of the shaft of the humerus. It is the longest segment of the artery and has 3 branches. Its major branch is the subscapular artery, which supplies the posterior axillary wall. A branch of the subscapular artery reaches the infraspinous fossa by passing through the **triangular space** of the upper arm. The triangular space is bounded laterally by the long head of the triceps muscle, superiorly by the teres minor muscle, and inferiorly by the teres major muscle. The last 2 branches are the anterior and posterior circumflex humeral arteries, which form an arterial network around the surgical neck of the humerus and are important arterial anastomoses around the shoulder joint.

Veins
(Figs 15–3 and 15–4)

The **axillary vein** is the most superficial major structure in the axilla. Following reflection inferiorly of both the costocoracoid membrane and the pectoralis minor muscle, it is immediately noted by the operating surgeon. With the arm moderately abducted and externally rotated, the axillary vein tends to block the axillary artery. The axillary vein begins at the lower border of the teres major muscle with the confluence of veins accompanying the brachial artery. The vein then joins with the basilic vein and continues medially as the axillary vein. It climbs to the border of the first rib, at which point it becomes the subclavian vein. In 10–12% of cases, as a result of delayed union of its tributary veins, the axillary vein may appear as a double or triple vein during its course through the axilla. In such cases, axillary dissection is obviously more difficult. Considerable venous blood drains into the most superior portion of the axillary vein via the **cephalic vein,** which runs in the deltopectoral cleft, pierces the costocoracoid membrane, and joins the axillary vein just inferior to the first rib. The medial cord of the brachial plexus and the median, ulnar, and pectoral nerves lie between the axillary vein and the axillary artery.

➠ *Cephalic vein as landmark. The cephalic vein serves as a landmark which identifies the first portion of the axillary artery. If the cephalic vein is followed through the costocoracoid membrane, it crosses the superior segment of the artery and then ends in the axillary vein.*

➠ *Preservation of cephalic vein. Care must be taken not to injure the cephalic vein during radical mastectomy, since it may have a major role in the adequacy of venous drainage of the upper extremity. This is particularly true if damage to the axillary vein below the level of the entrance of the cephalic vein should occur.*

Lymphatics

The axillary lymph nodes and the abundant axillary lymphatic channels play an important role in the diagnosis and treatment of infection and cancer of the anterolateral chest wall, the breast, the upper lateral abdominal wall, the scapular region, and the entire upper extremity.

About 15–40 axillary nodes and multiple lymphatic channels lie embedded in the fatty areolar tissue of the axillary space. The nodes are fairly large (2–8 mm in diameter) even in health. The channels are intimately related to the important venous structures in the axilla, particularly the axillary vein.

Axillary abscesses. Abscesses within the true confines of the axillary space, superior to the deep fascia of the axillary base, are usually secondary to the breakdown of suppurating axillary lymph nodes. They may become large enough to bulge outward through to the axillary floor, or they may protrude superiorly into the root of the neck. Incisions for drainage of deep axillary abscesses should be placed between and parallel to the anterior and posterior axillary folds to avoid injury to the lateral thoracic and subscapular vessels.

Resection of axillary lymph nodes. In performing radical mastectomy, the surgeon must incise the costocoracoid portion of the clavipectoral fascia and reflect it inferiorly along with the pectoralis minor muscle before the axillary contents can be properly inspected. Nodal dissection ordinarily starts with the highest node of the axilla, which is usually located just inferior to the first rib. In modified radical mastectomy, the pectoralis minor is usually retracted medially in order to provide access to the highest axillary nodal area.

Location of axillary lymph nodes. Since most of the lymphatic channels and nodes in the axilla lie in intimate relationship to the adventitia of the axillary vein and its major tributaries, the venous sheaths of these vessels have in the past been stripped during the course of axillary dissection for malignant neoplastic diseases. With the development of less radical surgical procedures for breast carcinoma, this practice has largely been abandoned.

For descriptive purposes, the axillary nodal areas are best divided into 5 groupings (Fig 14–3).

A **lateral group** consisting of 3–8 nodes lies both medial and dorsal to the third portion of the axillary vein. These nodes drain most of the upper extremity. Efferent drainage from the lateral group is into the central apical nodes.

The **pectoral nodes** (3–8 in number) stud the area along the course of the lateral thoracic artery and lie both along the lateral border of the pectoralis major muscle and deep to this border. They drain much of the chest wall, receive most of the primary drainage from the entire breast, and drain the abdominal wall above the level of the umbilicus. Pectoral node efferents drain into the central and apical axillary nodes.

The **subscapular nodes** (3–6 in number) lie close to the subscapular vessels and the thoracodorsal nerve on the central surface of the subscapularis muscle. Afferents to this group of nodes drain lymph from the skin and muscular areas of the posterior chest wall, the scapula, and the dorsal surface of the neck. There is also some direct drainage from the lateral area of the breast to the subscapular nodes. The subscapular nodes send their efferents to the central axillary nodes.

The **central group** of axillary nodes (4–6 in number) lie deep to the axillary fascia embedded in axillary fat. These nodes are usually the largest of the axillary group. Their afferents bring some lymph directly from the breast and from the upper extremity, but most of the lymph that reaches these nodes comes from the 3 groups described above. Central group efferents drain into the apical nodes of the axilla.

The **apical nodes** (6–10 in number) are the most superior lymph glands of the axilla. They surround the axillary vein superior to the pectoralis minor tendon. The afferent lymphatics are derived from all other axillary lymph areas. Additional afferents to this group are lymphatics accompanying the cephalic vein and lymphatics draining the upper inner quadrants of the breast. From the highest of the apical nodes, a narrow lymphatic trunk runs superiorly and medially, carrying all of the lymph that has drained into the apical axillary nodes. This trunk is called the subclavian lymphatic trunk. The trunk empties into the junction of the subclavian and internal jugular veins. There is also a direct connection between the apical nodes of the axilla and the farthest nodes of the deep chain of cervical lymph nodes (supraclavicular nodes).

Nerves

The medial, lateral, and posterior cords of the brachial plexus are arranged about the first and second portions of the axillary artery in the positions suggested by their names. The terminal branchings of the cords are arranged about the third portion of the axillary artery.

16

The Pleura

EMBRYOLOGY

The mediastinum originates from an aggregate of mesenchyme that is midline in position and lies dorsal and superior to the primitive coelomic cavity. Some of this mesenchymal tissue is carried laterally and inferiorly by the growth of the lung buds to become the visceral pleura. The mesothelium of the thoracic wall (derived from somatic mesoderm) becomes the parietal pleura.

The mass of midline mesenchyme is divided by further lung growth and descent. It is separated from the inner wall of the thoracic cavity and becomes a midline compartment lying between the 2 pleural compartments.

GROSS ANATOMY
(Figs 16–1 and 16–2)

The pleura is the thin mesothelial membrane that covers the lung surfaces, lines the pulmonary interlobar fissures, lines the inner surface of the chest wall, covers the superior surface of the diaphragm, and forms a reflected covering over the structures that lie in the mid thorax. Each lung is invaginated into and sealed within a sac of pleural membrane, the 2 pleural sacs being separated by the contents of the centrally placed mediastinum.

Each pleural sac has an inner or visceral layer and an external or parietal layer. The space (potential) between the 2 pleural layers is called the pleural cavity. The free surfaces of the pleura are shiny and moist. Under normal circumstances, the serous pleural surfaces secrete a small amount of fluid that serves to lubricate the surfaces and allow free movement between the parietal and visceral layers.

The pleural surfaces that are related to the lung surfaces—the visceral pleura—are tightly attached to the underlying organ. The pleural surfaces attached to the superior surface of the diaphragm and to the inner wall of the thorax—the parietal pleura—are tightly attached to the parietal structures that lie deep to them (endothoracic fascia).

Pleura that covers the lungs and lines the interlobar fissures is called the pulmonary visceral pleura. The pleura that lines the inner thoracic wall and covers the superior surface of the diaphragm is called (respec-

tively) the costal parietal and diaphragmatic parietal pleura. The pleura that covers the median surface of the pleural sacs is called the mediastinal parietal pleura.

➤ *Pleural friction rub. (Fig 16–1.) When the pleural surfaces, which normally are smooth and glistening and moistened by pleural fluid, become inflamed, they are roughened by fibrin deposits and as a consequence a "friction rub" may be heard early in the course of pleurisy upon auscultation over the area of inflammation. Later, adherence of the pleural surfaces or the presence of intervening fluid or air abolishes the pleural friction rub.*

➤ *Percussion flatness. Flatness to percussion over the pulmonary area of the thorax suggests the presence of fluid in the interpleural space. Fluid may be due to pleural inflammation or neoplasia; may be secondary to circulatory insufficiency; or may be a neighborhood reaction due to a process below the diaphragm.*

➤ *Examination of pleural fluid. (Fig 16–2.) Needle aspiration (thoracentesis) is an excellent diagnostic aid in patients with pleural effusion. Note the amount and gross appearance of fluid withdrawn from the space. Pleural fluid should always be examined for the presence of malignant cells. About 250 mL of pleural fluid must be present before a fluid level will be noted on x-ray; fluid is seen first in the phrenicocostal sinus (S curve of Ellis).*

➤ *Pneumothorax. (Figs 16–3 and 16–4.) Pneumothorax is the presence of air in the pleural cavity. Air may enter the pleural space secondary to the parietal or the visceral pleura. The most common cause of pneumothorax is spontaneous rupture of an emphysematous bleb. Normally, a significant pneumothorax is followed by partial or complete lung collapse, the extent of the collapse depending upon lung elasticity, the presence of lung adhesions to the thoracic wall, and the amount of pleural air present.*

Spontaneous pneumothorax usually responds readily to tube drainage with an underwater seal.

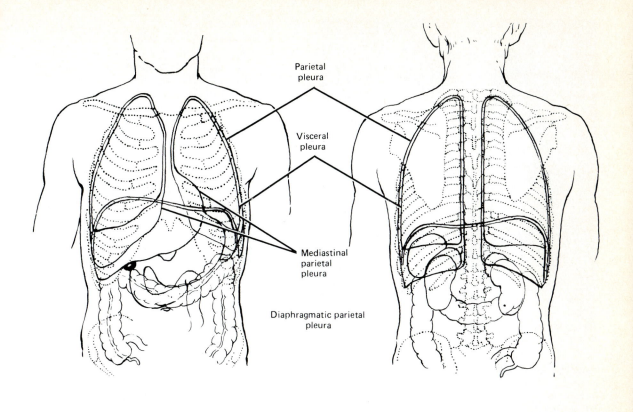

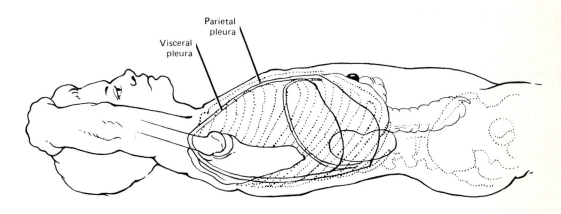

Figure 16–1. Pleural surfaces. (Adapted from Netter, in Popper H: *Ciba Clinical Symposia* 7:5:136.)

➠ ***Bronchopleural fistula.*** *If the pneumothorax persists, a bronchopleural fistula should be suspected. If, after a reasonable interval (7–10 days), the fistula fails to close, a thoracotomy with operative closure of the fistula should be done.*

➠ ***Tension pneumothorax.*** *Tension pneumothorax is a condition in which a break in the lung surface or in the parietal pleura creates a one-way valve-like action that allows air to pass into the pleural space but not out of it. At each inspiration, there is an increase in the amount of air in the pleural space. As intrapleural pressure increases, the lung collapses, and the central mediastinal structures are pushed against the contralateral lung, severely diminishing the patient's thoracic air space. Treatment consists of tube thoracostomy and water seal drainage. If the process continues, surgical closure of the site of entrance of air into the pleural cavity is required.*

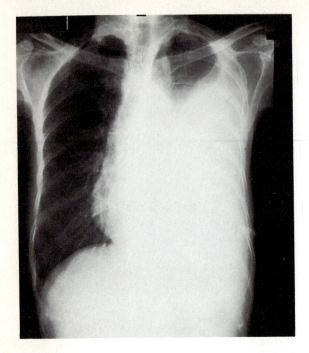

Figure 16–2. Malignant pleural effusion (carcinoma of lung). (Reproduced, with permission, from Way LW [editor]: *Current Surgical Diagnosis & Treatment,* 7th ed. Lange, 1985.)

➡ ***Hemothorax.*** *Hemothorax is the presence of blood in the pleural space. The blood varies in amount from several milliliters to as much as 1–2 L. Since superficial lung bleeding is usually self-contained, the major cause of a large hemothorax is bleeding from a ruptured intercostal or internal thoracic vessel. Air may be present in the pleural cavity along with the blood, a condition known as hemopneumothorax.*

➡ ***Empyema.*** *(Fig 16–5.) Pus in the pleural cavity often follows pulmonary suppurative infection and may result from sepsis secondary to a penetrating chest wound. It may involve the entire pleural cavity or it may become encapsulated ("loculated") and involve only a localized area of the pleural cavity. If a pulmonary lesion breaks into the pleural cavity, the pleural space may contain both air and pus (pyopneumothorax). The opening from the lung into the pleural cavity (bronchopleural fistula) will cause an air fluid level in the cavity.*

➡ ***Thoracentesis.*** *(Fig 16–6.) The presence of major amounts of air, blood, serous fluid, pus, or any combination of these substances in the pleural cavity usually calls for its removal. This may be accomplished by needle thoracentesis; by insertion of a chest tube into the pleural cavity via an intercostal space; or by resection of a rib followed by open pleural drainage. Failure to remove fluid may cause the lung to*

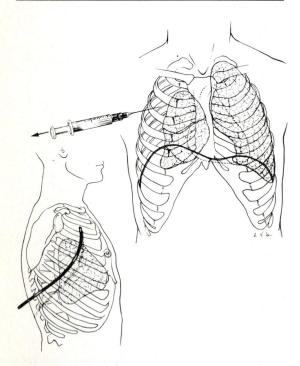

Figure 16–3. Relief of pneumothorax by immediate decompression with a needle introduced through the second anterior intercostal space. (Reproduced, with permission, from Way LW [editor]: *Current Surgical Diagnosis & Treatment,* 7th ed. Lange, 1985.)

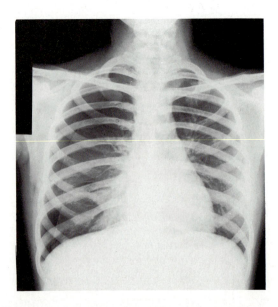

Figure 16–4. Spontaneous pneumothorax on right side. (Reproduced, with permission, from Way LW [editor]: *Current Surgical Diagnosis & Treatment,* 7th ed. Lange, 1985.)

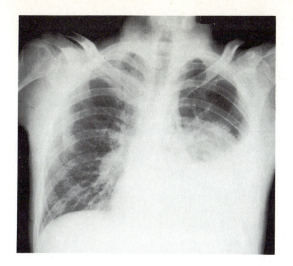

Figure 16–5. Streptococcal empyema. (Reproduced, with permission, from Way LW [editor]: *Current Surgical Diagnosis & Treatment,* 7th ed. Lange, 1985.)

be covered by a resistant fibrous membrane that inhibits expansion, later requiring lung decortication.

➡ **Site of chest tube insertion.** *The second interspace in the anterior axillary line is the usual site of the insertion of a tube into the pleural cavity for removal of air. The extracorporeal end of the tube is placed under a water seal with controlled suction to prevent air from being sucked back into the pleural cavity.*

SEGMENTS OF THE PARIETAL PLEURA

The parietal pleura is divided into 4 segments.

The **costal segment** covers the inner surface of the anterior, lateral, and posterior thoracic walls. The pleura is closely attached to the endothoracic fascia.

The costal pleura passes laterally from the deep surface of the mid sternum, covering the inner surfaces of the costal cartilages, ribs, and intercostal spaces. In the middorsal thorax, it covers the thoracic sympathetic trunk and ganglia, the lateral surface of the vertebral bodies, and part of the ventral surface of the vertebral bodies. In the posterior thorax, close to the vertebral bodies, the right and left costal pleura are separated only by a narrow 3-cm interval, the width of the posterior mediastinum.

The **diaphragmatic segment** of the parietal pleura is reflected from the costal segment onto the superior surface of the diaphragm. In this position it is tightly attached to the diaphragmatic layer of the endothoracic fascia.

That portion of the pleura which covers the apex of the lung and rises superiorly into the lower neck is called the **cupula** or **dome of the pleura,** or the **cervical pleura.** (See below.)

The **mediastinal pleura** forms the lateral boundary of the mediastinal viscera and the medial border of the lungs.

Posteriorly, as it leaves the anterolateral surfaces of the lower thoracic vertebral bodies, the pleura is reflected onto the posterolateral surface of the pericardium. It then continues to pass ventrally and covers the posterior surface of the root of the lung. From there, a triangular section of pleura moves inferiorly toward the superior surface of the diaphragm. This becomes the posterior layer of the pulmonary ligament. From the posterior surface of the lung root, the pleura also moves to cover the costal surface of the lung from apex to base, invaginating into the interlobar fissures. Medially, the pleura covers the mediastinal surface of the lung and the anterior surface of the root of the lung. From there, the pleura also continues inferiorly toward the diaphragm as the anterior layer of the pulmonary ligament. Superior to the level of the lung root, the mediastinal pleura passes from the vertebral column to the deep surface of the sternum.

Ventrally, the parietal pleura extends down to the costal cartilage of rib 7, laterally in the midaxillary line on the left side to the inferior border of rib 10, and laterally on the right side to the superior border of rib 10; posteriorly, it descends to the 12th rib and occasionally as far as vertebra L1.

Cupula of the Pleura

The cupula of the pleura rises through the superior thoracic inlet up to 4–5 cm above the anterior end of the first rib. This segment of the pleura is reinforced anteriorly by a domelike (Sibson's) fascia, which arises anteriorly from the inner surface of the first rib and is connected dorsally to the transverse process of C7.

Costophrenic Sinus

The costophrenic sinus is present bilaterally as a result of the reflection of the pleura from the lateral chest wall onto the superior surface of the diaphragm. In normal respiration the thin lateral edge of the lung does not reach the line of pleural reflection, the costal and diaphragmatic pleurae are not separated by lung and are in direct contact; the small space between them is called the pleural costophrenic sinus.

A similar situation prevails in the midline of the anterior thorax posterior to the sternum and the cartilages of the ribs. In this area, the thin anterior edge of the lung fails to reach the line of pleural reflection; the space between the 2 pleural layers with no intervening lung is called the costomediastinal sinus.

The line of reflection of the right costal pleura leaves the chest wall and reaches the superior surface of the diaphragm anteriorly, near the seventh sternocostal joint. It then passes inferiorly and cuts across the tenth rib at about the midaxillary line. From this point it runs dorsally in the direction of the inferior process of vertebra T12. The reflection of the left pleura from the chest wall onto the diaphragm pro-

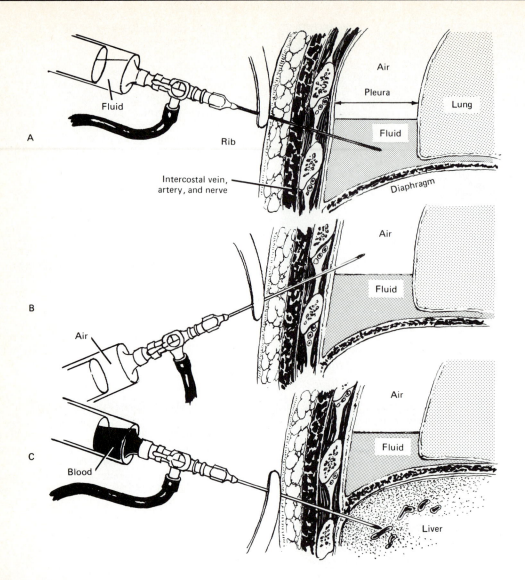

Figure 16–6. Technique of thoracentesis. **A:** Successful tap, with fluid obtained. Note the position of the needle with relation to the intercostal bundle, and the use of the clamp to steady the needle at skin level. **B:** Air is obtained as the needle is shifted upward. **C:** A bloody tap results from excessively low position of the needle with puncture of the liver. (Reproduced, with permission, from Mills J et al [editors]: *Current Emergency Diagnosis & Treatment,* 2nd ed. Lange, 1985. Redrawn from GE Lindskog and AE Liebow.)

ceeds along the sixth costal cartilage because of the position of the heart. It is reflected about 1–2 cm farther inferiorly than the pleura on the right side.

➡ ***Pleural reflections.*** *Familiarity with the levels of the pleural reflections, particularly with relationship to the superior surface of the diaphragm and to the 11th and 12th ribs, is of great help in pleural aspiration. It is also important in renal, suprarenal, and perirenal surgery, so that the pleural cavity will not be opened when a section of the 12th rib is removed to facilitate exposure and ease of operation.*

The pulmonary ligament consists of the 2 pleural investing layers, which cover the anterior and posterior surfaces of the root of the lung, extending inferiorly between the mediastinal surfaces of the lung and the pericardium to the superior surface of the diaphragm. As the 2 mesenterylike layers of pleural fold reach the diaphragm, they terminate in a free crescentic border that tends to hold the lower lung to some extent in apposition to the diaphragm.

➡ ***Mobilization of pulmonary ligament.*** *Release of the pulmonary ligament from its attachment to the diaphragm is necessary in order to mobi-*

lize the lower lung lobes. The procedure is a relatively avascular one, since no major vessels lie in the pulmonary ligament. Mobilization also allows for better visualization of the superior diaphragmatic surface and of the inferior thoracic esophagus and vagus nerves in the lower thorax.

BLOOD VESSELS, LYMPHATICS, & NERVES

The arterial supply to the pleura is derived from the internal thoracic, intercostal, musculophrenic, thymic, pericardial, pulmonary, and bronchial arteries. The venous drainage from the pleural surfaces roughly parallels the route of the arteries and eventually reaches the superior vena cava.

The pleural lymphatics are divided into 2 groups; those draining the parietal and those draining the visceral pleura. The parietal lymphatics may drain into the sternal nodes, the diaphragmatic nodes, or the posterior mediastinal nodes. The visceral pleural lymphatics drain into the superficial efferents that drain the lung tissues per se.

The nerve supply to the pleura comes from a variety of sources. Fibers derived from the phrenic, vagus, intercostal, and sympathetic nerves supply the parietal pleura. The visceral pleura is supplied by the vagus and the sympathetic trunk via the pulmonary plexuses that lie near the hilum of the lung.

➠ *Referred pain secondary to pleural irritation. The site of referred pain secondary to inflammation or irritation of the parietal pleura often gives a clue to the segment of pleura involved. When the costal pleura is irritated, pain is usually present in the chest wall over the area of irritation. Irritation of the diaphragmatic pleura can cause neck or shoulder pain on the ipsilateral side (phrenic supraclavicular reflex arc). When the most peripheral areas of*

the diaphragmatic pleura are irritated, pain is usually referred to the lower thoracic and lumbar regions of the back. Pleural pain secondary to basal pneumonia or to cancer of the lower lobe of the lung that involves the pleura is often referred to the abdomen and may mimic the pain of acute abdominal disease. The increase of thoracic or abdominal pain on deep inspiration suggests a pleuritic origin of the pain, as does the presence of concomitant shoulder and neck pain. However, inflammation below the diaphragm will also cause neck and shoulder pain.

➠ *Pain associated with pleural tumors. Tumors of the mesothelial type often originate in the pleura. If they involve the parietal pleura, they usually cause considerable thoracic cage pain.*

➠ *Pleural disease secondary to chest trauma. Trauma to the rib cage, the intercostal spaces, or the sternum will often result in pneumothorax, hemopneumothorax, or tension pneumothorax.*

➠ *Combined abdominothoracic wounds. Abdominothoracic wounds often pass through the pleural cavity. If a penetrating missile or weapon carries pathogens, empyema often results.*

➠ *Chylothorax. Injury to the thoracic duct with associated pleural injury will result in a chylous collection primarily in the left pleural cavity (chylothorax).*

➠ *Decortication of the lung. Decortication of the lung involves the removal ("peeling") of a thickened and adherent parietal pleura that has become "plastered" against the visceral pleura of the lung. The procedure can allow expansion and aeration of the involved lung.*

The mediastinum is the area situated in the center of the thoracic cavity bounded superiorly by the thoracic inlet, inferiorly by the diaphragm, anteriorly by the sternum and the costal cartilages, and posteriorly by the thoracic vertebrae and by their transverse processes. The mediastinum contains the viscera of the thorax (except the lungs and pleura) and the major thoracic nerves, blood vessels, and lymphatics.

The variations in shading in Fig 17–1 divide the mediastinum into a small superior segment and a larger inferior one that is further subdivided into (1) an anterior segment, which lies between the anterior surface of the pericardium and the sternum; (2) a middle segment, which contains the heart and pericardium; and (3) a posterior segment, which lies dorsal to the heart and the pericardium and ventral to the thoracic vertebrae and their transverse processes.

THE SUPERIOR MEDIASTINUM
(Figs 17–2, 17–3 and 17–4)

The superior mediastinum extends from the thoracic inlet to the pericardial sac and from the manubrium ventrally to vertebrae T1–4 dorsally. On either side, the superior mediastinum is bounded by the mediastinal pleura of the upper lung segments. Within the superior mediastinum are the thymus gland (Fig 17–3), the brachiocephalic (innominate) artery, the left common carotid artery, the left subclavian artery, the right and left brachiocephalic (innominate) veins, the arch of the aorta, the superior mediastinal lymph nodes, the superior vena cava, the left recurrent laryngeal nerve, the thoracic esophagus and trachea, the thoracic duct, the inferior segments of the 2 longus colli muscles, and the origins of the sternothyroid and sternohyoid muscles.

⟹ *Operations involving the superior mediastinum. Tumors of the thymus or of the parathyroid and thyroid glands are on occasion found in the superior mediastinum. Operations on the great vessels in this area are performed* to relieve pressure upon adjacent viscera, to stop hemorrhage, and to correct vascular anomalies. Stenoses and aneurysms of the great vessels and malignant, traumatic, and congenital lesions of the trachea and esophagus in the superior mediastinum often require operative management.

The superior mediastinum may be approached surgically by a low cervical incision, by median sternotomy, or by high intercostal thoracotomy. The approach that usually provides the best exposure to the mediastinum is median sternotomy. This approach gives optimal exposure of the ascending aorta, the aortic arch, the brachiocephalic vessels, the left common carotid and subclavian arteries, and the great veins as well as good exposure of mediastinal thyroid, parathyroid, and thymic tumors.*

⟹ *Mediastinoscopy and its complications. An endoscope introduced into the lower neck deep to the cervical fascia and sternohyoid muscles and advanced down the anterior surface of the trachea allows inspection of the superior mediastinum down to the bifurcation of the trachea. Biopsy of the superior pretracheal and paratracheal nodes may be done via this approach. Great care must be exercised to avoid injury to the innominate veins and other great vessels; to the pleura; and, on the left side, to the thoracic duct.*

THE THYMUS

1. EMBRYOLOGY

The primordial thymus forms from the epithelium of the ventral wing of the distal extremity of the third pharyngeal pouch. The primordia on each side break away from the pharyngeal wall and move inferiorly and medially along with the primordia of the inferior parathyroid glands. Each of the 2 primordia fuse together when they reach the anterosuperior wall of the thorax. Embryonal fragments may become embedded in the thyroid gland or on occasion may persist

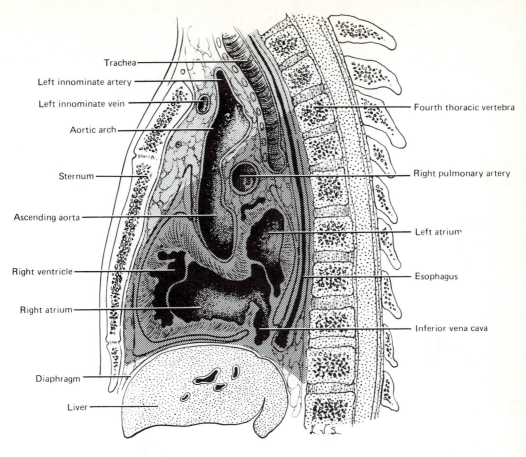

Figure 17–1. Divisions of the mediastinum.

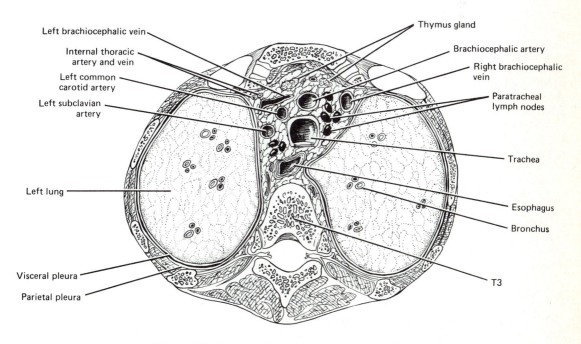

Figure 17–2. Cross section of the superior mediastinum.

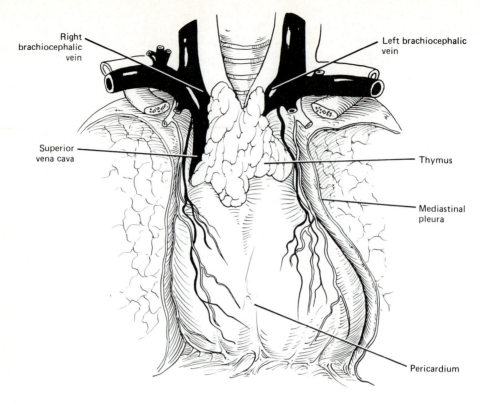

Figure 17–3. The thymus.

as cervical thymic rests along the course of the descent of the thymus.

The thymus continues to enlarge from birth to early puberty; it then degenerates, leaving only fragments of tissue just dorsal to the sternum and ventral to the heart and great vessels.

Anomalies. Congenital thymic aplasia with absence of the parathyroid glands (**DiGeorge's syndrome**) results from failure of the third and fourth pharyngeal pouches to differentiate into thymus and parathyroid glands.

Accessory thymic tissue—discrete segments of persisting tissue in the neck—is often associated with failure of descent of one of the inferior parathyroid glands.

Because of the combined descent of the parathyroid and thymic tissues, parathyroid tissue—normal, adenomatous, or hyperplastic—may be found in the fatty remains of the thymus.

2. ANATOMY

The thymus is a bilobate structure enclosed within a connective tissue capsule. It weighs about 12 g at birth and increases to about 30–40 g just before puberty. Then it begins to regress until adulthood, at which time it is usually difficult to locate. In adult-hood, it has the appearance of a fine fibrous tissue network whose meshes are filled with fat and an occasional lymphocyte. At first it occupies a position in the lowest segment of the neck and in the upper midline segment of the superior mediastinum. It consists mainly of lymphoid tissue. It has no known glandular function.

Each lobule is made up of a cortex and a medulla. The cortex is made up almost completely of small lymphocytes. The medulla is made up of the typical thymic cells called Hassall's corpuscles, which are arranged in a cellular reticulum; the medulla contains only a few lymphocytes.

➠ *Tumors of the thymus. Tumors are uncommon in the thymus gland, though there is perhaps an association between thymoma and myasthenia gravis (30% of cases). When tumors do occur, the enlarged thymus usually lies ventral to the aortic arch and the base of the heart. Thus, thymic tumors can initiate pressure upon the superior vena cava or the long left brachiocephalic vein.*

The thymus normally extends from the level of the thyroid (third tracheal ring) to the level of the third costal cartilage. In the neck, it lies ventral to the lowest cervical tracheal ring and deep to the origins of the sternohyoid and sternothyroid muscles, the lowest thyroid artery, and the manubrium. In the mediastinum, it lies just ventral to the great vessels of the superior mediastinum and those of the pericardial sac.

3. BLOOD VESSELS, LYMPHATICS, & NERVES

The thymus is supplied by the inferior thyroid artery and by branches of the internal thoracic arteries. Venous drainage is into the left brachiocephalic vein and the inferior thyroid veins.

Lymphatic flow from the thymus is into the tracheobronchial and superior mediastinal nodes.

The gland derives its nerve supply from the cervical and upper thoracic autonomic trunks and a few vagal fibers.

THE GREAT VESSELS OF THE NECK & THORAX (Figs 17–5 and 17–6)

1. EMBRYOLOGY (Fig 17–4)

Early Fetal Structures

As a result of the rotation of the cardiogenic plate and the fusion of the endocardial heart tubes, there is an arching of the cranial portions of the primitive dorsal aortas. The arched portion becomes the first of the pharyngeal aortic arches. As the more caudal of the pharyngeal arches develop, the aortas contribute one branch to each, 6 in all, but in the human all 6 arch arteries are never present at the same time. All aortic arches except the fifth and parts of the first and second develop into adult structures. The aortic arches arise from the aortic sac, which is the most distal part of the truncus arteriosus. The arteries lie in the mesenchyme of the branchial arches and end in the dorsal aortas.

Adult Structures

A. The First and Second Arches: The first aortic arch persists in part as the maxillary artery, while the second aortic arch (hyoid, stapedial) disappears except for part, which becomes the carotico-tympanic artery. Sometimes the stapedial artery persists when it traverses the 2 limbs of the stapes.

B. The Third Arch: The third aortic arch persists as the common carotid and the first part of the internal carotid arteries, while the external carotid artery is probably an outgrowth from it. Anomalies of the third aortic arch are uncommon. They include variations in the origins of the common carotids and their branches. Third arch arteries may substitute for the fourth arch artery when it is missing.

C. The Fourth Arch: The fourth aortic arch on the left forms part of the definitive aortic arch; on the right it forms the most proximal part of the right subclavian artery. Coarctation of the aorta is an important anomaly of the left arch. Double aortic arch results when the right dorsal aorta maintains its connection with the left dorsal aorta.

D. The Fifth Arch: The fifth aortic arch is transient and disappears.

E. The Sixth Arch and the Distal Aortas: The sixth aortic arch (pulmonary arch) on the right forms the proximal segment of the right pulmonary artery. On the left it forms the ductus arteriosus and the left pulmonary artery. The right dorsal aorta normally disappears. The left dorsal aorta forms the descending aorta. The anomalies include patent ductus arteriosus and persistence of right dorsal aorta. Persistent distal right dorsal aorta forms part of an abnormal right subclavian artery.

2. ANATOMY

The transverse aortic arch begins near the second right sternocostal joint. After rising about 1 cm, it arches to the left and passes ventral to the trachea. Upon reaching the left border of the trachea, the arch moves slightly farther dorsally and then turns inferiorly. Its inferior course parallels the left border of the fourth dorsal vertebra. At the level of the fourth thoracic vertebra, the aortic arch becomes the descending thoracic aorta. In its early course, its superior border rises to about 3 cm inferior to the top of the manubrium.

The aortic arch is situated just dorsal to the pleura, the anterior lung margins, and the thymus. As the arch runs dorsally and to the left, it is crossed ventrally by 4 nerves that descend into the thorax from the cervical region. From right to left, these are the phrenic nerve; the superior cardiac branches of the vagus nerve; the superior cardiac nerve (a branch of the left sympathetic trunk); and the main left vagal trunk. Just after the left vagus crosses the aortic arch to lie on the left side of the descending aorta, it gives off the left recurrent laryngeal nerve. Inferior to the aortic arch is the bifurcation of the pulmonary artery; the left major stem bronchus; the ligamentum arteriosum, connecting the bifurcation of the pulmonary artery with the inferior surface of the aortic arch; and finally the ascending segment of the left recurrent laryngeal nerve. Superior to the aortic arch are the innominate artery, the left common carotid artery, and the left subclavian artery, all of which arise from the superior surface of the arch and at their sites of origin lie dorsal to the long left brachiocephalic vein.

⤷ *Aortic arch lesions involving the left recurrent laryngeal nerve. Aneurysms and aortitis of the*

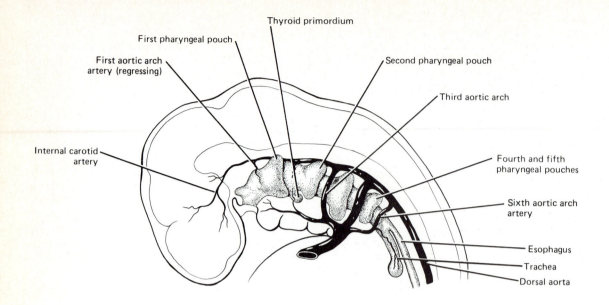

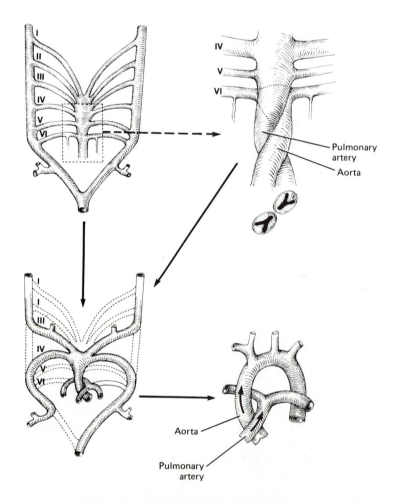

Figure 17–4. Embryology of major vessels.

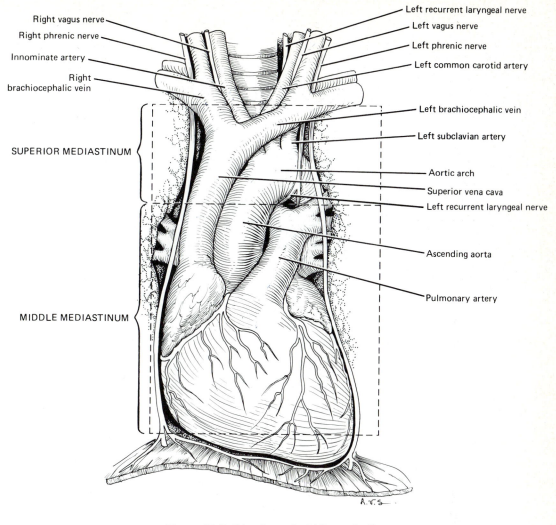

Figure 17–5. Superior and middle mediastina.

arch of the aorta may involve the left recurrent laryngeal nerve as it passes immediately dorsal to the arch. Involvement of the nerve may result in voice changes or a brassy cough. Endoscopic findings of changes in the degree of movement and tension of the left vocal cord help to make the diagnosis of recurrent laryngeal nerve entrapment. Aneurysms of the innominate artery, of the aortic arch, and of the upper descending thoracic aorta also present in the superior mediastinum. These lesions can be managed successfully by surgery.

Arteries
(Figs 17–5 and 17–6)

The largest vessel leaving the aortic arch is the **innominate artery,** which arises near the level of the second right costal cartilage and ascends in a slightly dorsal direction up to the right sternoclavicular joint, behind which it bifurcates into the right common carotid and the right subclavian artery. Ventral to the innominate artery, between it and the dorsal surface of the manubrium, are the tendons of origin of the right sternohyoid and sternothyroid muscles, the thymic remnants, and the long left brachiocephalic vein. Dorsal to the artery is the trachea, which is crossed from left to right by the artery as it ascends. To the right of the artery are the right brachiocephalic vein and superior vena cava, the right phrenic nerve, and the apical pleura of the right lung. In about 10% of individuals, the lowest thyroid artery arises from the innominate trunk and runs superiorly on the ventral surface of the trachea toward the isthmus of the thyroid gland.

The thoracic segment of the **left common carotid artery** arises from the most superior part of the arch of the aorta on a plane dorsal to the left brachiocephalic

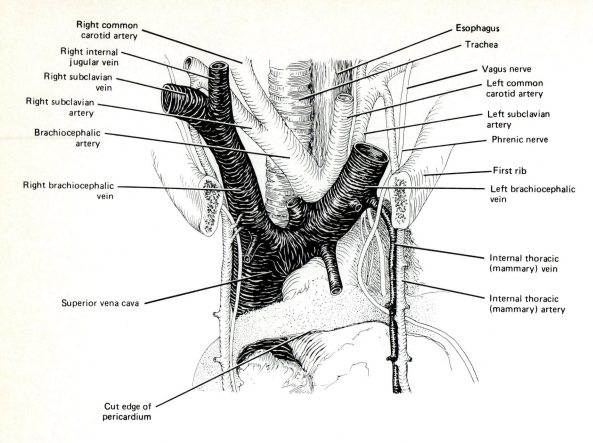

Right common carotid artery
Right internal jugular vein
Right subclavian vein
Right subclavian artery
Brachiocephalic artery
Right brachiocephalic vein
Superior vena cava
Cut edge of pericardium

Esophagus
Trachea
Vagus nerve
Left common carotid artery
Left subclavian artery
Phrenic nerve
First rib
Left brachiocephalic vein
Internal thoracic (mammary) vein
Internal thoracic (mammary) artery

Figure 17–6. Superior mediastinum and root of the neck.

artery. It rises through the superior mediastinum to the level of the left sternoclavicular joint, where it becomes a cervical vessel. The anterosuperior segment of the left lung and its covering pleura and the left sternohyoid and sternothyroid muscles lie ventral to the artery, as do also the thymus and the left brachiocephalic vein. Posterior to the left common carotid artery lie the trachea, the esophagus, the thoracic duct, and the left recurrent laryngeal nerve. The left vagus and phrenic nerves lie to the left of the artery. The left subclavian artery lies just dorsal and slightly to the left of the left common carotid artery.

The thoracic course of the **left subclavian artery** begins on the superior surface of the left side of the aortic arch at the level of the disk between T3 and T4. Its origin from the arch is more dorsal than that of the left common carotid. It runs superiorly, paralleled by the left phrenic, vagus, and cardiac nerves, all of which lie on a plane ventral to the artery. Lying ventral and to the right of the artery is the left common carotid artery, while the left brachiocephalic vein also lies ventral to the artery and crosses it from left to right. Dorsally, the left subclavian artery is related to the left side of the esophagus, the thoracic duct, the left superior thoracic ganglion of the sympathetic trunk, the left recurrent laryngeal

nerve, and the upper lobe of the left lung and its covering pleura. As the left subclavian artery ascends to the upper limits of the superior mediastinum, the esophagus and the thoracic duct gradually become related to its right lateral border.

In 90% of individuals, the **lowest thyroid artery** (arteria thyroidea ima) arises from the superior surface of the aortic arch to the right of the origins of the left common carotid and subclavian arteries. It runs superiorly on the anterior surface of the tracheal rings to the isthmus of the thyroid gland.

Veins
(Figs 17–5 and 17–6)

The 2 large **brachiocephalic veins** are formed at the right and left sides of the base of the neck by the union of the internal jugular and subclavian veins. The right and left brachiocephalic veins run from the base of the neck into the superior mediastinum and unite to the right of the midline to form the superior vena cava.

The **right brachiocephalic vein,** the shorter of the 2 veins, is formed dorsal to the medial end of the right clavicle. It moves directly inferiorly to the level of the inferior border of the first rib cartilage, where it joins with the left brachiocephalic vein. It lies to the right of the innominate artery and on a more superficial plane. The phrenic nerve lies close to the right side of the vein as the 2 structures cross the apex of the right lung. Joining the right brachiocephalic vein are the right vertebral vein, the right internal thoracic vein, and the right inferior thyroid vein.

The **left brachiocephalic vein,** which crosses the anterosuperior mediastinum obliquely from left to right, is about 3 times as long as the right brachiocephalic vein (about 5–6 cm). It begins dorsal to and close to the medial half of the left clavicle. Ventral to the vein are the manubrium and the origins of the left sternohyoid and sternothyroid muscles and thymic remnants. All these structures are interposed between the dorsum of the sternum and the vein. Lying dorsal to the vein in its relatively long oblique course across the superior mediastinum are the left common carotid artery, the subclavian artery, the brachiocephalic artery, and the left vagus and phrenic nerves. Joining the left brachiocephalic vein are the left inferior thyroid vein, the left vertebral vein, and the left internal thoracic vein. The left highest (suprema) intercostal vein occasionally also joins the left brachiocephalic vein. The left brachiocephalic vein terminates to the right of the midline by joining with the right brachiocephalic vein to form the superior vena cava.

The **2 inferior thyroid veins** (see Chapter 9) descend from the inferior poles of the thyroid gland, coming to lie deep to the sternothyroid muscles on the ventrolateral surfaces of the trachea. The left vein joins the left brachiocephalic vein in the superior mediastinum. The right inferior thyroid vein runs obliquely to the right in its superior mediastinal course. It crosses the ventral surface of the innominate artery and empties into the right brachiocephalic vein just before that vein merges with its mate to form the superior vena cava. The inferior thyroid veins receive blood from veins that drain the inferior half of the thyroid gland and additional venous drainage from the esophagus, the trachea, the thymus, the larynx, and the parathyroid glands.

The **internal thoracic (mammary) veins** run parallel and immediately adjacent to the internal thoracic arteries (venae comitantes). They receive blood from the pericardiophrenic, upper mediastinal, thymic, anterior intercostal, perforating, and sternal veins. They empty into the right and left brachiocephalic veins in the superior mediastinum.

The **superior vena cava** is short and stubby, formed by the junction of the 2 brachiocephalic veins, near the level of the first intercostal space, just lateral to the right sternal border. The vein moves inferiorly, close to the right border of the sternum, to the level of the second intercostal space, where it empties into the right atrium of the heart. Just superior to the atrial entrance, the vein is covered by the fibrous pericardial sac. The right lung and its covering pleura lie just anterior to the superior vena cava. Posterior to the superior vena cava are the right vagus nerve and the structures that make up the hilum of the right lung. To the right of the superior vena cava is

the right phrenic nerve, and to its left are the beginnings of the ascending aorta and the innominate artery. The superior vena cava is joined by the azygos vein just before it enters the pericardial sac.

➡ *Central venous pressure measurements. A catheter introduced into the superior vena cava via the subclavian vein and attached to a manometer at heart level gives an excellent reading of central venous pressure. Such a catheter may also be used for intravenous feedings.*

➡ *Catheter sampling of brachiocephalic venous blood for parathyroid hormone. Catheter sampling of blood from the inferior thyroid and brachiocephalic veins, for assay of parathyroid hormone content, may help locate parathyroid adenomas in the superior mediastinum. This type of mediastinal tumor usually lies in close relationshp or actually within the thymus gland. However, parathyroid tumors can take up almost any position in the superior mediastinum.*

➡ *Pressure of a low-lying thyroid gland upon the brachiocephalic veins or superior vena cava. Retrosternal thyroid tissue may be present either because of too low descent of the embryonic thyroglossal tract or because of growth inferiorly of an adenoma of a normally positioned thyroid gland. The presence of retrosternal thyroid tissue makes surgery upon the thyroid gland technically more difficult. Thyroid tissue ectopic in the mediastinum can almost always be removed via the cervical route without a sternal splitting incision. Low-lying thyroid tissue may press upon the superior vena cava, the left brachiocephalic vein, or both. Rarely, an aberrant segment of thyroid slips inferiorly, dorsal to the left brachiocephalic vein, and reaches the posterior mediastinum. Such tissue is difficult to remove via a cervical incision and thoracotomy is usually needed.*

TRACHEA & ESOPHAGUS
(Fig 17–7)

Trachea

The mediastinal segment of the trachea is located in the midline, dorsal (in order) to the manubrium, the thymic remnants, the left brachiocephalic vein, the left common carotid and subclavian arteries, and the aortic arch. Lying dorsal and slightly to the left of the superior mediastinal tracheal segment is the esophagus. To the right of the trachea lie the mediastinal pleura of the right lung and the right vagus nerve. To the left of the trachea lie the left recurrent nerve, the aortic arch and 2 of its branches, the left common carotid and subclavian arteries.

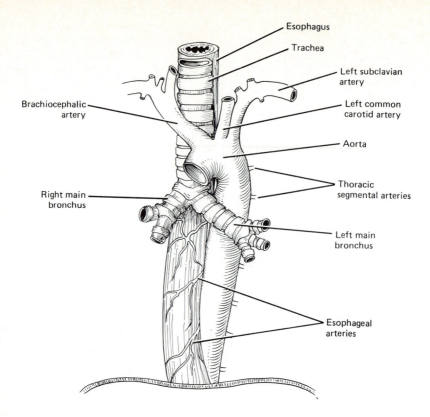

Figure 17–7. Relationships of the trachea, esophagus, and major bronchi in the superior mediastinum.

The mediastinal trachea is supplied by branches of the inferior thyroid arteries, and its venous return usually parallels the inferior thyroid veins. Branches from the vagus, the left recurrent nerve, and the thoracic sympathetic chain supply the thoracic trachea.

➠ *Mediastinitis following tracheal or esophageal perforation. Infection of the superior mediastinum may follow severe neck infections, endoscopic perforations of the trachea or esophagus, and penetrating wounds of the upper chest. Mediastinitis is now rare because of the use of antibiotics and early surgical treatment of endoscopic perforations and penetrating wounds.*

Esophagus

The superior mediastinal segment of the esophagus lies dorsal and slightly to the left of the trachea, between the trachea ventrally and the upper thoracic vertebrae dorsally. It continues inferiorly by passing to the right of the aortic arch and enters the posterior mediastinum, where it first runs along the right side of the descending aorta. To the left of the esophagus in the superior mediastinum are the left border of the aortic arch, the left subclavian artery, and the left lung apex, with its covering pleura. In the acute angle between the esophagus and the trachea is the left recurrent branch of the vagus nerve. To the right side of the esophagus are the right lung and pleura and the azygos vein.

➠ *Trauma to the superior mediastinum. Penetrating or nonpenetrating wounds of the superior mediastinum are common in high-speed decelerating injuries. In such circumstances the possibility of injury to the great vessels and to the upper trachea and esophagus must be seriously considered despite the protection afforded these structures by the sternum and anterior rib cage. Since trauma to the mediastinal structures may have lethal consequences, early diagnosis is essential—by angiography and serial x-rays in doubtful cases.*

➠ *Perforation of the trachea or esophagus. Traumatic perforation of the trachea or esophagus in the superior mediastinum may lead to mediastinitis and subcutaneous emphysema. Early thoracic exploration and drainage are mandatory if there is subcutaneous air on palpation or free mediastinal air on x-ray.*

Lymphatics

The superior sternal nodes (internal mammary nodes), the highest intercostal nodes, the superior mediastinal segments of the major thoracic duct, and the right thoracic duct all lie within the superior mediastinum.

The **superior sternal nodes** lie deep within the anterosuperior chest wall close to the sternal terminations of the upper 4 anterior interspaces. They lie alongside the internal thoracic (mammary) artery and veins. They drain the inner quadrant of the ipsilateral breast and are usually larger in the female than in the male. They also drain the ventrolateral abdominal wall (upper third) and the diaphragmatic surface of the liver. They usually drain via a single small trunk into the junction of the internal jugular and subclavian veins.

➡ *Scalene lymph node biopsy. The "scalene fat pad" just anterior to the lower segment of the anterior scalene muscle contains internal jugular lymph nodes that communicate with the superior sternal nodes and the bronchomediastinal nodes. Biopsy of these nodes may be of value in the diagnosis of intrathoracic and deep chest wall disease.*

The **highest intercostal nodes** are close to the posterior terminations of the intercostal spaces and closely related to the posterior intercostal vessels. They drain the superior posterior chest wall. On the left, they drain into the major thoracic duct; on the right, into the right thoracic duct.

The **major thoracic lymphatic duct** enters the superior mediastinum near the level of T4. It lies dorsal to the esophagus and to the left of the midline. It lies dorsal to the aortic arch and the left subclavian artery. It continues superiorly between the esophagus and the upper lobe of the left lung to the root of the neck. As it proceeds, it receives efferent lymphatic flow from almost all of the mediastinal lymph nodes and from the posterior intercostal lymph nodes of the upper 4 left intercostal spaces.

➡ *Thoracic duct injury. The thoracic duct may be injured in left-sided superior mediastinal surgery and secondary to left-sided upper thoracic trauma. If the injury is recognized when it occurs, the duct should be ligated to prevent chylothorax.*

The **right bronchomediastinal lymphatic trunk** enters the right superior mediastinum at the level of the fourth interspace. It runs superiorly to empty into the junction of the right subclavian and internal jugular veins or into the right lymphatic duct. It drains the upper 4 right posterior interspaces.

The **right lymphatic duct** receives lymph from the right side of the thorax, the right lung, the right heart, and the superior surface of the liver via the right bronchomediastinal duct; it empties into the right subclavian vein.

Nerves
(Fig 17–8)

The **vagus nerves** pass through the superior mediastinum.

The **right vagus nerve** enters the superior mediastinum by crossing ventral to the subclavian artery. At the inferior margin of the artery, it gives off its recurrent laryngeal branch. In the superior mediastinum, the vagus moves to the left, passing dorsal to the left brachiocephalic vein to lie alongside the right margin of the trachea, which it follows to the level of the lung hilum.

The **left vagus nerve** enters the superior mediastinum between the left common carotid and subclavian arteries. It lies deep to the left brachiocephalic vein and ventral to the left border of the aortic arch. It then moves posteriorly to lie between the descending aorta and the left pulmonary artery just distal to the ligamentum arteriosum and continues inferiorly to the level of the lung hilum.

The **left recurrent (inferior) laryngeal nerve** branches from the left vagus nerve just as the vagus passes anterior to the aortic arch. It runs superiorly and medially. Near the ligamentum arteriosum it moves deep to the aortic arch to lie alongside the left lateral border of the trachea. It reaches the root of the neck by running in the left tracheoesophageal groove.

➡ *Injury to the left recurrent laryngeal nerve in the superior mediastinum. In 4 areas of the superior mediastinum, the left inferior laryngeal nerve is prone to injury by trauma or lesions of neighboring structures: (1) Near a patent ductus arteriosus, it may be injured during surgical closure of the ductus; (2) if superior mediastinal lymph nodes contain cancer, the nerve may be compressed by the nodes; (3) on the dorsal surface of the aortic arch, the nerve may become involved in an aneurysm or syphilitic aortitis; and (4) trauma may occur by virtue of its relationships to the upper left lobe of the lung. In its position dorsal to the aortic arch, it must be identified and retracted away from the operative field in surgery upon that vessel.*

Late cancer of the upper lobe of the left lung may involve the left recurrent laryngeal nerve and cause left vocal cord paralysis and concurrent vocal changes. Pancoast's syndrome is arm and shoulder pain usually combined with Horner's syndrome on the same side. Vocal cord palsy occurs less frequently. It is

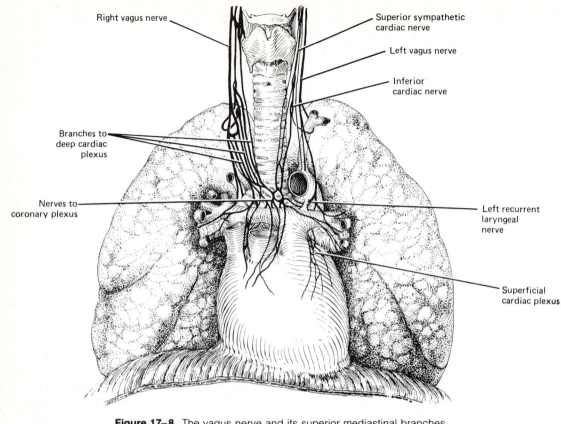

Figure 17–8. The vagus nerve and its superior mediastinal branches.

caused by cancer of the lung apex infiltrating the brachial plexus, the cervical sympathetic chain, and occasionally the recurrent laryngeal nerve.

The inferior cardiac branches of the right vagus nerve leave the vagus as it lies alongside the trachea. On occasion, however, they may arise from the right inferior laryngeal nerve low in the neck. On the left side, the inferior cardiac nerves arise from the left recurrent laryngeal nerve at various points along that nerve's course. Both right and left inferior cardiac

nerves terminate in the deep segment of the cardiac plexus.

The right and left **phrenic nerves** enter the superior mediastinum after crossing ventral to the first part of the subclavian artery. They then cross the origin of the internal mammary artery obliquely as that vessel leaves the inferior surface of the first part of the subclavian artery. The 2 phrenic nerves cross over the dome of the pleura in their descent to lie ventral to the lung hilum. In the superior mediastinum, the phrenic nerves give off pleural and pericardial branches. On the ventral surface of the lung hilum, the phrenic nerves are easily located.

The Inferior Mediastinum (& Heart)

18

The inferior mediastinum (Fig 18–1) extends from the plane of the superior border of the pericardial sac to the level of the diaphragm and is divided into anterior, middle, and posterior divisions.

I. THE ANTERIOR INFERIOR MEDIASTINUM

Arteries & Veins

The internal thoracic (internal mammary) arteries are the major vessels in the anterior inferior mediastinum. The arteries lie dorsal to the medial ends of the costal cartilage of ribs 1–6. Below the level of the third costal cartilage and continuing to the level of the diaphragm, the internal thoracic artery rests directly upon the fibers of the transverse thoracic muscle. Accompanying the artery are a pair of venae comitantes that terminate superiorly in the brachiocephalic veins. The internal thoracic artery gives off anterior mediastinal branches as follows:

The **pericardiophrenic artery** is a long, slender vessel that runs inferiorly along with the phrenic nerve. Both are between the mediastinal pleura and the pericardial sac. The artery finally reaches the superior surface of the diaphragm, which it helps to supply, and there it joins with the inferior phrenic and musculophrenic arteries. In its descent it gives off minor branches to the pericardial sac.

Small **mediastinal branches** supply the fatty tissues and lymph nodes of the anterior inferior mediastinum and the superior segment of the ventral portion of the pericardial sac. The mediastinal vessels branch from the ventral surface of the internal thoracic artery.

Small **sternal branches** supply the dorsal surface of the sternum and the transverse thoracic muscle.

Anterior **intercostal branches** supply the superior 5 or 6 anterior intercostal spaces.

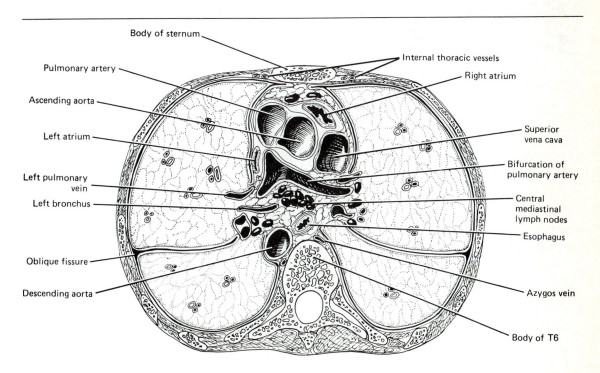

Figure 18–1. Cross section of the inferior mediastinum at the level of T7.

231

Perforating branches supply the breasts and the muscles, skin, and subcutaneous tissues of the anterior chest wall. These branches exist only in the superior 5 or 6 anterior intercostal spaces and are quite large in the second, third, and fourth interspaces in the female, particularly during the later months of pregnancy. Close to the lateral border of the sternum, they pass forward through the internal intercostal muscle and the anterior intercostal membrane.

The **internal thoracic (mammary) artery** terminates by dividing into the musculophrenic and superior epigastric arteries that supply the diaphragm and the upper half of the anterolateral abdominal wall, respectively.

Ventral to the internal thoracic artery lie the cartilages of the third to sixth ribs, the endothoracic fascia, the transverse thoracic muscle, the internal intercostal muscle, and the anterior intercostal membranes. The upper 6 intercostal nerves lie ventral to the internal thoracic vessels.

Lymph Nodes

The parietal lymph nodes of the anterior inferior mediastinum may be divided into 2 groups: sternal and diaphragmatic.

The **sternal lymph nodes** lie alongside the internal thoracic artery close to the anterior termination of the intercostal spaces. Afferent flow to these glands is from the breast, the anterolateral abdominal wall (upper third), the deep structures of the anterior thoracic wall, and the superior surface of the liver. Efferent flow is superior in direction, with delivery of lymph fluid into the subclavian vein, thoracic duct, or via the right thoracic duct.

The **diaphragmatic nodes** are usually 1–3 in number and lie on the posterior aspect of the base of the xiphoid process. They receive lymph from the superior surfaces of the liver and the anterior segment of the diaphragm. They discharge their lymph superiorly into the sternal nodes.

II. THE MIDDLE INFERIOR MEDIASTINUM

THE HEART

EMBRYOLOGY

Early Development
(Fig 18–2)

In the embryo of 19 days, splanchnic mesenchymal cells appear ventral to the pericardial coelomic aggre-gate and form 2 parallel longitudinal columns (cardiogenic cords). The cardiogenic cords become canalized. The 2 tubes fuse to form a single heart tube. Mesenchyme about the tubes begins to form the myoepicardial mantle. The inner segment of the (endocardial) tube becomes the endothelial lining of the heart. The surrounding mantle develops into the myocardium and epicardium. The heart tube elongates and the bulbus cordis, atrium, and ventricle appear, as do the truncus arteriosus and sinus venosus.

Anomalies of cardiac position are ectopia cordis and dextrocardia.

Fifth & Sixth Weeks

The bulbus cordis grows more rapidly than other primitive cardiac segments. Consequently, the heart tube flexes upon itself and becomes first U-shaped, then S-shaped.

During the fifth fetal week the bulbus cordis and all of the truncus arteriosus are divided by a septum, resulting in the formation of 2 channels, the aorta and the pulmonary trunk.

Partitioning of the atrioventricular canal, the atrium, and the ventricle is complete by the sixth fetal week. The atrioventricular canal is divided by the bulging endocardial cushions, which approach each other, fuse, and divide the canal into right and left areas. The primary atrium is divided into right and left atria by the septum primum and the septum secundum.

Anomalies are persistent atrioventricular canal, tricuspid atresia, and ostium primum defect.

An oval opening, the foramen ovale, is present in the septum secundum and allows part of the blood entering the right atrium from the inferior vena cava to pass to the left atrium during fetal life. The foramen ovale closes shortly after birth, and the interatrial septum becomes complete.

Anomalies of the atrial septum include ostium secundum defect, common atrium, and premature closure of the foramen ovale.

Seventh Week
(Fig 18–3)

The primary (primitive) ventricle becomes the left ventricle, and the bulbus cordis becomes the right ventricle. The chambers are separated by the interventricular septum, in which there is initially an opening (interventricular foramen), but this usually closes by about the seventh fetal week. After truncobulbar septation is complete and the interventricular foramen is closed, blood from the right ventricle enters the pulmonary trunk and blood from the left ventricle enters the aorta.

Anomalies of these structures are common ventricle, interventricular, septal defect, tetralogy of Fallot, persistent truncus arteriosus, and transposition of the great arteries.

Final Development

The semilunar valves develop from 3 valve ridges of subendocardial tissue located at the openings of

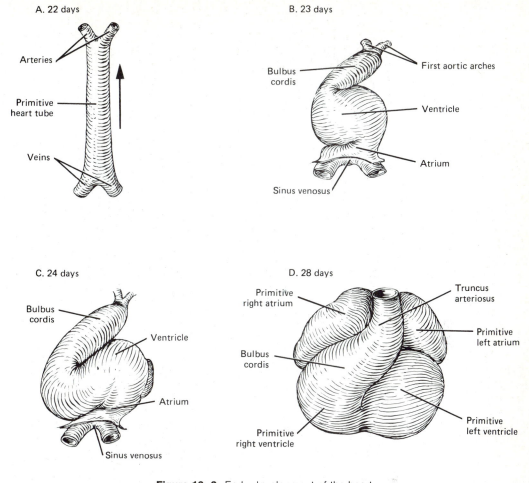

A. 22 days

Arteries

Primitive
heart tube

Veins

B. 23 days

Bulbus
cordis

First aortic arches

Ventricle

Atrium

Sinus venosus

C. 24 days

Bulbus
cordis

Ventricle

Atrium

Sinus venosus

D. 28 days

Primitive
right atrium

Truncus
arteriosus

Primitive
left atrium

Bulbus
cordis

Primitive
right ventricle

Primitive
left ventricle

Figure 18–2. Early development of the heart.

the aorta and the pulmonary trunk. The atrioventricular valves (tricuspid and mitral) are similarly formed from subendocardial tissues in the atrioventricular canals.

Anomalies of these structures are stenosis and atresia of the pulmonary valve and of the aortic valve.

➡ ***Obstructive congenital heart lesions.*** *The most common congenital obstructive lesions of the heart and great vessels are valvular stenosis of the aortic and pulmonary valves and coarctation of the aorta. Congenital tricuspid or pulmonary atresia occurs fairly often, but congenital mitral stenosis is quite rare.*

➡ ***Congenital heart lesions that*** **increase** ***pulmonary arterial blood flow.*** *These lesions are classified as follows: (1) atrial septal defect of the ostium secundum type, (2) atrial septal defect of the ostium primum type, (3) complete atrio-*

ventricular canal, (4) ventricular septal defect, (5) patent ductus arteriosus, and (6) persistent truncus arteriosus.

➡ ***Congenital heart lesions that*** **decrease** ***pulmonary arterial blood flow.*** *These lesions include tetralogy of Fallot, pulmonary atresia with intact ventricular septum, and tricuspid atresia.*

➡ ***Other congenital cardiac malformations.*** *Other congenital cardiac lesions are conotruncal malformation, transposition of the great arteries, double-outlet right or left ventricle, single ventricle, and cardiac malposition (dextrocardia, as in situs inversus totalis).*

➡ ***Diagnosis and treatment of congenital heart disease.*** *Most anomalies of the heart and the major thoracic vessels are amenable to repair by vascular and cardiac surgery. Abnormal openings between the atria and between the*

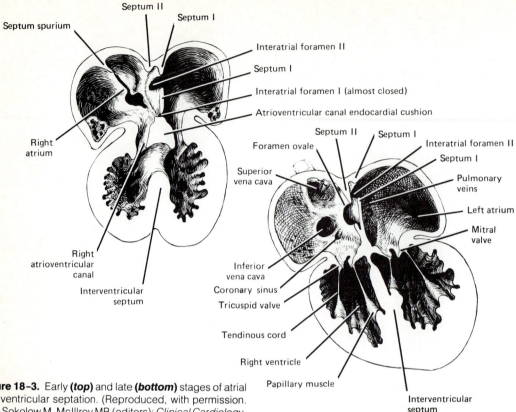

Figure 18–3. Early **(top)** and late **(bottom)** stages of atrial and ventricular septation. (Reproduced, with permission. from Sokolow M, McIllroy MB (editors): *Clinical Cardiology,* 3rd ed. Lange, 1981.

ventricles can be closed; abnormally placed great vessels exerting pressure upon adjacent vessels or upon mediastinal viscera can be re-positioned; and arteriovenous shunts such as exist with patent ductus arteriosus can be abolished. Such operative procedures have greatly reduced mortality and morbidity rates associated with the presence of cardiac and great vessel anomalies in infants and children and in adults as well. The use of both arteriograms and venograms is of great assistance in the diagnosis of cardiac anomalies. Cardiac catheterization with blood gas analysis of specimens taken from the various cardiac chambers and from the great vessels both leaving and reaching the heart is of great assistance in diagnosis of various forms and severity of congenital heart and thoracic vascular disease. The commonest combination of congenital cardiac defects that cause cyanosis in the newborn is tetralogy of Fallot. In this complex of anomalies, there is pulmonary stenosis, right ventricular hypertrophy secondary to the stenosis, interventricular septal defect, and an overriding aorta whose opening lies over the septal defect.

ANATOMY OF THE HEART

THE PERICARDIUM

The pericardium encloses the heart, the proximal segments of the great vessels at the base of the heart, and the terminal segment of the inferior vena cava. The sac consists of 2 layers: an outer fibrous layer and an inner serous layer. The outer fibrous layer is continuous with the middle layer of the deep cervical fascia. It merges with the adventitial layer of the major vessels. Inferiorly, it rests upon the middle leaflet of the central tendon of the diaphragm, and can be freed only by sharp dissection.

The inner serous layer of the pericardium is a single membranous sheet divided into an external parietal layer, which lines the inner surface of the outer fibrous pericardium; and the epicardium, which is the reflection of the inner (visceral) serous layer onto the myocardium. The (potential) pericardial space exists between the epicardium and the parietal layer of the serous pericardium. The space usually contains a small amount of serous fluid. The pericardial sac not only covers the cardiac ventricles and atria but also extends 1–3 cm up onto the great vessels leaving and entering the base of the heart.

The presence of the 2 serous membranes covering the surface of the heart allows the heart to move freely within its serous sac during both systole and diastole. The epicardial layer of the pericardium extends onto the great vessels and forms a pair of tubules. The pericardial tube that embraces the aorta and the pulmonary trunk is called the arterial mesocardium. That which covers the vena cava and the pulmonary veins is called the venous mesocardium.

Two major pericardial sinuses (Fig 18–4) lie within the pericardial sac. The **transverse pericardial sinus** in the posterior portion of the pericardial sac acts as a connection between the left and right sides of the pericardial cavity. It lies between the arterial and venous mesocardia. Ventral to it are the aorta and the pulmonary artery; dorsal to it are the left atrium, the right pulmonary artery, and the superior vena cava. The **oblique pericardial sinus** lies dorsal to the left atrium and ventral to the parietal serous pericardium. It is a U-shaped blind pocket in the posterior wall of the pericardial sac lined by the pulmonary veins and inferior vena cava.

The external fibrous pericardium is tough and loosely adherent to the structures with which it comes in contact: the manubrium (superior pericardiosternal ligament), xiphoid process (inferior pericardiosternal ligament), and vertebral column (pericardiovertebral ligament). It is tightly adherent to the central tendon of the diaphragm. Laterally, its mediastinal surfaces come in contact with the mediastinal parietal pleura. The phrenic nerve lies between the mediastinal pleura and the fibrous pericardium. The pleural cavity partially encircles the pericardial sac, a segment of the cavity lying between the sac and the anterior chest wall. A small triangular area of pericardium to the left of the thoracic midline at the level of the inferior margin of the sternal body and deep to the fourth and fifth costal cartilages is not covered by lung and pleura. This area is dull rather than resonant to percussion, and there a needle may be passed extrapleurally for drainage of the pericardial sac (Fig 18–5).

⇒ *Management of pericarditis. Pericarditis is an inflammatory process that involves the visceral and the parietal layers of the pericardium and sometimes also the myocardial surface. It may be caused by bacterial or viral infections, rheumatic fever, or uremia. Pericarditis may lead to cardiac tamponade or constrictive pericarditis. Unrelieved constrictive pericarditis results*

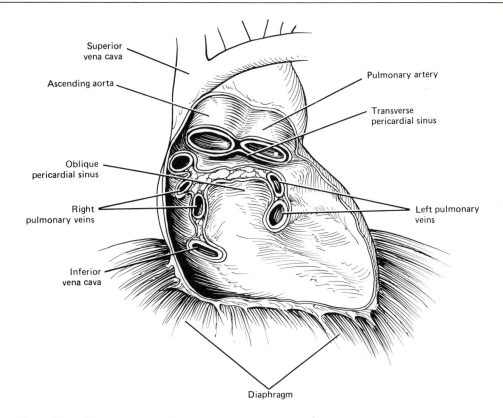

Figure 18–4. The posterior pericardium with the heart removed, showing the 2 pericardial sinuses.

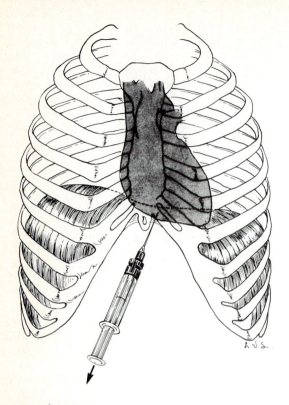

Figure 18–5. Aspiration of pericardial tamponade. (Reproduced, with permission, from Way LW [editor]: *Current Surgical Diagnosis & Treatment,* 7th ed. Lange, 1985.)

eventually in congestive heart failure, hepatomegaly, ascites, and peripheral edema. Pericardial effusion produces narrowed pulse pressure, muffled heart sounds, and an enlarged cardiac area of dullness to percussion. X-rays show an enlarged cardiac shadow, and pericardial tap reveals the presence and nature of the effusion. Constrictive pericarditis and cardiac tamponade usually result in distention of the neck veins, more pronounced on inspiration.

Surgical management of pericarditis consists of (1) pericardiocentesis for relief of cardiac tamponade; (2) open pericardial drainage for acute suppurative pericarditis; and (3) pericardiectomy for chronic constrictive pericarditis. In some instances, open pericardial biopsy is required to distinguish between chronic constrictive pericarditis and cardiomyopathy.

The dorsal surface of the fibrous pericardium is in intimate relationship with structures confined within the posteroinferior mediastinum. These include the major bronchi, the esophagus, the thoracic duct, the descending aorta, and the azygos and hemiazygos veins.

EXTERNAL ANATOMY
(Figs 18–6 to 18–13)

The heart normally lies dorsal to the sternum and the third to sixth left costal cartilages. At the level of the right third costal cartilage, the normal adult heart usually extends about 1 cm to the right of the sternal border; at the same level, it protrudes about 2.5 cm to the left of the left sternal border. At the level of the sixth right interspace, the right border of the heart is at the chondrosternal junction; at the level of the left fifth interspace, the apex of the heart is about 8.5 cm to the left of the left sternal border. These relationships may vary markedly in cardiac disease.

The heart is usually divided into an apex, a base, an anterior (sternocostal) surface, and a posterior (diaphragmatic) surface. Normally in adults, the heart is 10–12 cm long, 7.5–9 cm wide, and 5–7 cm thick. In the adult male, the normal heart weighs 275–360 g; in the adult female, 225–275 g.

Sulci

The surface of the heart exhibits 3 grooves, or sulci. The transverse (atrioventricular) sulcus, also called the coronary sulcus, forms a complete circle around the heart and separates the atria from the ventricles. The 2 longitudinal (interventricular) sulci separate the 2 ventricles and are known as the anterior and posterior longitudinal interventricular sulci. All 3 sulci contain fat, and the nutrient coronary vessels of the heart provide clues to the location of the cardiac chambers.

Heart Wall

The wall of the heart is made up of 3 layers: an external epicardium, a central myocardium, and an internal endocardium.

The **epicardium** is the visceral layer of the pericardium and is composed of mesothelial cells. Lying between the epicardium and the myocardium is a layer of connective tissue. This fibroelastic layer contains adipose tissue and the cardiac blood vessels and nerves.

The **myocardium** consists of cardiac muscle whose fibers show the typical cardiac cross-striated fibrils. On histologic section, the muscle tissue closely resembles striated skeletal muscle except that the fibers are only one-third as wide as those of striated skeletal muscle. The cardiac muscle fibers have a centrally placed nucleus and are rich in sarcoplasm. Cardiac muscle also contains intercalated disks that appear on histologic section as deeply staining lines which cross the muscle fibers and are positioned between the muscle nuclei.

The **endocardium** lines the interior of the heart. On its surface, there is a thin layer of squamous endothelial cells continuous with the endothelial lining of the great vessels. The endocardial connective tissue is thin and transparent over the ventricular walls but thicker in the atria, particularly in the areas of valve

Figure 18–6. Surface projection of heart valves.

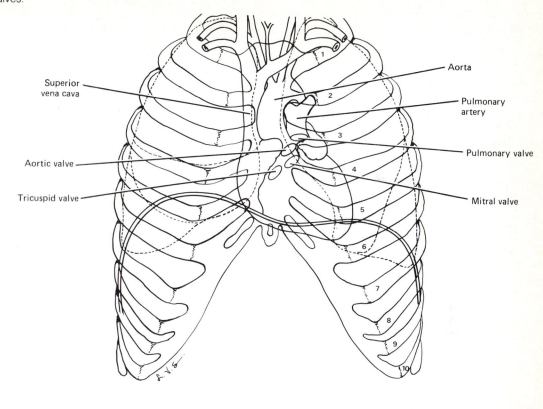

Figure 18–7. Anterior view of the heart. (Reproduced, with permission, from Sokolow M, McIllroy MB [editors]: *Clinical Cardiology*, 3rd ed. Lange, 1981.)

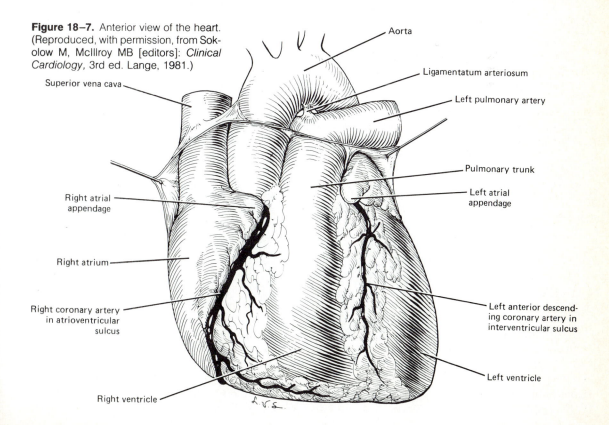

attachment. Endocardial connective tissue contains elements of the cardiac conduction system, a few areas of smooth muscle, and several small arteries and veins.

Apex & Base
(Figs 18–8 and 18–9)

The **apex of the heart** is directed inferiorly and to the left. It is completely covered by the medial surface of the left lung and pleura.

The **base of the heart** is intimately related to the great vessels. The base comprises the superior cardiac border and faces superiorly, dorsally, and to the right. It consists primarily of the left atrium, a segment of the right atrium, and the great arteries and veins that enter and leave the heart. Superiorly, it is bounded by the bifurcation of the pulmonary artery; inferiorly, by the coronary sulcus. Its right border is the sulcus terminalis; its left border is the oblique vein of the left atrium. Lying dorsal to the cardiac base are thoracic vertebrae T5–8, and between the vertebrae and the cardiac base are the esophagus, the thoracic duct, and the descending aorta.

Surfaces & Borders

The **sternocostal surface** of the heart is bounded on the right by the right atrium and on the left mainly by the left ventricle. The greatest part of the sternocos-tal surface is formed by the right ventricle. The sternocostal surface is crossed obliquely from left to right by the coronary sulcus superiorly and the anterior interventricular sulcus inferiorly.

➠ *Diagnosis and treatment of blunt and penetrating injuries to the heart. Trauma to the anterior chest wall, the diaphragm, or the upper abdomen may cause pericardial or cardiac injury, often accompanied by pericardial effusion. Blunt injury to the heart often occurs as a result of compression of the thorax by the steering wheel or the dashboard of an automobile. The extent of injury may vary from localized myocardial contusion to actual cardiac rupture. Such an injury is often accompanied by avulsion and tearing of the sternal and anterior costochondral fibers of the diaphragm. Blunt nonpenetrating cardiac injury may lead to the following clinical symptoms and findings: chest pain, pericardial friction rub, tachycardia, an increase in the heart size on percussion, and various cardiac murmurs and arrhythmias. Hemopericardium with associated cardiac tamponade usually follows cardiac rupture or tearing of the coronary vessels. Pericardial effusion must always be suspected and treated early.*

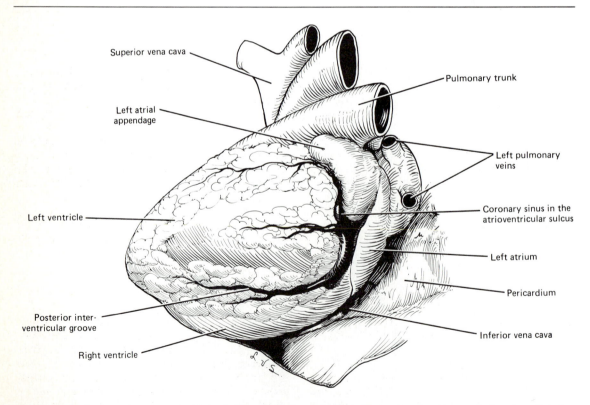

Figure 18–8. The heart viewed from the left side with the apex raised. (Reproduced, with permission, from Sokolow M, McIllroy MB [editors]: *Clinical Cardiology,* 3rd ed. Lange, 1981.)

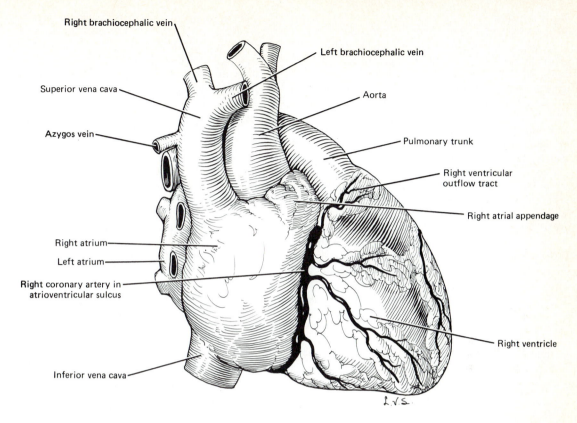

Figure 18–9. The heart viewed from the right side. (Reproduced, with permission, from Sokolow M, McIllroy MB [editors]: *Clinical Cardiology,* 3rd ed. Lange, 1981.)

In the absence of clear signs and symptoms of heart trauma following the traumatic event, electrocardiography may help in reaching the proper diagnosis.

Penetrating chest stab or missile wounds are frequently seen at large emergency centers. Pericardial lacerations secondary to stab wounds tend to seal rapidly, thus leading to pericardial tamponade. Gunshot wounds usually leave a large pericardial opening and cause diffuse myocardial damage and massive bleeding into the pleural spaces. Penetrating cardiac wounds may involve injuries to single or multiple valves, to the papillary muscles, and to the interventricular and interatrial septa. Infectious pericarditis may follow penetrating pericardial wounds. Myocardial lacerations are closed with sutures placed so as not to shut off or diminish the flow in the coronary arteries or impair the conduction system of the heart.

The **diaphragmatic surface** of the heart, which rests directly on the central tendon of the diaphragm, is composed of both right and left ventricles. The coronary sulcus separates the diaphragmatic surface from the base of the heart, and the posterior interventricular sulcus crosses the diaphragmatic surface obliquely from superior to inferior. This surface of the heart tends to be flattened by the pressure exerted by the diaphragm.

The long **right border of the heart** reaches from the superior vena cava to the cardiac apex. It is bounded superiorly by the lateral margin of the right atrium and inferiorly by the lateral border of the right ventricle.

The **left border of the heart** is formed mainly by the left ventricle and a small segment by the left atrium. The left border presents a gentle curve with the convexity facing to the left.

INTERNAL ANATOMY

The interior of the heart is divided into 4 cavities: 2 large, thick-walled ventricles and 2 smaller, thin-walled atria. The interventricular septum (between the 2 ventricles) and the interatrial septum (between the 2 atria) divide the entire heart into right and left halves. The right half occupies mainly an anterior thoracic position and the left half mainly a posterior thoracic position.

Right Atrium
(Figs 18–10 and 18–11)

The right atrium is larger than the left, but its wall is thinner. It is made up of a pair of cavities: a main cavity (sinus of the venae cavae) and a hollow appendix (the right atrial appendage).

The sinus of the venae cavae makes up the right side of the right atrial cavity. It is situated between the openings of the superior and inferior venae cavae and the atrioventricular opening. Its wall is continuous with the walls of the veins.

The right atrial appendage has the shape of a dog's ear as a cul-de-sac. It lies between the superior vena cava and the right ventricle. A ridge on its inner surface marks its junction with the sinus of the venae cavae. Its internal surface has parallel ridges that indicate the presence of underlying muscle bundles. These ridges are called the pectinate muscles.

Opening into the right atrial cavity are the orifices of the superior vena cava, the inferior vena cava, the coronary sinus, and the foramina venarum minimarum cordis (thebesian foramens). The superior vena cava, which returns blood from the superior segment of the body, opens into the superoposterior portion. Blood discharged from the superior vena cava is directed toward the atrioventricular opening.

The opening of the superior vena cava loops inferiorly and ventrally and lacks a valve. Blood that returns from the inferior segment of the body through the inferior vena cava empties into the sinus of the venae cavae at its lowest segment close to the interatrial septum. Its opening is larger than that of the superior vena cava and faces in the direction of the fossa ovalis. A crescentic fold attached to the left anterior edge of the opening ("valve of the inferior vena cava") is not a true valve, and in the adult it is probably nonfunctional. In the fetus, however, the "valve" helps to direct blood from the inferior vena cava into the left atrium via the patent foramen ovale.

The coronary sinus, which has a valve at its orifice, carries blood from the tissues of the heart. Its orifice lies between the inferior vena cava and the right atrioventricular opening. The thebesian foramens discharge blood directly into the right atrium. They are the orifices of small veins that reach the atrium directly from the myocardium.

Blood passes into the right ventricle from the right atrium by passing through the tricuspid opening.

The posterior wall of the right atrium is made up of the interatrial septum. An oval-shaped cup in the septal wall—the fossa ovalis—is the remnant of the foramen ovale of the embryonic heart.

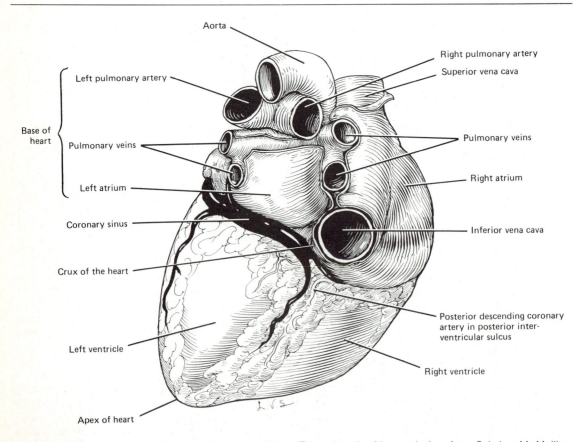

Figure 18–10. The heart viewed from below and behind. (Reproduced, with permission, from Sokolow M, McIllroy MB [editors]: *Clinical Cardiology,* 3rd ed. Lange, 1981.)

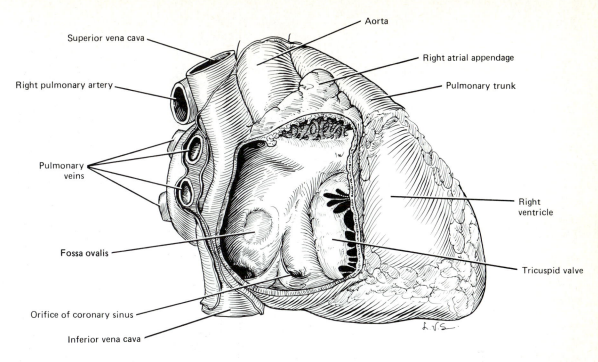

Aorta
Superior vena cava
Right atrial appendage
Right pulmonary artery
Pulmonary trunk
Pulmonary veins
Right ventricle
Fossa ovalis
Tricuspid valve
Orifice of coronary sinus
Inferior vena cava

Figure 18–11. View of the right heart with the right wall reflected to show the right atrium. (Reproduced, with permission, from Sokolow M, McIllroy MB [editors]: *Clinical Cardiology*, 3rd ed. Lange, 1981.)

Right Ventricle
(Fig 18–12)

The right ventricle occupies the major portion of the ventral (sternocostal) surface of the heart. It is bounded on the right by the coronary sulcus and on the left by the anterior longitudinal sinus. Its superior area, the infundibulum, merges into the pulmonary arterial trunk. Inferiorly, its margin forms the acute cardiac angle. The right ventricular myocardium is only one-third to one-half as thick as that of the left ventricle, and it is thickest superiorly.

The cavity of the right ventricle normally contains 80–90 mL of blood. An oval orifice about 4 cm wide represents the right atrioventricular ostium. Circling the ostium is a thick connective tissue ring. The ring is guarded by the tricuspid valve, whose 3 cusps project into the right ventricle. The cusps are of unequal size, with the largest one positioned anteriorly and the smallest one posteriorly. The cusps are triangular, with the bases of the triangles facing their area of attachment, while the apexes project into the cavity of the ventricle. Each cusp is composed of fibrous tissue that is thick centrally and thin laterally. The atrial surface of each cusp is lined with endocardium. The ventricular surface of each cusp is attached to the chordae tendineae. During ventricular systole, the chordae tendineae and the papillary muscles prevent atrial regurgitation by holding the cusps of the tricuspid valve in place.

The chordae tendineae are thin, strong fibrous cords that run superiorly from the muscular walls of the right ventricle and are attached to the edges, apexes, and inferior surfaces of the leaflets of the tricuspid valve. They vary in length and girth and are about 18–22 in number.

The papillary muscles are projecting strands of ventricular muscle whose apexes give attachments to the chordae tendineae. The larger anterior papillary muscle projects from the ventral and septal walls of the ventricle and gives attachments to the chordae tendineae running to the anterior and posterior cusps of the tricuspid valve. The posterior papillary muscle is composed of several segments that arise from the posterior wall of the right ventricle and give attachments to the chordae tendineae of the posterior and lateral septal cusps. The trabeculae carneae cordis are cylindric muscle columns that take origin from the inferior three-quarters of the interior of the ventricle. Some of the trabeculae appear as ridges in the myocardial wall; some extend a short distance into the lumen of the ventricle; and others form the papillary muscles described above. In most hearts, a muscle bundle called the septomarginal band or moderator band passes from the interventricular septum to the base of the anterior papillary muscle. It carries part of the right bundle branch of the heart's conduction system.

The conus arteriosus, the superior ventricular segment, is quite smooth, with no muscular projections. At the upper margin of the conus arteriosus, lying

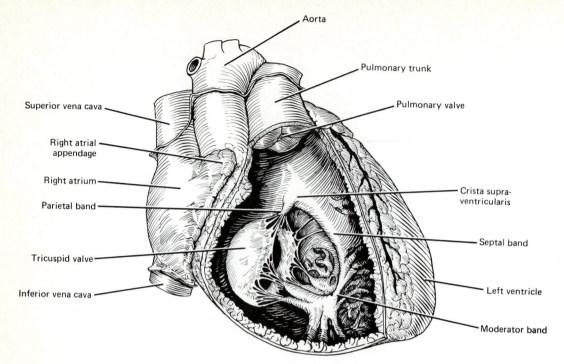

Figure 18–12. Anterior view of the heart with the anterior wall removed to show the right ventricular cavity. (Reproduced, with permission, from Sokolow M, McIllroy MB [editors]: *Clinical Cardiology,* 3rd ed. Lange, 1981.)

close to the ventricular septum and superior and to the left of the atrioventricular orifice, is the opening into the pulmonary trunk. This opening is guarded by the pulmonary valve, which is composed of 3 leaflets. The leaflets (cusps) consist of a central fibrous layer that is covered with the lining endocardium of the ventricle. The 3 cusps are designated right, left, and anterior. The cusps are semicircular, with the convexities of each cusp facing the ventricle and the concave aspects facing the pulmonary trunk. As a consequence, an increase in pressure in the pulmonary trunk brings the 3 cusps into apposition, preventing reflux into the right ventricle. Each pulmonary cusp has a nodule at the midpoint of its free margin; when the valve is closed, the point of contact between the cusps is at the point where the nodules touch.

➠ *Malfunctions of the tricuspid valve. Malfunctions of the tricuspid valve are much less common than aortic and mitral valve malfunctions. They are manifested by elevated venous pressure, hepatic enlargement, edema, and ascites. Operation is seldom indicated for tricuspid stenosis or insufficiency, as the condition usually responds well to medical management.*

Left Atrium

The left atrium is smaller than the right but possesses a thicker wall. It accounts for 85–90% of the base of the heart and also presents on the superior posterior cardiac surface. Ventrally, the aorta and the pulmonary trunk are interposed between the right and left atria. Dorsally, it is difficult to distinguish the line of atrial separation. Into the main cavity of the left atrium empty the 4 pulmonary veins, 2 on the left and 2 on the right, without valves. The smooth left atrial cavity empties into the left ventricle. The orifice is protected by the mitral valve. As in the right atrium, there is a depression in the wall of the interatrial septum, the remnant of the fetal foramen ovale.

The left atrial (auricular) appendage is narrowed where it joins with the major left atrial cavity. The appendage is in the shape of a narrow rectangle, and it curves around the base of the pulmonary trunk as it moves from dorsal to ventral. If one inspects the sternocostal aspect of the heart, only the tip of the left atrium is visible. The left atrial appendage lies atop the proximal segment of the left coronary artery.

Left Ventricle
(Fig 18–13)

The left ventricle comprises only a small segment of the sternocostal surface of the heart but makes up the apex of the heart and over half of the heart's diaphragmatic surface. Its walls are 2.5–3 times as thick as those of the right ventricle, and its cavity is longer and more pyramid-shaped than that of the right ventricle. The cavity of the left ventricle has 2

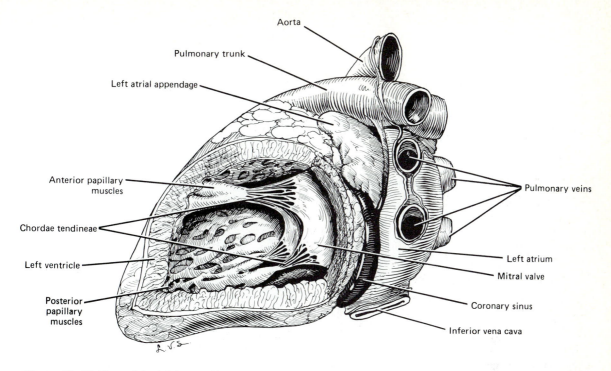

Figure 18–13. View of the left heart with the left ventricular wall turned back to show the mitral valve. (Reproduced, with permission, from Sokolow M, McIllroy MB [editors]: *Clinical Cardiology,* 3rd ed. Lange, 1981.)

orifices—the left atrioventricular opening, guarded by the mitral valve; and the aortic orifice, guarded by the aortic valve.

The mitral orifice, slightly smaller than the right atrioventricular orifice, is surrounded by a firm supporting ring of fibrous tissue. The mitral valve is bicuspid and extends inferiorly into the cavity of the left ventricle. The ventral cusp is larger. The chordae tendineae that attach to the valve cusps are fewer in number but stronger than the right ventricular chordae. The left ventricle contains 2 papillary muscles, one adherent to the dorsal wall of the ventricle and one to the ventral wall. These muscles are quite large, and their distal extremities are rounded; attached to the extremities are the chordae tendineae. The chordae from both the ventral and the dorsal papillary muscles attach to each of the 2 cusps of the mitral valve.

➠ *Mitral stenosis and mitral insufficiency. (Fig 18–14.) The diagnosis of advanced mitral stenosis is suggested by the presence of dyspnea and orthopnea, x-ray evidence of prominent superior pulmonary vessels, an enlarged left atrium, and an apical diastolic rumble. Advanced mitral insufficiency is characterized by a loud apical systolic murmur that radiates to the axilla, pulmonary congestion, a large left atrium, and left ventricular distention. Mitral stenosis is a disease of mechanical obstruction and responds well to surgical therapy. The best*

treatment for mitral insufficiency is replacement of the poorly functioning mitral valve.

The aortic valve is made up of 3 semilunar cusps: right posterior, left posterior, and anterior. Each cusp has its convexity facing the ventricular cavity and its concavity facing the aorta. In the middle of the free surface of the cusp is a fibrocartilaginous nodule (nodule of Arantius). Between the free surface of the cusps and the wall of the aorta are 3 pockets in the aortic wall, the aortic sinuses of Valsalva. The coronary arteries leave the aorta from the right posterior and left posterior sinuses of Valsalva.

➠ *Diagnosis and treatment of cardiac valvular disease. Valvular heart disease may involve a single valve or any combination of cardiac valves. The aortic and mitral valves are most commonly involved, the tricuspid valve less commonly. The valvular disease may be secondary to (1) congenital malformations; (2) infectious disease (rheumatic fever, syphilis); or (3) atherosclerosis. The valve may become stenotic, insufficient, or both. In aortic insufficiency, there is a left ventricular enlargement, and a diastolic murmur is heard along the left sternal border. In aortic stenosis, a systolic ejection type of murmur is heard in the right second interspace and is often transmitted supe-*

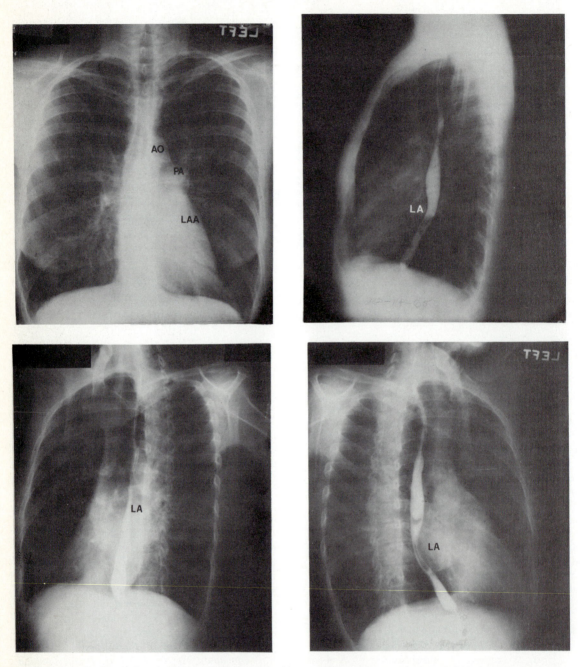

Figure 18–14. Cardiac series of chest x-rays of a 34-year-old woman with moderate mitral stenosis. Left atrial enlargement (LA) is seen on all views. The overall heart size is normal. **A:** Posteroanterior view. **B:** Lateral view. **C:** Left anterior oblique view. **D:** Right anterior oblique view. AO, aorta; PA, pulmonary artery; LAA, left atrial appendage. (Reproduced, with permission, from Sokolow M, McIllroy MB [editors]: *Clinical Cardiology,* 3rd ed. Lange, 1981.)

riorly to the neck vessels. In aortic stenosis, surgical replacement of the diseased valve should be done as soon as the disease becomes symptomatic. With aortic insufficiency, valve replacement should be done soon after the first episode of cardiac failure, since left ventricular function deteriorates rapidly.

THE CONDUCTION SYSTEM
(Fig 18–15)

The conduction system of the heart consists of the sinoatrial node, the atrioventricular node, the

atrioventicular bundle, and the final conducting fibers (Purkinje fibers). Each of these structures is composed of modified cardiac muscle that has greater conductivity than heart muscle generally. The atria and ventricles can contract spontaneously, but the conduction system initiates cardiac rhythm and transmits it to all areas of the heart.

Sinoatrial Node

The sinoatrial node is composed of a small portion of specialized heart muscle located at the point where the right atrium and superior vena cava meet. It initiates cardiac contraction and is thus the cardiac "pace-

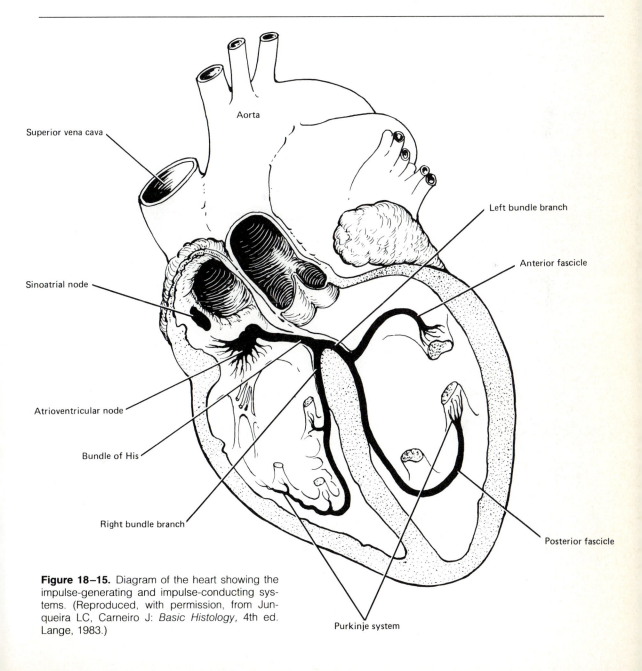

Figure 18–15. Diagram of the heart showing the impulse-generating and impulse-conducting systems. (Reproduced, with permission, from Junqueira LC, Carneiro J: *Basic Histology,* 4th ed. Lange, 1983.)

maker.'' It cannot be seen grossly but is easily identified in microscopic sections.

Atrioventricular Node

The atrioventricular node occupies a position in the right atrium near the opening of the coronary sinus. It is quite small and connected to the atrioventricular bundle.

Atrioventricular Bundle

The atrioventricular bundle (bundle of His) originates at the atrioventricular node and runs for about 2 cm along the atrial septum toward the left atrioventricular orifice. About halfway along its course, it divides into a right and a left branch to form an inverted Y across the most superior part of the ventricular septum. The right branch runs in a subendocardial position toward the apex of the heart, supplying all of the segments of the right ventricle. The left bundle branch makes its way into the fibrous septum and proceeds in a subendocardial position in the left ventricle to be distributed to the left ventricular musculature. Since each of the bundle branches tends to be ensheathed with fibrous connective tissue, they are usually grossly visible.

Purkinje Fibers

The terminal conducting fibers (Purkinje fibers) connect the nodal tissue with the cardiac muscle. They cannot be seen grossly, because they run in a subendocardial position to finally spread out within the ventricular musculature.

⏩ *Disorders of the cardiac conduction system. Cardiac conduction disturbances include (1) sinoatrial node dysfunction, (2) delay or interruption of impulse propagation (incomplete or complete heart block), and (3) abnormalities of the conducting pathways. Symptoms secondary to a conduction system disturbance may be due to low cardiac output, bradycardia, tachycardia, or asystole. The usual cause of conduction disturbances is idiopathic degeneration of the specialized conductive tissue of the heart. The disorders may also be due to myocardial infarction or ischemia secondary to coronary atherosclerosis. Conduction disorders are usually treated by electrical pacemaker implantation.*

BLOOD VESSELS, LYMPHATICS, & NERVES

Arteries

Arterial blood reaches the cardiac tissues via the 2 major coronary arteries, each of which arises from the base of the ascending aorta. The **right coronary artery** has its origin in the right aortic sinus of Valsalva and passes laterally to the right in the coronary sulcus, delivering branches to the right atrium and the right ventricle. It gives off a branch (called the marginal artery) that runs along the right border of the right ventricle. The main right coronary artery continues its course in the coronary sulcus to the posterior surface of the heart, where it merges with branches from the left coronary artery. On the posterior cardiac surface, the right coronary artery gives rise to a posterior descending branch which descends in the posterior longitudinal sulcus to anastomose with the descending branch of the left coronary artery.

The **left coronary artery** arises from the left aortic sinus of Valsalva and moves immediately to the left, lying at first between the left atrium and the pulmonary artery. It divides into 2 major branches. The left anterior descending coronary artery runs on the sternocostal surface of the heart to the anterior interventricular sulcus, where it descends to the apex of the heart. It supplies arterial blood to both ventricles. The second major branch of the left coronary artery, the circumflex branch, runs in the left coronary sulcus and almost reaches the posterior interventricular sulcus. It supplies arterial blood to the left atrium and left ventricle. It anastomoses with the corresponding branch of the right coronary artery.

⏩ *Coronary atherosclerosis. Coronary atherosclerosis is most common in older individuals. The sclerotic plaques impair myocardial blood flow, leading to ischemia and myocardial infarction. Atherosclerosis of the coronary arteries can induce angina pectoris and evidence of myocardial infarction on electrocardiography and serum enzyme studies. Complications are ventricular septal rupture and left ventricular aneurysm.*

Veins

The venous return from the heart is via 2 systems: the cardiac veins and the thebesian veins (venae cordis minimae). The **great cardiac vein** (vena cordis magna) begins at the cardiac apex and follows the anterior interventricular sulcus to the base of the ventricles. It then passes to the left in the coronary sulcus to end in the coronary sinus. It drains blood from both ventricles and the left atrium. The **small cardiac vein** (vena cordis parva) runs alongside the marginal coronary artery and then between the right atrium and right ventricle in the coronary sulcus to end in the coronary sinus. It drains blood from the posterior surface of the right atrium and right ventricle. The **middle cardiac vein** (vena cordis media) starts at the cardiac apex, rises in the posterior interventricular sulcus, and ends in the coronary sinus. The **posterior vein of the left ventricle** is found on the diaphragmatic surface of the heart. It too empties into the coronary sinus. The **oblique vein of the left atrium** runs on the posterior surface of the left atrium and ends in the coronary sinus. The **anterior cardiac** veins, 3–5 in number, drain blood from the anterior surface of the right ventricle and terminate in the right atrium. The **smallest cardiac veins** (thebesian veins; venae cordis minimae) begin in the myocardium and empty directly into either the cardiac atria or ventricles.

The **coronary sinus** is a short, wide vein located in the posterior segment of the coronary sulcus. It is covered by the muscle of the left atrium. It terminates in the right atrium in an orifice that lies between the orifice of the inferior vena cava and the atrioventricular orifice. It is fed by all of the cardiac veins except the anterior cardiac veins and the thebesian veins.

Lymphatics

Superficial and deep cardiac lymphatic plexuses empty into right and left thoracic lymphatic trunks and terminate in the tracheobronchial lymph nodes.

Nerves

The heart is supplied by the cardiac branches of the vagus nerve and by fibers from the sympathetic trunk joined in the cardiac and coronary plexuses. The vagal fibers are preganglionic, whereas the sympathetic fibers are postganglionic from the lower cervical and upper thoracic ganglia. The vagal fibers are cardiac inhibitors; the sympathetic fibers are cardiac accelerators.

THE GREAT VESSELS

THE ASCENDING AORTA

The ascending aorta and the pulmonary trunk are both ensheathed by the visceral pericardium. The ascending aorta varies in length from 4 to 6 cm. It begins at the superior margin of the semilunar valve, where it lies deep to the left half of the sternum near the third left costal cartilage. As it ascends, it moves to the right and reaches the level of the second right costal cartilage. In the superior mediastinum it becomes the aortic arch. Both the pulmonary artery and the right atrium lie ventral to the ascending aorta which is just superior to the semilunar valve. Dorsal to the ascending aorta are the left atrium and the right pulmonary artery. The superior vena cava and the right atrium lie to the right of the ascending aorta. The pulmonary trunk lies to its left. The right pleura, the anterosuperior portion of the right lung, and the fatty thymic remains lie between the ascending aorta and the dorsal surface of the sternum. The right and left coronary arteries are the only branches of the ascending aorta.

➠ *Aneurysms of the ascending aorta. Aneurysms of the ascending thoracic aorta are manifested by an enlarged ascending aortic silhouette and by angiographic evidence of an abnormally dilated vessel. Patients complain of chest pain that radiates to the back.*

THE INFERIOR SEGMENT OF THE SUPERIOR VENA CAVA

The inferior segment of the superior vena cava lies deep to the right second rib cartilage and the right second intercostal space and opens into the right atrium near the right third costal cartilage. As it approaches the heart, the superior vena cava is within the pericardial sac and is covered with serous pericardium. The anterosuperior portion of the right lung and its covering pleura lie ventral to the superior vena cava; dorsal to it lie the right vagus nerve and the root of the right lung. Along the right border of the superior vena cava lie the right phrenic nerve and the right pleura; the left side of the superior vena cava is related to the ascending aorta and the beginning of the innominate artery. At the point where the superior vena cava enters the pericardial sac, it receives the azygos vein and one or 2 small veins that drain the pericardium.

THE PULMONARY ARTERIAL TRUNK

The pulmonary arterial trunk carries poorly oxygenated blood from the heart to the lungs. It is a short vessel about 4–6 cm long and about 3.5 cm wide. It arises from the right ventricle and swings from right to left and from ventral to dorsal. It lies at first ventral and then slightly to the left of the ascending aorta. At about the level of the sixth thoracic vertebra, it divides into the right and left pulmonary arteries. The entire length of the pulmonary trunk is encased within the pericardial sac. The pleura and left lung separate the vessel from the second interspace. On the left side of the artery is the left atrial appendage and on its right side the right atrial appendage. The left coronary artery passes dorsal to the pulmonary trunk. Just superior to the point of bifurcation of the pulmonary trunk lies the cardiac plexus of nerves.

THE PULMONARY VEINS

Two pulmonary veins return to the heart from each lung, carrying oxygenated blood to the left atrium. They enter the pericardial sac soon after leaving the hilum of the lung, and each vein then opens separately into the left atrium. After the veins have entered the pericardial sac, only their ventral surfaces are ensheathed by the serous pericardium. The 2 right pulmonary veins lie posterior to the superior vena cava and the right atrium. The 2 left pulmonary veins lie ventral to the descending thoracic aorta.

➠ *Diagnostic aids in cardiac disease. Accurate diagnosis of cardiac disease is essential in order to make correct decisions about management. Cineradiography and cardiac catheterization are of great help in identifying cardiac disease amenable to operative treatment. Quantitative assessment of obstructive processes, regurgi-* *tant flow, ventricular ejection, pulmonary hypertension, and coronary artery patency also help determine the need for cardiac surgery.*

➠ *Cardiac tumors. Cardiac tumors are rare. Myxomas account for about 75% of all benign cardiac neoplasms; most of the malignant tumors are sarcomas. Metastatic carcinoma, sarcoma, and melanoma occasionally involve the heart or pericardium.*

Posterior Mediastinum

19

The posterior mediastinum (Fig 19–1) is the narrow area that lies just ventral to the plane of the vertebral column (T5–12) and dorsal to the pericardial sac. The dorsal segment of the dome of the diaphragm lies lower than the pericardial sac. The posterior segment of the vault of the diaphragm forms the ventral boundary of the posterior mediastinum, which is bounded laterally on either side by the mediastinal pleura.

Lying within the posterior mediastinum are the descending thoracic aorta and its branches; the azygos vein, the hemiazygos vein, and the accessory hemiazygos vein; the thoracic sympathetic chain and its ganglia; the greater splanchnic, lesser splanchnic, and least splanchnic nerves; the vagus nerves; the termination of the thoracic trachea and its bifurcation into the 2 major stem bronchi; the thoracic esophagus; the thoracic duct; and multiple lymphatic channels and a large number of lymph node groupings. The posterior mediastinal compartment is filled with areolar tissue.

➠ *Lesions in the posterior mediastinum. The commonest space-consuming lesions found in the posterior mediastinum are (1) thoracic aortic aneurysms, (2) tumors of neurogenic origin, (3) meningoceles, (4) reduplication cysts of the lower esophagus, and (5) the contents of a posterior diaphragmatic hernia that have entered the posterior mediastinum through the pleuroperitoneal hiatus or through a tear of the posterior segment of the diaphragm.*

EMBRYOLOGY OF THE VENOUS SYSTEM

The vitelline veins carry blood from the yolk sac to the sinus venosus. They form a venous plexus in the vicinity of the duodenum, then enter the liver to become hepatic sinusoids.

The plexus about the duodenum becomes a single vein, the **portal vein.** The distal portion of the right vitelline vein becomes the **superior mesenteric vein,** and its proximal portion, the hepatic part of the **inferior vena cava.** The distal and proximal portions of the left vitelline vein disappear.

The umbilical veins return oxygenated blood from the placenta.

A channel is formed between the left umbilical vein and the right hepatocardiac channel, the ductus venosus, enabling much of the blood to bypass the sinusoidal plexus of the liver. The proximal part of the left umbilical vein and the entire right umbilical vein then disappear. The distal part of the left umbilical vein thus remains to carry blood back to the fetus.

After delivery, the left umbilical vein becomes the **ligamentum teres** and the ductus venosus the **ligamentum venosum** of the liver.

The common pulmonary vein first appears as an evagination of the posterior wall of the primitive atrium. The evagination grows into the dorsal mesocardium to a point near the primitive foregut from which the lung buds are developing. As the left atrium enlarges, the common pulmonary vein is incorporated into its wall, allowing usually 2 veins from the right and left lungs to open directly into the left atrium.

Development of the inferior vena cava is such a complicated process that **anomalies** are quite common: double inferior vena cava at the lumbar level; absence of the inferior vena cava, which is always associated with cardiac anomalies; persistent left superior vena cava; and double superior vena cava.

Abnormal pulmonary venous drainage includes veins emptying into the right atrium, the inferior vena cava, or a persistent left superior vena cava.

THE DESCENDING THORACIC AORTA

The descending thoracic aorta begins at T4 at the termination of the transverse aortic arch. It ends by passing through the aortic hiatus at T12. The descending thoracic aorta lies to the left of the midline of the vertebral column. It does not decrease in girth as it descends through the thorax, since its branchings are quite small. As it descends, it lies dorsal to the root of the left lung, the pericardium, and the esophagus; as it passes into the abdominal cavity, it lies dorsal to the decussating crura of the diaphragm and ventral to the vertebral column and to the hemiazygos and accessory hemiazygos veins. To its left are the left pleura and lung, and to its right the azygos vein and the thoracic duct.

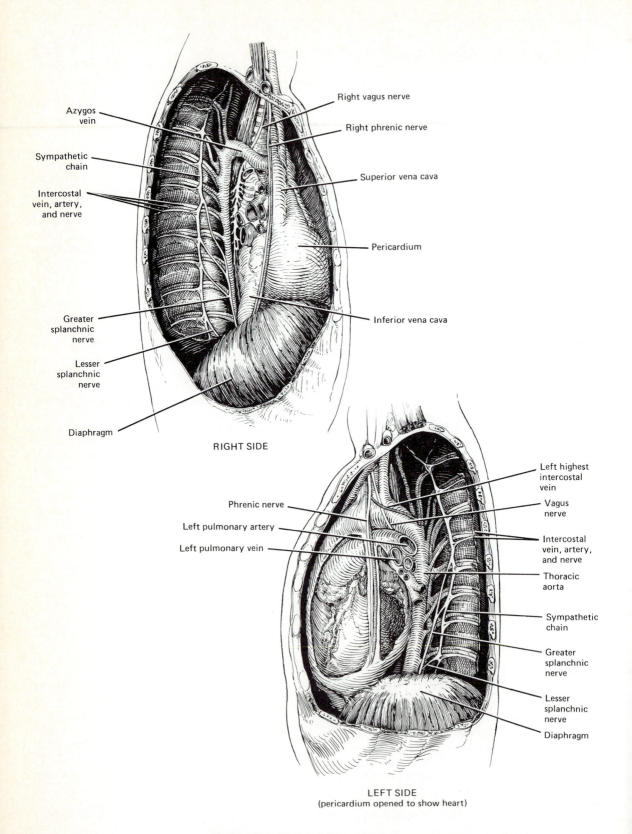

Azygos vein

Sympathetic chain

Intercostal vein, artery, and nerve

Greater splanchnic nerve

Lesser splanchnic nerve

Diaphragm

Right vagus nerve

Right phrenic nerve

Superior vena cava

Pericardium

Inferior vena cava

RIGHT SIDE

Phrenic nerve

Left pulmonary artery

Left pulmonary vein

Left highest intercostal vein

Vagus nerve

Intercostal vein, artery, and nerve

Thoracic aorta

Sympathetic chain

Greater splanchnic nerve

Lesser splanchnic nerve

Diaphragm

LEFT SIDE
(pericardium opened to show heart)

Figure 19–1. The posterior mediastinum.

➠ *Operative procedures upon the descending thoracic aorta. Plastic or replacement graft procedures upon the descending thoracic aorta are performed for coarctation of the aorta, syphilitic and atherosclerotic aneurysms, and dissecting aneurysms still within the thorax. Arteriographic studies are used to localize aneurysmal swellings of the ascending aorta and the transverse arch.*

BRANCHES OF THE DESCENDING THORACIC AORTA

The branches of the descending thoracic aorta are classified as visceral and parietal.

Visceral Branches

Pericardial branches that leave the aorta at heart level supply blood to the posterior surface of the pericardial sac.

There is usually one **right bronchial artery,** which may arise directly from the descending thoracic aorta or from the first right posterior intercostal artery or from the highest left bronchial artery. There are usually **2 left bronchial arteries.** The superior left bronchial artery arises from the thoracic aorta about 1 cm below the bifurcation of the trachea, while the inferior left bronchial artery arises from the thoracic aorta just inferior to the origin of the left main stem bronchus. The branches of the bronchial arteries run to and then onto the dorsal surface of the bronchi and supply the bronchi and the areolar tissue of the bronchi. They also send small twigs to the esophagus and to the peribronchial lymph nodes.

The 3–6 **esophageal arteries** arise from the anterior surface of the descending thoracic aorta. They run laterally and inferiorly to the thoracic esophagus, where they anastomose with esophageal branches of the inferior thyroid arteries and of the left inferior phrenic and left gastric arteries.

The small and variable **mediastinal branches** of the thoracic aorta supply the posterior mediastinal areolar tissue and lymph nodes.

Parietal Branches

The **posterior intercostal arteries** are usually arranged in 9 pairs—one arising from each side of the aorta. The arteries run to the inferior 9 intercostal spaces, while the 2 superior intercostal spaces receive blood from the descending branch of the costocervical division of the subclavian artery. The right posterior intercostal vessels are longer than those on the left and cross the anterior surface of the vertebrae. In their transverse course, the right posterior intercostal arteries lie dorsal to the esophagus, thoracic duct, and azygos vein, while ventral to them are the right lung and pleura. The shorter left intercostal arteries run posterolaterally along the left side of the vertebral column, covered by the left lung and pleura. The

superior 2 left intercostal arteries are crossed by the highest left intercostal vein, while the inferior 3 or 4 left intercostal arteries lie dorsal to the hemiazygos vein. Near the head of the ribs, both the right and the left posterior intercostal arteries are crossed ventrally by the thoracic sympathetic trunk, and the lowest posterior intercostal vessels are crossed also by the 3 descending splanchnic nerves.

The **subcostal arteries** run laterally and then ventrally below the lowest ribs. They are the most inferior of the segmental paired thoracic aortic branches. Accompanied by nerve T12, the subcostal arteries run dorsal to the kidney and ventral to the quadratus lumborum muscle. They pierce the posterior sheath of the transverse abdominal muscle and finally anastomose with the superior epigastric and lumbar arteries.

The small **superior phrenic arteries** arise from the thoracic aorta just prior to its passing through the diaphragm. They supply the superior surface of the diaphragm.

AZYGOS, HEMIAZYGOS, ACCESSORY HEMIAZYGOS, & HIGHEST INTERCOSTAL VEINS

Azygos Vein
(Figs 19–1 and 19–2)

The azygos vein arises in the retroperitoneum of the upper lateral abdomen near L1 and L2 as a branch of the right ascending lumbar vein. Almost immediately it passes through the aortic hiatus to the right side of the aorta. In the posterior thorax, it runs along the right border of the vertebral column, and at the level of T4 it arches anteriorly over the root of the right lung to terminate in the superior vena cava, just before that vein receives its pericardial covering. As the azygos vein ascends in the thorax, it lies to the right of the aorta and the thoracic duct and ventral to the posterior intercostal veins. The vein receives blood from the hemiazygos, esophageal, mediastinal, bronchial, pericardial, right subcostal, intercostal, and right bronchial veins.

Hemiazygos Vein

The hemiazygos vein takes its origin from the left ascending lumbar vein. The hemiazygos vein reaches the thorax by passing through the left crus of the diaphragm. It ascends in the posterior mediastinum along the left side of the vertebral column, and at the level of T9 it passes from the left to the right side, running posterior to the aorta, the esophagus, and the thoracic duct, to empty into the azygos vein. The hemiazygos vein receives blood from the lower 5 left intercostal veins, the left subcostal vein, and the accessory hemiazygos vein as well as from several small mediastinal and esophageal veins.

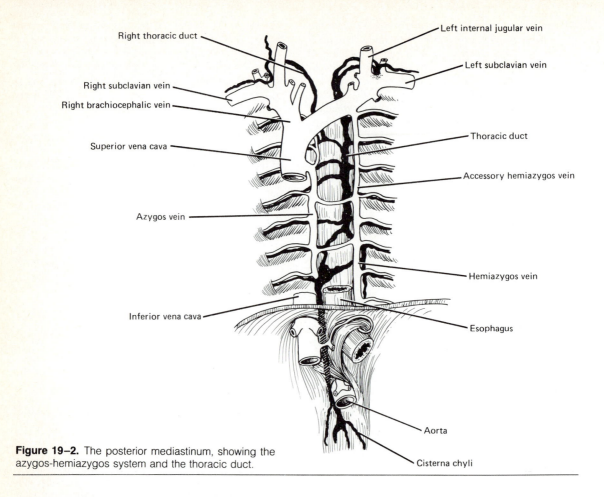

Figure 19–2. The posterior mediastinum, showing the azygos-hemiazygos system and the thoracic duct.

▥ *Collaterals of the azygos and hemiazygos venous systems. If there is extensive obstruction of the inferior vena cava (tumor mass, thrombus, ligation), the main vessels by which caval flow is carried superiorly are the azygos and hemiazygos veins, which have multiple connections with both the superior and inferior venae cavae.*

Accessory Hemiazygos Vein

The accessory hemiazygos vein lies solely within the thorax. It passes inferiorly from the level of T3 along the left side of the vertebral column and terminates by crossing the vertebral bodies at T8 to join the azygos vein, the hemiazygos vein, or both. It receives blood from the 2 or 3 highest intercostal veins and on occasion from the left bronchial vein.

Highest Intercostal Veins

The highest intercostal veins receive blood from the 3 highest posterior intercostal spaces. On the right, the highest intercostal vein courses caudally to join the azygos vein. On the left, the vein moves ventral to the aortic arch and the origin of the left common

carotid and subclavian arteries to terminate in the left brachiocephalic vein.

THE THORACIC COURSE OF THE RIGHT & LEFT VAGUS NERVES (Fig 19–3)

The thoracic pathways of the right and left vagus nerves are quite variable. The right vagus enters the thorax immediately after crossing ventral to the first segment of the subclavian artery. It passes dorsal to the subclavian vein and to the short right brachiocephalic vein and descends along the right wall of the trachea until it reaches the posterior surface of the root of the lung. At this point, it forms the posterior pulmonary plexus and a plexus upon the posterior surface of the esophagus. From this plexus, it sends communicating fibers to the left vagus. Upon leaving the esophageal plexus, the right vagus proceeds inferiorly as a single nerve that passes through the esopha-

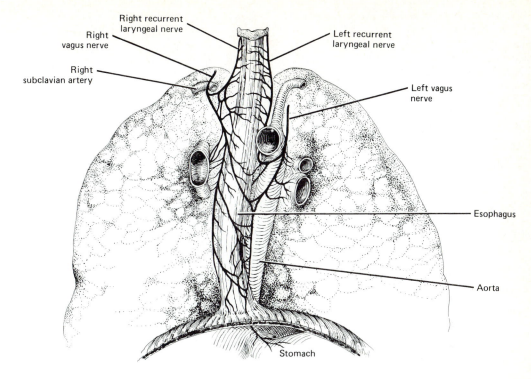

Figure 19–3. The right and left vagus nerves in the thorax.

geal hiatus of the diaphragm at T10, and then it is called the posterior vagus nerve.

The left vagus nerve enters the thorax between the left common carotid and subclavian arteries, dorsal to the long left brachiocephalic vein. It descends along the left margin of the arch of the aorta and finally comes to lie between the aorta and the left pulmonary artery at the level of the ligamentum arteriosum. There it gives off the left recurrent laryngeal nerve. It becomes related to the posterior surface of the root of the left lung, where it joins with the right vagus to form the posterior pulmonary plexus. It then breaks up into several cords that lie on the anterior surface of the esophagus, and it sends communicating fibers to the right vagus, which lies on the dorsal esophageal surface. The multiple cords of the left vagus unite to form the anterior vagus nerve, after passing through the esophageal hiatus into the abdominal cavity.

THORACIC PORTION OF THE SYMPATHETIC NERVOUS SYSTEM (Fig 19–1)

The thoracic sympathetic system consists of a series of ganglia and connecting cords, each ganglion corresponding in position to a thoracic spinal nerve. Adjacent sympathetic ganglia often fuse. In the upper thorax, the ganglia lie against the necks of the ribs; farther down, they lie in a more ventral position; the lowest thoracic ganglia lie alongside the lower thoracic vertebrae. The thoracic sympathetic trunk lies dorsal to the parietal pleura; the cords connecting the ganglia occupy a position between the pleura ventrally and the posterior intercostal vessels dorsally.

The branches that leave the thoracic sympathetic trunk are of 3 types: (1) The **gray rami communicantes,** which send several branches to the corresponding spinal nerves; (2) the **visceral branches,** which run to the pulmonary, cardiac, aortic, and esophageal plexuses; and (3) the 3 **splanchnic nerves,** which take their origin from the lower 6 thoracic ganglia and the first lumbar ganglion.

The **greater splanchnic nerve** is composed of fibers that arise from the fifth to ninth thoracic ganglia. The individual fibers of origin extend medially across the vertebral bodies and eventually join to form a single nerve that passes through the crus of the diaphragm and ends in the celiac ganglion. A small ganglion is placed on the body of the nerve at the level of T11 and T12. The visceral afferent fibers in the greater splanchnic nerve do not synapse in the celiac plexus but continue through the plexus from their origin in the various abdominal viscera. They carry painful impulses from the stomach, gallbladder, and small bowel.

The **lesser splanchnic nerve** arises from fibers

that originate in thoracic ganglia T10 and T11. The fibers join and form a single nerve that penetrates the diaphragm along with the greater splanchnic nerve to become part of the aorticorenal ganglion.

The **least splanchnic nerve,** a branch from either the lowest thoracic ganglion or from the lesser splanchnic nerve, accompanies the main sympathetic trunk as it passes from the thorax into the abdomen behind the median arcuate ligament of the diaphragm. The nerve terminates in the renal plexus.

ANATOMY OF THE TRACHEA & THE POSTERIOR MEDIASTINUM

THE TRACHEA
(Fig 19–4)

The trachea begins in the neck at C6, below the cricoid cartilage of the larynx, runs into the posterosuperior mediastinum and descends as far as the upper border of the fifth thoracic vertebra, where it divides into the 2 major stem bronchi. In its thoracic course, it is related on the right to the mediastinal pleura and the right vagus nerve and on the left to the left recurrent laryngeal nerve, the arch of the aorta, and the left common carotid and subclavian arteries. It is a midline structure except at the bifurcation, where it lies slightly to the right of the midline. Lying dorsal to the mediastinal trachea and slightly to its left is the superior segment of the thoracic esophagus. Lying directly dorsal to the trachea are the bodies of the upper thoracic vertebrae. At the tracheal bifurcation, the openings into the 2 main stem bronchi are separated by an elevated, sharp crest, the **carina.**

⮕ *Tracheal and bronchial injury. Penetrating wounds of the chest may involve the trachea, one or both main stem bronchi, the thoracic duct, and the esophagus. However, this is uncommon, since all of these structures lie deep within the posterior mediastinum. When such injuries do occur, there may be subcutaneous emphysema, esophageal spill, or chylothorax.*

THE MAJOR BRONCHI

Right Main Bronchus

The right main bronchus averages about 2.75–3 cm in length. It is wider and shorter than the left main bronchus and more vertical in position. It reaches the right lung at about the level of T5. The azygos vein passes dorsal and superior to the right main bronchus, while the pulmonary artery is first inferior

and then ventral to it. The right main bronchus terminates by dividing into 3 lesser bronchi, one for each lobe of the right lung. The upper lobe bronchus, which arises superior to the level of the pulmonary artery, is eparterial in position; the middle and lower lobe bronchi, which are given off below the level of the pulmonary artery, are hyparterial.

⮕ *Bronchoscopic examination of the mediastinal trachea. The bifurcation, the carina, the 2 main stem bronchi, and the lobar bronchi are examined as part of the diagnostic workup of patients with pulmonary disease. The bronchoscope may also be used for removal of aspirated foreign bodies and mucous plugs. Biopsy specimens may be taken, and bronchial washings may be collected for study of malignant cells, microbial pathogens, or parasites.*

Left Main Bronchus

The left main bronchus is 5–5.5 cm long and not as wide as the right major stem bronchus. From the tracheal bifurcation it moves to the left beneath the arch of the aorta. Lying dorsal to it are the esophagus, the thoracic duct, and the descending aorta. At its point of origin, it lies superior to the pulmonary artery; in mid course, it lies dorsal to the pulmonary artery; and before bifurcating, it lies inferior to the pulmonary artery. It divides into the upper lobe and lower lobe bronchi.

THE THORACIC ESOPHAGUS
(Fig 19–4)

EMBRYOLOGY

The esophagus begins to develop from the superior dorsal portion of the entodermal tube that lies just distal to the primitive pharynx and reaches to the dilatation of the foregut, which becomes the stomach. The esophagus lengthens with the growth of the embryo and as a result of inferior migration of the heart and pericardium and the increase in size and inferior movement of the lung buds, which develop from the ventral portion of the esophageal tube. During development, there is a short period of marked narrowing of the lumen of the esophagus; later, the width of the lumen is completely restored.

The anomalies include esophageal stenosis and atresia, tracheoesophageal fistula, enteric cyst or reduplication of the esophagus, and abnormally short esophagus with thoracic displacement of a portion of the stomach through the esophageal hiatus (rare).

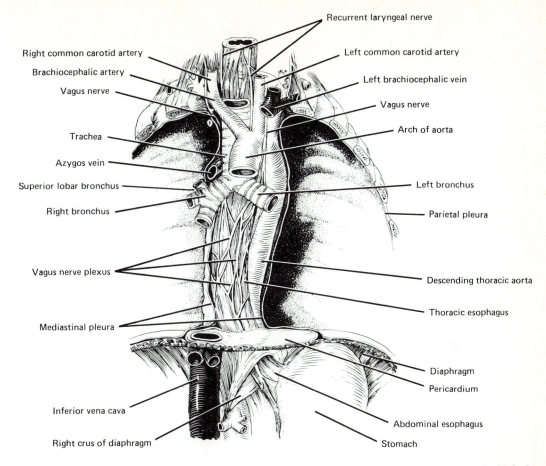

Figure 19–4. Anatomy of the esophagus and trachea. (Reproduced, with permission, from Way LW [editor]: *Current Surgical Diagnosis & Treatment,* 7th ed. Lange, 1985.)

GROSS ANATOMY

The esophagus lies in the posterosuperior mediastinum just to the left of the midline, dorsal and slightly to the left of the trachea, and ventral to the left of the vertebral column. It regains the midline at the level of T5 and comes to lie dorsal to and slightly to the right of the aortic arch. Then it lies immediately to the right of the descending thoracic aorta, but above the diaphragm it moves close to the left side of the aorta. It passes through the esophageal hiatus of the diaphragm at the level of T10.

➠ *Esophageal narrowing. There are 3 areas of anatomic esophageal narrowing: (1) at the level of C6, where the hypopharynx ends and the esophagus begins; (2) at the level of T5, where the tracheal bifurcation lies just anterior to the esophagus; and (3) at the level of T10, where the esophagus passes through the diaphragm. These normal narrowings must not be mistaken for pathologic narrowing due to tumor or other esophageal disease. Enlarge-*

ment of the left atrium, which lies just anterior to the midthoracic esophagus, may cause a pressure defect in the esophageal lumen seen on an x-ray taken during a thick barium swallow. Radiographic evidence of esophageal compression is also noted with (1) an anomalous right subclavian artery, which arises from the left side of the aortic arch; and (2) double aortic arch, where the esophagus and the trachea are both compressed.

➠ *Acquired esophageal fistula. In addition to congenital tracheoesophageal fistula, acquired esophageal fistula can occur secondary to (1) cancer of the esophagus, (2) cancer of the adjacent trachea or an adjacent bronchus, or (3) cancer in an adjacent mediastinal lymph node.*

Other Relationships of the Thoracic Esophagus in the Posterior Mediastinum

The trachea and left main bronchus, the superior arch of the diaphragm, and the pericardial sac, all lie ventral to the esophagus in the posterior mediastinum. Dorsal to the esophagus are the longus colli muscles, the vertebral bodies, the thoracic duct, the hemiazygos vein, and the right intercostal arteries. Below the level of the lung roots, the 2 vagus nerves have a close esophageal relationship. The right vagus is closely applied to its anterior surface. As the 2 vagus nerves descend, they form an intricate communicating plexus around the entire esophageal circumference.

Just above the diaphragm, the thoracic duct lies just to the right of the esophagus. Higher, at about T4 or T5, the thoracic duct passes dorsal to the esophagus and then continues upward just to the left of the esophageal tube.

The thoracic esophagus receives its arterial supply (1) from branches of the inferior thyroid artery; (2) directly from the aorta, via several esophageal branches; (3) from the bronchial arteries; (4) from branches of the left gastric artery; and (5) from the left inferior phrenic artery. Since the esophageal veins terminate in mediastinal veins that empty into the superior vena cava and into gastric veins that terminate in the portal venous system, there is in the submucosal layer of the lower thoracic esophagus an opportunity for an anastomotic anatomic portacaval venous shunting. Lymphatic drainage is into a rich plexus around the esophageal tube. The plexus empties into the posterior mediastinal nodes. A small amount of lymph empties into the tracheobronchial nodes.

The thoracic esophagus derives its nerve supply from the recurrent laryngeal branch of the vagus nerve, which supplies the striated muscle fibers that appear mainly in the upper third of the tube. Both the vagus and the thoracic sympathetic trunks supply nerve fibers to the smooth musculature.

➠ *Esophageal varices. Hypertrophy of or bleeding from the submucous plexus of the veins in the lower esophagus is presumptive evidence of portal hypertension secondary to either intra- or extrahepatic portal vein block.*

➠ *Esophagoscopy. The esophagoscope is of great assistance in the diagnosis of esophageal disease. It not only allows the clinician to inspect esophageal lesions directly—it also affords a means of measuring the length of the esophagus, taking biopsies, collecting washings for diagnostic examination, and removing esophageal foreign bodies.*

➠ *Mediastinitis secondary to esophageal perforation. Foreign body perforations of the esophagus, if not diagnosed early, may lead to fulminating mediastinitis. The perforation must be closed as soon as the diagnosis is made. Perforations of the esophagus secondary to peptic esophagitis, instrumentation, or cancer may result in mediastinitis or empyema.*

➠ *Strictures of the esophagus. Stricture of the esophagus is a common sequela of inflammatory disease, ingestion of caustics, or esophageal tumor. The most common sites of tumor formation are the levels of anatomic narrowing.*

➠ *Resection of the cardioesophageal junction. Resection of the lower esophagus and of the cardia of the stomach is performed for esophagogastric carcinoma or for a severe stricture of the gastroesophageal junction. Reconstruction usually consists of anastomosis of the lower esophagus to the stomach after mobilization of the stomach so it can be brought up into the thoracic cavity.*

THE THORACIC DUCT
(Thoracic Segment)
(Fig 19–2)

The thoracic duct reaches the posterior mediastinum by passing along with the azygos vein through the aortic hiatus of the diaphragm. Both structures are related to the right side of the aorta at the hiatal level. The duct then lies between the descending aorta and the azygos vein. In this position, the vertebral column, the right posterior intercostal arteries, and the hemiazygos veins lie dorsal to the duct. The pericardium, the heart, the superior surface of the diaphragm, and the esophagus lie ventral to the duct. At the level of T5, the thoracic duct passes dorsal to the esophagus to lie to the left of the esophagus. On the posterior surface of the esophagus, the thoracic duct is held tightly to the outer fibrous coat of the esophageal tube. The duct continues superiorly, dorsal to the aortic arch and the left subclavian artery, and in the lower neck is to the left of the midline. Then the duct arches above the level of the clavicle, moves ventral to the subclavian and vertebral arteries and the phrenic nerve, and empties into the angle formed by the junction of the left subclavian and internal jugular veins. In the thorax, the thoracic duct receives lymph from the superior lumbar nodes, from the posterior mediastinal nodes, and from the posterior intercostal nodes that drain the upper 7 left intercostal spaces.

➠ *Rupture of thoracic duct. Fractures of the thoracic vertebrae occasionally result in tears of the thoracic duct. This results in unilateral or bilateral chylothorax.*

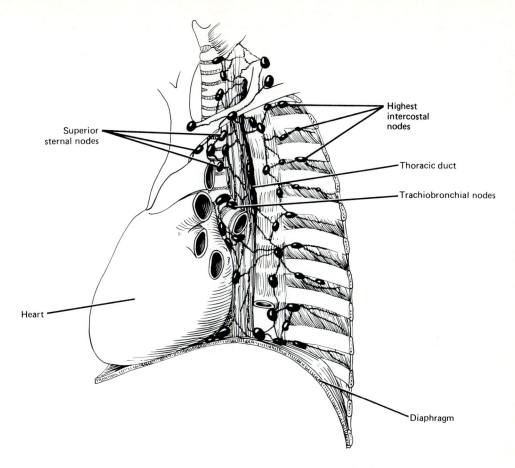

Figure 19–5. Lymph nodes in the posterior mediastinum.

POSTERIOR MEDIASTINAL LYMPH NODES (Fig 19–5)

The posterior mediastinal lymph nodes lie in apposition to both the esophagus and the descending aorta, dorsal to the pericardial sac. They drain the esophagus, the posterior surface of the pericardium, the posterior and mid segments of the diaphragm, and the superior convexity of the liver. Efferent lymph from the posterior mediastinal nodes flows in 2 directions—most of it into the thoracic duct but a small amount directly into the tracheobronchial nodes that lie in the midposterior mediastinum.

➠ *Lymphatic drainage from cancer of the esophagus. Lymphatic drainage from cancer of the esophagus is into the deep cervical chain of nodes in the lower neck and into gastric nodes lying below the diaphragm along the lesser gastric curvature.*

The lungs are the major organs of respiration. They lie within the thorax, one on each side, separated by the central mediastinal structures. The right lung is larger, weighing 625–650 g; the left lung weighs about 550 g. Lung weight varies with the amount of blood or serous fluid present at any given time. Each lung is roughly conical in shape and presents an apex, a base, 2 surfaces (costal and mediastinal), and 3 borders (inferior, anteromedian, and posterior). Lung tissue is light, buoyant, and elastic. The lung surface is normally shiny. Grossly, one can easily make out the polyhedral markings that outline the underlying lung lobules.

EMBRYOLOGY OF THE LARYNGOTRACHEAL TREE & THE LUNGS

The Laryngotracheal Tube

The laryngotracheal tube appears as an entodermal depression in the ventral wall of the foregut, just inferior to the hypobranchial eminence. The lateral walls of this depression fuse in the midline to form a tube. At first the tube is connected to the foregut; later, it is separated from the gut by the laryngotracheal septum.

The superior end of the tube becomes the larynx. The mid portion of the tube becomes the trachea. The 3-lobed right lung and the 2-lobed left lung develop from the terminal portion of the laryngotracheal tube.

Anomalies include tracheoesophageal fistula, congenital tracheal stenosis, congenital laryngeal septum, and blind ending of the trachea with absence of bronchi and lungs.

The Lung Buds

A lung bud develops from the most inferior segment of the laryngotracheal tube. Almost immediately it divides into 2 bronchial buds of entodermal origin. The buds lobulate peripherally, the right one into 3 lobules and the left one into 2 lobules. By the end of the sixth month, the pulmonary air sacs appear. Mesoderm surrounding the bronchial tree differentiates into cartilage. Muscle and blood vessels form a mesodermal framework around the entodermal bronchial tree.

Anomalies include agenesis of one lung or of a lung segment; abnormal divisions of the bronchial tree, with supernumerary lung lobes; ectopic lung lobes arising from the trachea or esophagus; and congenital lung cysts.

GROSS ANATOMY

SURFACE ANATOMY
(Figs 20–1 and 20–2)

The apexes of the lungs lie posterior to the middle third of the clavicle, and they rise 2–4 cm above the level of the clavicle to reach into the lower neck. The anteromedian border of the right lung reaches almost to the midsternal line. The anteromedian border of the left lung also reaches almost to the midsternal line, but on the left side the relationship to the sternum continues only to the level of the fourth costal cartilage, at which level the left lung is displaced laterally by the cardiac notch.

In full expiration, the lower border of each lung forms a gently curving line with a superior convexity, running from the level of the sixth sternocostal articulation to the level of T10. The line reaches the midclavicular line at the level of the sixth rib and the midaxillary line at the level of the eighth rib. The dorsomedian border of the lung lies 2.5 cm from the midline of the back and roughly parallels that line as it reaches from C7 superiorly to T10 inferiorly.

DIVISIONS OF THE LUNGS

Apex

The apex of the lung presents a smooth curved surface whose convexity protrudes superiorly into the lower neck 1.5–4.5 cm above the level of the sternal end of the first rib. The subclavian artery grooves the medial superior surface of the lung apex as the vessel arches into the neck.

Base

The base of the lung rests upon the convex superior surface of the diaphragm. The right lung base arches

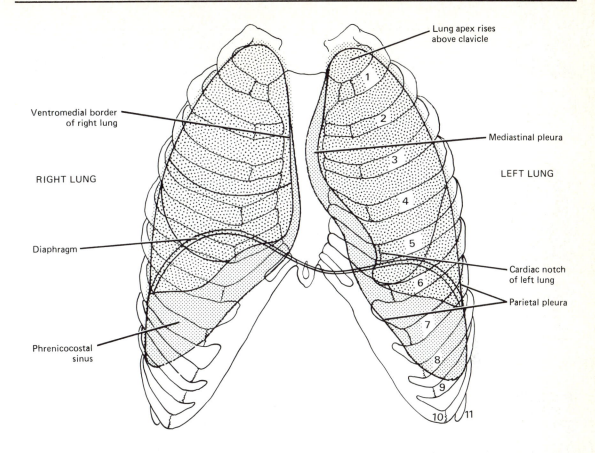

Figure 20–1. Surface anatomy of the lungs.

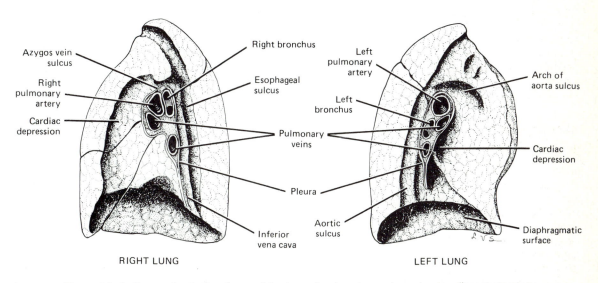

Figure 20–2. The mediastinal surfaces of the lung showing depressions due to adjacent structures.

higher than the left, since the liver elevates the diaphragm on the right side. Dorsolaterally, the base of the lung presents a thin, sharp edge that descends into the **costophrenic sinus** of the pleural cavity. The lung base is quite mobile, normally rising and falling 2–5 cm with expiration and inspiration (depending upon individual lung expansions).

Lung Surfaces
(Fig 20–2)

A. Costal Surface: The smooth costal surface of the lung is convex as it conforms to the anterior chest wall. The lung, lined by visceral pleura, is in close contact with the parietal pleural covering of the inner surface of the chest wall. On the surface of some lungs one can make out a stepladder pattern of shallow grooves formed by the pressure of the ribs. The costal surface of the lung descends slightly lower dorsally than ventrally.

The heart and great vessels leave impressions upon the mediastinal surfaces of the lung.

B. Mediastinal Surface: (Fig 20–2.) There is a deep cardiac depression on the medial surface of each lung into which the pericardial sac fits snugly. Superior and posterior to the cardiac depression is the hilum (or root) of the lung. The mediastinal surfaces of the right and left lungs differ.

1. Right lung—Just above the hilum of the right lung, there is a superiorly arching depression due to the pressure exerted by the azygos vein. Superiorly and laterally, a few centimeters below the apex of the right lung, is a depression that accommodates the superior vena cava and the right brachiocephalic vein. Extending inferiorly from the inferior border of the hilum of the right lung is the right pulmonary ligament. Posterior to both the lung hilum and the superior limit of the right triangular ligament is a groove that accommodates the esophagus. The groove is less well marked inferiorly as the esophagus moves to the left in order to pass through the esophageal hiatus of the diaphragm. Ventral to the lower half of the esophageal groove is a deep depression occupied by the inferior vena cava, which at this level has passed through the central tendon of the diaphragm but has not yet entered the right side of the pericardial sac.

2. Left lung—Just above the hilum of the left lung is a superiorly arching groove in which lies the transverse segment of the thoracic aorta. From the superior border of this furrow, a vertical groove runs farther superiorly in the direction of the lung apex; this is the depression made by the left subclavian artery. This groove is paralleled by a groove for the left brachiocephalic vein. Extending inferiorly from the inferior border of the hilum of the left lung is the left pulmonary ligament. Lying posterior to the left hilum and the left pulmonary ligament is the deep vertical depression created by the pressure of the descending thoracic aorta.

C. Borders of the Lung: Inferiorly, the lung border is quite thin and sharp as it separates the lung base from the costal surface of the lung. The inferior border of the lung only partially fills the phrenicocostal sinus laterally. As the inferior lung border moves medially, it loses its sharp edge and becomes rounded as it separates the base of the lung from the mediastinal surface of the lung.

Anteromedially, the lung border is thin and terminates sharply. This border of the lung covers a portion of the ventral surface of the heart and pericardium as it proceeds vertically. The anterior border of the left lung presents the so-called cardiac notching that allows the pericardium to come into contact with the bony posterior sternal surface just to the left of the midline of the thorax.

The posterior border of the lung is wide and well-rounded and fits into concavities on either side of the vertebral column.

Fissures & Lobes of the Lungs
(Fig 20–3)

A. Right Lung: The right lung presents 2 interlobar fissures that divide it into 3 major lobes: upper, middle, and lower. The **oblique fissure** of the right lung divides the lower lobe from the middle and upper lobes. The oblique fissure of the right lung is more vertical than that of the left lung. It begins at the angle of the fifth rib, follows that rib to the midaxillary line, and then moves anteriorly to end at the sixth costochondral junction in the midclavicular line.

The **horizontal fissure** divides the middle from the upper lobe in the right lung. It begins in the oblique fissure close to the posterior border of the lung and proceeds anteriorly to the fourth costal cartilage. The horizontal fissure is absent in about 10–15% of right lungs.

The wedge-shaped middle lobe is the smallest of the 3 lobes. The middle lobe includes the lower segment of the anterior border of the lung and the anterior segment of the lung base.

B. Left Lung: The oblique fissure divides the left lung into 2 lobes: upper and lower. The fissure reaches from the costal to the mediastinal surfaces. The superior arm of the left oblique fissure leaves the lung hilum and runs superiorly and dorsally on the mediastinal surface to about 5–6 cm below the lung apex. From this point, it runs inferiorly and ventrally on the costal surface to the lower border of the lung. It then traverses the mediastinal surface of the lung in a superior direction until it reaches the hilum. The oblique fissure of the left lung causes the apex, the anterior border, much of the costal surface, and about two-thirds of the mediastinal surface of the left lung to be part of the superior lobe. The left lower lobe—larger than the upper lobe—is made up of the greater portion of the lung base, over half of the costal surface, and nearly three-fourths of the vertebral segment of the medial surface of the lung.

The left lung has no horizontal fissure and **no** middle lobe. The **lingula** of the left lung is the homolog of the right middle lobe.

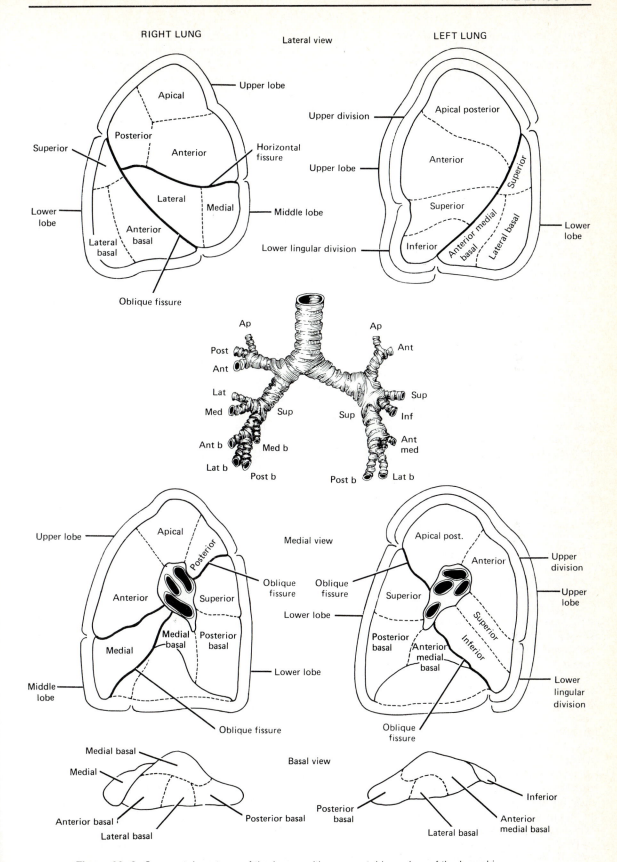

Figure 20–3. Segmental anatomy of the lungs, with segmental branches of the bronchi.

➠ *Penetrating wounds of the lung. Pneumothorax, hemopneumothorax, tension pneumothorax, and hemorrhage from the lung or its hilar vessels may follow trauma to the thoracic wall, pleura, and lung. Peripheral wounds of the lung are usually less serious than those that involve the lung hilum. Bleeding from the lung periphery is usually self-contained and seldom serious. Hilar bleeding may be life-threatening. Hemothorax is more often secondary to injury to a major intercostal vessel than to lung tissue injury.*

➠ *Treatment of bronchopleural fistula. Peripheral injury with involvement of a small bronchus, causing a bronchopleural fistula and permitting escape of air from the lung into the pleural cavity, may result in tension pneumothorax. Treatment consists of inserting a tube into the thorax and applying suction to evacuate pleural air. If that is not successful in fully expanding the lung after a reasonable period of time (10–14 days), thoracotomy and operative closure of the bronchial leak are required.*

Roots of the Lungs

The roots of the lungs are made up of several structures surrounded by mediastinal connective tissue and covered by a reflection of the mediastinal pleura. The structures of the lung roots include the pulmonary artery, the pulmonary veins, the major stem bronchi, the bronchial arteries and veins, the pulmonary nerve plexuses, pulmonary lymphatic channels, and the bronchial lymph nodes. The lung root lies posterior to the cardiac depression and is nearer to the posterior than to the anterior lung border. The root of the right lung lies posterior to the right atrium and superior vena cava; superior to it is the arch of the azygos vein. The root of the left lung lies anterior to the descending aorta and inferior to the arch of the aorta.

Ventral to the roots of both lungs are the phrenic nerve, the pericardiophrenic artery, and the anterior division of the pulmonary nerve plexus. The vagus nerve and the posterior division of the pulmonary nerve plexus lie posterior to the lung root. Running inferiorly to the diaphragm, from each lung root, are the anterior and posterior leaves of the pulmonary ligament. The pulmonary veins are the most anterior structures of the lung roots, while the bronchi are the most posterior. The pulmonary artery lies between the veins and the bronchi. This anteroposterior relationship of the major lung root structures holds for the roots of both right and left lungs. The superior and inferior relationships of the lung root structures vary on the right and left sides. On the right side, the upper lobe bronchus is the most superior of the lung root structures, and the pulmonary artery lies just below it. The bronchi to the middle and lower lobes lie inferior to the pulmonary artery. The pulmonary vein is the most inferior of the right lung root

elements. On the left side, the pulmonary artery is the most superior of the lung root structures; the main stem bronchus lies in a slightly more inferior position; and the pulmonary veins are the lowest structures making up the left lung root.

The Bronchopulmonary Segments (Fig 20–3)

Diagnosis and therapy of lung lesions have been greatly improved by the concept of the lung as a single organ that can be divided into bronchopulmonary segments by the bronchial branchings. By definition, a bronchopulmonary segment is an area of lung to which a specific bronchial branching provides aeration.

➠ *Pulmonary resection. The major problem encountered by the surgeon in segmental pulmonary resection is identification of arterial, venous, and bronchial structures running to the individual segment to be resected. This may be difficult owing to abnormalities of bronchovascular anatomy.*

The bronchopulmonary segments are named according to their position in the lung lobes, and each minor bronchus leading to such a segment takes its name from the segment it supplies.

A. Right Lung:

1. The right upper lobe is made up of 3 bronchopulmonary segments: apical, posterior, and anterior.

2. The right middle lobe is made up of 2 segments: lateral and medial.

3. The right lower lobe is made up of 5 segments: one superior and 4 basilar (medial, anterior, lateral, and posterior).

B. Left Lung:

1. The left upper lobe has 2 divisions: a superior division that is similar to the right upper lobe and an inferior lingular division that is similar to the right middle lobe.

a. The superior division of the left upper lobe is made up of 3 segments: apical, posterior, and anterior.

b. The inferior division of the left upper lobe is made up of 2 segments: superior and inferior.

2. The left lower lobe is made up of 4 segments: one superior and 3 basilar (anteromedial, lateral, and posterior).

The Bronchi

Major bronchial branchings are named for the parts of the lung they aerate.

The **right major stem bronchus** leaves the trachea more vertically than the left. It has a wider lumen and is 2.5–3 cm shorter than the left. It reaches the right hilum at the level of T5 and divides into 3 minor bronchi, each supplying a lobe of the lung. The upper lobe bronchus lies above the level of the pulmonary artery, whereas the bronchi to the middle and lower lobes divide below the level of the pulmonary artery. The bronchus to the right upper lobe segments has 3 divisions, each named for the bronchopulmonary segments it aerates. The bronchus to the right middle lobe has 2 branches; the right lower lobe bronchus, after giving off a branch to the superior segment of the lower lobe, divides into 4 minor bronchi, one for each of the basilar segments of the right lower lobe.

The **left major bronchus** is 4.5–5.5 cm long and is narrower than the right. After leaving the tracheal bifurcation, it passes beneath the arch of the aorta and to the left, on a plane anterior to the esophagus, thoracic duct, and descending aorta. At first it is superior to the pulmonary artery, then behind it, and finally inferior to it. The branch to the left upper lobe divides into 2 minor bronchi called the superior and inferior divisions of the upper lobe bronchus. The superior division has branches for the anterior segment and the apical posterior segment of the upper lobe. The inferior division has superior and inferior segmental bronchi, which aerate the lingular portion of the upper lobe. The bronchus for the lower lobe gives off a bronchus for the superior segment and then further divides into 3 branches for the 3 basilar segments.

➤ *Postoperative pulmonary atelectasis. Atelectasis is a common postoperative complication. Small areas of a lobe, an entire major lobar segment, a complete lobe or an entire lung may collapse. The usual cause is failure of the patient to cough thick bronchial mucus loose from the bronchial lumen. Early ambulation, deep breathing exercises, and coughing help to prevent postoperative atelectasis. On occasion, bronchial aspiration through a catheter or bronchoscope may be required to initiate proper bronchial toilet, so that the collapsed lung can expand. Atelectasis may also follow compression of a bronchus by a neighboring inflammatory or malignant process; or it may follow plugging of the bronchial lumen by tumor or an aspirated foreign body.*

➤ *Radiographic signs of atelectasis. The principal radiographic signs of massive atelectasis are (1) elevation of the ipsilateral diaphragm and interspace narrowing on the ipsilateral side; (2) shift of mediastinal structures, particularly the trachea, to the ipsilateral side of the chest and (3) increase in density of the collapsed lung.*

➤ *Bronchiectasis. Bronchiectasis is a pathologic entity in which there is a chronic dilatation of all or a portion of the bronchial tree. It may follow infection or aspiration of a foreign body, or it may be idiopathic. Pneumonitis is common in the areas served by the affected bronchi, as dilated bronchi fail to properly move bronchial secretions toward the trachea where they can then be removed by coughing.*

➤ *Carcinoma of the lung. Carcinoma involving the pleura is manifested by pain and bloody pleural effusion. Bronchial obstruction by the tumor often causes atelectasis or pneumonitis distal to the obstruction. If the tumor spreads into the neighboring mediastinum, it may cause pressure upon the left recurrent laryngeal nerve, the phrenic nerves, the esophagus, the thoracic duct, or the pericardial sac. The malignant process commonly results in formation of a lung abscess, often with cavitation. A lung abscess or pneumonic area that does not clear with routine therapy always arouses a suspicion of lung cancer.*

BLOOD VESSELS, LYMPHATICS, & NERVES
(Fig 20–4)

Arteries

The **pulmonary arterial trunk** carries oxygen-poor blood from the right heart to the lungs. It is a stubby vessel, 5–6 cm long, which takes its origin from the right ventricular conus. After leaving the conus it moves obliquely dorsally and to the left, passing at first anterior to and then slightly to the left of the ascending aorta. As it reaches the inferior border of the arch of the aorta, it bifurcates into right and left pulmonary arteries. Like the proximal segment of the ascending aorta, it is entirely ensheathed by the visceral layer of the pericardium.

The **right pulmonary artery** pursues a slightly longer course and has a larger lumen than the left pulmonary artery. After leaving the area of pulmonary bifurcation, it moves to the right, posterior to both the aorta and the superior vena cava but anterior to the right main stem bronchus. As it reaches the lung, it bifurcates into a small anterior trunk and a larger interlobar trunk. The anterior trunk supplies the superior lobe of the right lung, while the interlobar trunk supplies the right middle and inferior lobes.

The anterior trunk bifurcates into superior and inferior divisions, the superior division dividing into an apical bronchopulmonary segmental artery and a posterior segmental artery. The inferior division of the anterior trunk continues as the anterior segmental artery.

The **interlobar trunk** runs in the fissure between the upper and middle lobes to the point where the middle lobe artery branches from it. The middle lobe artery gives origin to the lateral and medial segmental arteries. The lateral segmental artery gives rise to anterior and posterior branches, while the medial segmental artery gives rise to superior and inferior branches.

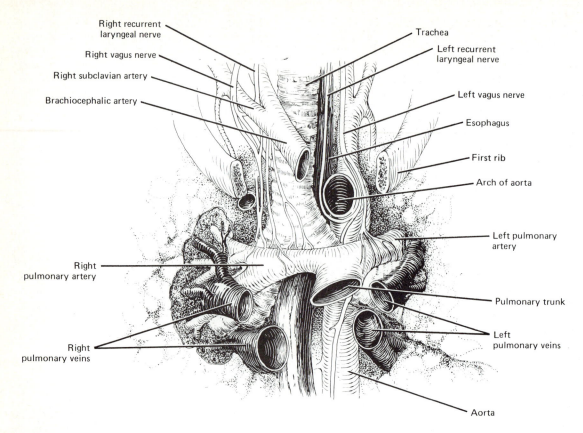

Figure 20−4. Superior mediastinum; relationships of the pulmonary arteries and veins. (Reproduced, with permission, from Way LW [editor]: *Current Surgical Diagnosis & Treatment,* 7th ed. Lange, 1985.)

The **left pulmonary artery,** which in fetal life gives rise to the ductus arteriosus, is smaller and shorter than its fellow on the right side. Its superior surface is attached to the inferior surface of the arch of the aorta by the ligamentum arteriosum, by the ascending left recurrent laryngeal nerve lying just to the left of the ligament, and by the cardiac autonomic nerve lying slightly farther to the left. As it reaches the root of the left lung, the left pulmonary artery forms an arch over the left major bronchus. It then passes dorsal to the bronchial divisions. It has no superior trunk, and its branches to the upper lobe are the apical segmental artery, the posterior segmental artery, and the anterior segmental artery, all of which arise high on the main trunk of the left pulmonary artery. The artery continues inferiorly as though it were an inferior trunk; however, the continuation is called the left interlobar artery. From the left interlobar artery will branch the posterior segmental artery, the lingular artery, and the superior and basal segmental arteries to the lower lobe.

As the right and left pulmonary arteries break up into their peripheral branches, they run along with the peripheral branches of the bronchi.

➠ *Pulmonary embolism. Pulmonary embolism may follow a surgical procedure or may occur as a complication of acute or chronic disease. The pulmonary artery is an end artery with little or no collateral circulation, and it carries to the lungs all of the blood that has been returned to the right heart via the vena caval system. Blockage by an embolus of a major pulmonary artery usually causes almost immediate death.*

If one or more of the peripheral divisions of the artery are blocked, the area served by the blocked divisions may become devascularized and infarcted. A greater or lesser degree of pulmonary insufficiency usually follows the larger peripheral infarctions. The use of body scans and radioactive isotopes to visualize the infarcted areas helps in the diagnosis and prognosis of pulmonary embolism.

The **bronchial arteries** supply the lung parenchyma. There is usually one bronchial artery for the right lung and 2 for the left lung. All 3 bronchial arteries are branchings from the anterior surface of the descending aorta, although one or more may arise as a branching from the upper intercostal vessels. The bronchial arteries supply the bronchial glands, the bronchial walls, the interlobar areolar tissue, and the thoracic esophagus. The bronchial arteries and their branches lie directly upon the dorsal surfaces of the bronchi.

Veins

There are **2 pulmonary veins** that return oxygenated blood from the lungs to the left atrium. Small lobular veins unite to form larger lobular veins, which join to form the lobar veins, 3 of which drain the right lung while 2 drain the left lung. The right middle lobe vein unites with the upper lobe vein to form a single vein just near the heart. Consequently, despite the fact that the right lung has 3 lobes, it has only 2 pulmonary veins entering the heart.

As they lie incorporated within the lung roots, the superior pulmonary veins lie inferior and anterior to the pulmonary arteries. The inferior veins draining the lower lobes as they lie in the lung hilum are posterior to the upper lobe veins and are the most inferior of the hilar structures. Both the superior and the inferior pulmonary veins run a very brief course before they enter the pericardium to open into the superior segment of the left atrium. As they pass from the lung hilum to the left atrium, the left pulmonary veins pass anterior to the descending aorta, while the right pulmonary vein passes posterior to the right atrium and the superior vena cava.

Within the parenchyma of the lung, the lobar and lobular veins do not accompany the bronchi or the arterial divisions to the lung segments. Rather, the veins lie either superficially, in close relationship to the pleura, or between the individual bronchopulmonary segments.

The **bronchial veins** are formed near the root of the lung and proceed as a single channel to empty the right side into the azygos vein and on the left side into the highest intercostal vein or the accessory hemiazygos vein. They collect venous blood from the perihilar area. The amount of blood carried by the bronchial veins is quite limited, since most of the blood brought to the lungs by the bronchial arteries is returned by the pulmonary veins.

Lymphatics

The lung lymphatics begin in a superficial pulmonary plexus, lying just under the pleura and in a deep pulmonary plexus closely associated with the segmental pulmonary vessels and bronchi. Minor radicals of the deep lymphatic plexus are in the submucous coats of the bronchi and in a peribronchial position. The deep lymph vessels enter the tracheobronchial nodes. The superficial lymphatics eventually reach nodes in the hilum alongside the pulmonary vessels. Except for small communicating vessels at the hilum, there is no junction between the superficial and deep lymphatic plexuses of the lung. Efferent lymphatics leaving the tracheobronchial nodes terminate in the right and left bronchomediastinal lymphatic trunks.

➠ ***Hilar dissection of bronchial lymph nodes.** Enlarged bronchial lymph nodes (due to infection or cancer) usually lie in the hilar angle between the pulmonary venous and pulmonary arterial branchings. The presence of these enlarged nodes makes hilar dissection and the identification of hilar structures tedious and time-consuming during pulmonary surgery. The hilar nodes are usually involved in late bronchiogenic carcinoma, and they become involved secondary to chronic long-standing pulmonary infections.*

➠ ***Pulmonary metastases. (Figs 20–5 and 20–6.)** Metastatic cancer may reach the lung either by the bloodstream or by lymphatic channels. Metastases are usually multiple at the time of diagnosis, but a single metastasis to the lungs is not rare. The metastases may produce all of the signs and symptoms associated with primary lung cancer.*

Nerves

Branches from the anterior and posterior pulmonary plexuses supply the lungs. The branches are made up of a combination of vagal and sympathetic fibers. Upon reaching the hilum, the nerve fibers run peripherally along with the major bronchi and the bronchial branchings, and supply efferent fibers to the bronchial musculature and afferent fibers to the mucous membrane of the bronchi. Some afferent fibers are also supplied to the lung alveoli.

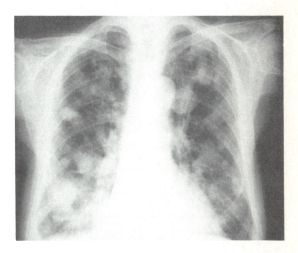

Figure 20–5. Adenocarcinoma of the kidney. Chest film showing metastases to lung. Note typical "cannonball" lesions. (Reproduced, with permission, from Smith DR [editor]: *General Urology*, 11th ed. Lange, 1984.)

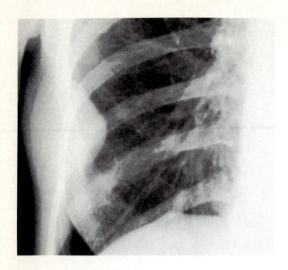

Figure 20–6. Rib metastasis and extrapleural mass from leiomyosarcoma of the uterus. (Reproduced, with permission, from Way LW [editor]: *Current Surgical Diagnosis & Treatment,* 7th ed. Lange, 1985.)

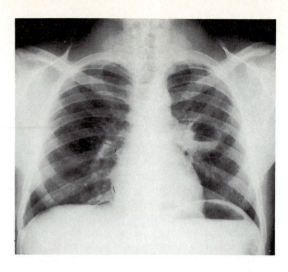

Figure 20–7. Lung abscess involving the superior segment of the left lower lobe. (Reproduced, with permission, from Way LW [editor]: *Current Surgical Diagnosis & Treatment,* 7th ed. Lange, 1985.)

⟶ *Lung abscesses. (Fig 20–7.) Lung abscess may result from necrosis of lung tissue following microbial infection. Abscesses commonly form after aspiration or pulmonary infarctions. Specific antibiotic therapy usually prevents abscess formation and promotes early cure. If the abscess does not resolve with adequate antibiotic therapy and becomes chronic, lobar or segmental lung resection may be required for cure. A chronic lung abscess that does not resolve with adequate antibiotic therapy should arouse a suspicion of lung cancer.*

⟶ *Diagnosis of lung disease. Standard diagnostic measures for evaluation of the thoracic surgical patient are (1) anterior, posterior, oblique, and lateral chest x-rays; (2) CT scans; (3) bronchoscopy for direct examination, biopsy of lesions, and the collection of bronchial washings to be examined for malignant cells and for culture; (4) bronchography for delineation of the bronchi; (5) angiocardiography; (6) scalene lymph node biopsy; (7) mediastinoscopy; and (8) needle biopsy of lesions.*

The Diaphragm

21

The diaphragm is the musculomembranous septum that separates the thoracic cavity from the abdominal cavity. Its contractions result in diaphragmatic descent and an increase in the size of the thoracic cavity, with consequent inspiratory assistance. It is shaped like a dome with a right and a left vault, separated by a depression upon which rests the heart. During respiration, the height of the diaphragm is continually changing. Normally, the right vault rises higher than the left, pushed up by the right lobe of the liver. In forced expiration, the right vault is depressed to the level of the fourth costal cartilage anteriorly, while the left vault reaches to the level of the fourth interspace. Diaphragmatic position is a function of 3 major factors: (1) elastic recoil of pulmonary tissue; (2) visceral pressure upon the diaphragm from the abdominal side; and (3) contraction of the musculature of the anterolateral abdominal wall, which increases intra-abdominal pressure.

The vault of the diaphragm curves superiorly in 2 planes—from right to left in a transverse plane and from ventral to dorsal in a ventrodorsal plane. The peripheral portions of the diaphragm are muscular; the central portion is membranous and tendinous.

EMBRYOLOGY
(Fig 21–1)

Mesenchymal tissue that originates high in the cervical region forms the septum transversum and ultimately forms most of the central tendon of the diaphragm. **Anomalies:** Partial or complete absence of a leaf of the diaphragm (usually posterolateral), reduplication of the diaphragm (very rare), and eventration of the diaphragm.

The superior segment of the dorsal mesentery of the foregut forms that portion of the diaphragm that lies just dorsal to the esophagus plus the crura of the diaphragm.

Mesodermal tissues arising from the posterolateral costal walls and from the pericostal fascia posterior to the level of the primitive kidney buds form parts of the posterolateral portions of the diaphragm and a small portion of the domes of the diaphragm, as well as the sternal fibers and most of the costochondral fibers. **Anomalies:** Abnormal enlargement of one or both sternocostal triangles (foramens of Morgagni).

The pleuroperitoneal membranes form a segment of the posterolateral portion of the diaphragm and

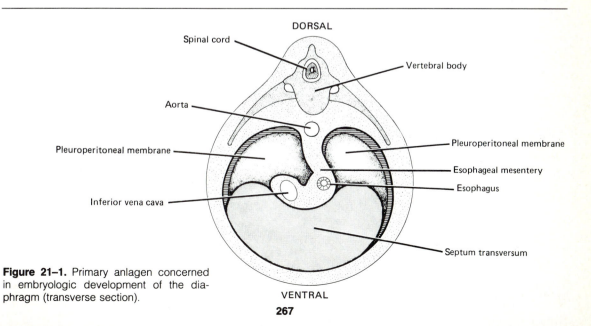

Figure 21–1. Primary anlagen concerned in embryologic development of the diaphragm (transverse section).

thus create a partition between the thoracic and abdominopelvic cavities. Failure of closure of one or both pleuroperitoneal hiatuses results in congenital diaphragmatic hernia. Abnormal enlargement of the esophageal hiatus may also occur.

GROSS ANATOMY
(Fig 21–2)

MUSCLES & TENDONS

The **sternal fibers** of the diaphragm arise as 2 muscular slips about 5 cm wide from the posterior surface of the xiphoid process. The slips run only a short distance before they insert into the anterior mid portion of the central tendon of the diaphragm.

The **costochondral fibers** of the diaphragm arise from the inner surfaces of the cartilages of the lower 6 ribs, interdigitating with the most superior fibers of insertion of the transverse abdominal muscle. Inser-

tion of the costochondral fibers is into the anterior and anterolateral surfaces of the central tendon of the diaphragm. The most lateral of the costochondral fibers are longer and arch higher, particularly on the right side, than do the more medial fibers.

The **posterolateral fibers** of the diaphragm are divided into 3 groups: (1) the crura, (2) fibers arising from the medial lumbocostal arches (internal arcuate ligament), and (3) fibers arising from the lateral lumbocostal arches (external arcuate ligament).

The **right crus** of the diaphragm arises from the anterior longitudinal ligament of the vertebral column, just ventral to the bodies of L1, L2, and L3, directly from these vertebrae and from their intervertebral disks. The crus is tendinous and narrow at L3 but gradually becomes more muscular and wider as it ascends. At the level of T12, the right crural muscular fibers pull away from the anterior surface of the vertebral column to form the right half of an arch of muscular fibers lying just ventral to the vertebral column at T12 (Fig 21–3).

The right crural fibers eventually decussate with the fibers of the left crus and come to lie on the left of the midline. On the left side of the vertebral column, at the level of T10, they split and allow passage of

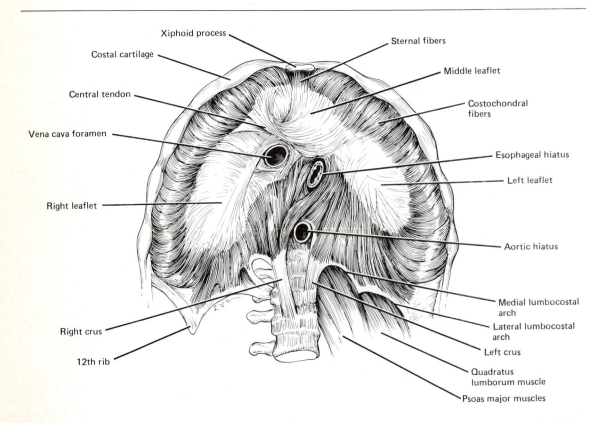

Figure 21–2. The inferior surface of the diaphragm. (Modified and reproduced, with permission, from Way LW [editor]: *Current Surgical Diagnosis & Treatment,* 7th ed. Lange, 1985.)

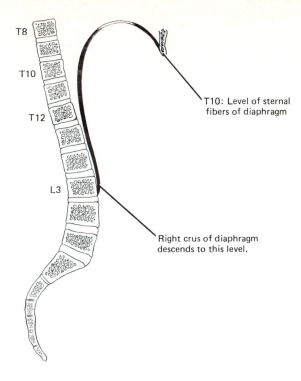

T8

T10

T12

L3

T10: Level of sternal
fibers of diaphragm

Right crus of diaphragm
descends to this level.

Figure 21–3. Lateral view of the diaphragm, showing levels of origin of anterior and posterior fibers.

the thoracic esophagus. They then continue their course to insert into the left midposterior surface of the central tendon of the diaphragm.

The **left crus** of the diaphragm arises from the anterior longitudinal ligament lying ventral to the bodies and intervertebral disks of L1 and L2. It is tendinous at its origin and becomes muscular. At T12, it pulls away from the anterior surface of the vertebral column and crosses to the right side to form the left side of the aortic hiatal arch. The left crus then decussates with the fibers of the right crus and ventrally inserts into the right midposterior surface of the central tendon of the diaphragm. As the fibers of the right and left crura move ventrally to decussate ventral to T12, they leave a triangular space. The thoracic aorta, the azygos vein, and the thoracic duct pass through this space behind the diaphragm. The 2 converging crural arches are united just prior to their decussation by a fairly well defined tendinous arch, the arcuate ligament. It originates from the medial borders of each crus, the fibrous edges joining to form the arcuate ligament at the apex of the ventral pullaway of the crura from the vertebral column. Following the decussation of the crural fibers, they fan out, become thickly muscular, and join with the fibers originating from the 2 lumbocostal arches to form the complete posterior muscular area of the diaphragm.

The **medial lumbocostal arch** is a fibrotendinous structure that crosses the ventral surface of the psoas

major muscle at the level of L1. Medially, it arises from the lateral tendinous margin of the adjacent crural fibers of the diaphragm and from the side of the body of L1. Laterally, it attaches to the lateral tip of the transverse process of L1. A group of muscular fibers arise from this arch and run superiorly and anteriorly to insert into the posterior surface of the central tendon of the diaphragm just lateral to the insertion of the crural fibers.

The **lateral lumbocostal arch** is a fibrous tendon that extends across the upper ventral surface of the quadratus lumborum muscle. It is attached medially to the transverse process of L1 and laterally to the tip and margin of the twelfth rib. From this arch, muscular fibers run superiorly and ventrally to insert into the dorsolateral surface of the central tendon of the diaphragm, just lateral to the fibers arising from the medial lumbocostal arch.

The **central tendon** of the diaphragm is a thin but very strong aponeurosis occupying the central portion of the vault of the diaphragm. It lies much closer to the ventral than to the dorsal surface. As a consequence, the posterior fibers of the diaphragm, as they rise to insert into the central tendon, are longer than the ventral fibers. The mid portion of the central tendon lies just inferior to the heart. The central tendon is so intimately blended with the base of the pericardial sac that it is extremely difficult to dissect the tendon away from the sac. The fibers of the central tendon interlock in a closely woven pattern, which gives great strength to what appears to be a thin membrane. All of the muscular fibers of the diaphragm insert into its central tendon.

Lying between the muscular fibers of the superior surface of the diaphragm and the parietal pleura is the **endothoracic fascia.** Running between the muscle fibers of the undersurface of the diaphragm and the subdiaphragmatic peritoneum is the less well-defined subdiaphragmatic fascia. As these 2 fasciae approach the esophageal hiatus, they fan out and insert into the fibrous outer coat of the esophageal tube both above and below the diaphragm. These insertions into the esophagus of the thoracic and abdominal lining fasciae together form the **phrenoesophageal ligament** of the esophagus. This ligament plays a role both in the causation and surgical repair of esophageal hiatus hernia.

ANATOMIC RELATIONSHIPS

Structures Passing Posterior to the Diaphragm

The aorta, the azygos vein, and the thoracic duct pass posterior to the diaphragm through the **aortic hiatus.** This is a triangular opening whose base is the anterior surface of T12 and whose 2 sides are formed by the diaphragmatic crura (Fig 21–4). The triangular space lies slightly to the left of the midline. The anterior (apical) border of the hiatus is bounded by the median arcuate ligament of the diaphragm.

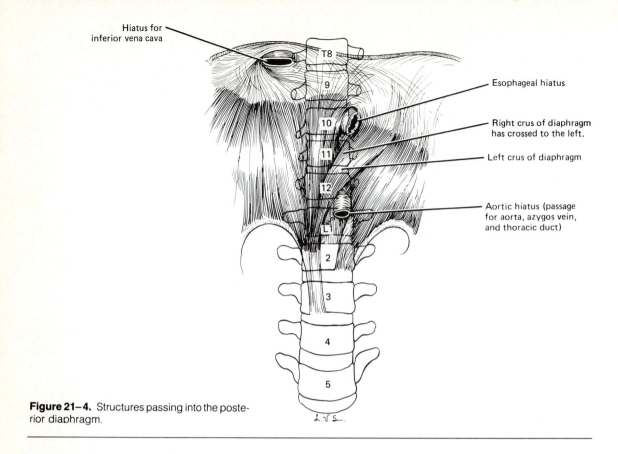

Figure 21–4. Structures passing into the posterior diaphragm.

The aorta traverses the space just to the left of the vertebral midline and is related ventrally to the arcuate ligament of the diaphragm and the thick, ropy conglomeration of the celiac plexus and ganglia.

Two small apertures dorsal to the right crus of the diaphragm usually transmit the right greater, lesser, and least splanchnic nerves as they run from thorax to abdomen. Two small apertures lying dorsal to the left crus of the diaphragm transmit the hemiazygos vein and the left greater, lesser, and least splanchnic nerves, but sometimes they pass through the aortic hiatus. The ganglionated thoracic sympathetic chain enters the abdominal cavity behind the diaphragm, lying dorsal to the medial lumbocostal arch. There is sometimes an aperture between the adjacent fibers of the right medial and lateral lumbocostal arches. When this aperture is present, the upper dorsal surface of the right kidney is separated from the right parietal pleura only by fatty areolar tissue. In such cases, the kidney may project superiorly into the chest, appearing in an x-ray film as a thoracic structure.

The **esophageal hiatus** is situated in the posterior muscular portion of the diaphragm at the level of T10 just to the left of the midline and just anterior to the vertebral column, the aorta, and the celiac plexus. Its edges are formed by a split in the right crural diaphragmatic fibers after they have decussated and crossed to the left side. Anteriorly, where the esophagus fits tightly against it, the encircling hiatal

ring is fibrous and strong. Posteriorly, the margins of the hiatus are thin and abut a layer of fragile areolar tissue that separates the posterior hiatus from the celiac ganglion and the adventitia of the aorta. The esophageal hiatus transmits the esophagus, the 2 vagus nerves, some esophageal arteries and veins, some ascending branches of the left gastric artery, and some gastric veins draining the cardia and the lesser curvature of the stomach. The esophageal hiatus has a larger aperture than is required by the girth of the empty esophagus. Because it is located in the muscular portion of the diaphragm, the esophageal hiatus is more apt to dilate in response to pressure than an opening in the tougher, fibrous central tendon.

➠ *Esophageal hiatus hernias. Three mechanisms serve to prevent esophageal hiatus hernia and the peptic esophagitis that often results: (1) the pinchcock action of the diaphragm, (2) the encircling sling of right crural muscle fibers, and (3) the oblique angle at which the esophagus enters the cardia of the stomach with the creation of the so-called gastric mucosal flap.*

An intrinsic sphincter in the lower esophagus has not been demonstrated anatomically. However, a zone of "physiologic contraction" in the lower third of

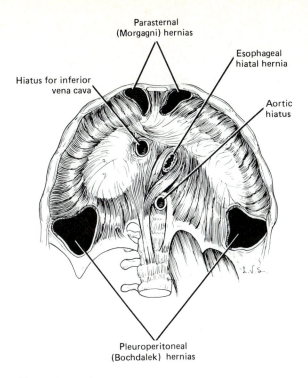

Figure 21–5. Commonest sites for diaphragmatic hernia (inferior view). (Modified and reproduced, with permission, from Way LW [editor]: *Current Surgical Diagnosis & Treatment,* 7th ed. Lange, 1985.)

the esophagus apparently causes intraesophageal pressure to exceed intragastric pressure.

The esophageal sphincteric action is assisted by the attachment of the phrenoesophageal ligament. This is a complex structure composed of both subdia-

phragmatic and endothoracic fascia. Its stronger upper leaf is attached to the physiologic sphincter zone of the lower esophagus. The weaker lower leaf of the ligament is attached to the upper third of the abdominal esophagus immediately below the diaphragm.

The hiatus for the **inferior vena cava** is located at the level of the disk between T8 and T9 in the central tendon of the diaphragm. The margins of the hiatus are sharp and fibrous. The hiatus transmits the inferior vena cava, whose walls are adherent to the margins of the opening, and on occasion some subphrenic branches of the right phrenic nerve. The undersurface of this hiatus is effectively plugged by the right lobe of the liver, so herniation through it is quite rare. The 2 or 3 major hepatic veins empty into the vena cava near the edges of the vena caval hiatus.

Parasternal (Morgagni Hernia) Structures Passing Anterior to the Diaphragm (Fig 21–5)

Anteriorly, on either side of the midline, there is a small opening between the sternal and costochondral fibers of the diaphragmatic origin. These intervals, the foramens of Morgagni, transmit the superior epigastric branches of the internal mammary arteries and some lymphatics that drain the anterior abdominal wall and the superior surface of the liver. Lymphatic flow via these lymphatics is in a superior direction to intrathoracic lymph nodes. These openings sometimes permit parasternal herniations.

➠ *Gastroesophageal hernia.* (*Fig 21–6.*) *The commonest esophageal hiatus hernia is the gastroesophageal* (*sliding*) *type, in which the nor-*

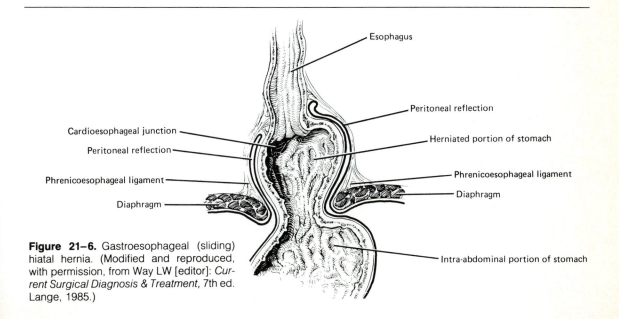

Figure 21–6. Gastroesophageal (sliding) hiatal hernia. (Modified and reproduced, with permission, from Way LW [editor]: *Current Surgical Diagnosis & Treatment,* 7th ed. Lange, 1985.)

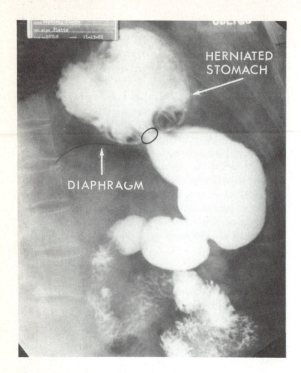

HERNIATED
STOMACH

DIAPHRAGM

Figure 21–7. Large sliding hiatal hernia. Diaphragmatic hiatus is circled. (Modified and reproduced, with permission, from Way LW [editor]: *Current Surgical Diagnosis & Treatment,* 7th ed. Lange, 1985.)

mal oblique cardioesophageal angle is lost as the cardia slides above the diaphragm. The superior movement stretches and thins the phrenoesophageal ligament and its attached parietal pleura and peritoneum. This results in displacement of the inferior esophageal "physiologic sphincter" superiorly. In sliding gastroesophageal hernia, the esophagus always enters the stomach above the level of the diaphragm.

➠ **Esophageal hiatus hernia.** (Fig 21–7.) Once herniation through the esophageal hiatus occurs, the diagnosis depends upon radiologic examination, which may be quite difficult. A special examination with the patient in the Trendelenburg position may be necessary. Radiologic diagnosis depends upon identifying a portion of the stomach above the level of the diaphragm. If the radiologist is able to demonstrate an accompanying reflux of barium into the distal esophagus, the diagnosis is made more clear.

➠ **Paraesophageal hernia.** (Fig 21–8.) Paraesophageal hernia is a less common esophageal hiatus hernia. The lower esophagus retains its normal anatomic relationships; a portion of the fundus or at times a sizable segment of the stomach herniates through the esophageal

hiatus into the thoracic cavity and comes to lie alongside the left border of the lower esophagus. The phrenoesophageal ligament is not stretched. Incarceration or obstruction of the herniated stomach may occur.

➠ **Indications for repair.** Indications for repair of esophageal hiatus hernia include peptic esophagitis (which is refractory to medical treatment), chronic ulceration of the lower esophagus, perforation of the lower esophagus, hemorrhage from an ulcerated esophagus, and stricture and obstruction of the lower esophagus due to longstanding chronic inflammation.

Relationships of the Diaphragm to Structures Superior to It

The superior surfaces of the diaphragm are intimately related to the visceral pleura of the bases of the lower pulmonary lobes. Lying between the visceral pleura of the lung bases and the parietal pleura covering the superior diaphragmatic surface is the pleural cavity. The endothoracic fascia separates the muscular fibers of the superior surface of the diaphragm from the basilar parietal pleura.

Laterally in the costophrenic angles, the parietal pleura does not descend to the base of the costophrenic sinus. As a consequence, there is an extrapleural portion of the diaphragm that is directly related to the lower chest wall without intervening pleura and lung.

➠ **Importance of diaphragmatic relationships in combined thoracicoabdominal injuries.** Thoracicoabdominal wounds may be extrapleural, pleural, or pneumopleural. Because of the diaphragmatic relationships in the costophrenic angles (above), it is possible to explore and even drain the liver from above the level of the diaphragm via the costophrenic sinus without entering the pleural cavity. In like fashion, penetrating thoracicoabdominal injuries may enter the abdominal cavity extrapleurally.

The inferior surface of the pericardial sac is tightly fused to the central tendon of the diaphragm. As a consequence, the pericardium, the pericardial cavity, and the diaphragmatic surface of the heart itself are in direct relationship to these portions of the diaphragm, varying with the size and configuration of the heart. The central portion of the superior surface of the diaphragm is related to the inferior portion of the mediastinum as follows: (1) anteriorly, to the inferior anterior mediastinum and its contents (terminal segments of internal thoracic vessels, a few lymph nodes); (2) centrally, to the central mediastinum and its contents (heart, pericardium, and related structures); and (3) posteriorly, to the inferior posterior mediastinum, which contains the great vessels, the

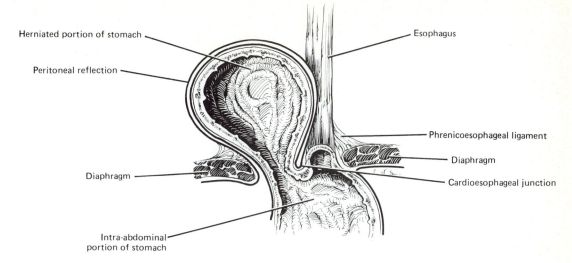

Figure 21–8. Paraesophageal hernia. (Modified and reproduced, with permission, from Way LW [editor]: *Current Surgical Diagnosis & Treatment,* 7th ed. Lange, 1985.)

lymph trunks and nerves of the lower thorax, and to the inferior segment of the thoracic esophagus.

⟶ ***Lacerations of the diaphragm.*** *Lacerations of the diaphragm may result from blunt nonpenetrating lower thoracic or upper abdominal trauma (steering wheel injuries) or from penetrating injuries. Lacerations or disruptions may be easily overlooked at the time of thoracic or abdominal exploration, especially when more dramatic injuries to major organs dominate early management. Untreated lacerations of the diaphragm may result in immediate or delayed diaphragmatic hernia.*

Relationships of the Diaphragm to Structures Inferior to It

The entire inferior and posterior surfaces of the diaphragm, with the exception of those portions related to the bare area of the liver and to the posterior surfaces of the kidneys, duodenum, and pancreas, are covered with parietal peritoneum. The right and left lobes of the liver occupy the entire right two-thirds of the diaphragmatic cupula. Beyond the left lobe of the liver, the diaphragm is related (from left to right) to the abdominal esophagus, the cardia of the stomach, the fundus of the stomach, the spleen, and the splenic flexure of the colon.

The posterior muscle fibers of the diaphragm descend lower than do its anterior muscle fibers. As a consequence, the posterior muscular fibers of the diaphragm (the right and left crura) become directly related to the posterior surfaces of the descending, transverse, and ascending duodenum and to the posterior and superior surfaces of the pancreas as that organ crosses the mid portion of the abdominal cavity.

BLOOD VESSELS, LYMPHATICS, & NERVES

Arteries

The **musculophrenic artery** is a terminal branch of the internal mammary artery. After its origin at the level of the sixth anterior intercostal space, the musculophrenic artery runs laterally along the superior surface of the diaphragm to the lowest posterior intercostal space. It gives off branches to the 3 lowest anterior intercostal spaces, to the superior surface of the diaphragm, and to the pericardium. The vessel is a relatively large one, and bleeding from it can be copious in operative procedures upon the diaphragm. Generally, the posterior muscular segment of the diaphragm is more vascular than the anterior segment.

The **lower intercostal arteries,** both anterior and posterior, supply both the anterior and posterior peripheral surfaces of the diaphragm. The anterior lower intercostals branch from either the internal mammary or the musculophrenic arteries; the lower posterior intercostals are branches of the thoracic aorta.

The **inferior phrenic arteries,** branches of the abdominal aorta or of the celiac artery, supply the undersurface of the diaphragm.

The **upper 2 lumbar arteries** supply the posterior portion of the undersurface of the diaphragm.

The **pericardiophrenic artery,** a branch of the internal mammary artery, accompanies the phrenic nerve to the diaphragm and supplies blood to the superior surface of the diaphragm and to the pericardium.

Veins

Venous return from the diaphragm is into both the superior and inferior vena cava. From the superior surface of the diaphragm, venous flow is via the internal thoracic, azygos, and hemiazygos venous systems into the superior vena cava. Below the level of the diaphragm, flow is via the inferior phrenic vein and the highest lumbar veins into the inferior vena cava. The short right inferior phrenic vein empties directly into the inferior vena cava; the longer left inferior phrenic vein is usually a double structure, one branch joining with the left suprarenal vein and proceeding via the left renal vein to the inferior vena cava, while the other branch joins the inferior vena cava directly. The latter is close to the posterior surface of the left triangular ligament of the liver and must be watched for when the ligament is sectioned in order to mobilize the lobe and move it medially in surgery upon the left infradiaphragmatic area (vagotomy).

Lymphatics

The flow in lymphatics draining the diaphragm may proceed either superiorly, toward the thoracic cavity; or inferiorly, toward the abdominal cavity. Lymphatic channels and plexuses are most abundant where the pleura abuts the diaphragm, but also below the diaphragm in areas where the peritoneum is in contact with the diaphragmatic fibers. Those lymphatics above the level of the diaphragm join with the pleural lymphatics to run to nodes about the aorta and the inferior vena cava just above the level of the diaphragm. The infradiaphragmatic nodes anastomose with liver lymphatics and with lymphatics of the retroperitoneal areolar tissues.

➡️ *Diaphragmatic lymph flow. The ability of the diaphragmatic lymphatics to carry lymph both superiorly and inferiorly accounts for symptoms and signs both above and below the diaphragm when the inciting inflammation or tumor is present on only one side. In like manner, malignant cells may traverse the diaphragm in either a superior or inferior direction. As a consequence, tumor cells from the liver may pass into the thorax, and lung tumors may spread to the liver via the diaphragmatic lymphatics.*

Nerves

The **phrenic nerve,** the major nerve to the diaphragm, is 2 parts motor and 2 parts sensory. It arises from the cervical plexus (C3–5) and descends from the neck through the thorax to the superior surface of the diaphragm. Its sensory pathways carry impulses mainly from the central area of the diaphragm. When the phrenic nerve reaches the diaphragm, it divides into anterior and posterior branches, most of which penetrate the diaphragmatic musculature to be finally distributed to the abdominal surface of the structure.

Ten percent of people have an accessory phrenic nerve arising from the cervical plexus (C5). It descends in the neck and thorax lateral to the course of the major phrenic nerve on one or both sides. The nerve (when present) supplies mainly the lateral surfaces of the diaphragm. The posterior fibers of the diaphragm receive some sensory and motor innervation from the lower intercostal nerves (T9–11). Sympathetic fibers reach the diaphragm from the phrenic plexus, a branch of the celiac plexus. A few vagal fibers are also probably distributed to the diaphragm.

➡️ *Shoulder pain. Referred pain to the shoulder may occur in such pathologic conditions as inflammation of the lower lobe of the lung and cancer of the lower lung lobe involving the diaphragmatic pleura. It may also follow disease of the spleen, liver, gallbladder, and stomach, since segments of those organs are related to the undersurface of the diaphragm. The right lumbar gutter may carry irritative fluids from the lower abdomen to the right subdiaphragmatic area, with resultant right shoulder pain (eg, ruptured appendix, ruptured ectopic pregnancy, or ruptured ovarian follicle with resultant bleeding; ruptured sigmoid diverticulitis). The ascending pain fibers in the phrenic nerve are irritated and synapse in the cervical plexus, with the supraclavicular nerves supplying sensation to the shawl area of the shoulder.*

Embryology of the Gastrointestinal Tract

22

An entodermal tube suspended in the midline of the coelomic cavity by a complete dorsal mesentery and an incomplete superior ventral mesentery develops into the **foregut,** supplied by the celiac artery; the **midgut,** supplied by the superior mesenteric artery; and the **hindgut,** supplied by the inferior mesenteric artery.

The foregut develops into the esophagus, the stomach, and the first portion of the duodenum. **Anomalies** of these structures include tracheoesophageal fistula, atresia and stenosis of the esophagus, congenital short esophagus, thoracic stomach, and hypertrophic pyloric stenosis.

The midgut develops into the second, third, and fourth portions of the duodenum; the jejunum, ileum, cecum and appendix, and ascending colon; and the right three-fourths of the transverse colon. **Anomalies** include stenosis, atresia, or valve formation in the duodenum or jejunum; bowel diverticula; bowel reduplication; anomalies of midgut rotation and fixation; and anomalies of the vitellointestinal duct and its vessels.

The hindgut develops into the left one-fourth of the transverse colon, the descending colon, the sigmoid colon, and the rectum to the level of the anorectal line. **Anomalies** include mobile splenic flexure of the colon, mobile descending colon, abnormal length of the sigmoid colon, congenital reduplication and diverticula of the hindgut (rare), and Hirschsprung's disease of the left and sigmoid colon (megacolon).

INTRODUCTION

Our modern concept of the development, rotation, and fixation of the primitive gastrointestinal tract is in great measure due to the work of Norman Dott, an Edinburgh surgeon. His classic 1923 article, "Anomalies of Intestinal Rotation," established the basis for the diagnosis and treatment of the complex clinical problems of intestinal malrotation and malfixation.

Without knowledge of the normal development and evolution of the primitive gastrointestinal tract, the clinician might fail to recognize the precise nature of abnormalities and might overlook other anomalies that often accompany the presenting one. Because restoration of normal bowel continuity often depends on retracing the steps that led to bowel obstruction

resulting from the anomaly, the clinician must have a firm knowledge of the normal embryologic process of rotation and fixation of the intestinal tract.

THE PRIMITIVE GUT
(Fig 22–1; Table 22–1)

At the 5-mm (4-week) stage of embryonic life, the primitive gastrointestinal tract appears as a simple vertical entodermal tube suspended in the center of the coelomic cavity by a complete **dorsal mesentery** (posterior common mesentery) and an incomplete **ventral mesentery** (ventral mesogastrium). The dorsal mesentery, which attaches the tube to the posterior abdominal wall, extends the length of the gastrointestinal tract; the ventral mesentery extends only the length of the foregut, from the esophagogastric junction to the termination of the first portion of the duodenum.

Even at this extremely early (5-mm) stage of development, the primitive gastrointestinal tube is differentiated into 3 distinct segments by the 3 branches of the abdominal aorta that will supply them in postfetal life. The 3 branches are practically end arteries, with little or no collateral circulation to link them. The proximal branch, running from the abdominal aorta to the most proximal segment of the gut, the **celiac artery** (celiac axis), supplies the foregut. The middle branch of the abdominal aorta to the gut, the superior mesenteric artery, supplies the long central gut segment, or **midgut.** The distal branch, the inferior mesenteric artery, supplies the **hindgut.**

The disposition of the primitive gut in the 5-mm embryo during the fifth week of intrauterine development, before the first stage of rotation of the midgut loop, is as follows: The endodermal bud, which will form the liver, gallbladder, extrahepatic biliary tract, and a portion of the head of the pancreas, has issued from the ventral surface of the junctional area of foregut and midgut and has grown superiorly and ventrally into the **ventral mesogastrium,** spreading the 2 mesenteric leaves as it does so. The bud continues to pursue its way within the ventral mesogastrium in the direction of the **septum transversum,** the primitive mesodermal structure that is the forerunner of the diaphragm. The advancing segment of the bud, on reaching the septum transversum, invades it—having previously divided into 2 branches, each of which

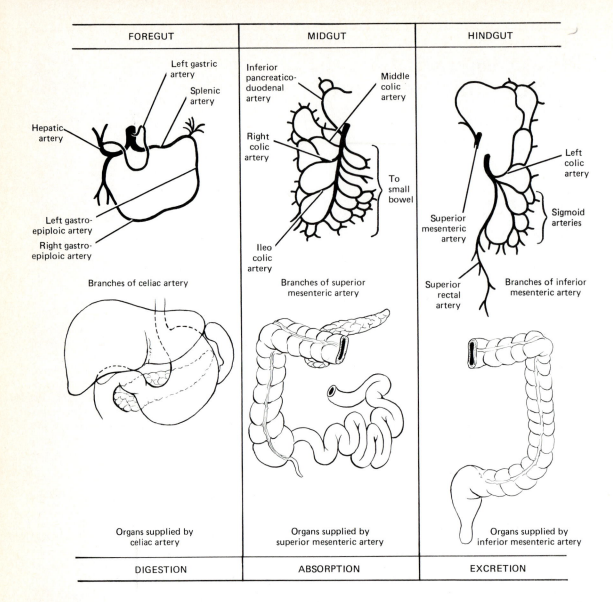

FOREGUT	MIDGUT	HINDGUT

Branches of celiac artery — Branches of superior mesenteric artery — Branches of inferior mesenteric artery

Organs supplied by celiac artery — Organs supplied by superior mesenteric artery — Organs supplied by inferior mesenteric artery

DIGESTION — ABSORPTION — EXCRETION

Figure 22–1. Diagram showing the branches of the abdominal aorta, which supplies the derivatives of the 3 primitive gut segments.

Table 22–1. Visceral derivation, arterial supply, and physiologic function of the abdominal gut.

Segment	Adult Extent	Arterial Supply	Primary Gut Function
Foregut	Abdominal esophagus, stomach, and first and second (proximal) portions of duodenum.	Celiac artery	Digestion
Midgut	Second (distal), third, and fourth portions of duodenum; all of the small bowel (jejunoileum); cecum and appendix; ascending colon; right three-fourths of the transverse colon.	Super mesenteric artery	Absorption
Hindgut	Left one-fourth of the transverse colon, descending colon, sigmoid colon, and all of the rectum down to the anorectal line.	Inferior mesenteric artery	Excretion

will form one of the 2 major lobes of the liver. Also during the 5-mm stage there issues from the dorsal surface of the junctional area of foregut and midgut, slightly above the level of issuance of the liver bud, the entodermal projection that will form a major portion of the head and all of the neck, body, and tail of the pancreas. The dorsal bud grows into the terminal segment of the dorsal mesogastrium and the adjoining superior segment of the mesoduodenum. The pressure of the enlarging mass of the developing pancreas, growing in the dorsal mesentery of the bowel, forces the distal segment of the foregut and the most proximal segment of the midgut to the right, initiating the C loop of the duodenal curvature.

The proximal segment of the midgut and that of the hindgut become fixed to the posterior abdominal wall, thus establishing a fixed narrow **duodenocolic isthmus** about which the first stage of rotation of the midgut will take place. The fixation of the proximal hindgut is not as firm as that of the distal foregut. This will allow for later left lateral and superior displacement of the hindgut.

The dominant organ in the abdomen of the embryo during the fifth week of intrauterine development is the rapidly growing liver, which soon fills the entire upper half of the abdomen down to the level of the umbilical orifice. The mobile midgut, suspended between the 2 posteriorly fixed points of the duodenocolic isthmus, has increased in length at an extremely rapid rate—far more rapidly than the growth of the **abdominal coelom**—with the result that there is no room for it in the abdominal cavity because of the great size of the liver. The enlarging, mobile midgut therefore herniates from the abdominal coelom into the ventrally connected **umbilical coelom.** The proximal segment of the herniated midgut loop, attached within the abdomen to the fixed first portion of the duodenum, faces superiorly; while the distal midgut segment, attached within the abdomen to the beginning of the hindgut, which will eventually be the left one-fourth of the transverse colon, faces inferiorly. The superior mesenteric artery runs from the abdominal aorta to the mesenteric border of the apex of the herniated midgut loop. The portion of the midgut loop that lies above the superior mesenteric artery is called the prearterial loop (cephalic limb); the portion below the artery is called the postarterial loop (caudal limb); and the mesenteries to the 2 loops are called the prearterial and postarterial mesenteries.

Projecting from the antimesenteric border of the apex of the herniated midgut loop is a diverticulum, the **yolk sac.** The yolk sac is connected to the lumen of the apex of the midgut loop by the **vitellointestinal duct** (yolk stalk). Branches from the most terminal segment of the superior mesenteric artery cross the surface of the midgut from its mesenteric to its antimesenteric border and then follow the course of the vitellointestinal duct out to the yolk sac, supplying arterial blood to the yolk sac and the vitellointestinal duct. Persistence of the vitellointestinal duct or the accompanying vitellointestinal vessels leads to (1)

Meckel's diverticulum of varying length and caliber and (2) patent or nonpatent vessels that cross the terminal ileum from the mesenteric surface to the antimesenteric bowel surface with progress on occasion to the deep umbilical surface, as may Meckel's diverticulum also. Both anomalies may lead to intestinal obstruction. Shortly thereafter, during the fifth week of intrauterine development, the yolk sac, the vitelline duct, and the vitellointestinal vessels normally disappear completely. By the end of the fifth week, the **cecal bud** appears on the antimesenteric border of the postarterial loop of the midgut just distal to the apex of the herniated bowel. The time of appearance of the cecum is of great significance in the normal evolution of midgut rotation.

⟶ *Role of the cecal bud in orderly midgut return. The timing of the appearance of the cecal bud on the antimesenteric border of the postarterial loop of the herniated midgut is of great importance to the orderly return of the midgut loop. If the umbilical orifice is of normal size, the postarterial loop and the superior mesenteric artery cannot return to the abdomen until the prearterial loop has returned, because the bulky cecum will catch on the edges of the umbilical orifice and thus prevent premature return of the postarterial loop. If the cecal bud appears on time but the umbilical orifice is larger or more lax than normal, the cecal bud and the postarterial loop obviously may return to the abdomen before either the prearterial loop or the superior mesenteric artery have done so. If the cecal bud appears too late, the postarterial loop may return before the prearterial loop even if the umbilical orifice is of normal size.*

By the time the first stage of midgut rotation begins, the midgut loop and the accompanying superior mesenteric vessels have herniated into the umbilical stalk; the vitellointestinal duct, the yolk sac, and its supplying vessels have regressed; and the liver, which fills the entire upper abdomen, is the dominant structure in the abdominal coelom.

THE FIRST (90-DEGREE) STAGE OF ROTATION OF THE MIDGUT LOOP (Fig 22–2)

The first stage of midgut rotation occurs between the fifth and tenth weeks of intrauterine development. It is brought about chiefly by descent of the rapidly enlarging liver and by the pressure exerted by the vitelline and umbilical veins running from the liver to the umbilicus. Pressure of these structures on the

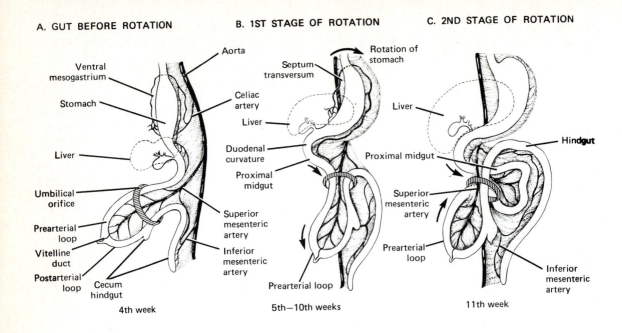

A. GUT BEFORE ROTATION

B. 1ST STAGE OF ROTATION

C. 2ND STAGE OF ROTATION

4th week

5th–10th weeks

11th week

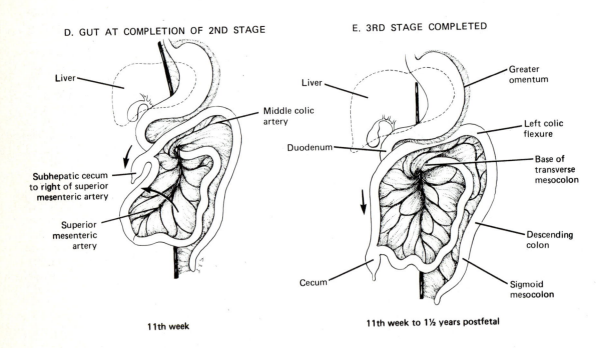

D. GUT AT COMPLETION OF 2ND STAGE

E. 3RD STAGE COMPLETED

11th week

11th week to 1½ years postfetal

Figure 22–2. Development and rotation of the gut.

prearterial loop at the point where it leaves the umbilical orifice to run to the umbilical stalk causes the prearterial loop to rotate 90 degrees counterclockwise to the right and the postarterial loop to rotate 90 degrees counterclockwise to the left. When this stage of rotation is complete, the prearterial loop lies to the right of the superior mesenteric artery instead of superior to it; whereas the postarterial loop, containing the cecal bulge, lies to the left of the superior mesenteric artery instead of inferior to it.

⯈ *Extroversion of cloaca. The first stage of rotation of the midgut loop is seldom interfered with. Extroversion of the cloaca is a rare anomaly associated with malrotation at this stage.*

THE SECOND STAGE OF ROTATION OF THE MIDGUT LOOP: RETURN OF THE MIDGUT TO THE ABDOMINAL CAVITY (Fig 22–2)

During the second stage of rotation, the herniated midgut loop normally proceeds in an orderly way to return from the umbilical stalk into the abdominal cavity. The movement usually requires 1 week and occurs between the tenth and 11th weeks of fetal life. The midgut loop is able to return to the abdominal cavity by the tenth fetal week because (1) liver growth has generally slowed, and the left side of the liver has actually diminished in size; and (2) the coelomic cavity has increased markedly in size. Slowing of growth of the left side of the liver leaves some unoccupied space in the left upper quadrant of the abdomen.

Return of Prearterial Loop

The prearterial loop of the midgut, which lies to the right of the superior mesenteric artery, is the first segment of the midgut to return to the abdomen. Its proximal segment is attached to the body wall at the future duodenojejunal junction. As the returning bowel leaves the umbilical stalk, it necessarily returns to the right side of the mid abdomen, where it lies just below the inferior surface of the right lobe of the liver.

As its more distal coils return to the abdomen, the prearterial midgut finds no room in the right mid abdomen because of the large size of the right lobe of the liver. Because the left lobe of the liver has become smaller, there is room in the left upper abdomen. Consequently, the coils of the prearterial loop move to the left horizontally and then superiorly on a plane deep to the superior mesenteric artery. The superior mesenteric artery remains in the umbilical stalk until the entire prearterial loop of midgut has returned to the abdominal coelom.

The returning prearterial coils of midgut, as they move superiorly and to the left, push the dorsally fixed beginning of the hindgut superiorly and to the left, thus positioning the splenic flexure in the left upper quadrant and the descending portion of the colon against the left abdominal parietes. The prearterial loop first fills the left upper quadrant and then spills obliquely across the abdomen from the left upper quadrant to the right pelvis, and then finally climbs superiorly on the right side of the abdominal cavity toward the liver via its most terminal coils. The final coil of prearterial midgut carries the superior mesenteric artery with it as it returns to the abdomen.

Return of Postarterial Loop

The postarterial loop, which in postfetal life will become the terminal segment of the ileum, the cecum, the vermiform appendix, the ascending colon, and the proximal three-fourths of the transverse colon, now returns to the abdomen. The segment of bowel attached to the terminal segment of the prearterial loop returns first and positions both itself and the adjacent cecum on a plane dorsal to the superior mesenteric artery, just inferior to the visceral surface of the right lobe of the liver.

The cecum and terminal ileum now rotate counterclockwise about the axis of the superior mesenteric artery from a position dorsal to the artery to a position to the left of it, then to a position ventral to it, and finally to a position to its right. The cecum and terminal ileum have now rotated 270 degrees around the axis of the superior mesenteric artery, placing the cecum in a subhepatic position to the right and ventral to the artery, paralleling the more medially situated descending duodenum.

The terminal portion of the postarterial loop (the transverse colon) crosses the abdomen from right to left on a plane ventral to the superior mesenteric artery to join the proximal hindgut that has been positioned in the left upper quadrant of the abdomen by the first of the returning coils of prearterial midgut.

Status at Completion of Second Stage

The second stage of rotation of the midgut is now complete, resulting in the following intra-abdominal positions of the returned midgut loop:

(1) The transverse (third) portion of the duodenum crosses dorsal to the superior mesenteric artery as it runs from right to left.

(2) The transverse colon crosses from right to left on a plane ventral to the superior mesenteric artery.

(3) The splenic flexure of the colon and the beginning of the descending colon have been pushed into the left upper lateral quadrant of the abdomen to lie just inferior to the left leaf of the diaphragm and just medial to the left upper abdominal parietes.

(4) The coils of the small intestine range in oblique fashion from the left upper abdomen to the right pelvis, from which they run superiorly to join the cecum in the right mid quadrant of the abdomen.

(5) There is no ascending colon at this time, the transverse colon taking off directly from the left lateral margin of the cecum to cross the abdomen toward the colon's splenic flexure.

⮕ *Orderly sequence of midgut return. The second stage of midgut rotation consists essentially of reduction (in orderly sequence) into the coelomic cavity of the physiologically herniated midgut loop. Abnormalities of the second stage of rotation are due to a departure from the orderly sequence of return.*

During the third stage of bowel development (see below), anomalies are due to complete or incomplete failure of fixation or abnormal fixation of one or more of the bowel segments. Errors during this stage lead to or predispose to a great variety of clinical syndromes. There may also be failure of normal elongation of any one or all of the colonic segments.

A. NONROTATION   B. REVERSE ROTATION   C. VOLVULUS

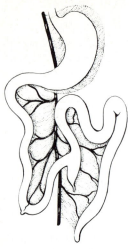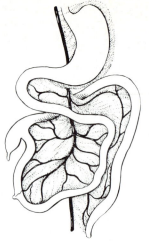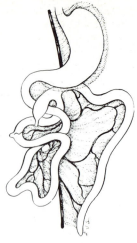

Cecum, ascending colon, and left colon all on left side of abdomen

Transverse colon passes deep to superior mesenteric artery

Short attachment of mesentery of small bowel with nondescent of cecum and ileocecal colic volvulus

Figure 22–3. Anomalies of rotation of the gut.

Nonrotation of the midgut loop. (*Fig. 22–3.*) *In this condition, the small bowel, on its return to the abdomen, lies chiefly to the right of the midline. The duodenum descends directly from the duodenocolic isthmus into the right lower quadrant of the abdomen, lying, as it descends, along the right side of the superior mesenteric artery. In such cases, the terminal ileum may cross the midline to reach a left iliac cecum, thus entering the cecum from right to left; or the terminal ileum may terminate in the midline in a pelvic cecum. In these 2 conditions, the entire colon is usually found on the left side of the abdomen, the ascending and descending colons paralleling each other. The abnormally situated loops of gut are usually fixed in position by one or more anomalous fibrous bands, usually the hepatoduodenal colic ligament. On occasion, the entire midgut loop is attached to the posterior abdominal wall, suspended from it by an extremely narrow pedicle (the earlier duodenal colic isthmus), and in such cases, the midgut loop is prone to volvulus. Nonrotation of the midgut is usually the result of a lax umbilical ring but may occasionally result from a late cecal appearance that allows the postarterial loop containing the cecum to reduce first. In such cases, the prearterial loop, on its return to the abdomen following the previous return of the postarterial loop, displaces the colon and superior mesenteric artery to the left of the midline.*

Reversed rotation of the midgut loop. (*Fig. 22–3.*) *As in nonrotation of the midgut loop, the postarterial loop, in cases of reversed rotation, reduces first, passing dorsal to the superior mesenteric vessels, which remain in the umbilical stalk. The portion of the postarterial loop destined to become the transverse colon passes to the left, dorsal to the superior mesenteric vessels, whereas the duodenum and small bowel, which develop from the prearterial loop, come to lie on a plane ventral to the superior mesenteric artery. Otherwise, the intestines are in their normal location.*

THE THIRD STAGE OF ROTATION & FIXATION OF THE BOWEL: STAGE OF ELONGATION & FIXATION (Fig 22–2)

Elongation and fixation of segments of the bowel take place between the 13th week of fetal life and the 17th month of postfetal life. This third and final stage in the process of movement and eventual fixation of the intestinal tract is one of differential growth and final positioning of the ascending colon; fixation of the root of the small bowel mesentery; and fixation of segments of the large bowel to the dorsal abdominal wall, either by their mesentery or by their posterior surfaces.

Cecum

The cecum descends from its subhepatic position to reach its normal location in the mid portion of the right iliac fossa.

Ascending Colon

The ascending colon is formed by descent of the cecum and the resulting elongation of that portion of the colon just distal to the cecum. It may vary markedly in length depending upon how far the cecum descends.

Obliteration of Mesenteries

The postarterial mesenteries—the mesenteries of the cecum, the ascending colon, the hepatic flexure, the splenic flexure, the descending colon, and the upper portion of the sigmoid colon—are obliterated by fusion with posterior parietal peritoneum.

Persistence of Mesenteries

The mesentery of the transverse colon persists as the transverse mesocolon and is fixed to the anterior mid surface of the pancreas. The length of transverse mesocolon from pancreatic fixation to the mesenteric border of the colon varies greatly.

The mesentery of the pelvic colon persists as the sigmoid mesocolon. Because the apex of the mesentery of the sigmoid colon does not always completely fuse with the posterior parietal peritoneum of the left pelvis, the failure of fusion forms a fossa, the intersigmoidal recess. The recess may serve as the nidus for an internal hernia.

ANOMALIES OF ROTATION & FIXATION

➠ *Malpositions of the cecum.* Early fixation of the subhepatic cecum by peritoneal fusion or by aberrant bands may cause maldescent or nondescent of this portion of the bowel. In such cases, the cecum and appendix may lie in a subhepatic or lumbar position. If the cecum descends too far, it will result in a pelvic cecum, and in such cases it will lie in intimate relationship with the pelvic organs (bladder, sigmoid colon, male or female generative organs, pelvic floor). A cecum that descends too far into the pelvis may give rise to "pelvic appendicitis." It also presents a problem in differential diagnosis because of its proximity to the genitals in the pelvis.

An undescended cecum may give rise to subhepatic appendicitis.

➠ *Abnormal fixation of the right colon and cecum.* This anomaly is fairly common. The circumferential degree of fixation as well as the length of fixation of the right colon and on occasion of the cecum to the posterior abdominal wall varies markedly. The right colon may at times be completely unfixed, while at other times the entire right colon may be fixed tightly to the posterior abdominal parietes. The mesentery of the right colon and hepatic flexure is the mesentery of the proximal portion of the postarterial midgut loop. The right colic mesentery normally disappears by becoming fixed to the posterior abdominal parietes. The mesentery is recreated in a right colon resection when the ascending colon is freed from the posterior abdominal parietes, from right to left, prior to its resection. If the right colic mesentery does not become fixed in position, the right colon swings free and is predisposed to volvulus. The cecum may be completely free and mobile, or it may be fixed to the posterior peritoneum of the abdominal wall as far inferiorly as its caput.

➠ *Surgical mobilization of right and left colon.* It is quite easy to mobilize a right or left colon fixed to the posterior abdominal wall if one stays in the proper cleavage planes. Mobilization must always be done from lateral to medial; no important structures are encountered at the initiation of mobilization, since they all lie deep to the posterior peritoneum (kidneys, ureters, testicular and ovarian vessels). To initiate mobilization, the parietal peritoneum in the lumbar gutters just lateral to the bowel is incised. The bowel, the 2 leaves of its fused mesentery, and the posterior peritoneum are elevated, care being taken to push the important retroperitoneal structures laterally.

➠ *Intussusception and volvulus.* A tightly fixed cecum and adjacent inferior segment of ascending colon predispose to intussusception of the ileocecal colonic segment and to right-sided sliding hernia formation. A poorly fixed or nonfixed cecum and lower ascending colon predispose to volvulus of the ileocecal colonic segment (Fig 22–3).

➠ *Abnormal fixations of the root of the mesentery of the small bowel to the posterior abdominal wall.* Fixation of the small bowel mesentery is normally along a line that reaches from just to the left of L2 to the midpoint of the right sacroiliac joint. The fixation may be markedly shortened (2.5–5 cm long). The fixation area may exhibit one or more of a series of openings between the mesentery and its fixation to the posterior peritoneum. Too short a fixation of the mesentery of the small bowel predisposes to total or partial midgut loop volvulus, a condition that usually occurs shortly after birth. Incomplete or poor fixation—or nonfixation—of the root of the small bowel mesentery to the posterior parietal peritoneum may lead to internal herniation of the mesentericoparietal type, the loops of bowel passing into a space bounded ventrally by small bowel mesentery and dorsally by retroperitoneum.

Symptoms secondary to defective rotation or fixation. *Disturbances of function of the gastrointestinal tract do not invariably follow abnormal bowel rotation or fixation. The great majority of persons with such anomalies probably lead normal lives, and their abnormalities of bowel position and fixation are usually discovered only during gastrointestinal x-ray examination, at surgery, or at postmortem examination. Even so, excessive bowel fixation may* cause signs and symptoms of bowel compression, bowel kinking, interference with bowel mobility and motility, and internal herniation. It may also predispose to intussusception. Poor bowel fixation may lead to ptosis, torsion, or volvulus. Abnormalities of small bowel embryonic development are frequently accompanied by stenosis, atresia, or valve formation in a bowel segment and by multiple abnormal bands that often cause bowel obstruction. Such embryonic errors are often associated with imperforate anus and errors of development of the cardiorespiratory center.

The Anterolateral Abdominal Wall

23

GROSS ANATOMY

The anterolateral abdominal wall is the anatomic area the physician must frequently inspect, percuss, auscultate, and palpate—and, if need be, breach—in order to diagnose intra-abdominal disorders and perform intra-abdominal procedures.

BOUNDARIES

The anterolateral abdominal wall is bounded superiorly, from medial to lateral, by the **xiphoid process** of the sternum, the joined seventh to tenth **costal cartilages,** and the surface of the tenth rib. Laterally, the region is bounded by a perpendicular line from the highest point on the **iliac crest** to the tenth rib (approximately the anterior axillary line). The line roughly marks the anterior border of the thoracolumbar fascia. Inferolaterally, the abdomen is bounded by the anterior segment of the iliac crest and farther medially by the **inguinal ligament.** Caudally, the boundaries are the 2 **pubic bones** and the **symphysis pubica.**

CLINICAL ZONES OR REGIONS
(Fig 23–1)

For precise orientation within the boundaries of the anterolateral abdomen, the area is divided into 9 regions by drawing 2 horizontal and 2 vertical lines upon the abdominal wall. The superior horizontal line crosses the abdomen between the lowest points on the tenth ribs. The inferior horizontal line connects the highest points on the 2 iliac crests. The 2 ventral lines are raised from the midpoint of each inguinal ligament to the point where they intersect the tenth rib. The midsuperior area is the **epigastrium;** the 2 lateral superior areas are the right and left **hypochondrium.** The 2 midlateral areas are the right and left **lumbar areas;** the central area between them is the **umbilical area.** The 2 inferolateral regions are the right and left **ilioinguinal areas;** the mid inferior area is the pubic or **hypogastric area.** The size and shape of these regions vary markedly with the habitus of the individual. For clinical reference purposes the abdomen is divided into quadrants: right and left upper and right and left lower. The lines dividing the quadrants are drawn horizontally and vertically through the umbilicus.

UMBILICUS

The umbilicus normally lies in the midline of the abdomen just above a line drawn between the 2 anterior superior iliac spines. The skin there is innervated by nerve T10, and the umbilicus is important in determining the level of spinal cord lesions. The umbilicus marks the lower end of the upper linea alba. Above the umbilicus, the linea alba is clearly discernible and up to 1 cm wide. Below the umbilicus, the linea alba is vague. Normally, the umbilicus is about halfway between the xiphoid process and the os pubis, but its position may vary by 4–5 cm in either direction.

LANDMARKS
(Fig 23–2)

The bony and cartilaginous ventrolateral abdominal landmarks are either visible or easily palpable. They are the xiphoid process supplied by nerve T5), the joined costal cartilages of ribs 7–10, the anterior segment of the tenth rib, the anterosuperior iliac spine, the crest of the iliac bone, the superior surface of the pubic bones, and the pubic symphysis. In most males it is easy to palpate the pubic tubercle 1 cm above and 2.5 cm lateral to the symphysis pubica. The tubercle is difficult to palpate in females. It is an important landmark in the diagnosis and surgical repair of groin hernias.

The linea semilunaris is a palpable line formed by the lateral border of the rectus abdominis muscle; it marks the site of blending of the sheaths of the flat abdominal muscles to form the sheaths of the rectus abdominis muscle. It starts just lateral to the symphysis pubica; then arches in a flat curve to end at the undersurface of the tenth rib. It is visible in thin, well-muscled individuals.

The tendinous intersections (inscriptions) of the rectus abdominis muscles are transverse fibrous bands that divide the muscle into 4–5 segments above the level of the umbilicus. When the rectus abdominis is tensed, the transverse intersections become visible as dimplings of the subcutaneous tissue and skin that overlie them.

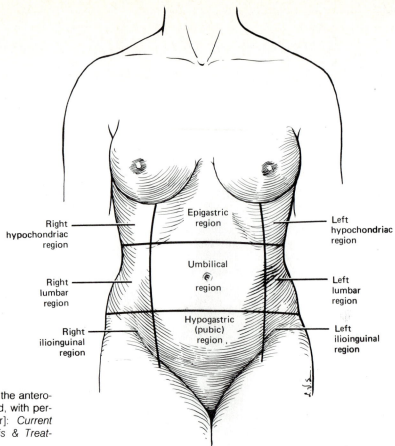

Figure 23–1. Regional divisions of the antero-lateral abdominal wall. (Reproduced, with permission, from Benson RC [editor]: *Current Obstetric & Gynecologic Diagnosis & Treatment,* 5th ed. Lange, 1984.)

LAYERS OF THE ANTEROLATERAL ABDOMINAL WALL

The anterolateral abdominal wall consists of 6 layers:

(1) Skin.

(2) Subcutaneous fascia:
   Superficial layers (Camper's fascia)
   Deep layer (Scarpa's fascia)

(3) Musculature:
   Lateral:
      External oblique
      Internal oblique (and cremaster)
      Transversus abdominis
   Medial:
      Rectus abdominis
      Pyramidalis

(4) Transversalis fascia (ventral lining fascia of the abdominal cavity)

(5) Preperitoneal areolar tissue and fat

(6) Peritoneum

Skin

The skin and subcutaneous tissues of the ventro-lateral abdominal wall lie loosely upon the underlying fasciae and abdominal musculature. Consequently, the skin and subcutaneous tissues can easily be raised from the underlying tissues—except at the umbilicus, where the skin is firmly attached to the umbilical scar.

➠ *Striae, ecchymoses, and discolorations of the abdominal skin. Depigmented striae are evidence of substantial weight loss or, in women, stretching during pregnancy. The distinctive purplish striae or Cushing's disease are usually noted laterally over the hips. The abdominal skin may show ecchymotic discolorations resulting from trauma or bleeding as a sequela of a blood dyscrasia. The site of the discoloration may give a clue to the intra-abdominal organ that may also have been injured. Periumbilical redness suggests anomalies of persistent omphalomesenteric or urachal tracts, or the presence of a foreign body deep in the umbilicus. A bluish periumbilical discoloration may be a late sign of pelvic bleeding from a ruptured ectopic pregnancy or a ruptured ovarian follicle cyst. In such cases, the pelvic blood travels*

Figure 23–2. Anatomic landmarks of the anterolateral abdominal wall.

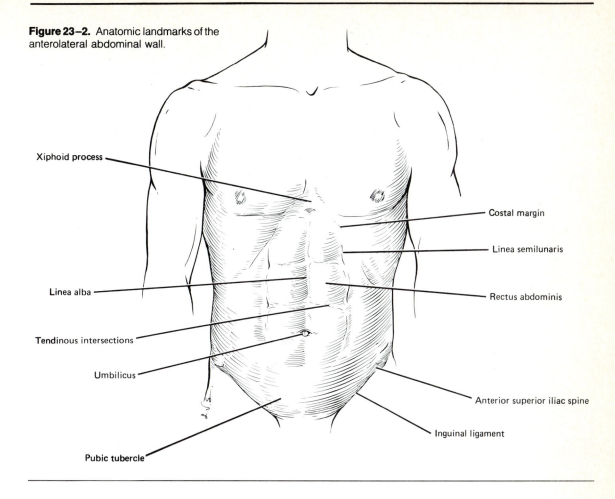

Xiphoid process

Costal margin

Linea semilunaris

Linea alba

Rectus abdominis

Tendinous intersections

Umbilicus

Anterior superior iliac spine

Inguinal ligament

Pubic tubercle

---

toward the umbilicus via the 3 peritoneally related umbilical ligaments (Cullen's sign).

Subcutaneous Fascia

A. Superficial Layer: The superficial layer of the subcutaneous (Camper's) fascia is of no clinical importance. It is a thin fibrous mesh filled with areolar fatty tissue. By fusing inferiorly in the midline with the deep layer of the subcutaneous fascia, it assists in formation of the dartos (tunica dartos) of the scrotum. Its fat-filled meshes give substance to the labia majora as the fascia sweeps over the os pubis and into the anterior perineum.

B. Deep Layer: (Fig 23–3.) The deep layer of the subcutaneous (Scarpa's) fascia is of major clinical importance. It begins at the upper fourth of the abdominal wall. It arises from the anterior sheaths of the rectus abdominis muscle and the linea alba; and laterally, from the external oblique muscle. The fascia descends over the lower three-fourths of the ventrolateral abdominal wall. It fuses laterally with the thoracolumbar fascia. Farther inferiorly, it fuses laterally with the external plate of the iliac crest at the anterosuperior spine of the ilium; and it attaches to the pubic tubercle. Between the anterosuperior iliac spine and

the pubic tubercle, the fascia crosses ventral to the inguinal ligament to reach the upper anterior thigh. The fascia fuses with the deep thigh fascia along a line 2.5 cm below and parallel to the inguinal ligament.

The deep layer of the subcutaneous fascia gradually thickens and becomes more distinct, reaching its greatest thickness in the ilioinguinal region of the abdominal wall. In the midline of the male, Scarpa's fascia extends over the os pubis onto the dorsum of the penis, the spermatic cord, and the scrotum. In the scrotum, it joins with Camper's fascia to form the tunica dartos of the scrotal wall. From the scrotum, Scarpa's fascia may be traced in the perineum to the ischial tuberosities, where it fuses with the urogenital diaphragm. In the perineum, it is known as Colles' fascia and becomes the superficial boundary of the superficial perineal pouch, which is the cleft between Colles' fascia and the perineal musculature. (See Chapter 38.) In the female, Scarpa's fascia continues over the os pubis to the labia majora and then in the perineum to the urogenital diaphragm as a thin, poorly defined fascia. As Colles' fascia passes dorsally in the perineum, it attaches to the inferior border of the ischiopubic rami.

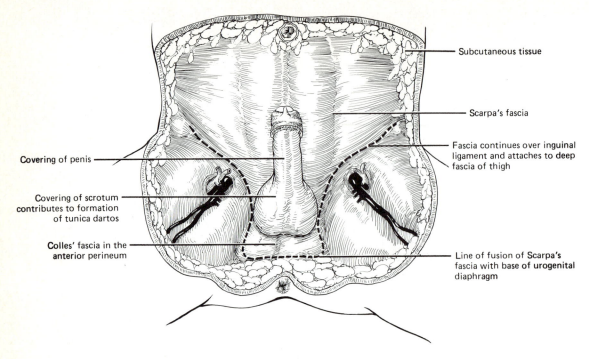

Figure 23–3. Scarpa's fascia, showing continuation into the anterior male peritoneum.

Labels on figure:
- Subcutaneous tissue
- Scarpa's fascia
- Fascia continues over inguinal ligament and attaches to deep fascia of thigh
- Covering of penis
- Covering of scrotum contributes to formation of tunica dartos
- Colles' fascia in the anterior perineum
- Line of fusion of Scarpa's fascia with base of urogenital diaphragm

⇨ *Urinary extravasation deep to Colles' fascia in the perineum. (Fig 23–4.) With rupture of the male urethra in the perineum, urine leaks into the perineal pouch, then escapes into the scrotum and penis and onto the anterolateral abdominal wall; there it will lie dorsal to the deep layer of the superficial fascia and ventral to the rectus abdominis and external oblique muscles. The extravasation will be limited by the attachments of Scarpa's fascia and Colles' fascia.*

Lateral Musculature

A. External Oblique Muscle: (Fig 23–5.) This is the most superficial of the lateral flat muscles of the abdominal wall. The muscle arises over the thorax from 8 fleshly digitations on the lower 8 ribs. The thoracic muscular fibers interdigitate with the fibers of the serratus anterior muscle on the fifth to eighth ribs and with the fibers of the latissimus dorsi muscle on the ninth to 12th ribs. The external oblique muscle is roughly quadrilateral; its fibers generally run vertically. Its most posterior fibers insert into the anterior half of the iliac crest and form the anterior border of the lumbar triangle (of Petit). The more medial and superior fibers abut the linea semilunaris. There, the muscular fibers cease and the anterior and posterior sheaths of the muscle join with the sheaths of the internal oblique and transversus abdominis muscles to form the anterior and posterior rectus sheaths, which insert into the linea alba.

The thick muscular fibers of the external oblique muscle become aponeurotic between the anterior superior iliac spine and the umbilicus. The aponeurosis is a thin, strong membrane whose fibers run caudally and medially, just deep to Scarpa's fascia, and cover the deeper structures of the ilioinguinal region.

The aponeurosis of the external oblique muscle is responsible for formation of the inguinal (Poupart's) ligament, the external inguinal ring and its intercrural fibers, the lacunar (Gimbernat's) ligament, the pectineal (Cooper's) ligament, the reflected inguinal ligament, and the external spermatic fascia.

The superficial or external inguinal ring is a roughly triangular opening in the aponeurosis of the external oblique, near the pubic spine. The apex of the ring points obliquely laterally and superiorly. In men, the ring is about 2.5 cm long from base to apex and about 1 cm wide at its base. In women, the opening is about one-third to one-half as large. The ring is bounded inferiorly by the lateral segment of the pubic crest and laterally and medially by the crura in the external oblique aponeurosis. The inferior crus (external pillar of the ring) is strong and is reinforced by the inguinal ligament. Above the apex of the external inguinal ring are a group of transverse fibers that reinforce the vertical fibers of the external oblique aponeurosis and prevent them from splaying out as a result of intra-abdominal pressure exerted down the inguinal canal. These are the **intracrural fibers** of the external oblique aponeurosis.

Through the subcutaneous inguinal ring pass the spermatic cord and ilioinguinal nerve in the male

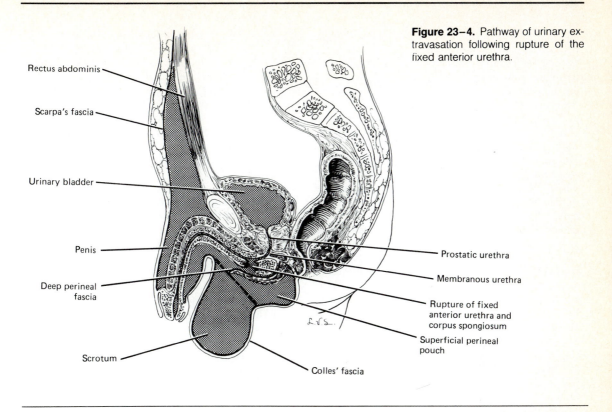

Figure 23–4. Pathway of urinary extravasation following rupture of the fixed anterior urethra.

Rectus abdominis

Scarpa's fascia

Urinary bladder

Penis

Deep perineal fascia

Scrotum

Colles' fascia

Prostatic urethra

Membranous urethra

Rupture of fixed anterior urethra and corpus spongiosum

Superficial perineal pouch

Figure 23–5. External oblique muscles of abdominal walls.

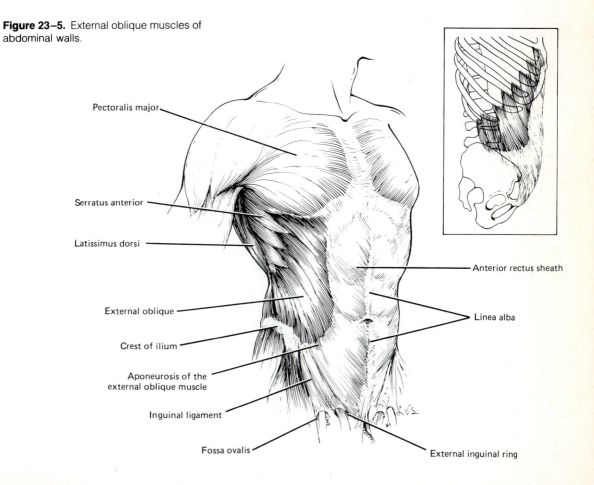

Pectoralis major

Serratus anterior

Latissimus dorsi

External oblique

Crest of ilium

Aponeurosis of the external oblique muscle

Inguinal ligament

Fossa ovalis

Anterior rectus sheath

Linea alba

External inguinal ring

and the round ligament of the uterus and the ilioinguinal nerve in the female. The ring is covered with the external spermatic fascia, derived from the external oblique aponeurosis and prolonged inferiorly as the outermost covering of the spermatic cord and the round ligament of the uterus.

The **inguinal ligament** extends from the anterosuperior iliac spine to the pubic tubercle. It is formed as the inferior edge of the aponeurosis of the external oblique muscle rolls upon itself to produce a cordlike structure. The ligament reaches toward the thigh, where it blends with the fascia lata. The lateral half of the inguinal ligament is thick and round; the medial half is flat and almost horizontal at the point where it is crossed by the spermatic cord or round ligament.

The **lacunar (Gimbernat's) ligament** (Fig 23–6) is that portion of the inguinal ligament which is reflected dorsally and laterally from the pubic tubercle. The triangular lacunar ligament is about 1.25 cm long, with the base of the triangle directed laterally. Its lateral margin (base) is concave and sharp, and along with fibers of the iliopubic tract of the transversalis fascia it forms the medial boundary of the femoral ring. The medial apex of the lacunar ligament abuts the pubic tubercle. The posteroinferior margin is attached to the pectineal line of the os pubis and is continuous with the pectineal fascia; the anterosuperior margin is attached to the undersurface of the inguinal ligament. The spermatic cord and the round ligament of the uterus rest upon the lacunar ligament just before they emerge from the superficial inguinal ring.

➡️ *Strangulation of femoral hernia. The sharp lateral crescentlike border of the lacunar ligament marks the level at which a femoral hernia is most apt to strangulate.*

An aberrant obturator artery, which in one of 7 persons arises from the external iliac or inferior epigastric rather than from the internal iliac artery, must run inferiorly to reach the obturator foramen. Thus, it runs on the inner surface of the lateral border of the lacunar ligament. Therefore it is not advisable to blindly cut the lateral border of the lacunar ligament ("artery of death") to free a strangulated femoral hernia.

The **pectineal (Cooper's) ligament** is a lateral extension of the inferior fibers of the lacunar ligament for about 3 cm along the pectineal line of the os pubis. It is reinforced by the posteriorly reflected fibers of the iliopubic band of the transversalis fascia. The ligament is usually flanked on each side by a small vein that can make placement of sutures in the ligament hazardous.

The **reflected inguinal ligament** consists of fibers of the inguinal and lacunar ligaments which are reflected deep to the external oblique aponeurosis, in the direction of the linea alba. The ligament ends about 2 cm above the os pubis and is of no clinical significance.

The external oblique muscle is supplied mainly by the eighth to 12th intercostal nerves and by the iliohypogastric and ilioinguinal nerves. The muscle compresses the abdominal cavity. Acting as a pair, the 2 external oblique muscles flex the spinal column. Acting alone, the muscle bends the spinal column ipsilaterally.

B. Internal Oblique Muscle: (Fig 23–7.) The internal oblique muscle lies deep to the external oblique and is thinner and smaller. Its fibers run predominantly in a transverse direction. The muscle

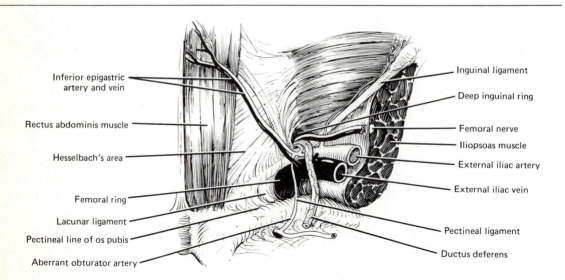

Figure 23–6. The inner surface of Hesselbach's area, with the peritoneum and transversalis fascia removed and the deep inguinal ring delineated.

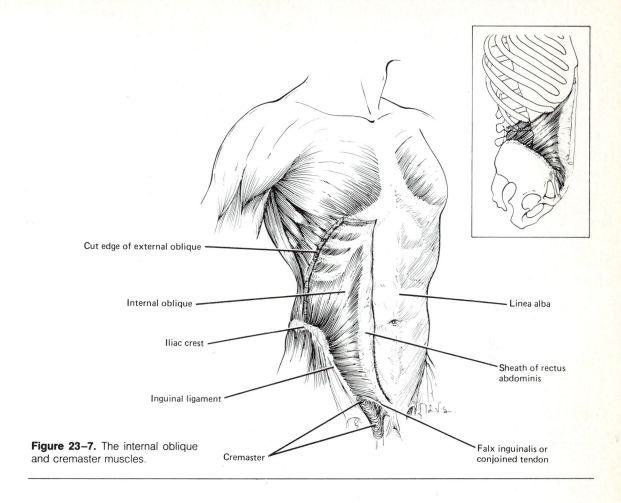

Figure 23–7. The internal oblique and cremaster muscles.

Cut edge of external oblique

Internal oblique

Iliac crest

Inguinal ligament

Cremaster

Linea alba

Sheath of rectus abdominis

Falx inguinalis or conjoined tendon

arises from the lateral half of the inguinal ligament, beginning at the **deep (internal) inguinal ring,** from the anterior two-thirds of the iliac crest, and from the **thoracolumbar fascia.** From these sites of origin, the fibers of the internal oblique diverge and insert as follows:

The fibers that arise from the **inguinal ligament** arch just above the deep inguinal ring and fuse (along the lateral border of the rectus abdominis muscle) with the descending fibers of the transversus abdominis muscle, then insert into the pubic crest. The tendons of insertion of the 2 muscles form the **conjoined tendon,** or **falx inguinalis.**

The fibers arising from the **iliac crest** pass either transversely or obliquely to become aponeurotic at the lateral border of the rectus abdominis muscle and aid in the creation of the rectus sheaths to insert into the linea alba (see rectus abdominis muscle).

The fibers most dorsal in origin—those from the **posterior segment of the iliac crest** and from the **posterior lamella of the thoracolumbar fascia**—insert into the cartilages of the seventh to 12th ribs. There they interdigitate with the intercostal muscles of the chest wall. The area just medial to the inguinal ligament, from a point two-thirds down the ligament

to the pubic tubercle, is not covered by fibers of the internal oblique muscle, thus weakening this area of the anterolateral abdominal wall (Hesselbach's area). The internal oblique muscle has the same innervation and function as the external oblique.

The cremaster muscle (Figs 23–7 and 23–8) is a thin structure whose separate muscle fibers are held together by a tight covering fascia. The muscle is derived from the lowermost fibers of the internal oblique muscle where that muscle comes in contact with the descending spermatic cord. This point is immediately after the cord has passed through the deep inguinal ring. The muscle fibers of the cremaster, with their intervening sustaining fascia, loop themselves along the descending spermatic cord. The longest loop reaches to the superior pole of the testis. The medial arm of each loop inserts into the pubic tubercle. The cremaster muscle and fascia become the outermost covering of the spermatic cord in the inguinal canal and the middle layer of the cord coverings after the cord has passed the superficial inguinal ring and acquired the external spermatic fascia. The cremaster muscle varies markedly in thickness; in females and in some males, it is mainly a fascial envelope. However, in most males it is thick and

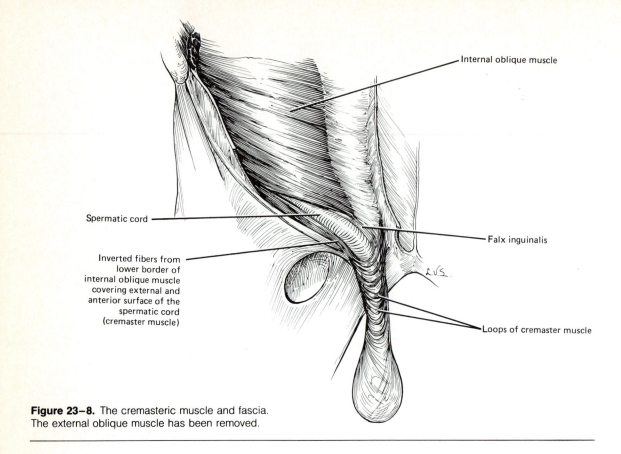

Figure 23–8. The cremasteric muscle and fascia. The external oblique muscle has been removed.

bulky enough to be an impediment during fascial repair of an inguinal hernia. The cremaster muscle and its fascia serve to pull the testis superiorly from the lower scrotum toward the external inguinal ring (cremaster reflex). The cremaster is supplied by the genital branch of the **genitofemoral nerve.**

▐➤ *Hernial sac covered by cremaster. The cremaster muscle and fascia must be routinely identified and then incised so that the underlying sac of an indirect inguinal hernia may be located, dissected free, and ligated at or above the level of the deep inguinal ring.*

C. Transversus Abdominis Muscle: (Figs 23–9 and 23–10.) This is the thinnest of the flat muscles of the anterolateral abdominal wall. Its fibers run mainly in a transverse direction. It is close to the internal oblique muscle, which lies ventral to it. The major vessels and nerves supplying the anterolateral abdominal wall run mainly in the plane between these 2 muscles. The muscle arises from the lateral third of the inguinal ligament; from the anterior three-fourths of the iliac crest; from the thoracolumbar fascia; and from the inner surfaces of the cartilages of the seventh to 12th ribs. At rib level, it interdigitates

with the anterolateral fibers of the diaphragm. It ends medially in a broad aponeurosis, the lowest fibers of which insert into the os pubis along with the lowest fibers of the internal oblique. The remainder of the aponeurosis of the transversus abdominis muscle passes horizontally toward the midline, assists in sheathing of the rectus abdominis, and inserts into the linea alba. The transversus abdominis muscle does not cover the weak area of the anterolateral abdominal wall (Hesselbach's area). The transversus abdominis plays little part in repair of an inguinal hernia except for that portion of the muscle that contributes to the falx inguinalis. The transversus abdominis is supplied by the eighth to 12th intercostal nerves and by the iliohypogastric and ilioinguinal nerves. It helps in contraction of the abdominal wall.

Medial Muscles

A. Rectus Abdominis Muscle: (Fig 23–10.) This muscle, one of the longest in the body, lies in the mid portion of the abdomen separated from its mate by the linea alba. The muscle is about 2½ times broader superiorly, near the costal margins, than inferiorly, at the os pubis. It is thicker in its suprapubic segment than in its costal segment. It arises from the os pubis and the symphysis pubica via a short tendon. It inserts into the anterior surfaces of the joined cartilages of the fifth to seventh ribs, into the lateral

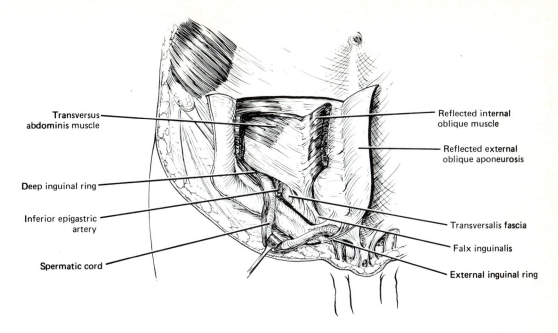

Transversus abdominis muscle

Deep inguinal ring

Inferior epigastric artery

Spermatic cord

Reflected internal oblique muscle

Reflected external oblique aponeurosis

Transversalis fascia

Falx inguinalis

External inguinal ring

Figure 23–9. The ilioinguinal region. The external oblique aponeurosis and internal oblique muscles have been sectioned and retracted both laterally and medially.

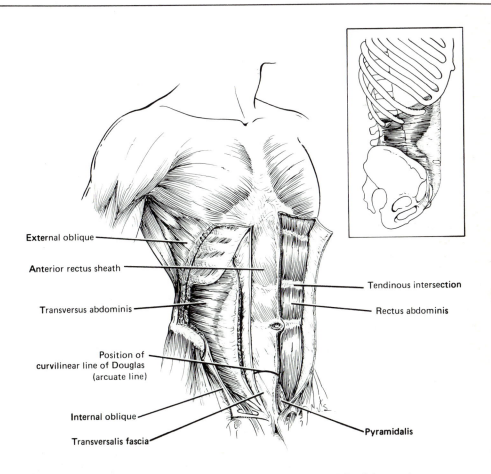

External oblique

Anterior rectus sheath

Transversus abdominis

Position of curvilinear line of Douglas (arcuate line)

Internal oblique

Transversalis fascia

Tendinous intersection

Rectus abdominis

Pyramidalis

Figure 23–10. The rectus abdominis and transversus abdominis muscles.

borders of the xiphoid process, and into the lowest segment of the body of the sternum.

Three or 4 fibrous bands, the **tendinous intersections,** cross the ventral surface of the muscle between the umbilicus and the xiphoid process. The intersections are attached to its ventral sheath and the most ventral fibers of the muscle. They divide the long, superior segment of the rectus abdominis into 3–5 segments and enhance the mechanical efficacy of the muscle. When the muscle contracts, the intersections are usually visible through the skin.

The rectus abdominis is enclosed in a sheath formed by the aponeuroses of all 3 of the flat lateral muscles of the anterolateral abdominal wall (Fig 23–11). Between the xiphoid process and the halfway point between the umbilicus and the os pubis, the anterior and posterior sheaths of the external oblique pass ventral to the rectus abdominis muscle. The sheaths of the internal oblique divide into 2 lamellae; one lamella passes ventral to the rectus to join with the 2 lamellae of the external oblique to complete the **anterior rectus sheath.** The posterior sheath of the internal oblique passes dorsal to the rectus abdominis along with the 2 fascial lamellae of the transversus abdominis muscle. Together these 3 sheaths form the **posterior rectus sheath.** At a point roughly halfway between the umbilicus and the os pubis, the posterior rectus sheath terminates in the line of Douglas, or arcuate line.

Below the line of Douglas, all fascial lamellae of the 3 flat lateral muscles run anterior to the rectus abdominis muscle, so that the rectus possesses only an anterior sheath below this level, its deep surface resting directly upon the underlying transversalis fascia.

⮞ *Lower abdominal rectus incisions. Since the inferior third of the rectus abdominis muscle rests directly upon the transversalis fascia, there is a weakness of lower abdominal rectus incisions owing to the absence in the wound closures of a strong posterior rectus sheath.*

The **anterior rectus sheath** is tightly applied to the ventral fibers of the muscle, whereas the posterior rectus sheath, where present, is not attached to the dorsal surface of the muscle. In the superior and mid abdomen, between the posterior sheath and the deep surface of the rectus abdominis muscle, lie the nerves and blood vessels supplying the muscle. Over the lower one-fourth of the abdomen, the vessels and nerves lie directly between the deep surface of the rectus abdominis muscle and the transversalis fascia. The rectus abdominis is supplied by the seventh to 12th intercostal nerves. The rectus abdominis flexes the inferior segment of the vertebral column and compresses the mid portion of the abdomen.

B. Pyramidalis: The pyramidalis, a small triangular muscle, occupies the lower mid portion of the abdomen. It lies anterior to the rectus abdominis but is contained within the anterior sheath of that muscle. The pyramidalis arises from the ventral surface of the os pubis and from the anterior pubic ligament and passes superiorly to end in a pointed extremity

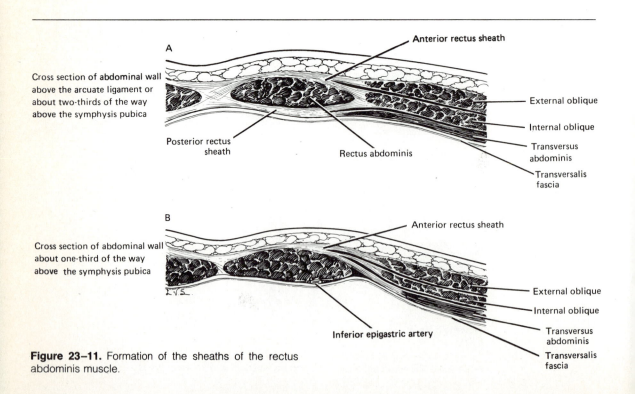

Figure 23–11. Formation of the sheaths of the rectus abdominis muscle.

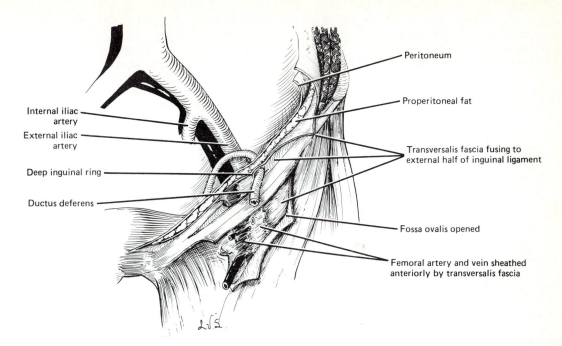

Figure 23–12. The transversalis fascia and its relationship to the medial and lateral halves of the inguinal ligament.

that inserts into the linea alba halfway between the os pubis and the umbilicus. The muscle frequently obscures the pubic tendons of origin of the rectus abdominis. The pyramidalis is supplied by branches of the 12th thoracic nerve. The muscle serves to tighten the linea alba.

⮕ *Pararectus abdominal incisions. Since the posterior surface of the rectus abdominis is not attached to the posterior rectus sheath or to the transversalis fascia, it allows the rectus abdominis to be displaced either laterally or medially in pararectus abdominal incisions.*

The **linea alba** is formed by the interlocking of the anterior and posterior sheaths of the rectus abdominis muscles as they meet in the midline of the abdomen. The line runs from the xiphoid process to the os pubis. In the upper abdomen, the linea alba is fibrous and about 1 cm wide. Just above the umbilicus, it narrows and becomes a thin fibrous line; below the umbilicus, it is hard to discern. Only the transversalis fascia and some fat separate the linea alba from the peritoneum of the upper anterolateral abdominal wall. In the upper abdomen, the linea alba provides a quick, relatively avascular approach to the abdominal cavity. It is perforated by many small nerves and a few minor blood vessels.

⮕ *Site of epigastric hernias. Above the umbilicus, the linea alba is frequently the site of epigastric*

hernias. These perforate the fascia either via the small foramens that serve as an exit for nerves or blood vessels or via a congenital weakness of a segment of the fascia. The areas of weakness are frequently multiple. They are more frequent to the left of the midline.

The Transversalis Fascia (Fig 23–12)

The transversalis fascia lies dorsal to the abdominal musculature and ventral to the preperitoneal fat. The fascia is thinner and less well developed in the upper abdomen; in the lower abdomen, it is a well-marked layer, particularly in the ilioinguinal region. It is directly continuous with the subdiaphragmatic fascia superiorly, the lumbar and iliacus fascia dorsally, and the endopelvic fascia caudally.

⮕ *Ilioinguinal region transversalis fascia. The transversalis fascia is the tissue of choice for the repair of direct inguinal and femoral hernias. In the ilioinguinal region, this fascia is both thick enough and lax enough to be used in hernia repair.*

In the ilioinguinal region, the transversalis fascia has an opening, the **deep inguinal ring.** The beginning of the passage through the anterior abdominal wall of the **processus vaginalis** peritonei and the gubernaculum testis or ovarii in the embryo is marked by the deep inguinal ring. After the embryonic descent of the testis or ovary, the deep inguinal ring is traversed by the **spermatic cord** in the male and the **round ligament of the uterus** in the female. The deep inguinal ring margins, unlike those of the superficial inguinal ring, are not easily defined from a ventral approach, since the transversalis fascia is prolonged onto the spermatic cord or the round ligament at the deep inguinal ring level. The prolongation becomes the internal spermatic or round ligament fascia. The deep inguinal ring lies at the midpoint of the inguinal ligament and about 1.25 cm medial and superior to the ligament. The ring is larger in males than females, thus predisposing males to indirect inguinal hernias. The ring is bounded superiorly, medially, and ventrally by the arching lowermost fibers of the internal oblique muscle and inferiorly and medially by the inferior epigastric artery and veins. The ring's lateral edge is formed by the transversalis fascia.

The transversalis fascia fuses with the deep surface of the lateral two-thirds of the inguinal ligament, thus lying ventral to the fascia covering the **iliopsoas muscle.** Over the medial third of the inguinal ligament, the transversalis fascia passes deep to the inguinal ligament and then appears on the ventral surface of the deep fascia of the upper thigh. In the upper thigh, the fascia lies ventral to the femoral vessels and the **femoral canal** and forms the ventral wall of the **femoral sheath.** The dorsal wall of the femoral sheath is formed by the **iliacus fascia.** The great vessels of the retroperitoneum pass dorsal to the inguinal ligament, deep to the transversalis fascia and superficial to the iliacus fascia. The transversalis and iliacus fasciae fuse with the sheaths of the femoral vessels, forming a triangular fascial cone, the apex of which is inferior and lies deep to the fossa ovalis

of the thigh, whereas the base is superior and lies deep to the medial third of the inguinal ligament.

The **iliopubic tract of the transversalis fascia** lies parallel to and just medial to the inguinal ligament. It is a fascial strip that inferiorly is reflected along the inner surface and the sharp lateral crescentic border of the lacunar ligament.

Preperitoneal Areolar Tissue & Fat

The preperitoneal fat lies deep to the transversalis fascia and superficial to the peritoneum of the anterolateral abdominal wall. It consists of adipose tissue held in the meshes of a loose network of connective tissue.

➡ *Surgery in obese persons. In obese persons, the preperitoneal fat layer makes abdominal incisions more difficult. The layer is a frequent site of accumulations of blood, serum, or pus after abdominal surgery. The poorly vascularized fatty tissue makes an excellent culture medium for bacteria.*

Peritoneum (Fig 23–13)

The peritoneum of the anterolateral abdominal wall lies deep to the preperitoneal fat and the transversalis fascia. As the peritoneal envelope spreads laterally in the region of the medial 2 cm of the inguinal ligament, it pulls away medially from the ligament by as much as 0.5 cm. This affords an extraperitoneal suprainguinal approach to retroperitoneal structures

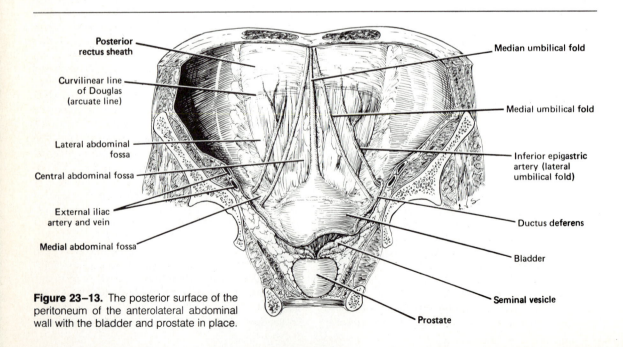

Figure 23–13. The posterior surface of the peritoneum of the anterolateral abdominal wall with the bladder and prostate in place.

Posterior rectus sheath

Curvilinear line of Douglas (arcuate line)

Lateral abdominal fossa

Central abdominal fossa

External iliac artery and vein

Medial abdominal fossa

Median umbilical fold

Medial umbilical fold

Inferior epigastric artery (lateral umbilical fold)

Ductus deferens

Bladder

Seminal vesicle

Prostate

related to the most medial segment of the inguinal ligament.

➡️ *Suprainguinal extraperitoneal approach for ligation of iliac vessels. Since the lateral limit of the peritoneal sac does not quite reach the lower one-fifth of the inguinal ligament, it is possible (1) to ligate the external iliac, inferior epigastric, or deep circumflex iliac vessels above the level of the inguinal ligament without entering the peritoneal cavity; (2) to use a suprainguinal approach for femoral hernia repair; and (3) to approach the ureter at the level of the pelvic brim without entering the peritoneal cavity.*

The deep surface of the parietal peritoneum of the anterolateral abdominal wall (Fig 23–13) presents 5 peritoneal folds. Three of the folds contain fibrous cords and 2 lateral folds contain the inferior epigastric vessels. The 3 cords run from the superior surface of the bladder to the umbilicus. The **median umbilical** fold covers the central cord and runs from the mid portion of the bladder fundus to the umbilicus. It is the remnant of the fetal urachus, the primitive connection between the bladder and the **allantois** of the **umbilical stalk.** The 2 lateral umbilical folds cover the remnants of the paired umbilical arteries of the fetal circulation. As fetal vessels, these arteries are continuations of the superior vesical branch of the internal iliac artery to the surface of the bladder, then to the umbilicus and into the umbilical stalk. After birth and the cutting of the umbilical cord, the segment of umbilical artery running from the bladder to the umbilicus persists as a fibrous cord, the lateral umbilical ligament.

➡️ *Urachal patency and urachal cysts. A patent urachus may leak urine at the umbilical level when the umbilical cord is cut at birth. Secretory transitional type epithelium may persist at single or multiple urachal levels, leading to the formation of urachal cysts, most often present at or just below the umbilical level. A possible patent urachus must be recognized and avoided in the making of lower midline incisions.*

The 3 peritoneal folds, running from the superior bladder surface to the umbilicus along with the inferior epigastric vessels, divide the deep surface of the peritoneum of the ilioinguinal area of the ventrolateral abdomen into 6 fossae, 3 on each side of the midline. There are 2 central abdominal fossae between the median and medial umbilical folds. These fossae lie deep to the strong rectus abdominis muscles. The medial abdominal fossae lie lateral to the lateral umbil-

ical ligaments but medial and inferior to the inferior epigastric vessels. The 2 medial fossae therefore lie dorsal to Hesselbach's area, the weak area of the ventrolateral abdominal wall through which pass direct inguinal hernias. The lateral abdominal fossae lie lateral and superior to the inferior epigastric vessels. These fossae contain the internal or deep inguinal ring, situated in the transversalis fascia one layer ventral to the peritoneum. The lateral fossae are the site of exit of indirect inguinal hernias from the abdominal cavity.

DESCENT OF THE TESTIS (Fig 23–14)

The descriptive anatomy of the anterolateral abdominal wall is complicated by the (apparent) fetal descent of testis and ovary and the effect of this descent on the structures of the ilioinguinal region.

During the **fourth month** of fetal life, the embryonic testis is situated in the lumbar region of the posterior abdominal wall, dorsal to the posterior peritoneum but ventral to the lumbar division of the abdominal lining fascia. The primitive testicular artery, a branch of the aorta, and the accompanying testicular veins, run to and from the superior pole of the testis to form a superior vascular pedicle called the **plica vascularis testis.**

By the **fifth month,** a herniation of the peritoneum occurs through the muscular and fascial layers of the ilioinguinal region. As the peritoneum herniates through the transversalis fascia, it forms the deep inguinal ring. Its further herniation and descent form the inguinal canal. Finally, the herniation pushes through the external oblique aponeurosis to form the superficial inguinal ring and then proceeds to the base of the scrotum. In so doing, the herniating sac of peritoneum, the **processus vaginalis peritonei,** forms a pathway through the ilioinguinal region's wall for the later descent of the testis by creating a peritoneal diverticulum stretching from the abdominal cavity to the scrotal base. Later in fetal life, the testis will descend dorsal to the diverticulum.

The position of the testis changes during the **sixth month** of fetal life. It still lies between the posterior peritoneum and the lining fascia of the posterior abdominal wall. It has, however, descended and now lies anterior to the mid portion of the iliacus muscle, resting ventral to the iliacus fascia but dorsal to the posterior abdominal peritoneum. In this position, it is approaching the preformed deep inguinal ring. The plica vascularis follows the course of the testis, lengthening as the testis descends. Preceding the testis in its descent and attached to its lower pole is a fibrous cord, the gubernaculum testis. The gubernaculum probably serves to keep the preformed **inguinal canal** open for testicular descent; it persists after birth as a short fibrous ligament that holds the lower pole of the testis loosely to the base of the scrotal sac. It is called the scrotal ligament in postfetal life (Fig 23–14).

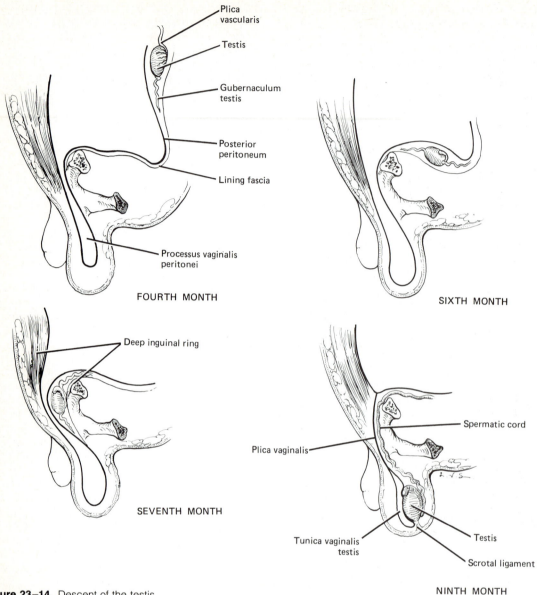

Figure 23–14. Descent of the testis.

By the **seventh month,** the testis has passed through the deep inguinal ring and has started its descent through the inguinal canal. Within the inguinal canal and throughout its subsequent descent, the testis will lie dorsal to the posterior layer of the **processus vaginalis peritonei** and ventral to the posterior fascial lining of the abdominal cavity.

During the **eighth month,** the testis traverses the inguinal canal, passing obliquely through the anterior abdominal wall in the ilioinguinal region. The testis and its following spermatic cord have both acquired 2 covering layers from the tissues of the anterolateral abdominal wall through which they have passed (internal spermatic fascia from the transversalis fascia and

cremaster muscle and fascia from the inferior edge of the internal oblique).

By the beginning of the **ninth month,** the testis normally has passed the external inguinal ring and taken its position at the base of the scrotum. The testes and spermatic cord acquire their third covering, the external spermatic fascia, from the external oblique muscle as they pass through the external inguinal ring.

Once the testis has reached the scrotum, the cavity of the processus vaginalis peritonei disappears as its anterior and posterior walls fuse to form the **plica vaginalis,** a minor component of the spermatic cord. There are 2 areas where a remnant of retained processus vaginalis peritonei is of importance. Distally in the scrotum, it normally persists as the tunica vaginalis testis. It may also persist as a slight dimple in the peritoneum just proximal to the internal inguinal ring. Failure of the 2 layers of the processus vaginalis peritonei to fuse properly is a factor in the occurrence of indirect inguinal hernia and also of hydrocele of the spermatic cord or of the testis.

➠ *Differential descent of testis, right and left sides. Descent of the testis and fusion and closure of the processus vaginalis peritonei progress more slowly on the right side of the abdomen than on the left, accounting for the higher incidence of right-sided indirect inguinal hernia. The right testis enters the scrotal sac about 1 week after the left. Therefore, when a left-sided indirect inguinal hernia is found, the physician must always suspect a possible right-sided indirect hernia as well.*

➠ *Improper testicular descent. Incomplete testicular descent, with the testis located within the abdominal cavity, at the internal inguinal ring, in the inguinal canal, or in a subcutaneous inguinal ring position, is called cryptorchidism. In this condition, the testis is found in an abnormally high location but is still placed between the posterior peritoneum and the posterior lining abdominal fascia. An ectopic testis is one that leaves the normal pathway of descent. It may be found in the thigh, within the anterolateral abdominal wall, ventral to the os pubis, within the peritoneal cavity, or in the retroperitoneum. In all these cases, the testis fails to lie in its normal position behind the posterior peritoneum and ventral to the posterior lining fascia.*

THE INGUINAL CANAL

By the end of the fourth month of fetal life, the future scrotal ligament—the gubernaculum testis—extends from the lower pole of the abdominal testis to the base of the scrotum. The ligament passes through the abdominal wall via the inguinal canal that forms around it. The processus vaginalis peritonei evaginates through the abdominal wall, following the course of the gubernaculum testis. Thus, the inguinal canal is the pathway through the anterior abdominal wall formed by the passage of both the **gubernaculum testis** and the processus vaginalis peritonei. Through it, the testis and spermatic cord pass from the abdomen to the scrotum. In males, the inguinal canal also contains the ilioinguinal nerve. In females, the canal is occupied by the **round ligament of the uterus,** passing to the **labia majora,** and by the ilioinguinal nerve.

The inguinal canal pursues an oblique downward course through the abdominal wall. The canal runs from the deep inguinal ring in the transversalis fascia to the superficial inguinal ring in the external oblique aponeurosis. The most immediate ventral relationship of the canal is to the external oblique aponeurosis. Once this fascia is opened, the inguinal canal is entered. The lowermost arching fibers of the internal oblique muscle cover the upper one-eighth of the inguinal canal ventrally. Dorsally, the major relationship of the inguinal canal is to the underlying transversalis fascia. The extreme lowermost segment of the canal is related dorsally to the conjoined tendon of the transversus and internal oblique muscles as they swing inferiorly to insert into the pubic tubercle.

THE SPERMATIC CORD
(Fig 23–9)

The spermatic cord forms in the preperitoneal tissues just dorsal to the deep inguinal ring. This area serves as the collecting station for the structures forming the cord. The cord then passes through the ring, down the inguinal canal, out the superficial inguinal ring, over the os pubis, and through the scrotal sac to the base of the sac, where it is attached to the superior pole of the testis. The left cord is uniformly longer and thicker than the right cord. The spermatic cord is composed of arteries, veins, lymphatics, nerves, fat, the ductus deferens, and the plica vaginalis peritonei.

Arteries

The largest of the cord arteries is the **testicular artery,** which arises as a paired branch of the abdominal aorta, given off just inferior to the renal arteries. It crosses ventral to the ureter and the psoas muscle but dorsal to the colon as it runs obliquely to the deep inguinal ring, where it joins with the other structures of the spermatic cord. It supplies the mid ureter, the testis, and the epididymis. The cremasteric (external spermatic) artery is a branch of the inferior epigastric artery. It joins the spermatic cord in the inguinal canal 0.35 cm distal to the deep inguinal ring and supplies the coverings of the cord. The **artery to the ductus deferens** can be a branch of either the superior or the inferior vesical artery. It joins the ductus deferens deep in the pelvis, where the duct rests upon the prostate before its junction with the seminal vesicles. The artery then follows the ductus, supplying it until it terminates in the testis. Tension exerted upon the ductus deferens can obliterate blood flow in this artery.

Veins

The testicular veins issue from the posterosuperior surface of the testis, receive branches from the epididymis, and form a complex venous plexus (pampiniform plexus) as they surround the cord. The testicular veins form the bulk of the spermatic cord. The plexus of testicular veins follows the ductus deferens and, usually just within the internal inguinal ring, channels into one or 2 testicular veins. The right vein empties into the inferior vena cava at an acute angle; the left vein joins with the left renal vein at a right angle.

▥▶ *Varicocele. When the testicular veins dilate and become tortuous, they form a varicocele of the spermatic cord. This is usually on the left. There is seldom a right-sided varicocele, probably because of the acute angular junction of the right testicular vein with the inferior vena cava.*

Lymphatics

The rich cord lymphatics accompany the testicular veins superiorly and drain primarily into the external iliac and hypogastric lymph nodes.

Nerves

The spermatic nerve plexus is derived from the abdominal sympathetic outflow as well as from nerves derived from the pelvic plexus that join the ductus deferens as it leaves the pelvis to become part of the spermatic cord nerve complex.

THE DUCTUS DEFERENS
(Fig 23–13)

The ductus deferens (vas deferens) (see also Chapter 39) is the superior continuation of the excretory duct of the epididymis. As a constituent of the spermatic cord, the ductus deferens runs in the inguinal canal to the internal inguinal ring, where it diverges from the other cord structures by curving around the lateral side of the inferior epigastric vessels. It then runs a retroperitoneal course toward the pelvis, where, on the posteroinferior surface of the bladder, it joins with the duct of the ipsilateral seminal vesicle to form the prostatic ejaculatory duct.

PLICA VAGINALIS

The plica vaginalis is the thin fibrous remnant of the processus vaginalis peritonei, present in the cord as an inconspicuous structure.

COVERINGS OF THE
SPERMATIC CORD

The internal spermatic fascia, derived from the transversalis fascia, covers the spermatic cord from the deep inguinal ring to the testis. It is thin and tightly attached to the overlying **cremaster muscle and fascia.** Derived from the internal oblique's lowermost arching fibers, the cremasteric layer covers the cord from a point just external to the deep inguinal ring to the superior pole of the testis. The outermost

covering of the cord is the external spermatic fascia, derived from the external oblique aponeurosis. This layer covers the cord only from the external inguinal ring to the testis.

FORMATION OF THE CANAL
OF NUCK IN THE FEMALE
(Descent of the Ovary)

During the third month of fetal life, the ovary lies between the peritoneum of the dorsal abdominal wall and the lumbar lining fascia. The fetal ovary has a gubernaculum attached to its caudal extremity. The gubernaculum of the ovary passes through the anterolateral abdominal wall dorsal to the processus vaginalis via the deep inguinal ring, the inguinal canal, and the superficial inguinal ring, finally to become attached to the subcutaneous tissues of the labia majora. The **gubernaculum ovarii** become attached to the superior lateral side of the developing uterus. The pathway through the anterolateral abdominal wall taken by the processus vaginalis and the gubernaculum ovarii is called the **canal of Nuck.** In its postfetal state, the gubernaculum ovarii becomes both the ovarian ligament, attaching the ovary to the uterus, and the round ligament of the uterus. The pathway taken by the round ligament of the uterus from the lateral wall of the uterus to the labia majora crosses the lateral pelvic wall and the external iliac vessels along its route to the internal inguinal ring. It hooks around the inferior epigastric vessels at the deep inguinal ring just before the ligament enters the inguinal canal.

On occasion, the ovary may show abnormal descent, lying ectopically along the course of the round ligament, within the totally or partially unfused processus vaginalis peritonei. When it is ectopic, the ovary may be found anywhere from the deep inguinal ring to the labia majora and may be palpable within the inguinal canal or within the labia majora. An ectopic ovary in the canal of Nuck is always accompanied by an indirect inguinal hernia. Hydroceles of the canal of Nuck are quite common.

▥▶ *Extra-abdominal ovary in the canal of Nuck. If an ovary lies extra-abdominally in the canal of Nuck, it must be repositioned in the abdominal cavity. If the ovary is congested and consequently too large to pass through the internal inguinal ring, the ring must be surgically enlarged for the replacement. The ring must then be repaired and reduced to normal size in order not to predispose to recurrence of an indirect inguinal hernia.*

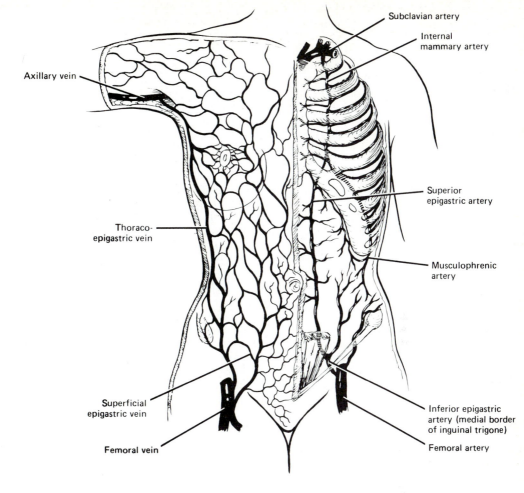

Figure 23–15. Arteries.

BLOOD VESSELS, LYMPHATICS, & NERVES OF THE ANTEROLATERAL ABDOMINAL WALL

Arteries
(Fig 23–15)

The **superior epigastric artery** is one of the 2 terminal branches of the internal mammary artery. It reaches the anterolateral abdominal wall after passing through the foramen of Morgagni, a hiatus between the sternal and costochondral fibers of the diaphragm. The artery then becomes related to the rectus abdominis muscle. It lies deep to the fibers of the muscle, between them and the posterior muscular sheath. The artery descends in this position, anastomosing at about umbilical level with the ascending branch of the inferior epigastric artery, with the anterior subcostal artery, and with the highest lumbar arteries.

The **inferior epigastric artery** arises from the external iliac artery just before that artery passes beneath the inguinal ligament to become the femoral artery. The artery runs toward the lateral border of the rectus abdominis muscle, in a plane deep to the transversalis fascia and superficial to the peritoneum. As it ascends, it forms the lateral superior border of Hesselbach's triangle since it lies immediately below the inferior arc of the deep inguinal ring. When the artery reaches the rectus abdominis muscle, it perforates the transversalis fascia and enters a plane between the rectus abdominis muscle and its posterior sheath. The artery then divides into ascending and descending branches. As the inferior epigastric artery lies against the inferior arc of the deep inguinal ring, the ductus deferens or the round ligament lies at first dorsal and then lateral to it as these structures enter the inguinal canal. Just medial to the deep inguinal ring, the inferior epigastric artery gives off the cremasteric artery, which supplies the coverings of the spermatic cord and the round ligament. In one of

10 individuals, the **obturator artery** is a branch of the inferior epigastric artery rather than the internal iliac artery.

The 3 **lower posterior intercostal arteries** and the **anterior subcostal artery** help to supply the superior lateral abdominal wall with blood.

The 4 **lumbar arteries** supply the mid and lower lateral abdominal wall.

The **deep circumflex iliac artery** arises from the external iliac artery opposite the origin of the inferior epigastric artery. It ascends obliquely, deep to the inguinal ligament, in a fibrous sheath formed by the junction of the iliacus and transversalis fasciae. It rises to the level of the anterosuperior iliac spine and then turns posteriorly along the inner surface of the crest of the ilium to its midpoint, where it pierces the transversus abdominis muscle and comes to lie between that muscle and the internal oblique muscle. In this position, the artery anastomoses with the **iliolumbar** and **gluteal arteries.**

➠ *Bleeding from a descending branch of the deep circumflex iliac artery. The deep circumflex iliac artery supplies the lower lateral abdominal wall and gives off a medial descending branch that tends to bleed in a McBurney appendectomy incision when the lower segment of the external oblique muscle is split superiorly.*

The superficial inferior epigastric, superficial external pudendal, and superficial circumflex iliac arteries are the most immediate branches of the femoral artery and supply the lower abdominal wall with superficial arterial circulation as they or their branches run superiorly across the superficial surface of the inguinal ligament.

➠ *Bleeding in hernia incisions. The superficial lower abdominal vessels that branch from the proximal femoral artery and vein are frequently the source of bleeding into the subcutaneous tissues when a groin incision is made for hernia repair.*

Veins
(Figs 23–15 and 23–16)

To understand the anatomy of the **superficial venous return** from the anterolateral abdominal wall, it is helpful to divide the area into 3 large segments and one small one. The 2 lateral areas of the superficial anterolateral abdominal wall are drained by many

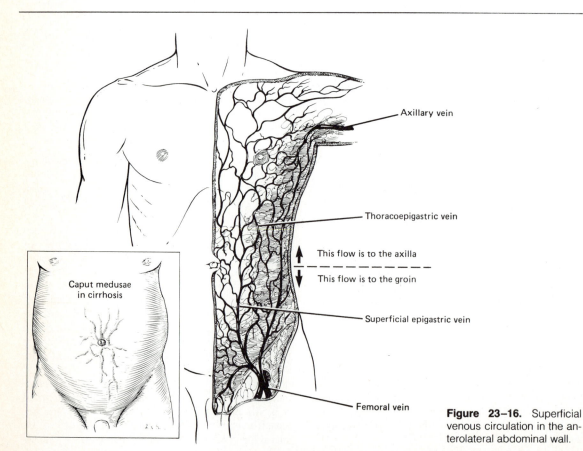

Caput medusae
in cirrhosis

Axillary vein

Thoracoepigastric vein

This flow is to the axilla

This flow is to the groin

Superficial epigastric vein

Femoral vein

Figure 23–16. Superficial venous circulation in the anterolateral abdominal wall.

large veins that run from groin to axilla. The flow in these lateral veins may be either (1) toward the axilla and then into the superior vena cava or (2) toward the groin and then into the inferior vena cava.

The superior central section above the umbilicus drains superficial venous blood into the superior vena cava via the azygos, hemiazygos, and internal thoracic system.

The lower central section, below the umbilicus, drains superficial venous blood inferiorly into the inferior vena cava, mainly via vessels that parallel the inferior epigastric artery and branches of the femoral artery.

A circular area around the umbilicus, about 6 cm in diameter, drains its superficial venous blood centrally toward the umbilicus and then into small veins that empty into one or 2 paraumbilical veins running in the base of the **falciform ligament of the liver.** These veins eventually enter the portal venous circulation.

In many people, both in health and in disease, many of these superficial venous pathways are visible; consequently, the direction of flow in them is easily checked. Changes in normal directional flow are important in some pathologic conditions.

⇒ *Reversal of flow in the superficial abdominal veins. When flow in the superior vena cava is blocked as a result of trauma or the presence of a thoracic tumor mass, superficial venous flow in the mid supraumbilical area reverses direction and moves toward the groin and the inferior vena cava. When the inferior vena cava is blocked, flow from the lower mid abdomen moves superiorly toward the axilla and then to the superior vena cava. With an intra-or extrahepatic block of the portal venous flow, the hepatic venous flow reverses direction and some blood passes into the umbilical vein. The paraumbilical subcutaneous veins dilate and become tortuous, and their blood flows away from the umbilicus toward the caval system to form a caput medusae. This is a frequent late sign in cirrhosis of the liver.*

Venous return from the deep anterolateral abdominal wall is via veins that parallel their arterial counterparts (chiefly the superior and inferior epigastrics). These veins eventually empty into the inferior or superior vena caval systems.

Lymphatics
(Fig 23–17)
Lymphatic return from the deep anterolateral abdominal wall follows the pathways of deep venous return. Lymph vessels that parallel the inferior epigastric vessels empty into the **external iliac nodes,** as do lymphatic vessels that parallel the deep circumflex

iliac vessels. The lumbar veins are closely allied with lymph channels that empty into the **lumbar nodes.** The upper abdominal wall is drained by lymphatics that flow into the **retrosternal group of lymph nodes** and then through the **mediastinal group of nodes** and channels. The superior abdominal wall also sends lymph into the nodes of the axillary chain.

The superficial tissues of the abdominal wall drain to the **subpectoral and axillary nodes** superiorly and to the **subinguinal nodes** inferiorly. There is a paucity of cross-midline drainage by lymphatics.

Nerves
(Fig 23–18)
The nerve supply to the anterolateral abdominal wall is a segmental one via the lower 6 intercostal nerves and the iliohypogastric and ilioinguinal nerves from the lumbar plexus. The abdominal wall nerves run primarily between the internal oblique and transversus abdominis muscles to terminate within the rectus abdominis.

The **iliohypogastric nerve,** a branch of nerves L1 and T12, appears first near the crest of the ilium. There it perforates the transversus abdominis muscle to lie between it and the internal oblique. Its anterior cutaneous branch eventually pierces the internal oblique muscle and becomes subcutaneous by perforating the external oblique aponeurosis about 2.5 cm above the superficial inguinal ring, where it is distributed to the skin of the hypogastric area of the abdomen. The lateral cutaneous branch of the nerve passes through both oblique muscles above the iliac crest and innervates a portion of the skin of the buttock along with the 12th thoracic nerve.

The **ilioinguinal nerve,** also a branch of nerves T12–L1, perforates the transversus abdominis muscle about 1.5 cm closer to the anterosuperior iliac spine than the iliohypogastric nerve. It pierces the internal oblique muscle, and deep to the external oblique aponeurosis it accompanies the spermatic cord or the round ligament through the inguinal canal. It emerges from the external inguinal ring to be distributed to the skin of the upper inner thigh, the skin of the root of the penis and the upper scrotum in males, and the skin covering the pubis and labia majora in females.

⇒ *Location of ilioinguinal nerve. Identification of the ilioinguinal nerve in the inguinal canal and its relationship to the external inguinal ring are important in the performance of a hernioplasty and also in making a low McBurney incision for appendectomy. For purposes of local anesthesia, the ilioinguinal nerve is found 1.5 cm medial to the anterosuperior spine of the ilium along a line running from the anterior iliac spine to the umbilicus. The needle is passed dorsally to the level of the transversus abdominis muscle, and the area is then infiltrated with local anesthetic.*

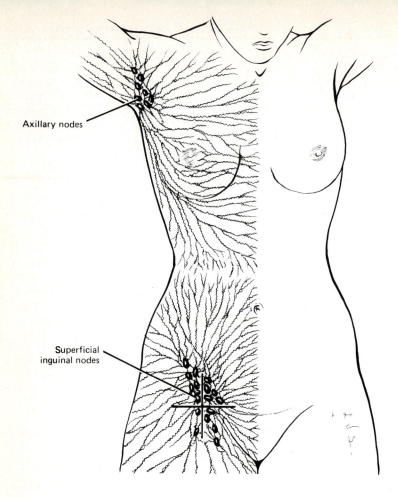

Axillary nodes

Superficial
inguinal nodes

Figure 23–17. Lymphatics of abdominal wall. Only one side is shown, but contralateral drainage occurs, ie, crosses midline to the opposite side.

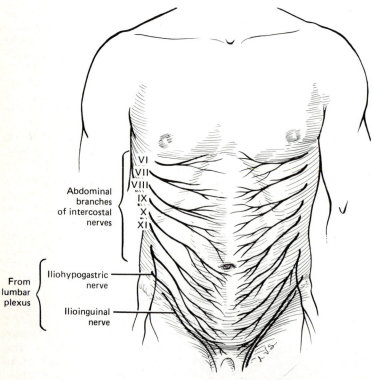

VI
VII
VIII
IX
X
XI

Abdominal
branches
of intercostal
nerves

From
lumbar
plexus

Iliohypogastric
nerve

Ilioinguinal
nerve

Figure 23–18. Nerve supply to the anterolateral abdominal wall.

The genital branch of the **genitofemoral nerve** descends dorsal to the spermatic cord in the inferior third of the inguinal canal. It supplies the cremaster muscle and the skin of the upper scrotum. Its fibers arise from nerves L1 and L2.

The cutaneous area at the level of the xiphoid process is supplied by nerve T5; the paraumbilical cutaneous area is supplied by nerve T10; and the suprapubic cutaneous area is supplied by nerve T12.

HERNIAS

➠ ***Indirect inguinal hernia.*** *(Figs 23–19 and 23–20.) An indirect inguinal hernia leaves the abdominal cavity via the deep inguinal ring in the transversalis fascia and descends inferiorly, ventrally, and medially, through the inguinal canal, toward the external inguinal ring and the scrotal sac or labia majora. It is a herniation into the spermatic cord because of improper fusion of the processus vaginalis peritonei, which lies within the cord coverings. Above the level of the external ring, the hernia is termed incomplete. Once it reaches or passes the external ring, it is a complete hernia. In the male, the hernia reaches the scrotal sac it is called a scrotal hernia.*

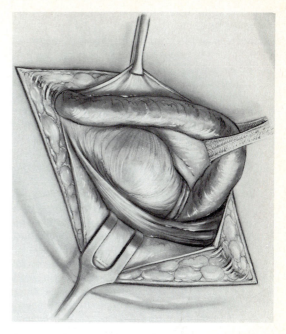

Figure 23–20. Indirect inguinal hernia. Inguinal canal opened, showing spermatic cord retracted medially and indirect hernia peritoneal sac dissected free to above the level of the internal inguinal ring. (Reproduced, with permission, from Way LW [editor]: *Current Surgical Diagnosis & Treatment,* 7th ed. Lange, 1985.)

The congenital indirect inguinal hernia may be noticed at birth or at any time up to the fifth year of life. It may present at any level from the deep inguinal ring to the base of the scrotal sac. If the hernia is incomplete, it is frequently associated with hydrocele of the spermatic cord or of the tunica vaginalis testis and frequently with an undescended testis.

The most common occupants of an indirect inguinal hernial sac are the omentum, small bowel, and large bowel; infrequently the uterine tube and ovary; and rarely the bladder.

The diagnosis of an indirect inguinal hernia is usually not difficult. The bulge of the peritoneal sac and its contents is usually visible or palpable as a protrusion in the groin, within the inguinal canal, at the external inguinal ring, over the anterior surface of the os pubis, or within the scrotal sac. It is occasionally difficult to differentiate between a direct and an indirect inguinal hernia. A direct inguinal hernia seldom passes the level of the external inguinal ring and thus is almost never a scrotal hernia. A lipoma of the spermatic cord can simulate the presence of an indirect hernial sac. A femoral hernia usually protrudes at a level below the line of the inguinal ligament, but it may come to lie above the level of the inguinal ligament. One should always attempt to differentiate indirect inguinal hernias from (1) a hema-

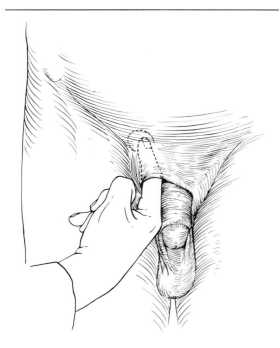

Figure 23–19. Insertion of a finger through the upper scrotum into the external inguinal ring. (Reproduced, with permission, from Way LW [editor]: *Current Surgical Diagnosis & Treatment,* 7th ed. Lange, 1985.)

toma in the inguinal region; (2) a varix of the lower abdominal or upper thigh veins; (3) an abscess in the groin from suppurating lymph nodes; (4) a noninflammatory swelling of groin lymph nodes; (5) a psoas abscess; and (6) hydrocele of the spermatic cord.

Repair of indirect inguinal hernia. The major principles in repair of all indirect inguinal hernias are (1) locating the indirect hernial sac after opening the cord coverings; (2) clean dissection of the sac to a level well superior to the deep inguinal ring, and complete freeing of the many adjacent structures that may be attached to the hernial sac replacing in the abdomen any organ or part found in the sac; (3) maintaining traction on the peritoneal sac so that it can be ligated as high as possible; and (4) tightening of the transversalis fascia about the enlarged deep inguinal ring, to prevent recurrent indirect hernia. Only when Hesselbach's area shows signs of weakness (in people with debilitating illness, in the elderly with poor tissues) is a concomitant plastic procedure for repair of the weak area of the ilioinguinal region carried out.

The recurrence rate in the surgical repair of indirect inguinal hernia averages 2–4%. Indirect hernia in infancy and childhood should have a recurrence rate of less than 1%.

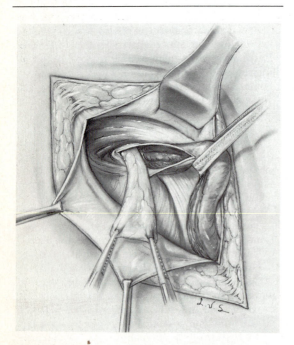

Figure 23–21. Direct inguinal hernia. Inguinal canal opened and spermatic cord retracted inferiorly and laterally to reveal the hernia bulging through the floor of Hesselbach's triangle. (Reproduced, with permission, from Way LW [editor]: *Current Surgical Diagnosis & Treatment,* 7th ed. Lange, 1985.)

Direct inguinal hernia. (Fig 23–21.) A direct inguinal hernia is one that pushes ventrally straight through Hesselbach's area, the weak area of the ilioinguinal region of the anterior abdominal wall. The hernia leaves the abdomen through the central abdominal fossa, at the lateral border of the rectus abdominis muscle and inferior and medial to the inferior epigastric vessels. The hernia is almost always acquired. Direct inguinal hernia is due to a developed weakness in the fascia of the floor of the inguinal canal (transversalis fascia) and increases with advancing age. It is infrequent in children and young adults. The bladder is a common component within its sac. Direct inguinal hernia almost never descends past the level of the subcutaneous inguinal ring and seldom appears in the scrotum.

On occasion, a direct inguinal hernia will break through the overlying thinned-out transversalis fascia and become strangulated. Sometimes a direct hernia will change its direction so that differentiation from an indirect inguinal hernia becomes more difficult. A finger placed over the deep inguinal ring may keep an indirect inguinal hernia from descending; thus, if a bulge appears, it will be a direct inguinal hernia.

Surgical repair of direct inguinal hernia. The surgeon must strengthen Hesselbach's area. The hernial sac is usually not opened but is depressed dorsally. The prime tissue used in repair is transversalis fascia, a plentiful supply of which nearly always lies deep to the rectus abdominis muscle. A direct hernia is frequently accompanied by a small asymptomatic indirect inguinal hernia, and the spermatic cord must always be opened and carefully inspected to avoid the presence of an indirect hernia after direct hernia repair. Bilateral direct hernia repair in adults should not be performed at one sitting. Recurrence and morbidity rates are significantly higher with this practice. Bilateral indirect hernia repair in children, however, is the rule.

Direct inguinal hernia has a higher recurrence rate than indirect inguinal hernia, and the rate rises with each successive attempt at repair. Initial repair of direct inguinal hernia has a recurrence rate of 6–8%. If a direct hernia recurs more than once, the transversalis fascia and its iliopubic tract are of poor quality and the surgeon must often depend on prosthetic material (Marlex [polypropylene] mesh) to reinforce the weak Hesselbach's area.

Sliding inguinal hernia. (Fig 23–22.) Sliding inguinal hernia constitutes about 2% of all inguinal hernias, mainly indirect hernias. By definition, a sliding hernia is one in which the

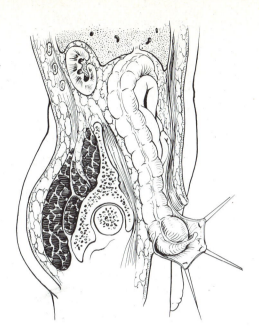

Figure 23–22. Right-sliding hernia. The cecum, appendix, and lower ascending colon occupy the sac and form the posterior portion of the circumference of the sac. The sac has been opened anteriorly to show the cecum forming a part of the posterior sac wall. (Reproduced, with permission, from Way LW [editor]: *Current Surgical Diagnosis & Treatment,* 7th ed. Lange, 1985.)

visceral peritoneum covering a segment of the bowel or bladder forms a portion of the wall of the hernial sac. On the right side, cecum and lower ascending colon form a portion of the sac wall, whereas on the left side, the sigmoid colon forms a portion of the sac wall. A sliding hernia becomes possible because of (1) the degree of posterior fixation of the large bowel, (2) the proximity of the segment of large bowel that herniates to the deep inguinal ring, and (3) an enlarged deep inguinal ring.

As a result of physiologic aging or chronic debilitating disease, the cecum and ascending colon, if partially fixed posteriorly, may slide inferiorly on the tissues of the posterior abdominal wall to the level of the deep inguinal ring and enter the inguinal canal as a sliding hernia. On the left side of the abdomen, an abnormally low position of the sigmoid colon permits sliding of this colonic segment down to (and into) the left internal inguinal ring, the 2 leaves of the sigmoid mesentery opening to allow the wall of the sigmoid colon to present as all or part of the apex of the hernial sac.

Sliding hernia—seldom diagnosed before surgery—is an affliction of aged or debilitated patients. It is more common in men than in women and is more frequent on the left than on the right side. The diagnosis should always

be considered when a large hernia appears suddenly in the scrotal sac. Barium enema showing a large segment of colon in a scrotal sac is suggestive of sliding hernia. Strangulation and obstruction of the bowel are uncommon.

➠ ***Repair of sliding hernia.*** *The surgeon must be careful not to enter the bowel that forms a portion of the circumference of the hernial sac. Repair on the left side consists of replacing the bowel and reapproximating the leaves of the sigmoid mesentery whose opening has allowed the bowel to slide inferiorly. On the right side, repair consists of bowel reduction and as high a sac ligation as possible.*

Anatomy of the Femoral Region (Fig 23–23)

The femoral triangle in the superoanterior thigh is bounded superiorly by the inguinal ligament, laterally and inferiorly by the sartorius muscle, and medially by the adductor longus muscles. The superficial fascia of the upper thigh is continuous with Camper's fascia of the lower abdomen and consists of a network of fine areolar tissue with varying amounts of fat in its meshes. Camper's fascia crosses the inguinal ligament to reach the upper anterior thigh, where it covers the fossa ovalis and is firmly attached to its borders. It is perforated by numerous blood and lymphatic vessels ("fascia cribrosa"). Scarpa's fascia, the deep layer of the superficial fascia of the anterior abdominal wall, also crosses ventral to the inguinal ligament as it passes onto the upper thigh. It attaches to the deep fascia of the thigh along a line 2 cm below and parallel to the inguinal ligament.

The deep fascia of the thigh is tough and thick. In the upper lateral thigh, it swings superiorly and medially to attach to the crest of the ilium, the iliac spine, and the entire length of the inguinal ligament; most medially, it inserts into the os pubis. The medial swing of the thick lateral superior portion of the fascia lata places a crescent-shaped segment of the fascia ventral to the femoral vessels and the femoral canal. It also constitutes the superior and lateral borders of the fossa ovalis.

The medial segment of the deep fascia of the upper thigh covers the adductor group of muscles. It is thin, passes dorsal to the sheath of the femoral vessels, and forms the medial and inferior margins of the fossa ovalis. Thus, the fossa ovalis exists between the 2 fasciae as they move toward each other. The aperture is placed in the upper medial thigh about 2.5 cm below the medial end of the inguinal ligament. The fascia cribrosa covers the aperture and must be removed before the edges of the opening can be seen.

The femoral artery and vein pass deep to the inguinal ligament as they run from the abdomen to the

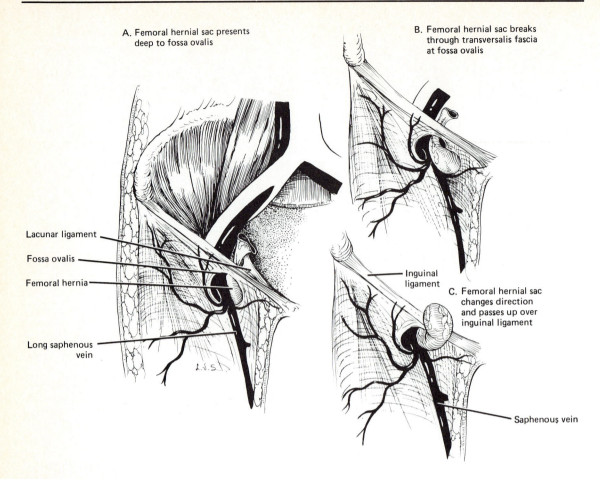

A. Femoral hernial sac presents deep to fossa ovalis

B. Femoral hernial sac breaks through transversalis fascia at fossa ovalis

Lacunar ligament

Fossa ovalis

Femoral hernia

Long saphenous vein

Inguinal ligament

C. Femoral hernial sac changes direction and passes up over inguinal ligament

Saphenous vein

Figure 23–23. Route taken by femoral hernia in its descent. (Reproduced, with permission, from Way LW [editor]: *Current Surgical Diagnosis & Treatment,* 7th ed. Lange, 1985.)

thigh. They carry with them a cone of the great lining fascia of the abdomen. The cone is formed ventrally by the transversalis fascia and dorsally by the iliacus fascia. The base of the cone lies deep to and parallel to the medial third of the inguinal ligament. The fascial cone fuses with the walls of the enclosed femoral artery about 4 cm below the inguinal ligament and with the walls of the femoral vein about 2 cm below the inguinal ligament.

The femoral canal lies medial to the femoral vein on the anteromedial surface of the thigh. The canal begins at the level of the inguinal ligament and ends just deep to the superior border of the fossa ovalis. It is bounded ventrally by transversalis fascia and dorsally by iliacus fascia, laterally by the femoral vein, and medially by the lacunar ligament and the transversalis fascia.

➪ *Femoral hernia. Femoral hernia is an acquired hernia, more common in women than in men. Women are probably more prone to develop*

femoral hernia for the following reasons: (1) the wider flare of their iliac crests results in a longer inguinal ligament and a wider femoral ring; (2) the increased abdominal pressure during pregnancy upon the inferior medial portion of the pelvic peritoneal envelope; and (3) the laxity of the inguinal, sacroiliac, sacrotuberous, and pubic symphyseal ligaments that occurs just before parturition. The ligaments never quite regain their normal strength and tension following pregnancy.

Femoral hernia comprises about 8–10% of all hernias in the groin. Any factor increasing intra-abdominal pressure causes the femoral ring to dilate. As shown in Fig 23–23, a femoral hernia descends inferiorly and slightly laterally through the femoral canal to a point below the upper border of the fossa ovalis, where the transversalis fascia blends with the iliacus fascia to close off the femoral canal. When the hernia reaches the closed end of the femoral canal, it breaks out ventrally through the transversalis fascia and the fossa ovalis, eventually to lie in a subcutaneous subinguinal position in the upper thigh. The commonest occupant of a femoral hernial sac is omentum, which is frequently incarcerated within loops of a small bowel and bladder.

Repair of femoral hernia. For repair of simple uncomplicated femoral hernia, the incision should generally be suprainguinal. The transversalis fascia is identified as it passes through the femoral ring. It is teased back through the femoral ring. The sac is dissected free, the excess sac is cut away, and the base of the sac is transfixed at peritoneal level. A McVay type of repair is done, the transversalis fascia being sutured to Cooper's ligament, reinforcing the inferior portion of the floor of the inguinal canal and effectively closing the femoral ring.

Femoral hernia is prone to strangulation because of (1) the resistant character of the structures forming the femoral ring; (2) extrusion of the hernia through the transversalis fascia, which may leave a tight neck about the hernia; and (3) the sharp superior border of the fossa ovalis, which lies just above the advancing hernia. The many directional changes taken by the hernia as it continues to protrude also favor strangulation.

Epigastric hernia. (Fig 23–24.) An epigastric hernia protrudes through the linea alba in the midline of the anterolateral abdominal wall, above the level of the umbilicus.

About 3–5% of persons have epigastric hernias. Epigastric hernia is 3 times more common in men than in women and is most common between the ages of 20 and 50 years.

The most common finding associated with epigastric hernia is the presence of a subcutaneous mass noted close to the midline above the level of the umbilicus. Most such masses are painless and unsuspected by the patient and are frequently found only on routine abdominal examination. The smaller hernias usually contain only preperitoneal fat, and such hernias are prone to incarcerate and strangulate.

Repair of epigastric hernia. If the epigastric hernia is symptomatic or is more than 0.5 cm in diameter, operative treatment is advised. A liberal vertical incision is preferable to a transverse one, as it allows searching for the multiple epigastric hernias that are occasionally present. Intraperitoneal herniating structures are reduced, but no attempt is made to close the peritoneal sac.

Littre's hernia and Spigelian hernia. Littre's hernia and Spigelian hernia are 2 rare types

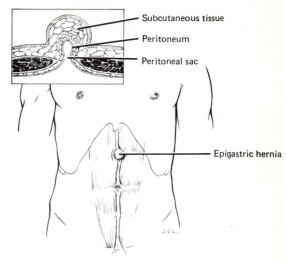

A. Cross section of herniation of peritoneal sac through the linea alba

— Subcutaneous tissue
— Peritoneum
— Peritoneal sac

— Epigastric hernia

B. Epigastric hernia occurring in the linea alba above the umbilical level

Figure 23–24. Epigastric hernia. (Reproduced, with permission, from Way LW [editor]: *Current Surgical Diagnosis & Treatment,* 7th ed. Lange, 1985.)

of hernia that leave the abdominal cavity via the ventrolateral abdominal wall.

Littre's hernia (diverticular hernia) leaves the abdominal cavity through one of the "weak" areas of the anterolateral abdominal wall (internal inguinal ring, Hesselbach's triangle, femoral ring) with a Meckel's diverticulum as the sole occupant of the hernial sac. It occurs more often on the right side, is most often present as a femoral hernia, and appears most often in men.

Spigelian hernia is a spontaneously occurring anterolateral hernia through the linea semilunaris at the point where sheaths of the 3 lateral abdominal flat muscles all join to form the anterior rectus abdominis sheath. This point in the abdominal wall is anatomically weak because it is where the line of Douglas is crossed by the linea semilunaris. The medially turning superior branch of the inferior epigastric artery, which reaches the rectus abdominis at this point, further weakens the area because at this point the vessel passes through the transversalis fascia to lie deep to the rectus muscle.

Incisional hernias through the anterolateral abdominal wall. Incisional hernias through the anterolateral abdominal wall account for 7–12% of all hernioplasties performed in large

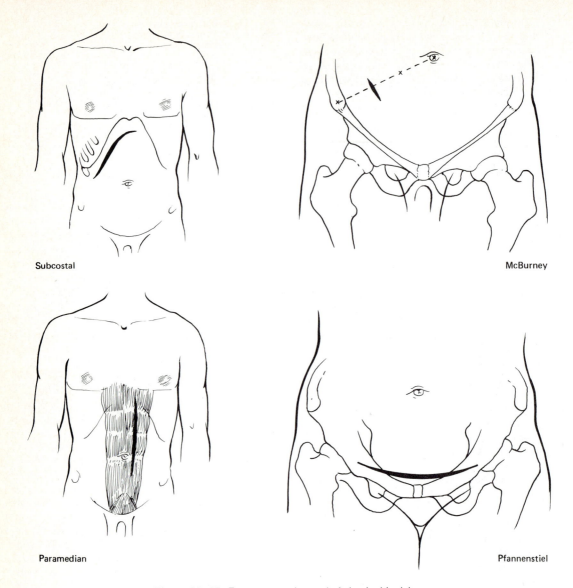

Subcostal

McBurney

Paramedian

Pfannenstiel

Figure 23–25. Four commonly used abdominal incisions.

general hospitals. *Despite significant advances in operative technique, improved suture material, better pre- and postoperative care, use of reinforcing and "bridging" materials, antibiotics, etc, this type of hernia persists and does not seem to be significantly decreasing in frequency. The increasing proportion of older people requiring abdominal surgery contributes to the persistent high incidence of this type of hernia.*

Many factors contribute to the occurrence of an incisional hernia. The factors most often responsible for incisional hernia are as follows: (1) The age of the patient. (2) General debility of patients. (3) Obesity. (4) Postoperative wound infection. (5) The type of incision.

(6) Postoperative pulmonary complications. (7) The placement of drains or colostomy or iliostomy openings in the primary operative wound.

*The ultimate in wound weakness is complete or partial **dehiscence**—a breakdown of all layers of the closure. A final breakthrough at skin level leads to **evisceration**. Both of these conditions call for prompt operative management.*

In contrast to the wound that almost immediately dehisces or eviscerates is one that shows no immediate postoperative indications of discomfort or drainage but suddenly or gradually weakens either throughout its entire length or in a specific area. This is due to complete or partial collapse of the peritoneal or the fascial closure of the wound. Clinically, this wound will show an incisional bulge with or without pain when the patient coughs or otherwise raises the intra-abdominal pressure. These hernias gradually increase in size and may become painful. The incidence of incarceration and strangulation of intraperitoneal contents in an incisional hernia is relatively high.

➭ **Repair of incisional hernias.** *Incisional hernias should be closed as soon as possible if the patient is well enough to undergo major surgery. Except for very large hernias, a good fascial closure can usually be carried out. Marlex mesh is used for control of very large hernial gaps where the usual fascia-to-fascia closure would necessarily be under tension.*

➭ **Types of incisions in the anterolateral abdominal wall.** *(Fig 23–25.)*
A. Upper abdominal incisions related to the rectus abdominis and its sheaths:
1. Incision through the linea alba–The fatty tissues of the falciform ligament of the liver may have to be divided for good exposure.
2. Muscle splitting upper rectus abdominis incision–The anterior sheath of the rectus abdominis is incised, and the muscle fibers are split vertically. The area is extremely vascular and the procedure time-consuming. With this incision, it is difficult to preserve the peripheral branches of the nerves supplying the rectus abdominis.
3. Paracostal or oblique subcostal incision–This incision is made about 3 cm below and parallel to the inferior costal border. Generally, it is possible to stay within the confines of the sheaths of the rectus abdominis. It should not be used if the patient has an acute costal angle with a long narrow epigastrium.
4. True transverse upper abdominal incisions–These incisions give excellent exposure for surgery of the abdomen above the level of the umbilicus. They are poor incisions for use in emergency abdominal explorations, since they are difficult to extend superiorly and inferiorly.
B. Muscle splitting or gridiron incisions of the lateral abdominal wall: The most popular of these incisions is the McBurney incision, which is made in the ilioinguinal region. An oblique incision is made in the skin of the abdomen, and the external oblique muscle and aponeurosis are opened along the line of their fibers. The fibers of the internal oblique and the transversus abdominis muscles are spread transversely in the line of their fibers.
C. Lower abdominal incisions: The anatomic features of lower abdominal vertical rectus incisions: (1) below the umbilicus, the linea alba appears only as a thin fibrous band; (2)

the rectus abdominis lacks a posterior sheath below the point halfway between the umbilicus and the os pubis; and (3) the lower portion of the rectus abdominis is complicated by the presence of the pyramidalis muscle. As in the upper abdomen, these incisions may be midline, muscle-splitting, or pararectus.
D. Transverse lower abdominal incisions: These are of 2 major types.
1. Pfannenstiel incision–This is a transverse skin incision just within the pubic hairline. The anterior sheath of the rectus abdominis is incised transversely, and the 2 rectus bodies are retracted laterally.
2. Cherney incision–This is a curvilinear transverse incision with its concavity facing superiorly. It begins about 7 cm medial to the anterosuperior iliac spine and drops down to a level just above the symphysis pubica. The anterior sheath of the rectus abdominis muscle is opened transversely, and the lower flap of the sheath is dissected inferiorly toward the pubis. The tendons of origin of the rectus muscle are transected, and the rectus muscle is then retracted superiorly. The peritoneum is opened first above the bladder level. Closure must be carefully done to prevent wound weakness. The rectus tendons are reapproximated, the anterior rectus sheath is closed, and the remainder of the wound is closed in layers. Closure takes time, but the exposure gained in this incision is excellent.

THE UMBILICAL AREA
(Fig 23–26)

The umbilicus is a depressed scar in the central abdomen, indicating the site of fusion of the layers of the ventral abdominal wall after severance of the umbilical cord. The area is of interest because of the frequent occurrence of various types of congenital or acquired anomalies.

EMBRYOLOGY

During the fourth and fifth weeks of embryonic development, the apex of the midgut loop, which is physiologically herniated into the umbilical stalk, communicates with the yolk sac via the vitellointestinal duct. The vitellointestinal vessels—branches of the ileocolic artery, the terminal segment of the superior mesenteric artery—accompany and supply the duct and the yolk sac. The vitellointestinal vessels must cross the midgut to reach its antimesenteric border and then continue along with the duct.

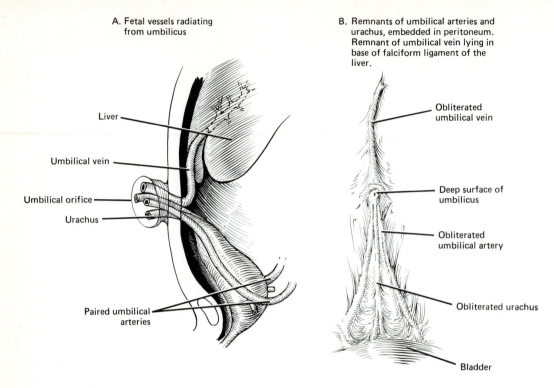

A. Fetal vessels radiating from umbilicus

Liver

Umbilical vein

Umbilical orifice

Urachus

Paired umbilical arteries

B. Remnants of umbilical arteries and urachus, embedded in peritoneum. Remnant of umbilical vein lying in base of falciform ligament of the liver.

Obliterated umbilical vein

Deep surface of umbilicus

Obliterated umbilical artery

Obliterated urachus

Bladder

Figure 23–26. The umbilicus in the fetus and in the adult.

The allantois, formed as a prolongation of the lower end of the primitive alimentary tube, also presents in the umbilical stalk and communicates via the urachus with the primitive bladder. Three major blood vessels connect the fetal and maternal circulations and run through the umbilical stalk. These are the paired umbilical arteries and the single umbilical vein.

By the beginning of the fourth month of fetal life, the herniated midgut has returned to the abdomen and the anterolateral abdominal wall has normally contracted about the umbilical orifice. The vitellointestinal vessels, the yolk sac, and the vitellointestinal duct have disappeared. The urachus has atrophied into a fibrous cord. By the fourth month, the umbilical ring contracts into a small orifice through which pass only the paired umbilical arteries and the umbilical vein.

Following birth, these vessels atrophy and appear as 3 fibrous cords on the deep surface of the peritoneum of the anterior abdominal wall.

A small crust remains at the spot at which the umbilical cord has been ligated and cut. This crust, at the abdominal cutaneous level of cord transection, heals and epithelializes rapidly. Scarring takes place deep to the epithelialized area, and the urachus and the umbilical vessels draw the epithelialized area against the circumference of the umbilical ring. The superior arc of the umbilical ring is generally fused less tightly than the inferior arc and is the site for development of most umbilical hernias. The umbilical depth varies markedly, from an orifice flush with the surrounding skin to one that is almost 1 cm deep.

➠ *Umbilical orifice lesions. A deep umbilicus may harbor a small fecal leak from a partially open vitellointestinal duct or a leak of urine from a severed patent urachus. A palpable mass in the abdominal wall just deep to the umbilicus suggests the presence of a urachal or vitellointestinal cyst. A chronic red eczematous rash around the umbilical orifice suggests the presence of a foreign body in the umbilical cavity.*

➠ *Omphalocele and hernia into the umbilical cord. (Fig 23–27.) A true omphalocele has the following characteristics: (1) improper development and faulty approximation of the central abdominal muscles surrounding the umbilicus; (2) a poorly developed abdominal coelomic (peritoneal) cavity; and (3) complete or partial non- or malrotation of the bowel.*

There is no proper umbilicus in omphalocele. Instead, there is a broad funnel-shaped defect into which the midgut has herniated, along with its supporting mesentery.

At the time of birth, a true omphalocele may or may not be related to the size of the abdominal defect. The hernia is covered with translucent membranes (peritoneum, Wharton's jelly, and amnion), and the hernia con-

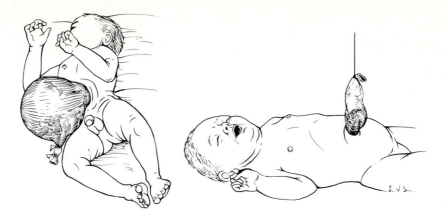

A. Omphalocele   B. Hernia into the umbilical cord

Figure 23–27. Omphalocele and hernia into the umbilical cord.

tents are usually visible through the membranes. If the hernial sac has ruptured before delivery, the herniating viscera are reddened, thickened, and covered with fibrin and occasionally with meconium.

Nonrotation or malrotation of the bowel is nearly always present, associated anomalies of the intestine or the cardiopulmonary system are common. Omphalocele is often associated with prematurity.

With herniation into the umbilical cord, a small hernia is present in the umbilical stalk along with a marked defect in the anterior abdominal wall. Most of the intestine and the abdominal organs lie within the normal abdominal cavity. Membrane rupture and midgut volvulus are infrequent complications.

Gastroschisis. Congenital protrusion of intraabdominal contents occurs here through a defect in the inferior anterolateral abdominal wall other than the umbilical orifice. The hernia in gastroschisis is not covered by a sac, and the defect in the abdominal wall has smooth edges. The hernia is noticed immediately after delivery. The defect is more common in males than in females (2:1) and in premature than in term deliveries. The defect is most commonly to the right of the umbilicus (6:1). The average size of the defect is 3–5 cm. The condition is often accompanied by congenital stenosis or atresia of segments of the extruded bowel.

Infantile umbilical hernias. These occur as a result of imperfect healing of the scar of the umbilical orifice. The defect involves a widened and thinned-out linea alba at the umbilical level. The greatest width of the defect lies in the transverse plane. The hernia opening is

usually smaller than 1–2 cm. Most of these herniations are easily reducible, and complications are rare. Nearly all defects less than 1 cm in diameter close spontaneously by the end of the second year of life. All defects larger than 2 cm in diameter, particularly in females, require closure. Taping of the orifice is of little value. Occasionally, painful incarceration of omentum demands operative intervention despite the small size of the orifice.

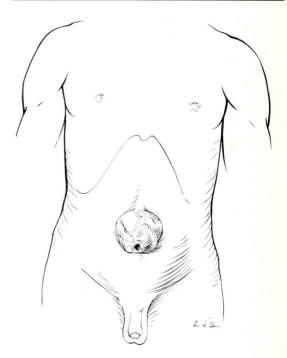

Figure 23–28. Adult umbilical hernia.

➤ ***Umbilical hernias in adults.*** *(Fig 23–28.) Adult umbilical hernias are due to gradual yielding of the cicatricial tissue. The hernia usually presents at the superior arc of the ring, its weakest area. It occurs in females about 10 times as frequently as in males. Predisposing factors are multiple pregnancies with prolonged labor, ascites accompanying cirrhosis, obesity, and long-standing, large intra-abdominal tumor masses. Umbilical hernias in adults show no tendency toward spontaneous closure. The larger hernias are covered by a thin peritoneal sac, and the hernia appears to be subcutaneous. The hernial sac usually contains an omental mass, but also segments of small and large bowel. Adult umbilical hernias frequently strangulate and require emergency surgery. When diagnosed, an umbilical hernia in an adult should be repaired promptly to avoid emergency surgery.*

I. THE POSTEROLATERAL ABDOMINAL WALL

The posterolateral abdominal wall is a roughly square area bounded above by the lower borders of the tenth, 11th, and 12th ribs; below by the postero-superior margin of the iliac crests; and laterally by a line drawn vertically from the highest segment of the iliac crest to the tenth rib, approximately in the midaxillary line. The area is divided into halves by the vertebral column.

➠ *Importance of posterior abdominal wall. The posterior abdominal wall assumes major clinical importance because of the frequent incisions made through it to approach organs in the retroperitoneal region of the abdominal cavity: the kidney, the adrenals, and the ureter. An abscess originating in the retroperitoneum may point subcutaneously in the posterolateral abdominal wall. The area is a frequent site of both blunt and penetrating trauma. On occasion, hernias will present in this area, usually as a complication of surgical incisions. Muscle strains in the area are common and disabling, particularly if accompanied by vertebral fractures.*

GROSS ANATOMY

Topographic Anatomy

The incomplete 12th rib is of clinical importance in procedures related to the posterolateral abdominal wall. The acute angle formed by the 12th rib as it leaves the vertebral column is called the costovertebral angle.

➠ *Costovertebral angle. Kidney-punch tenderness in the costovertebral angle is suggestive of renal, perirenal, or subdiaphragmatic disease. A swelling in the angle suggests abscess or tumor of a retroperitoneal organ.*

The spinous processes of the lumbar vertebrae are usually easily palpable and assist in relating areas of the posterior abdominal wall to the important structures in the retroperitoneum. The spine of L1 is at the takeoff of the superior mesenteric artery from the abdominal aorta. The spinal cord ends at the level of the spine of L2. The spine of L2 is at the level of both the cisterna chyli and the **duodenojejunal flexure.** The abdominal aorta bifurcates at the level of the spine of L4. The inferior vena cava begins at the level of the spine of L5.

The costodiaphragmatic reflection of the parietal pleura is bounded along a line reaching from the tenth rib in the midaxillary line to the lower border of the 12th thoracic vertebra.

➠ *Costodiaphragmatic pleural reflection. Because the costodiaphragmatic reflection of the parietal pleura passes inferior to the 11th and 12th ribs, the pleural space may be inadvertently entered when posterior abdominal wall approaches are used for nephrectomy, suprarenalectomy, or posterior drainage of a subphrenic abscess. This is particularly true if the 11th and 12th ribs are partially resected to facilitate exposure. The surgeon must consider the risk of entering the pleural cavity when working on the medial half of the 12th rib and on the medial three-fourths of the 11th rib. A pleural opening may cause pneumothorax or empyema.*

The kidneys and the upper ureters are closely related to the posterolateral abdominal wall. The hilum of each kidney lies close to the level of the spine of L1 and about 5 cm lateral to the midline. The superior pole of the left kidney rises to the level of the tenth rib, whereas its inferior pole is at about the level of the spine of L2. The right kidney is about 2 cm lower than the left kidney, and one or both kidneys may have abnormally increased mobility. Knowledge of the relationships of both kidneys to the posterolateral abdominal wall aids in planning the site for needle biopsy of the organ. The ureter in the abdomen usually descends from the kidney hilum about 5 cm lateral to the midline, running from the level of the spine of L1 to the level of the posterosuperior spine of the ilium.

TISSUE LAYERS

The skin and superficial tissues of the posterolateral abdominal wall present little of anatomic or clinical importance. The superficial fascia covering the area is thin and difficult to dissect as a separate layer.

DEEP FASCIA
(Fig 24–1)

The deep fascia of the posterolateral abdominal wall is called the **thoracolumbar (lumbodorsal) fascia.** The fascia arises from the spinous processes and supraspinal ligaments of all lumbar vertebrae, from the medial and lateral sacral crests, and from the iliac crest. The fascia passes laterally, splitting to invest the erector spinae group of muscles. The dorsal layer of the split becomes the dorsal layer, and the ventral layer becomes the ventral layer of the thoracolumbar fascia. At the lateral border of the erector spinae muscles, the 2 layers of the thoracolumbar fascia join, fuse, and continue their course laterally and ventrally as the single-layered fascia of origin of the transversus abdominis and internal oblique muscles.

MUSCULATURE
(Figs 24–1, 24–2, and 24–3)

The muscles of the posterolateral abdominal wall are divided into 3 layers: superficial, middle, and deep.

Superficial Layer
(Fig 24–2)

The superficial layer consists of 2 muscles. The **latissimus dorsi** is a large triangular muscle that covers all of the lumbar region and the lower lateral half of the thoracic region of the back. It arises mainly from the dorsal layer of the thoracolumbar fascia, which connects the muscle to the spinous processes of the lower thoracic, lumbar, and sacral vertebrae. It also arises from the iliac crest and from the lower 3 ribs. It runs obliquely toward the shoulder region. It covers the upper seven-eighths of the posterior abdominal wall and the inferior half of the posterolateral thoracic wall. After passing under the inferior border of the teres major, it inserts into the base of the intertubercular groove of the humerus by means of a 6-cm-long quadrilateral tendon. The muscle extends, adducts, and rotates the arm medially and draws the shoulder posteriorly and inferiorly. It is supplied by the thoracodorsal nerve.

Vertical fibers of the **external oblique muscle,** which run from the lateral segments of the lower ribs to the iliac crest, are the most lateral muscular fibers of the superficial layer of the posterolateral abdominal wall. Lying lateral to the latissimus dorsi is **Petit's inferior lumbar triangle,** bounded laterally by the external oblique muscle, medially by the latissimus dorsi muscle, and inferiorly by the crest of the

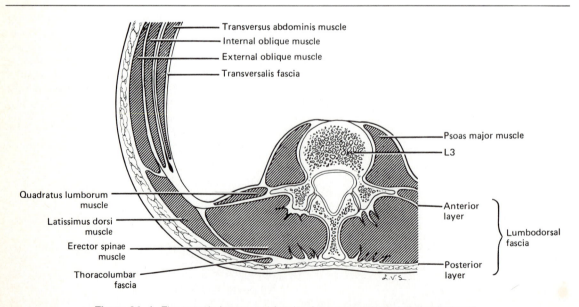

Transversus abdominis muscle
Internal oblique muscle
External oblique muscle
Transversalis fascia

Psoas major muscle
L3

Quadratus lumborum muscle
Latissimus dorsi muscle
Erector spinae muscle
Thoracolumbar fascia

Anterior layer
Lumbodorsal fascia
Posterior layer

Figure 24–1. The muscle layers and fascia of the posterolateral abdominal wall.

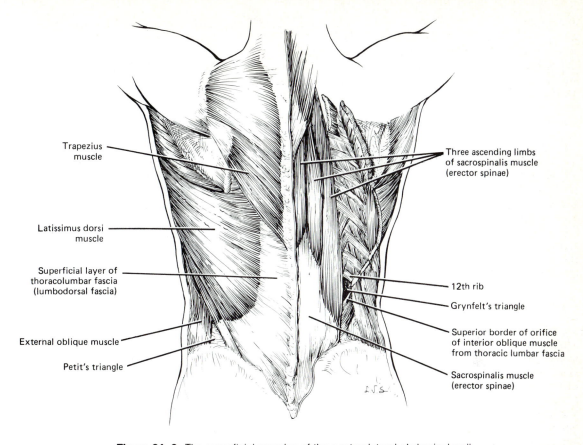

Trapezius
muscle

Latissimus dorsi
muscle

Superficial layer of
thoracolumbar fascia
(lumbodorsal fascia)

External oblique muscle

Petit's triangle

Three ascending limbs
of sacrospinalis muscle
(erector spinae)

12th rib

Grynfelt's triangle

Superior border of orifice
of interior oblique muscle
from thoracic lumbar fascia

Sacrospinalis muscle
(erector spinae)

Figure 24–2. The superficial muscles of the posterolateral abdominal wall.

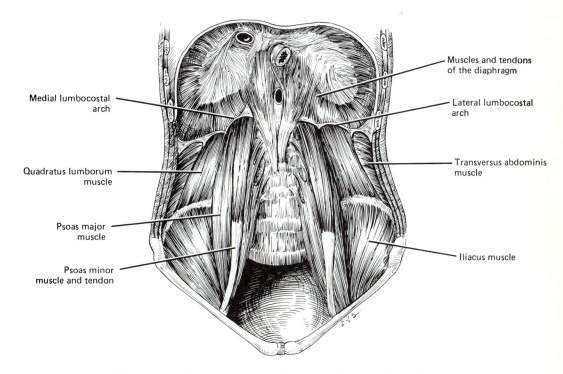

Medial lumbocostal
arch

Quadratus lumborum
muscle

Psoas major
muscle

Psoas minor
muscle and tendon

Muscles and tendons
of the diaphragm

Lateral lumbocostal
arch

Transversus abdominis
muscle

Iliacus muscle

Figure 24–3. The deep muscles of the posterior abdominal wall.

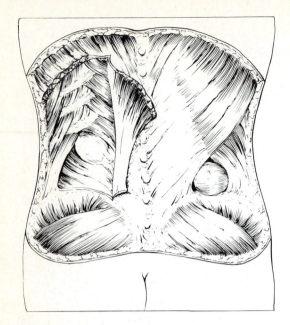

Figure 24–4. Anatomic relationships of lumbar or dorsal hernia. (Adapted from Netter.) On the left, lumbar or dorsal hernia into space of Grynfelt. On the right, hernia into Petit's triangle (inferior lumbar space).

ilium. The floor of the triangle is the internal oblique muscle.

➡ *Petit's triangle. (Fig 24–4.) Petit's lumbar triangle lies inferior to the usual site of genitourinary surgical incisions in the posterolateral abdominal wall. Spontaneous herniations of retroperitoneal contents occasionally make their way through this triangle, but postoperative herniations do not present in the triangle.*

Middle Layer
(Fig 24–2)

The middle layer of the posterolateral abdominal wall consists of 2 muscles: The lumbar group of **erector spinae (sacrospinalis) muscles** are the great extensors of the lumbodorsal segment of the vertebral column. They lie on either side of the spinous processes of the lumbar vertebrae. The fibers are completely covered dorsally by the latissimus dorsi. The muscles are sheathed by the ventral and dorsal layers of the thoracolumbar fascia. All lumbar erector spinae muscles function together as a single muscle. There is a superficial group, whose fibers run laterally as they ascend alongside the lumbar spine; and a deeper group, whose fibers run medially as they ascend. The superficial group includes the 3 long columns of muscle into which the erector spinae divides as it reaches the upper lumbar region; the iliocostalis, the longissimus, and the medial column. The deep

group is composed solely of the multifidus muscles. All of the lumbar erector spinae muscles are supplied by branches of the dorsal primary divisions of the spinal nerves.

The most posterior fibers of the **internal oblique muscle** arise from the fused ventral and dorsal layers of the thoracolumbar fasciae. The configuration of the muscles in this mid layer of the posterolateral abdominal wall is responsible for formation of the superior or surgical lumbar space of Grynfelt. The base of the space is formed by the lateral segment of the 12th rib. The space is bounded posteriorly by the erector spinae muscles and laterally by the internal oblique muscle close to its origin in the thoracolumbar fascia. The triangle lies superior and medial to the inferior lumbar triangle and is covered by the latissimus dorsi muscle. The floor of the triangle is the transversus abdominis aponeurosis.

➡ *Grynfelt's triangle. (Fig 24–4.) The superior lumbar triangle of Grynfelt is the usual route used for a posterior approach to the kidneys, suprarenal glands, and upper ureters. On occasion, postoperative herniations make their way to the surface through this triangle, and a perirenal or a subphrenic abscess may point through it.*

Deep Layer
(Fig 24–3)

The deep muscles of the posterolateral abdominal wall lie dorsal to the posterior peritoneum of the abdominal cavity, the posterior lining abdominal fascia, and the retroperitoneal organs. From medial to lateral, the muscles of this layer are the (1) psoas major, (2) psoas minor, (3) iliacus, (4) quadratus lumborum, and (5) that portion of the transversus abdominis muscle that forms the posterolateral abdominal wall.

The **psoas major muscle** arises from the anterior border of the body of T12, from the transverse process of T12, and also from all 5 lumbar vertebrae. Its fleshy body lies just lateral to the bodies of these vertebrae. It also arises from the surfaces of the bodies and intervertebral disks of T12–L4. It is a long roughly fusiform muscle, which passes inferiorly and slightly laterally. As it crosses the lesser pelvic brim, it becomes tendinous. The psoas major tendon receives most of the descending fibers of the iliacus muscle just above the insertion of the psoas tendon into the lesser trochanter. The psoas major is the great flexor of the hip joint; it also flexes the lumbar vertebrae and moves them laterally. Crossing the ventral surface of the psoas major muscle at the level of L1 is the tendinous medial lumbocostal arch.

➡ *Psoas abscesses. (Fig 24–5.) The psoas major muscle runs from the lumbar vertebrae inferi-*

orly to the lesser trochanter of the femur. This is the pathway along which lumbar vertebral abscesses or abscesses secondary to Crohn's disease of the ileum reach the inguinal ligament. Such an abscess may be palpated or visualized in the groin either just below or just above the ligament. The psoas abscess may be mistaken for an inguinal or femoral hernia, a saphenous varix, or adenitis of the supra- or infrainguinal lymph nodes.

The **psoas minor muscle** is long and thin and lies ventral to the medial portion of the psoas major. It arises from the lateral surfaces of T12 and L1 and from the intervening disk and runs inferiorly to insert by a long flat tendon into the pectineal line of the pelvis and the adjacent iliacus fascia. In about 30% of people, the muscle is absent. The psoas minor assists in flexion of the lumbar vertebrae. Both the psoas major and the psoas minor muscles are supplied by ventral rami from the lumbar plexus (L1–3).

The **iliacus,** a thin triangular muscle, occupies most of the iliac fossa. It arises from the bed of the iliac fossa, from the iliac crest, and from the base of the sacrum. Its fibers narrow to an apex, and near the inguinal ligament they insert into the tendon of the psoas major muscle. The iliacus assists the psoas major muscle in flexion of the hip joint. The combined iliacus and psoas major muscles and their tendons pass under the lateral half of the inguinal ligament as they course to their insertion on the lesser trochanter. The iliacus is supplied by branches from the femoral nerve (L2, 3).

The **quadratus lumborum** is a square, central muscle of the deep layer of the dorsolateral abdominal wall. It occupies the area between the psoas muscles and the tendon of origin of the transversus abdominis. It arises from the iliac crest and inserts into about half of the inferior surface of the 12th rib and into the transverse processes of lumbar vertebrae L1–4. Crossing the ventral surface of the quadratus lumborum muscle is the fibrous lateral lumbocostal arch, which runs from the tip of the transverse process of L1 to the tip of the 12th rib. From this arch arise the most lateral of the posterior fibers of the diaphragm. The quadratus lumborum is supplied by branches from T12 to L2. It draws the 12th rib toward the pelvis and the lumbar vertebrae toward the ipsilateral side.

The **transversus abdominis** arises from the fused ventral and dorsal layers of the thoracolumbar fascia lateral to the lateral border of the erector spinae muscles. (See Chapter 23 for a more complete discussion of this muscle.)

Deep Fascia

External to the dorsal peritoneum but ventral to the deep layer of the dorsal abdominal wall muscles are the lumbar and iliacus fasciae. Lying ventral to

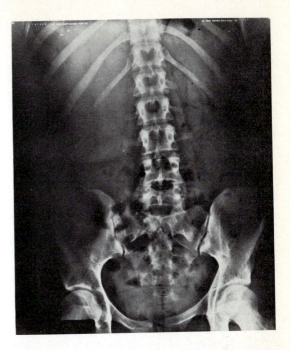

Figure 24–5. Obliteration of the psoas shadow on the right by a subhepatic abscess. (Reproduced, with permission, from Way LW [editor]: *Current Surgical Diagnosis & Treatment,* 6th ed. Lange, 1983.)

these 2 fasciae but dorsal to the posterior peritoneum are the important visceral and vascular structures of the retroperitoneum.

II. THE RETROPERITONEUM

GROSS ANATOMY

The retroperitoneum is the segment of the abdominal cavity that lies dorsal to the posterior peritoneum and ventral to the dorsal lining fascia. It contains portions of the gastrointestinal tract, the kidneys and ureters, the suprarenal glands, the **abdominal aorta** and its branches, the **inferior vena cava** and its tributaries, the **lumbar plexus** and its most immediate branches, the **abdominal sympathetic chain** and its ganglia, the great complex of retroperitoneal lymph channels and lymph nodes, and the **cisterna chyli.** The anatomy of the kidneys, ureters, and suprarenal glands will be discussed in Chapter 37.

BLOOD VESSELS, LYMPHATICS, & NERVES

Arteries
(Fig 24–6)

The abdominal aorta begins at the aortic hiatus of the diaphragm at the level of T12 and extends inferiorly about 9.5–10.5 cm to the level of L4, where it bifurcates into the right and left common iliac arteries.

➠ *Visualization of the abdominal aorta. In the past, the aorta was visualized by injecting dye into the aorta via a dorsal cutaneous puncture at L1 or L2. This is now done by inserting a catheter into the femoral artery at the groin and advancing to the proper level for visualization of the aorta and its branches.*

Dorsally, the abdominal aorta is closely related to the left side of the lumbar vertebral bodies and the left crus of the diaphragm. To the right side of the aorta is the inferior vena cava. The left lumbar sympathetic chain and its ganglia lie just lateral to the aorta, a position that usually does not impair its surgical removal. In contrast, the right lumbar sympathetic chain lies dorsal to the inferior vena cava, a position that makes both viewing and operating on

the chain difficult. Ventrally, the 2 most important relationships of the abdominal aorta are (1) to the root of the mesentery of the small bowel containing the superior mesenteric vessels and many lymphatics, and (2) to the transverse and ascending portions of the duodenum. The root of the mesentery of the small bowel crosses the ventral surface of the aorta obliquely from left to right and must be displaced superiorly to expose the upper abdominal aorta. The third and fourth portions of the duodenum lie ventral to the aorta just above the level of origin of the renal arteries. (See Chapter 26.) The left renal vein crosses the ventral surface of the aorta on its way to the hilum of the left kidney.

➠ *Pressure from abdominal aneurysm. An expanding fusiform abdominal aortic aneurysm may impinge upon and erode the left lateral surfaces of the lumbar vertebrae, but this is less common than erosion of thoracic vertebrae by a saccular aneurysm of the thoracic aorta.*

➠ *Injury to inferior vena cava during aortic surgery. The abdominal aorta and the inferior vena cava are so close together in the lower abdomen that the vena cava or left common iliac vein is easily injured in surgery for treatment of an abdominal aneurysm below the level of the kidneys. Consequently, the sac of the aneurysm is not removed but merely opened.*

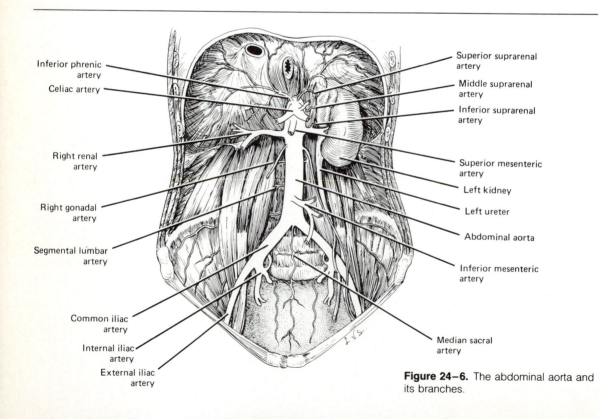

Inferior phrenic artery
Celiac artery
Right renal artery
Right gonadal artery
Segmental lumbar artery
Common iliac artery
Internal iliac artery
External iliac artery

Superior suprarenal artery
Middle suprarenal artery
Inferior suprarenal artery
Superior mesenteric artery
Left kidney
Left ureter
Abdominal aorta
Inferior mesenteric artery
Median sacral artery

Figure 24–6. The abdominal aorta and its branches.

➠ ***Relationship of the transverse and ascending duodenum to the aorta.*** *The transverse duodenum lies just ventral to the abdominal aorta close to the site of most aneurysms. These aneurysms may rupture directly into the transverse duodenum. If the anastomosis of the superior segment of the aorta to the prosthesis used to replace the diseased aorta should rupture, the blood may pour directly into the transverse duodenum, causing massive upper gastrointestinal hemorrhage.*

Arteries

The dorsolateral region of the abdominal wall is supplied segmentally by the subcostal and lumbar arteries, branches of the lower thoracic and abdominal segments of the aorta.

The abdominal aorta gives off several branches. The visceral branches of the abdominal aorta (from superior to inferior) are the celiac, the superior mesenteric, the middle suprarenal, renal, testicular or ovarian, and inferior mesenteric arteries. The parietal branches of the abdominal aorta (from superior to inferior) are the inferior phrenic arteries, the 4 paired segmental lumbar arteries, and the median sacral artery.

Veins
(Fig 24–7)

The **inferior vena cava** is the large collecting vein that carries blood returning from the legs, perineum, pelvis, kidneys, suprarenal glands, and lower half of the abdominal walls back to the heart. The vena cava lies in the retroperitoneum parallel to and 1.5–2 cm to the right of the abdominal aorta. It begins at the level of L5, just to the right of the right common iliac artery, and is formed by the junction of the left and right common iliac veins. The inferior vena cava leaves the abdomen through its hiatus in the right leaf of the central tendon of the diaphragm at the level of T8. Dorsal to the right lateral border of the inferior vena cava is the right lumbar sympathetic chain and its ganglia. Also dorsal to the inferior vena cava are the right lateral surfaces of the lumbar vertebral bodies and their transverse processes and the medial edge of the right psoas major muscle. Near the junction of the inferior vena cava and the renal veins, the right crus of the diaphragm intervenes between it and the abdominal aorta. At the level of the epiploic foramen, the inferior vena cava lies deep to the posterior boundary of the lesser peritoneal sac. Thus, the inferior vena cava at the epiploic foramen level is separated by 2 layers of peritoneum from the portal vein that lies just ventral to the epiploic foramen between the 2 layers of the hepatoduodenal ligament. Just below the diaphragm, the inferior vena cava lies very close to the dorsal surface of the liver and forms the left border of the bare area of the liver. Immediately after passing through the caval diaphragmatic hiatus, the cava enters the pericardial sac.

Venous flow returns from the posterolateral abdominal wall via venous plexuses that lie external to the vertebral column or lie within the vertebral canal. The venous plexuses external to the vertebral

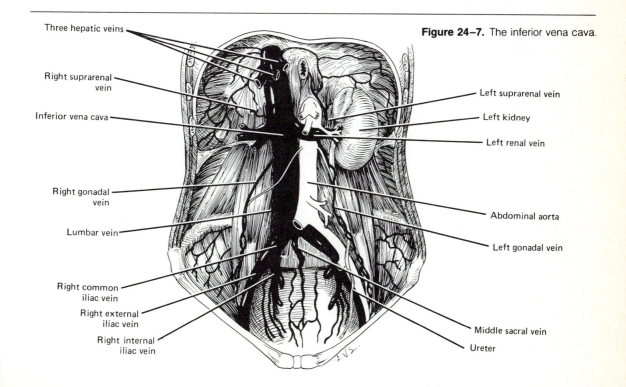

Figure 24–7. The inferior vena cava.

Three hepatic veins

Right suprarenal vein

Inferior vena cava

Right gonadal vein

Lumbar vein

Right common iliac vein

Right external iliac vein

Right internal iliac vein

Left suprarenal vein

Left kidney

Left renal vein

Abdominal aorta

Left gonadal vein

Middle sacral vein

Ureter

canal drain into the lumbar veins that empty into the inferior vena cava. Veins within the vertebral canal drain into the **intervertebral veins** that pass outward from the vertebral canal along with the spinal nerves. These veins join with the external vertebral veins, and the combined venous blood drains first into the **lower intercostal, lumbar,** and **lateral sacral veins** and then into the inferior vena cava.

⟶ *Role of the vena cava in the passage of emboli. The inferior vena cava is the major pathway of venous emboli from the lower extremity, the pelvis, the perineum, and the posterolateral abdominal wall to the right heart and thence to the lungs. Ligation, plication, or placement of an umbrella filter in the inferior vena cava is done in an attempt to block the upward passage of emboli. Surgical interruption or diminution of caval flow must be done at a level below the entrance of the renal veins into the inferior vena cava. The gonadal venous flow into the left renal vein or the inferior cava should be interrupted when pelvic and perineal sites for the formation of emboli are suspected. This is particularly important on the left side, where the gonadal veins empty directly into the left renal vein.*

⟶ *Hyperalimentation via the vena cava. During the past decade, indwelling catheters have been placed in the superior (via the subclavian vein) and inferior vena cava (via the femoral vein) to be used for the infusion of high-caloric nourishment and other supplements into the patient unable to take nourishment by mouth.*

⟶ *Vascular complications of surgical procedures on the lumbar intervertebral disks. Surgical procedures on the upper lumbar intervertebral disks via the posterior approach may, if the surgeon proceeds too far ventrally, injure the lower aorta, the inferior vena cava, or the common iliac artery or vein. Such iatrogenic vascular trauma may result in severe retroperitoneal hemorrhage that is extremely difficult to control by the dorsal approach.*

The inferior vena cava receives visceral and parietal venous tributaries. Blood from the lower extremities is carried by the 2 external iliac veins; blood from the pelvis and the perineum is carried by the internal iliac veins. The internal and external iliac veins join to form the common iliac veins. The 2 common iliac veins join to form the inferior vena cava. The inferior vena cava drains blood from the dorsolateral abdominal wall by 4 paired lumbar veins. From the inferior surface of the diaphragm it receives the right inferior phrenic vein directly; the left inferior phrenic vein may drain directly or via the left suprare-

nal or left renal vein. From the viscera of the retroperitoneum, the inferior vena cava receives blood from the long left renal vein and the short right renal vein. It receives a direct right suprarenal vein, and the left suprarenal venous return is via left renal veins. The inferior vena cava also drains some small ureteral veins, the middle and the inferior rectal veins of the perineum. The anorectal junction is one of the areas of portocaval anastomosis. On the right side, the gonadal veins join the right side of the inferior vena cava at an oblique angle; on the left side, they join with the left renal vein at a right angle.

The 3 or 4 short hepatic veins that empty directly from the liver into the inferior vena cava at the level of the diaphragm are described in Chapter 31.

Lymphatics
(Fig 24–8)

Many lymphatic chains and lymph nodes are placed in the retroperitoneum. The large, preaortic nodes lie close to the ventral surface of the abdominal aorta. They are divided into the celiac, superior mesenteric, lumbar, and iliac inferior mesenteric lymphatic plexuses. The lymphatics draining the cutaneous areas of the dorsolateral abdominal wall drain primarily into the inguinal nodes.

The lymphatics of the stomach, liver, pancreas, and spleen drain into the deep nodes of the **celiac plexus,** as do several connecting channels from the superior mesenteric chain of nodes.

The **superior mesenteric nodes** are divided into the (1) mesenteric, (2) ileocolic, and (3) mesocolic nodal groups. They drain the small bowel, the cecum, the appendix, the ascending colon, the right three-fourths of the transverse colon, and the adjacent mesenteries. They receive lymphatic drainage from the pancreas and the spleen. Lymph channels ascend from the inferior to the superior mesenteric nodes.

The **inferior mesenteric nodes** drain the left side of the colon, the sigmoid colon, and the upper three-fourths of the rectum and the adjacent mesenteries of these segments of the large bowel.

Retroperitoneal lymphatics and nodes lie on either side of the midline at lumbar height, called the right and left lumbar lymphatic chains. The lumbar lymphatic nodes and vessels lie in lateral aortic, preaortic, and retroaortic positions. The left lumbar chain parallels the left border of the abdominal aorta and lies dorsal to that vessel. These nodes receive drainage from the left iliac nodes. The right and left lumbar nodes drain upward into the cisterna chyli. The right lumbar chain of nodes is closely related to all surfaces of the inferior vena cava. These nodes are fed by the right external iliac and hypogastric nodes and are of particular importance in the spread of cancer from the right testis.

⟶ *Lymphangiography of retroperitoneal lymphatics. The retroperitoneal lymphatics play an important role in the upward spread of pri-*

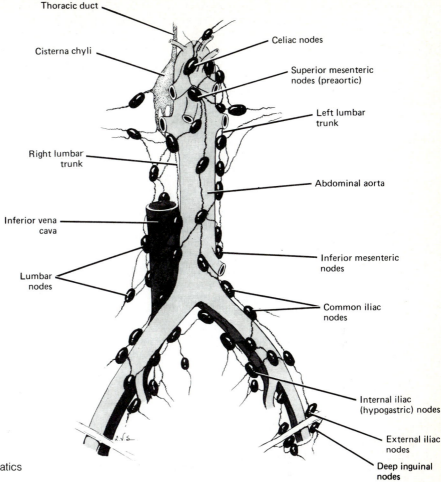

Figure 24–8. The lymphatics of the retroperitoneum.

mary malignant disease from the lower extremities, pelvis, perineum, and external genitalia. The ability of the surgeon to completely dissect and remove all lymphatic channels and nodes in the lower and mid retroperitoneal areas has greatly increased the survival rate in such cases. Lymphangiography and CT scanning permit imaging of the retroperitoneal lymphatic system and ascertain both the level of spread and the primary sites of malignancies, as well as to assess the possible benefits of retroperitoneal lymphatic dissection.

Lymphatic drainage from the **left kidney** empties into the left lumbar nodal group at the level of the left renal vein. Lymphatic drainage from the **right kidney** is into the right renal nodes interspersed among the right renal vessels close to the right kidney hilum. Drainage from the **suprarenal glands** is into the highest group of lumbar nodes, which lies just inferior to the origin of the celiac artery.

⟶ **Retrograde lymphatic flow into the suprarenal lymphatics.** The connections between the posteroinferior mediastinal lymphatics and the lymphatics draining the suprarenal glands are of clinical importance. There may be retrograde lymphatic extension from the lungs to the suprarenals in cancer of the lung and in pulmonary tuberculosis. Such retrograde extension may result in destruction of the suprarenals by tumor or infections (Waterhouse-Friderichsen syndrome).

The lymphatics that drain the **testes** flow superiorly as a frequently anastomosing set of small vessels accompanying the pampiniform plexus of veins in the spermatic cord. On the right side, they terminate in nodes lying in the angle formed by the junction of the right renal vein with the inferior vena cava. On the left side, testicular lymph flows to the para-aortic nodes just below the level of the left renal vein. A small amount of lymph from the left testicle runs to the inferior mesenteric nodes. Occasionally, a small amount of left testicular lymph follows the vas deferens into the pelvis and enters the left external iliac nodes.

➠ **Surgery for cancer of left testis.** *The pattern of left testicular lymphatic drainage demands that all primary nodal areas reached by the lymph be removed, along with removal of the para-aortic nodes as high as the level of the left renal vein (radical lymph gland dissection for cancer of the left testicle).*

Lymphatic drainage from the **ovaries** closely follows the superior course of the ovarian veins. On the left, the lymph empties into nodes lying about the aorta at the level of the renal vein; on the right, it empties into nodes along the inferior vena cava at the level of the right renal vein.

The **cisterna (receptaculum) chyli** is the large lymphatic sac into which drain the major lymphatic trunks that run superiorly in the retroperitoneum. It lies on the ventral surface of L2 and the right crus of the diaphragm, dorsal and to the right of the abdominal aorta. It is formed mainly by the junction of the right and left lumbar lymphatic trunks with the major intestinal lymphatic trunks. The thoracic duct leaves the superior margin of the cisterna chyli and passes through the right side of the aortic hiatus of the diaphragm into the thoracic cavity.

➠ **Injury to the cisterna chyli.** *The cisterna chyli or the abdominal segment of the thoracic duct (or both) may be injured by trauma to the abdominal walls. Chylous ascites may ensue. Because the cisterna chyli lies directly on L2, any sudden convulsive flexion or extension of the vertebral column close to this level may result in rupture of this lymphatic structure.*

Nerves
(Fig 24–9)

The **lumbar plexus** is the massive complex of the primary spinal nerves and their branchings that occupies the lumbar retroperitoneum. It lies ventral to the transverse processes of the lumbar vertebrae

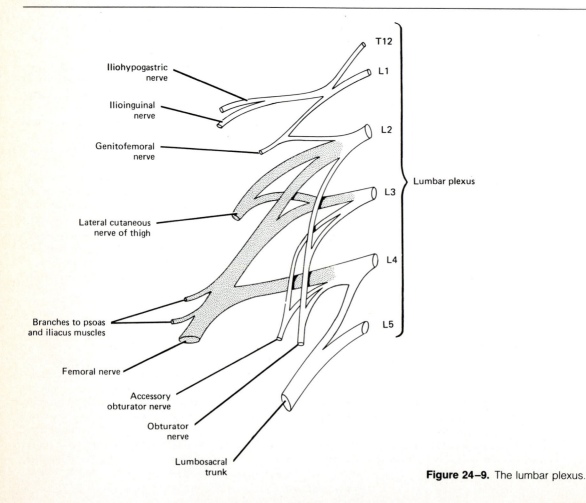

Figure 24–9. The lumbar plexus.

and either within or just dorsal to the psoas major muscle. The plexus results from union of the ventral primary divisions of lumbar spinal nerves L1–4 plus a twig from T12, which joins with L1. Nerve L1, joined by the small branch from T12, divides into superior and inferior divisions. The superior division gives rise to the ilioinguinal and iliohypogastric nerves; the inferior division, joined by a twig from L2, forms the genitofemoral nerve. Nerves L2, L3, and L4 each divide into a small ventral and a large dorsal branch. All 3 ventral divisions join to form the obturator nerve. Of the dorsal divisions of L2 and L3, the 2 smaller branches join to form the lateral femoral cutaneous nerve, while the 2 larger branches join the dorsal branch of L4 to form the femoral nerve. A large segment of the fourth lumbar nerve joins with the fifth lumbar nerve to form the lumbosacral trunk. The iliohypogastric, ilioinguinal, and genitofemoral nerves supply the lower lateral portion of the anterolateral abdominal wall; the lateral femoral cutaneous, obturator, and femoral nerves supply motor and cutaneous innervation to the anterior medial and lateral thigh. In about 20% of people, a small accessory obturator nerve is present. It arises from the anterior divisions of L3 and L4, crosses the superior pubic ramus, and supplies the pectineus muscle that adducts, flexes, and medially rotates the thigh. The genitofemoral nerve innervates the cremaster muscle and the scrotum and vulva and the upper inner surface of the thigh.

⇒ *Anesthesia of ilioinguinal and iliohypogastric nerves. The ilioinguinal and iliohypogastric branches of the lumbar plexus are the specific nerves that must be anesthesized in order to perform hernioplasty under local anesthesia. The local anesthetic is delivered to these nerves along a line running from the anterosuperior iliac spine to the umbilicus. The ilioinguinal nerve lies one fingerbreadth medial to the anterosuperior iliac spine, while the iliohypogastric nerve lies one fingerbreadth farther medially along that line.*

⇒ *Ilioinguinal and iliohypogastric nerve damage during appendectomy. During appendectomy, care must be taken not to cut the ilioinguinal or iliohypogastric nerves and not to retract them too strongly, because this may lead to painful neuroma or muscular weakness of the right inguinal region of the abdominal wall.*

⇒ *Obturator nerve branches to hip and knee joint. The obturator branch of the lumbar plexus gives branches to the hip and knee joint. As a consequence, pain from a diseased hip joint will often be referred to the area of the medial surface of the knee joint. Thus, in cases of pain around either the knee or the hip, both*

joints must be thoroughly checked for disease. Obturator neurectomy performed intrapelvically may be done for the relief of painful neuritis. Obturator neuritis is characterized by adductor spasm and pain referred to the upper anterior and medial surfaces of the thigh.

The **lumbar sympathetic chain** (Fig 24–10) enters the upper retroperitoneum posterior to the medial lumbocostal arch and comes to lie just lateral to the vertebral bodies on the ventral surface of the psoas major muscle, which separates the chain from the transverse processes of the lumbar vertebrae. Inferiorly, the lumbar sympathetic chain is continuous with the pelvic sympathetic chain. There are 2–5 lumbar sympathetic ganglia. The first lumbar ganglion lies at the level of the medial lumbocostal arch and is not easily accessible at operation. The left lumbar chain lies just lateral to the abdominal aorta; the right chain is hidden behind the inferior vena cava. The second lumbar ganglion is usually the largest of the group, relatively constant in position, and thus it serves as a landmark. The fifth lumbar sympathetic ganglion is usually hidden behind the common iliac artery and vein. The chain is responsible in great part for maintenance of vascular tone of the vessels of the pelvis and lower extremities.

⇒ *Surgery on the lumbar sympathetic chain. The usual approach to the lumbar sympathetic chain and its ganglia is via a midlateral abdominal muscle-splitting incision that allows the surgeon to enter the retroperitoneum via an extraperitoneal route. The chain may also be approached via the anterior transperitoneal route. The lumbar sympathetic ganglia most often removed are the second, third, and fourth, along with the intervening segments of the lumbar sympathetic chain. Lumbar sympathectomy is an adjuvant procedure in vasospastic disease of the lower extremities. It is also used occasionally for relief of causalgia and hyperhidrosis in the lower extremity or perineum. Its use as a primary vascular procedure has diminished markedly.*

The branches of the lumbar sympathetic chain are the gray rami communicantes that pass through the celiac plexus, and the lumbar splanchnic nerves.

In the retroperitoneum are many complicated nerve plexuses consisting of a mixture of sympathetic and parasympathetic fibers. Several of these plexuses are extensive, and nearly all of them are clustered around the major blood vessels of the retroperitoneum. The fibers from the plexuses accompany the distal branches of the retroperitoneal vessels to the terminal areas supplied by them.

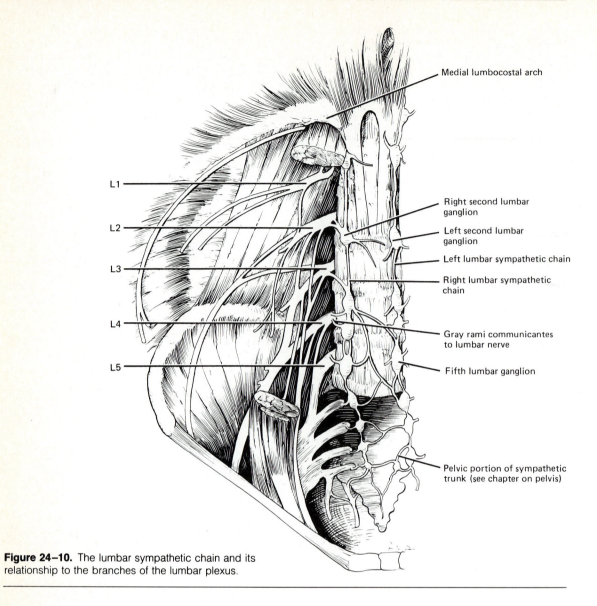

Figure 24–10. The lumbar sympathetic chain and its relationship to the branches of the lumbar plexus.

The major autonomic plexus is the **celiac plexus.** It lies on the ventral surface of the abdominal aorta at the level of L1 and is composed of 2 large ganglia and a maze of nerve fibers closely allied to the origins of the celiac and superior mesenteric arteries. The celiac plexus lies just anterior to the arcuate ligament of the diaphragm.

⇒ *Use of arcuate ligament in retention of reduced sliding hiatus hernia. Since the thick, ropy celiac autonomic nerve plexus lies just anterior to the arcuate ligament of the diaphragm, the 2 structures are used jointly for placement of fixation sutures for the Hill repair (posterior gastropexy) of sliding esophageal hiatus hernia.*

Many **secondary autonomic plexuses** (Fig 24–11) originate in the celiac plexus and lie in the retroperitoneum close to the major branches of the abdominal aorta.

(1) The **phrenic plexus,** whose fibers accompany the inferior phrenic arteries and add to the nerve supply of the diaphragm.

(2) The **hepatic plexus,** from which fibers accompany the hepatic artery to the liver.

(3) The **splenic plexus,** with fibers accompanying the splenic artery to the spleen.

(4) The **superior gastric plexus,** from which fibers run with the left gastric artery to the stomach.

(5) The **suprarenal plexus,** which receives fibers both from the phrenic plexus and from the greater splanchnic nerve and sends preganglionic sympathetic fibers to the medulla of the suprarenal gland.

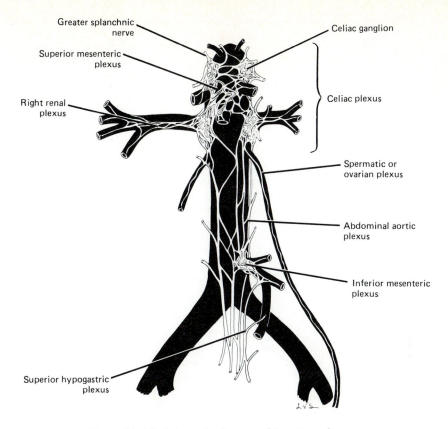

Figure 24–11. Autonomic plexuses of the retroperitoneum.

(6) The **renal plexus,** which receives fibers from the aorticorenal plexus, the lesser splanchnic nerve, and the celiac plexus and whose fibers run with the renal artery to the kidney.

(7) The **spermatic plexus** in the male and the **ovarian plexus** in the female, whose fibers accompany the testicular and ovarian arteries to the testes, ovaries, uterine tubes, and uterus.

(8) The **superior mesenteric plexus,** an inferior portion of the celiac plexus, whose fibers run with the superior mesenteric artery to all areas supplied by that vessel.

(9) The **inferior mesenteric plexus** surrounds and runs with the inferior mesenteric artery to the areas supplied by the artery.

(10) The **superior and inferior hypogastric plexuses,** which lie ventral to the terminal aorta and the common iliac arteries. The fibers run to the vessels and viscera of the pelvis.

The stomach is the dilated portion of the alimentary tube situated between the abdominal esophagus and the duodenum. It begins at the cardia, which normally lies to the left of the vertebral column at the level of the disk between T10 and T11, and ends by becoming the first portion of the duodenum, which lies to the right of the right diaphragmatic crus at the level of L1.

EMBRYOLOGY
(Fig 25–1)

During the fourth week of fetal life, the stomach first appears as a widened area of the foregut. It is first positioned in the cervical region but gradually descends through the thorax to take its final intra-abdominal position. To arrive at its final position, it first rotates 90 degrees around a vertical axis. As a result of this rotation, the dorsal mesogastrium moves to the left, the movement creating the omental bursa. As a result of a second gastric rotation around an anteroposterior axis, the pyloric segment of the stomach moves to the right and superiorly while the proximal portion moves to the left. The gastric cavity then runs from superior left to inferior right.

Failure of complete descent of the proximal foregut from the cervical area results in the anomaly known as thoracic stomach. Congenital hypertrophic pyloric stenosis may also occur. Rare anomalies include congenital diverticula of the stomach and enteric cysts of the stomach.

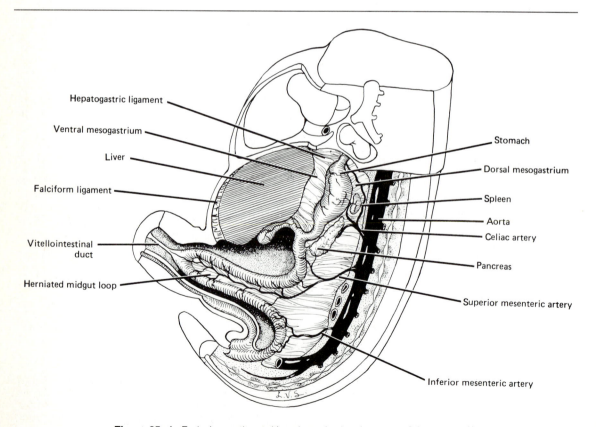

Figure 25–1. Early (seventh week) embryonic development of the stomach.

Labels: Hepatogastric ligament, Ventral mesogastrium, Liver, Falciform ligament, Vitellointestinal duct, Herniated midgut loop, Stomach, Dorsal mesogastrium, Spleen, Aorta, Celiac artery, Pancreas, Superior mesenteric artery, Inferior mesenteric artery

GROSS ANATOMY

SIZE, SHAPE, & POSITION OF THE STOMACH
(Fig 25–2)

Gastric shape and size are extremely variable and are modified by many factors, including the state of gastric physiologic activity; the amount and character of the gastric contents, individual eating habits, changes in the position and tension of the surrounding viscera and of the adjacent gastric supporting ligaments; and the presence of gastric disorders such as linitis plastica or acute gastric dilatation.

Normally, the stomach is positioned mainly in the left hypochondrium and the epigastrium, but its position may vary markedly, either as a physiologic anatomic difference or as a result of disease. The anatomic factors that tend to maintain the stomach in its normal position are the following: (1) attachment of the stomach to the relatively immobile abdominal esophagus; (2) attachment to the relatively immobile distal half of the first portion of the duodenum; (3) the suspensory action of the hepatogastric ligament; (4) the supporting sling action of the transverse colon and transverse mesocolon, on which the stomach normally rests; (5) the arterial supply to the stomach from the relatively immobile celiac artery; (6) intra-abdominal pressure, which pushes the small intestine upward against the greater curvature of the stomach; (7) the **gastrosplenic ligament,** which connects the

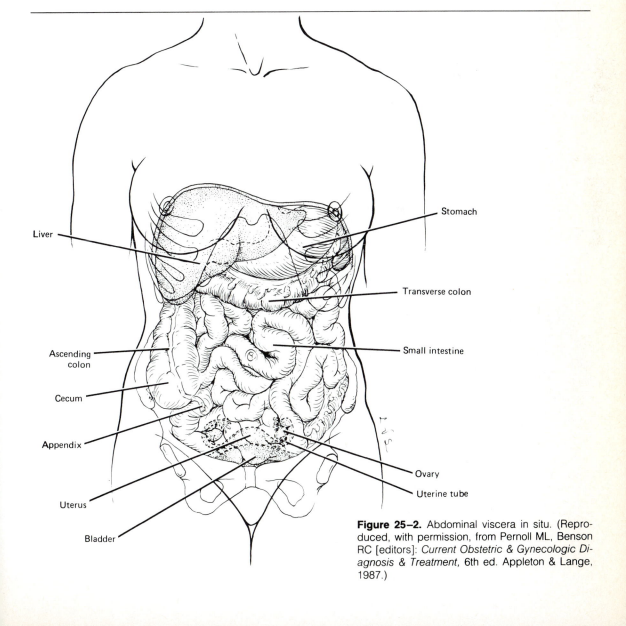

Figure 25–2. Abdominal viscera in situ. (Reproduced, with permission, from Pernoll ML, Benson RC [editors]: *Current Obstetric & Gynecologic Diagnosis & Treatment,* 6th ed. Appleton & Lange, 1987.)

stomach to the relatively fixed spleen; and (8) the position and movement of the left leaf of the diaphragm, with particular regard to its sucking action on the adjacent **gastric fundus.**

DIVISIONS OF THE STOMACH
(Fig 25–3)

The stomach is divided into 8 anatomic areas.

Lesser Curvature

The lesser curvature of the stomach begins at the right inferior border of the abdominal esophagus and follows the esophagogastric curve to the right to the superior border of the pylorus; it is suspended by the hepatogastric ligament and faces superiorly and to the right.

⟹ *Mallory-Weiss syndrome affecting gastric lesser curvature. The area of the lesser curvature of the stomach just distal to the gastro-*

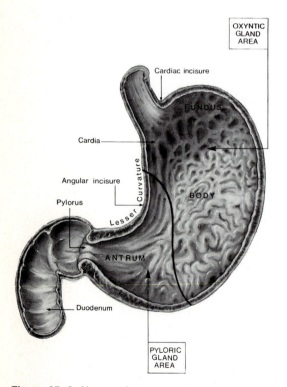

Figure 25–3. Names of the parts of the stomach. The line drawn from the lesser to the greater curvature depicts the approximate boundary between the oxyntic gland area and the pyloric gland area. No prominent landmark exists to distinguish between antrum and body (corpus). The fundus is the portion craniad to the esophagogastric junction. (Reproduced, with permission, from Way LW [editor]: *Current Surgical Diagnosis & Treatment*, 7th ed. Lange, 1985.)

esophageal junction is the site of mucosal and submucosal tears and bleeding in Mallory-Weiss syndrome. The tears are usually due to prolonged forceful vomiting, most commonly in alcoholics.

Greater Curvature

The greater curvature of the stomach is about 4 times as long as the lesser curvature. It begins at the left inferior border of the abdominal esophagus and follows the curve of the fundus and the convexly curving lower border of the gastric body to the right to the inferior surface of the pylorus. It faces inferiorly and to the left, except for its fundal surface, which faces superiorly, dorsally, and to the left.

Cardia

The cardia is the portion of the stomach in immediate juxtaposition to the abdominal esophagus. It therefore includes the proximal portion of the lesser curvature and the lower segment of the ascending portion of the gastric fundus. Palpation of the cardia reveals a marked difference in texture as compared to that of the lower esophagus. The cardia feels firm and resistant, whereas the lower esophagus is soft and spongy. The left free border of the hepatogastric ligament reaches the lesser curvature just below the esophagogastric junction. The left gastric artery reaches the lesser curvature by passing through the posterior layer of the gastrohepatic ligament close to the cardia of the stomach and the left free border of the ligament.

Fundus

The fundus of the stomach begins where the left termination of the esophagus meets the left segment of the cardia at an acute angle, the **cardiac incisure** of the stomach. The fundus rises from the cardiac incisure to a point beneath the left cupula of the diaphragm, rising as high as the fifth costal cartilage. When the fundus is fully expanded, it exerts pressure through the thin overlying diaphragm on the heart and on other adjacent mediastinal organs. The left side of the fundus is actually the superior segment of the greater curvature. The fundus is composed of layers of muscle (circular, longitudinal, and oblique) (Fig 25–3).

⟹ *Pressure of dilated gastric fundus on the diaphragm and the supradiaphragmatic structures. The pressure exerted by a dilated gastric fundus against the undersurface of the left leaf of the diaphragm is responsible for many gastric, cardiac, and pulmonary symptoms, all of which are usually promptly relieved by mechanical emptying of the stomach. The fundus may be dilated by gas, fluid, or food, singly or in any combination.*

Body

The body of the stomach is its largest subdivision, extending on the lesser curvature from the cardia to the superior border of the **angular incisure** (gastric notch), and on the greater curvature from the base of the fundus to a point below the angular incisure. The body comprises the central two-thirds of the stomach and is the part responsible for the elaboration of hydrochloric acid by its lining parietal cells. The angular incisure is formed by a pinching of both the lesser and greater curvature surfaces. It marks the termination of the gastric body and the beginning of the pyloric vestibule.

Pyloric Vestibule

The pyloric vestibule runs from the termination of the gastric notch (angular incisure) to the beginning of the pyloric antrum (sulcus intermedius gastricus). It is represented by a narrowing of the gastric lumen (by about two-thirds). It is about 5 cm long.

Pyloric Antrum

The pyloric antrum is the short thickened area of the stomach that begins about 3–4 cm proximal to the pylorus at the termination of the vestibule and runs to the right as far as the pylorus. It secretes gastrin, which stimulates the elaboration of acid in the gastric body.

Pylorus

The pylorus—the most distal segment of the stomach—is situated at the junction of the stomach and duodenum and is surrounded by a greatly thickened ring of gastric circular smooth muscle, the pyloric sphincter. The pyloric vein (of Mayo) lies at the serosal level on the anterior surface of the pylorus, and because of its relative anatomic constancy it acts as a landmark for the pyloric region. The pyloric ring is the narrowest segment of the gastric lumen. The right border of the hepatoduodenal ligament reaches the superior surface of the first part of the duodenum just distal to the pylorus.

⇢ *Enlargement of the gastric outlet by pyloroplasty.* (Fig 25–4.) *Heinecke-Mikulicz pyloroplasty, a method of enlarging the gastric outlet at the expense of the pyloric ring, is performed through a longitudinal incision over the ventral surface of the pylorus, 2.5 cm long on the duodenal side and 5 cm long on the gastric side of the pyloric ring. This allows the duodenal bulb to be explored. The longitudinal incision is then closed in a transverse direction, widening the pyloric aperture. The procedure is frequently used for improving emptying of the stomach after vagotomy. It is often the first step in the treatment of bleeding duodenal ulcer. The surgeon can inspect the bleeding ulcer and ligate it with sutures under direct vision before closing the pyloric lumen. Many surgeons pre-*

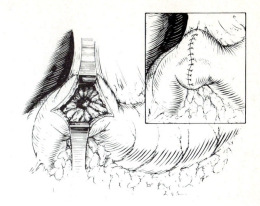

Figure 25–4. Heinecke-Mikulicz pyloroplasty. A longitudinal incision has been made across the pylorus, revealing an active ulcer in the duodenal bulb. The insert shows the transverse closure of the incision that widens the gastric outlet. The accompanying vagotomy is not shown. (Reproduced, with permission, from Way LW [editor]: *Current Surgical Diagnosis & Treatment,* 7th ed. Lange, 1985.)

fer pyloroplasty in combination with vagotomy as the first procedure of choice in treating an uncomplicated but medically intractable duodenal ulcer.

GASTRIC RELATIONSHIPS
(Figs 25–5 and 25–6)

Anterior Relationships

Anteriorly, the stomach is related to the free peritoneal cavity.

⇢ *Indications for gastrostomy. Gastrostomy was used during the first half of the 20th century to feed patients suffering from proximal stomach cancer or from any stricture blocking the gastric lumen. It was used also as a bypass procedure for obstructions of the lower esophagus. It is still used as an emergency procedure for feeding a patient with an obstructed esophagus. Gastrostomy also serves as a temporary bypass for patients suffering from caustic esophageal burns or severe esophageal spasm and in cases of congenital esophageal atresia. After a definitive curative procedure, the gastrostomy tube may be removed and the gastric opening allowed to close. Gastrostomy is occasionally used in place of a nasogastric tube in the elderly, the very young, and patients who have an anticipated prolonged and stormy postoperative course. Being able to feed a patient intravenously has greatly limited the indications for gastrostomy.*

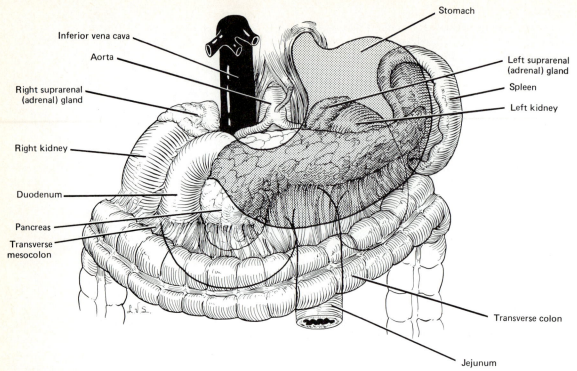

Inferior vena cava

Aorta

Right suprarenal
(adrenal) gland

Right kidney

Duodenum

Pancreas

Transverse
mesocolon

Stomach

Left suprarenal
(adrenal) gland

Spleen

Left kidney

Transverse colon

Jejunum

Figure 25–5. Gastric relationships. The stomach is made transparent to show its posterior relationship to the pancreas, spleen, and transverse mesocolon.

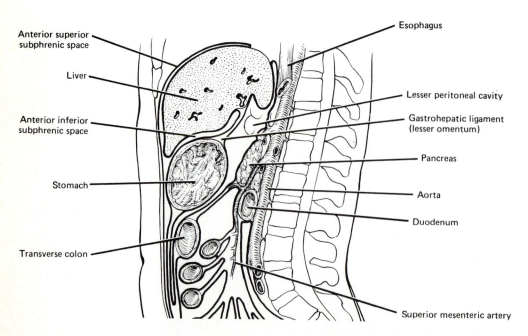

Anterior superior
subphrenic space

Liver

Anterior inferior
subphrenic space

Stomach

Transverse colon

Esophagus

Lesser peritoneal cavity

Gastrohepatic ligament
(lesser omentum)

Pancreas

Aorta

Duodenum

Superior mesenteric artery

Figure 25–6. The peritoneal reflections and location of the lesser peritoneal cavity.

Posterior Relationships

Posteriorly, the stomach is related to the enclosed peritoneal cavity. The entire posterior surface of the stomach constitutes the lower half of the anterior wall of the lesser sac. Posterior to the lesser sac lies the pancreas, with the splenic vessels running on its superoposterior surface. The pancreas is separated from the lesser sac and the stomach by the posterior peritoneum of the abdominal cavity, which covers its anterior surface. In health, the lesser sac is merely a potential space, since the peritoneum of the posterior surface of the stomach lies directly on the posterior peritoneum that covers the pancreas.

➠ *Relationship of posterior surface of stomach to lesser sac. Since the posterior surface of the stomach forms the anterior wall of the potential cavity of the lesser sac and the pancreas lies posterior to it, pancreatic pseudocysts and lesser sac abscesses tend to push the stomach anteriorly. The anterior displacement can usually be seen in a lateral x-ray view of the stomach. The posterior wall of the stomach is usually adherent to the pancreas after an attack of pancreatic inflammation.*

Relationships of the Lesser Curvature

The lesser curvature of the stomach is continuous with the lower right border of the abdominal esophagus. The superior surface of the lesser curvature is related to the inferior border of the hepatogastric ligament, which runs from the porta hepatis to the lesser gastric curvature and consists of an anterior and a posterior layer of peritoneum. The 2 layers form the upper half of the ventral boundary of the lesser peritoneal sac. Just superior to the left half of the lesser curvature of the stomach, lying between the 2 layers of the hepatogastric ligament, are the terminal branches of the left gastric artery. The right gastric artery, a branch of the hepatic artery, lies on the right half of the superior surface of the lesser curvature. The left and right gastric arteries complete the lesser curvature circulation. The visceral surfaces of the right and left lobes of the liver often lie directly on the superior ventral surface of the stomach (the lesser curvature), partially hiding it from view.

Relationships of the Greater Curvature

The greater omentum hangs from the greater curvature of the stomach. Between the greater curvature and the transverse colon are the 2 descending anterior layers of the greater omentum, known as the gastrocolic ligament. This ligament contains between its 2 layers, close to the curvature of the stomach, the left and right gastroepiploic vessels. The transverse colon and transverse mesocolon together from a shallow bed upon which the posteroinferior surface of

the greater curvature rests. The colonic bed separates the stomach from the transverse duodenum, the duodenojejunal flexure, and the most proximal loops of small intestine as they confine the stomach to the supramesocolic compartment of the abdomen.

➠ *Mobilization of the right side of the greater gastric curvature. In mobilizing the right side of the greater gastric curvature to facilitate gastric resection or pyloroplasty, one should bear in mind the frequent relationship of the middle colic artery and its major branches to the subpyloric area of the stomach. If ligated, the loss of these vessels may occasionally cause gangrene of the mid transverse colon despite the presence of the marginal artery (of Drummond).*

Relationships of the Fundus

The fundus of the stomach is related laterally to the spleen and to the gastrosplenic ligament, which contains between its 2 layers the short gastric (recurrent) branches of the splenic artery. Since the spleen is relatively fixed in position by the lienorenal and phrenicolienal ligaments, the attachment of the spleen to the gastric fundus serves to fix the fundus in the left upper abdominal quadrant of the abdomen. The thin gastrophrenic ligament passes from the fundus of the stomach to the left leaf of the diaphragm just to the left of the abdominal esophagus. The ligament is formed by the junction of the ventral and dorsal peritoneal surfaces of the stomach. The fundus of the stomach is related to the descending left surface of the diaphragm and consequently to the mediastinal structures just superior to it.

Relationships of the Pylorus

The posterior surface of the pylorus is closely related to the descending gastroduodenal artery and its duodenal branches and to the common bile duct. The lower margin of the epiploic foramen lies just above the upper margin of the pylorus. The middle colic artery running in the transverse mesocolon is frequently held in close relationship to the lower margin of the pylorus.

➠ *Close relationship of the posterior surface of the pylorus to the common bile duct and gastroduodenal artery. Both posterior duodenal disease and disease of the pancreatic head can draw the common bile duct and the descending gastroduodenal artery closer together. The relationship of bile duct to artery becomes of great importance during gastric resection for a posterior duodenal ulcer or in suture ligation of branches of the gastroduodenal artery for a bleeding duodenal ulcer. Jaundice following these procedures is usually due to obstruction*

*of the common bile duct by edema or ductal
ligation. To make sure of the relationships of
the common bile duct to the gastric pylorus
and the first portion of the duodenum, a catheter
should be introduced into the supraduodenal
portion of the common bile duct and threaded
down into the duodenum in order to help ascertain by palpation the retroduodenal course of
the duct.*

Peritoneal Relationships

The stomach is covered with peritoneum except
over the narrow areas where the gastric vessels run
in the greater and lesser omenta on the greater and
lesser curvatures and in a small triangular space on
the posterosuperior surface of the fundus, the takeoff
site of the gastrophrenic ligament. The peritoneum
that covers the stomach begins superior to the lesser
curvature by separation of the inferior 2 layers of
the hepatogastric ligament. The 2 layers leave the
stomach below the greater curvature to form the 2
anterior layers of the greater omentum.

LAYERS OF THE GASTRIC WALL

Outer Serous Coat

The outer serous coat of the wall of the stomach
is derived from the 2 layers of peritoneum of the
hepatogastric ligament that upon reaching the lesser
curvature split to encircle the stomach. The serous
coat covers the entire gastric circumference except
for a narrow strip along the greater and lesser curvatures, where the greater and lesser omenta attach to
the stomach. At these locations, the 2 layers of the
covering gastric serous coat leave a small triangular
space through which pass the nutrient vessels to the
stomach.

Muscular Coat
(Fig 25–7)

The muscular coat (muscularis externa) of the
stomach lies deep to its serous covering. It consists
of 3 sets of smooth muscle fibers: longitudinal, circular, and oblique. The **longitudinal fibers** are the most
superficial and are arranged in 2 groups. The first
group is continuous with the longitudinal muscle of
the esophagus and runs distally along the lesser curvature of the stomach. The second group of longitudinal
fibers is primarily related to the greater gastric curvature and runs from fundus to pylorus. The **circular
group** begins at the fundus of the stomach and passes
from left to right, completely enclosing the stomach
as it passes distally. The circular fibers are most abundant at the pylorus, where they thicken to form the

pyloric sphincter. The circular fibers of the stomach
are continuous with the circular fibers of the esophagus
but are quite sharply distinct from the circular fibers
of the duodenum.

The **oblique gastric fibers** are few in number
and lie deep to the circular muscle. They are limited
mainly to the cardia.

Submucous Layer

The submucous (areolar) layer of the stomach consists of loose areolar tissue that connects the mucous
and muscular layers. Between the mucosa and the
submucosa is a thin layer of smooth muscle, the muscularis mucosae, composed of an inner circular layer
and an outer longitudinal layer. This layer is of
importance in gastric surgery, since it holds sutures
quite well.

Mucous Membrane

The mucous membrane of the stomach is soft,
thick, and velvety and moves freely on the adjacent
submucosal layer. The mucous membrane is thin at
the cardia but thickens as it approaches the pylorus.
When the stomach contracts, the gastric mucosa is
thrown into folds or rugae that are plicated longitudi-
nally and are particularly marked near the pylorus
and along the greater curvature.

➭ *Changes in gastric rugae in disease. Gastric
rugae tend to be obliterated in gastric distention
by food, fluid, or air. The rugae are markedly
accentuated in hypertrophic gastritis (Méné-
trier's disease), a rare cause of dyspepsia and
gastric bleeding. The rugae are flattened out
in atrophic gastritis associated with pernicious
anemia.*

The epithelium of the gastric mucosa consists of
a single layer of tall columnar epithelial cells. Goblet
cells are occasionally present also. At the cardioesophageal juncture, there is an abrupt change from
stratified squamous epithelium of the esophagus to
gastric columnar epithelium.

The ducts of the gastric glands are lined with columnar epithelium. The mucosa of the stomach presents 3 types of glands, each named for the geographic
area in which it is situated. The **cardiac glands,**
situated about the cardiac opening of the stomach,
may be either compound racemose or simple tubular
in type. The **fundal glands** occupy the fundus and
most of the body of the stomach. In the fundal glands
are zymogen or chief cells and eosinophilic parietal
cells. The short-tubed **pyloric glands** occupy the pylorus and the proximally adjacent narrowed channel
of the stomach.

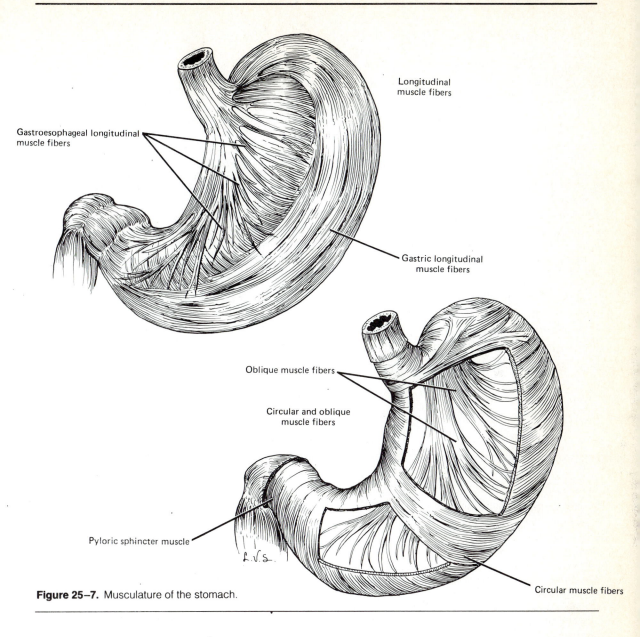

Figure 25–7. Musculature of the stomach.

BLOOD VESSELS, LYMPHATICS, & NERVES

Arteries
(Fig 25–8)

The stomach develops completely from the fetal foregut and thus is supplied by the foregut artery, the **celiac artery.** This artery usually arises from the aorta as its first ventral abdominal branch. On occasion, the celiac artery arises at the level of the diaphragm; in about 5% of persons, it arises from the lower thoracic aorta just above diaphragmatic level. The celiac artery is a short, stubby trunk about

0.75 cm long that runs in a ventral direction and promptly divides into its 3 major branches: the left gastric, the common hepatic, and the splenic arteries. In about 15% of persons, the inferior phrenic arteries also branch from the celiac artery.

➠ *High origin of the celiac artery. A supradiaphragmatic takeoff of the celiac artery can lead to compression of the celiac artery against the arcuate ligament of the diaphragm, since the artery must descend through the aortic hiatus to enter the abdomen. This compression may be a factor in the origin of so-called upper abdominal angina.*

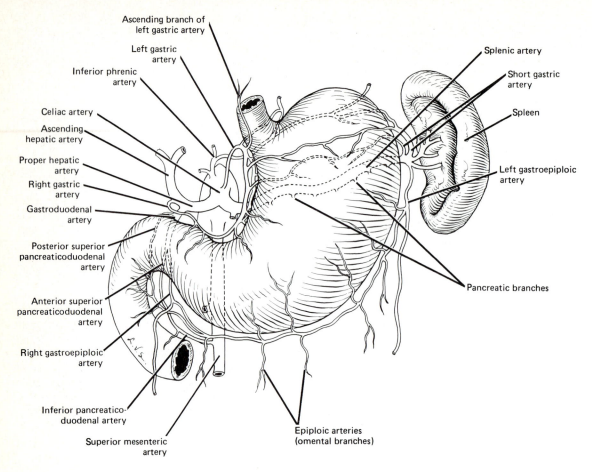

Figure 25–8. Arteries of the stomach.

The **left gastric artery** is the smallest branch of the celiac artery. It runs to the left, dorsal to the posterior peritoneum, and reaches the left free border of the gastrohepatic omentum just below the gastroesophageal junction. At this point, the artery runs ventrally and comes to lie between the 2 layers of the gastrohepatic omentum just superior to the lesser curvature of the stomach. On reaching the lesser gastric curvature, it divides into its 3 terminal branches: the cardioesophageal artery and the 2 descending lesser curvature branches, one ventral and one dorsal. The **cardioesophageal branch** runs superiorly from the cardia, supplying the abdominal esophagus and the lowermost thoracic esophagus. It terminates by anastomosing with the lower thoracic esophageal arterial branches from the thoracic aorta. The **descending gastric branches** of the left gastric artery run from left to right along the lesser curvature, the anterior branch supplying the anterior surface and the posterior branch the posterior surface of the lesser curvature. The 2 arteries terminate by anastomosing with the right gastric branches of the hepatic artery near the middle of the lesser curvature.

In about 15% of individuals, the left gastric artery gives off a major **hepatic branch** where it reaches the lesser curvature.

The left gastric artery tends to limit superior and left lateral mobility of the superior end of the stomach.

➠ *Left gastric arterial supply to the left lobe of the liver. A branch of the left gastric artery may carry all of the arterial blood to the left lobe of the liver. This vessel, when present, runs in the left free border of the gastrohepatic omentum and must be searched for and preserved in surgery near the gastric cardia and in procedures in which the entire gastrohepatic omentum is to be transected.*

➠ *Limited mobility of left gastric artery. The left gastric artery, because it limits motion of the left side of the lesser curvature, may have to be sacrificed in procedures in which the stomach must be moved either superiorly or laterally.*

The **common hepatic artery** is the second largest branch of the celiac artery. It runs inferiorly and to the right, dorsal to the posterior peritoneum of the lesser sac toward the pylorus. Just superior to the lower margin of the epiploic foramen (foramen of Winslow) it comes to lie between the 2 layers of the hepatogastric omentum. At this point, it divides into its 2 terminal branches, the ascending hepatic artery and the descending gastroduodenal artery.

The **right gastric artery** arises from the common hepatic artery above the pylorus, near the point at which the hepatic artery divides into its ascending hepatic and descending gastroduodenal branches. On occasion it may arise from the most proximal portion of the gastroduodenal artery. The right gastric artery descends to the pyloric end and then passes from right to left along the lesser gastric curvature between the 2 layers of the lesser omentum. It terminates by anastomosing with the posterior descending branches of the left gastric artery to complete the lesser curvature gastric circulation.

The **gastroduodenal artery** is a large vessel that arises from the common hepatic artery just superior to the pylorus. It runs obliquely dorsal to the most proximal segment of the duodenum. In its descent, it lies to the left of the common bile duct, also a retroduodenal structure. At the superior border of the pylorus, the gastroduodenal artery and the common bile duct are about 1.5 cm apart, but they gradually move closer together, and at the inferior margin of the first portion of the duodenum they are only 4–5 mm apart. After supplying the superior duodenal artery to the superior surface of the duodenum and the retroduodenal artery to the dorsal surface of the first part of the duodenum, the gastroduodenal artery divides into 3 terminal branches: the right gastroepiploic artery and the anterior and posterior superior pancreaticoduodenal arteries.

The **right gastroepiploic artery** runs from right to left along the greater curvature between the 2 layers of the greater omentum (gastrocolic ligament). When it reaches the midpoint of the greater curvature, it anastomoses with the left gastroepiploic artery, a branch of the inferior polar branch of the splenic artery. This anastomosis completes the arterial circulation of the greater curvature. Close to the pylorus, the right gastroepiploic artery is in close contact not only with the subpyloric region of the greater curvature but also with the middle colic artery and some of its branches to the transverse colon. This is because the transverse mesocolon is drawn superiorly toward the subpyloric region of the stomach by a congenital peritoneal band. The right gastroepiploic artery supplies the right half of the greater curvature and the right half of the greater omentum.

➠ *Preservation of gastroepiploic circulation to the greater omentum. Care must be taken to preserve the gastroepiploic arterial branches to the greater omentum to avoid omental infarc-*

tion. Omental infarction occurs because the supplying arteries are end arteries. Omental infarction close to a gastrojejunal anastomotic area may be one of the causes of a malfunctioning stoma.

The 2 **superior pancreaticoduodenal arteries** (anterior and posterior) descend between the left border of the descending duodenum and the head of the pancreas. The anterior vessel runs on the anterior surface of the head of the pancreas; the posterior vessel supplies the deep surface of the pancreatic head. The 2 arteries supply the head of the pancreas, the upper half of the descending duodenum, the posterior and inferior surfaces of the pylorus, and the first portion of the duodenum. The arteries terminate by anastomosing with the inferior pancreaticoduodenal branches of the superior mesenteric artery and with pancreatic branches of the splenic artery.

➠ *Arterial supply to the duodenum. The region of the pancreatic head is extremely vascular. The many branches of the superior pancreaticoduodenal arteries that lie between the pancreatic head and the left border of the descending duodenum make this area of the bowel a "no-man's land" for operative procedures. The duodenum will become ischemic if it is removed from the pancreas.*

The **splenic artery** is the widest, longest, and most tortuous branch of the celiac artery. It passes horizontally to the left, behind the peritoneum of the lesser sac past the pancreas. The splenic vein lies just inferior to the splenic artery. The artery passes from right to left ventral to the upper rim of the left kidney. Just proximal to the hilum of the spleen, the artery divides into its terminal branches. As the artery traverses the upper posterior border of the pancreas, it gives off many short branches to the neck, body, and tail of the pancreas. The branches anastomose with one another and also with branches of the pancreaticoduodenal arteries.

The **short gastric branches of the splenic artery** are given off from the superior terminal branch of the vessel just before entry into the spleen (superior polar branch). There are usually 5–7 short gastric arteries; they pass from left to right between the 2 layers of the gastrosplenic ligament to supply the superior margin of the gastric greater curvature and all of the gastric fundus.

The **left gastroepiploic artery** is usually a branch of the inferior terminal branch (inferior polar artery) of the splenic artery, being given off just before entry into the spleen. The left gastroepiploic artery runs from left to right between the 2 anterior layers of the greater omentum about 0.5 cm below the greater curvature. It terminates by anastomosing with the right gastroepiploic artery near the middle of the greater curvature.

⇛ *Gastric area of decreased circulation. Since the mid portions of the ventral and dorsal surfaces of the stomach are less well supplied with blood than the gastric curvatures, they are the sites of choice for openings into the stomach.*

Veins
(Fig 25–9)

The gastric veins roughly parallel the gastric arteries, particularly those along the greater and lesser curvatures. Venous blood leaving the stomach eventually reaches the portal vein via pathways that either empty directly into the portal vein or reach the portal vein via the splenic or superior mesenteric venous trunks.

The **short gastric veins** in the gastrosplenic ligament and the **left gastroepiploic veins** in the left half of the gastrocolic omentum usually empty into the splenic vein. The short gastric veins drain the gastric fundus and the left superior surface of the greater curvature; the left gastroepiploic vein drains

the left side of the greater curvature and the left side of the greater omentum. The **right gastroepiploic vein** runs in the right half of the gastrocolic omentum and drains the right side of the greater curvature and the right side of the greater omentum. It usually empties into the superior mesenteric vein just before that vein joins the splenic vein to form the portal vein.

The **pancreaticoduodenal veins** accompany their corresponding arteries and join either the right gastroepiploic vein or the superior mesenteric vein.

The **left gastric (coronary) vein** drains the anterior and posterior surfaces of the entire lesser curvature; it runs from right to left along that curvature between the 2 layers of the hepatogastric ligament; it finally reaches the gastric cardia just below the esophageal hiatus in the diaphragm. There it receives blood from the veins draining both the inferior segment of the thoracic esophagus and the abdominal esophagus. The left gastric vein then runs from left to right, dorsal to the lesser sac, and eventually terminates in the portal vein.

A few lesser curvature veins in the region of the gastroesophageal junction run superiorly into the lower thorax and there anastomose with the lower thoracic esophageal veins, whose flow leads into the superior vena cava. As a result, the gastroesophageal

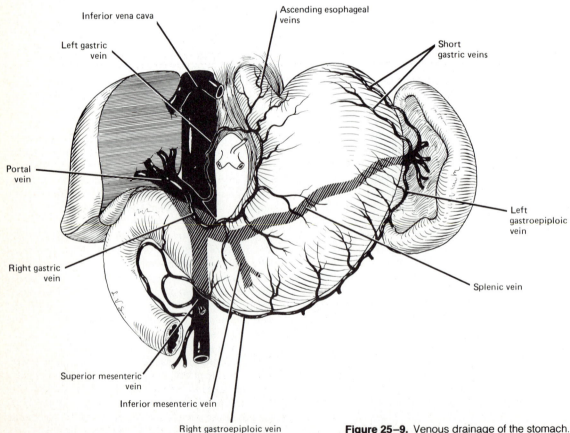

Figure 25–9. Venous drainage of the stomach.

junction becomes one of the main areas of anatomic portacaval venous anastomosis.

▥➡ ***The cause of esophageal varices.** Because venous blood from the gastroesophageal junction can discharge into either the portal or the superior caval system of veins, gastroesophageal varices frequently occur as a result of portal hypertension. These varices are prone to bleed quite easily, and bleeding from this source is one of the prime causes of massive upper gastrointestinal hemorrhage.*

The portal vein, formed by the junction of the superior mesenteric and splenic veins, begins just dorsal to the junction of the head and neck of the pancreas. The inferior mesenteric vein, bringing venous blood from the left side of the colon and the upper and mid rectum, may empty into the splenic vein or superior mesenteric vein or into the angle formed by the junction of these 2 veins as they meet to form the portal vein. The portal vein drains venous blood from the inferior mesenteric vein and from the stomach, the duodenum, the entire small bowel, the right colon, and the mid portions of the colon, spleen, and pancreas. Venous currents entering the portal vein from the superior mesenteric and splenic veins generally do not mix very much. The splenic venous blood passes mainly to the left lobe of the liver, whereas most blood from the superior mesenteric vein passes to the right lobe of the liver.

Lymphatics
(Fig 25–10)

The small lymphatic channels in the submucosa of the stomach anastomose freely, forming a dense submucosal lymphatic plexus. This plexus communicates with the gastric intermuscular lymphatics that eventually drain into a subserosal lymphatic network. The subserosal lymphatic network drains into larger lymphatics that accompany the 4 major arteries on the greater and lesser curvatures. The submucosal lymphatics of the stomach and esophagus join freely with each other, facilitating spread of gastric cancer to the adjacent lower esophagus. The gastric submucosal lymphatics rarely anastomose with those of the duodenum. Duodenal carcinoma secondary to gastric carcinoma is extremely rare.

Primary gastric lymphatic drainage is into nodes in the hepatogastric ligament just above the lesser curvature and into nodes just below the greater curvature in the superior segment of the greater omentum (gastrocolic ligament).

Secondary drainage of gastric lymph is from the nodes related to the greater and lesser gastric curvatures into nodes alongside the superior segment of the abdominal aorta, the deep celiac group of nodes.

▥➡ ***Poor prognosis in operative treatment of gastric cancer.** Since the celiac lymph nodes are*

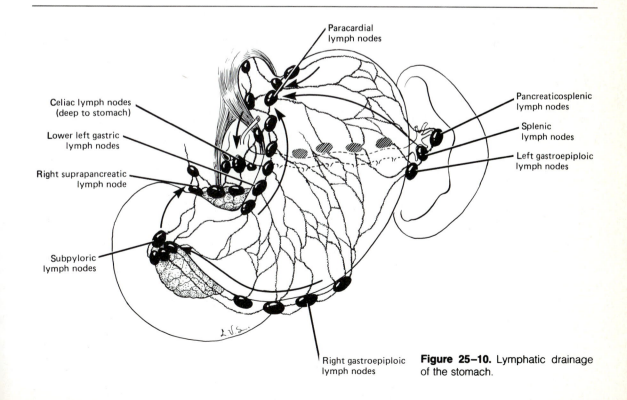

Paracardial lymph nodes

Celiac lymph nodes (deep to stomach)

Lower left gastric lymph nodes

Right suprapancreatic lymph node

Subpyloric lymph nodes

Pancreaticosplenic lymph nodes

Splenic lymph nodes

Left gastroepiploic lymph nodes

Right gastroepiploic lymph nodes

Figure 25–10. Lymphatic drainage of the stomach.

so deeply situated and so hard to identify during operation, they cannot be completely resected in surgery for gastric cancer. This accounts in part for the poor prognosis following gastric cancer surgery.

The routes taken by the gastric lymph as it proceeds to the deep celiac group of nodes are as follows: (1) Channels from the lesser curvature and the cardia pass via the superior gastric nodes that lie along the course of the left gastric artery to reach the celiac nodes. (2) Channels from the fundus and the superior segment of the greater curvature follow the course of the short gastric and left gastroepiploic arteries to reach the celiac nodes. Lymph draining from nodes in the splenic hilum and from the pancreaticosplenic nodes joins with the short gastric lymph to flow eventually into the deep celiac group of nodes. (3) Channels draining the right half of the gastric curvature accompany the right gastroepiploic artery and run primarily into the subpyloric and superior gastric nodes and from there into the deep celiac nodes. (4) Channels from the superior pyloric area drain into both the deep hepatic and deep celiac nodes.

From the **deep celiac group of nodes,** lymphatic channels pass to the subdiaphragmatic group of nodes situated just below the diaphragm and superior to the takeoff of the celiac axis from the abdominal aorta. Lymphatic drainage from the subdiaphragmatic

nodes passes upward above the diaphragm into the posteroinferior mediastinal nodes. Lymph nodes in the region of the cardia may drain upward into para-esophageal nodes that drain farther superiorly into the great thoracic lymph trunks. Virchow's node, in the left supraclavicular area of the neck, receives lymph from the gastric cardia via this route.

Nerves
(Fig 25–11)
The stomach is supplied by branches of the **vagus nerve** and by sympathetic nerve fibers from the **celiac plexus.** The right and left vagi enter the abdomen through the esophageal hiatus. Just above the diaphragm, the vagi lie right and left alongside the esophagus. Upon entering the abdominal cavity, the left vagus lies anterior and the right vagus posterior to the abdominal esophagus. The left (anterior) vagus lies close to the right anterior surface of the abdominal esophagus. The right vagus lies posterior to and to the right of the abdominal esophagus in the areolar tissue of the left free border of the gastrohepatic omentum.

The right vagus divides high on the stomach into a celiac branch, which runs on the posterior surface of the stomach to join the celiac plexus, and a gastric branch (the posterior nerve of Latarjet), which runs on the posterior surface of the stomach parallel to and just below the lesser gastric curvature.

The left vagus divides into a hepatic branch and

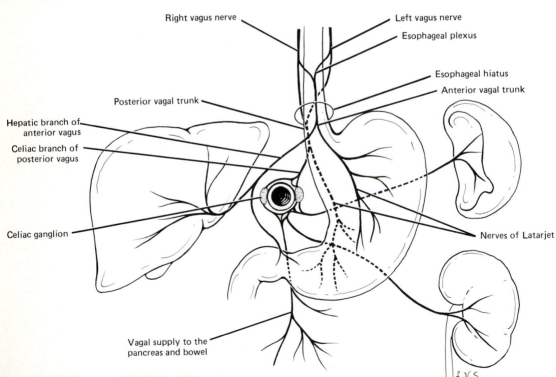

Figure 25–11. Diagram of distribution of the vagus nerve.

a gastric branch. The gastric branch (the anterior nerve of Latarjet) runs on the anterior gastric wall, parallel to the lesser curvature, and about 2 cm below it. It terminates by a crow's foot distribution of its most distal fibers to the pyloric antrum.

➧ *Parietal cell (highly selective) vagotomy. When highly selective vagotomy is performed, the 2 nerves of Latarjet are preserved: only their branches to the upper two-thirds of the stomach are sectioned. Thus, innervation of the antrum is left intact, obviating the need for a gastric drainage procedure. In simple selective vagotomy, the vagal celiac and hepatic branches are preserved but the nerves of Latarjet are sectioned. In such cases, pyloroplasty is usually performed as an adjunctive procedure to facilitate gastric emptying. Sympathetic fibers from the celiac plexus reach the stomach via the gastric arterial supply.*

➧ *Vagotomy: physiologic basis and techniques. Since the vagus nerve controls gastric secretion and motility, bilateral vagotomy results in diminished gastric acid secretion and reduced gastric motility. Currently, vagotomy seems to be indicated (1) as a definitive procedure when combined with limited gastric resection for the treatment of gastric and duodenal ulcer; (2) when combined with pyloroplasty, as a defini-tive procedure for duodenal ulceration; (3) when combined with pyloroplasty and oversewing of the bleeding ulcer area, as a means of treating bleeding duodenal ulcer; and (4) for gastrojejunal stomal ulceration with or without hemorrhage.*

Bilateral vagotomy for gastric disease calls for mobilization and elongation of the abdominal esophagus by downward traction. This downward displacement stretches the vagus nerves and makes them easier to visualize and palpate. An opening is then made into the right free border of the gastrohepatic ligament where it reaches the cardia. All nerve trunks and fibers that are branches of the right vagus running to the esophagus and the cardia are then located and interrupted.

Section of the vagi results in gastric dilatation, diminution of gastric tone, slower and weaker gastric peristalsis with increased gastric emptying time, and marked lowering of gastric acid secretion. A gastric emptying procedure, either gastrojejunostomy or pyloroplasty, should always be done along with the vagotomy. Today, highly selective vagotomy is more frequently employed. Selective vagotomy and highly selective vagotomy are preferable, because total vagotomy may disturb pancreatic, biliary, and small and large bowel function and cause chronic indigestion or diarrhea.

The duodenum, the most proximal portion of the small bowel, begins at the gastric pylorus and ends at the duodenojejunal flexure. It is about 25 cm long and consists of 4 segments: superior, descending, transverse, and ascending.

EMBRYOLOGY
(See also Chapter 22.)

The duodenum develops from the distal end of the foregut and the proximal segment of the midgut.

Anomalies

Duodenal anomalies may be characterized generally as anomalies of fixation (duodenum inversum, or M-shaped duodenum), length (short or long duodenum), size (megaduodenum), or position (duodenum may pass inferiorly into the right lower abdomen, or the transverse segment may lie ventral to the superior mesenteric artery). Stenosis, atresia, or duodenal valve formation may occur, as well as enteric cysts and diverticula. (Figs 26–1 and 26–2.)

GROSS ANATOMY
(Figs 26–3 and 26–4)

The duodenum is the C-shaped most proximal portion of the small bowel. It is situated farther posteriorly than any other portion of the small bowel, and its second and third segments are retroperitoneal. Except for its most proximal segment, the duodenum is a fixed structure, whereas all other portions of the small bowel are mobile and suspended by a mesentery. The excretory ducts of the liver and pancreas discharge into the duodenum, because the embryonic duodenum serves as the site of origin of these 2 organs.

As in the remainder of the small bowel, the coats of the duodenum are a serous outer coat, a muscular coat of both longitudinal and circular smooth muscle, a submucosa, and an inner mucosal layer with a thin layer of muscularis mucosae. However, the duodenum has certain histologic features not shared with the remainder of the small intestine.

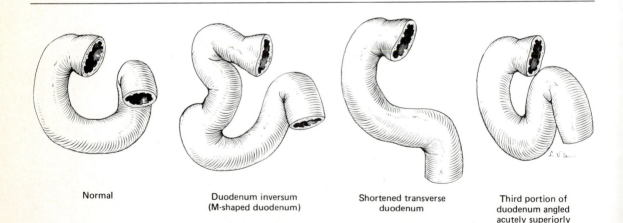

Normal   Duodenum inversum (M-shaped duodenum)   Shortened transverse duodenum   Third portion of duodenum angled acutely superiorly

Figure 26–1. Variations in shape of the duodenum.

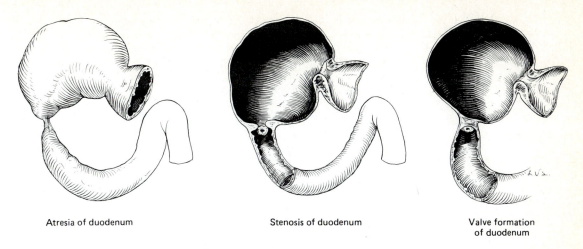

Atresia of duodenum   Stenosis of duodenum   Valve formation
of duodenum

Figure 26–2. Congenital obstruction of the duodenum.

The descending, transverse, and ascending segments of the duodenum contain large circular valve-like folds known as Kerckring's folds, or circular folds (plicae circulares), composed of submucosa and mucosa, that project 5–10 mm into the lumen of the bowel. The submucosal core of the fold is rigid, so that the folds do not disappear when the bowel becomes distended. The presence of the folds gives the second, third, and fourth segments of the duodenum a toughness and firmness not present in the

remainder of the small bowel. Knowledge of the presence of the circular folds is of importance in the x-ray diagnosis of duodenal disease.

SEGMENTS OF THE DUODENUM

The **first (superior) segment** of the duodenum is divided into proximal and distal portions. The proximal portion is about 2.5 cm long and runs superiorly

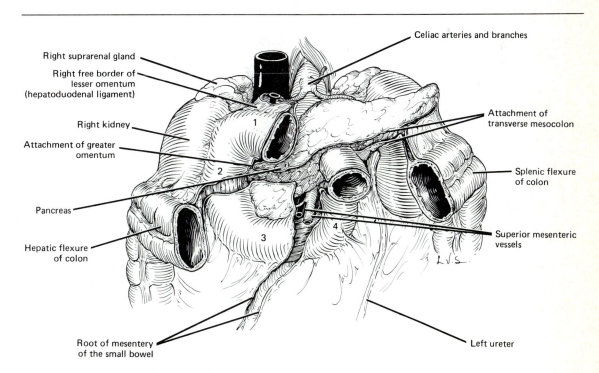

Figure 26–3. Duodenal relationships. 1 = superior segment; 2 = descending segment; 3 = transverse segment; 4 = ascending segment.

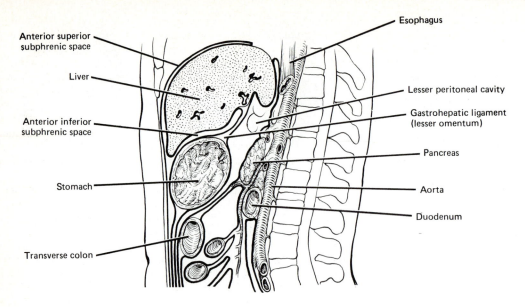

Figure 26–4. The peritoneal reflections and the location of the lesser peritoneal cavity.

and dorsally after leaving the pylorus. It rises as high as vertebra T12. There it comes in contact with the gallbladder and the visceral surface of the right lobe of the liver. Like the distal end of the stomach, this segment of the duodenum is entirely covered with peritoneum and is consequently quite mobile. The right free border of the hepatogastric ligament, known as the hepatoduodenal ligament, attaches to it and suspends the superior surface of this duodenal segment. The right free border of the greater omentum is attached to its inferior surface; thus, this segment of the duodenum has a double mesentery. The epiploic foramen (of Winslow), the entrance into the lesser omental sac, lies immediately above this duodenal segment; the gastroduodenal branch of the hepatic artery and the common bile duct pass posterior to this segment of the bowel.

⊫➡ *Disorders involving the first segment of the duodenum. The proximal duodenal segment is a frequent site of peptic ulceration. Primary gallbladder inflammation may cause the gallbladder to adhere to the proximal duodenum, and stones may then pass directly from the gallbladder, the cystic duct, or the common bile duct into the proximal duodenal lumen, on occasion leaving an open cholecystoduodenal fistula. These are more common in the second portion of the duodenum, but they also occur in the first portion.*

⊫➡ *Relationship of the first segment to the transverse colon. Because the first segment of the duodenum lies in the supramesocolic compartment, anterior perforation of an ulcer in this*

portion of the duodenum releases liquid or air into the supramesocolic compartment of the greater peritoneal cavity. The fluid may remain there for 2–24 hours, so that early symptoms and findings are epigastric, right hypochondriac, or right subphrenic in location. Spilling of fluid then commonly occurs into the right hepatorenal pouch (of Morison) and from there into the right lumbar gutter. The usual presenting symptoms are generalized pain and board-like rigidity of the abdomen.

*The presenting symptoms and signs of posterior penetration or perforation of an ulcer of the first segment of the duodenum differ according to whether the proximal or distal portion is involved. With involvement of the **proximal portion,** the manifestations and the routes of drainage are usually the same as in anterior perforations. Occasionally, there may be a perforation through which fluid passes directly into the lesser sac via the epiploic foramen.*

*With posterior penetration through an ulcer in the **distal portion** of the first segment, fluids usually enter the pancreas or retroperitoneal tissues. The fluid may move upward to the bare area of the liver via the retroperitoneal tissues. Penetration of the pancreas frequently causes boring lumbodorsal pain, intensified at night when the stomach is empty and hypersecreting. The pain is similar to that of pancreatitis or pancreatic cancer.*

The distal portion of the first segment of the duodenum is about 3 cm long. At its sharp angle of departure from the ascending first segment of the duodenum, it appears on x-ray studies as a 3-cornered cap. The distal portion of the first segment of the duodenum is covered only anterolaterally by peritoneum and is fixed by a fusion fascia to the posterior abdominal peritoneum. In addition, it is fixed to the right lateral abdominal wall by its anterolateral peritoneal covering. Posteriorly and medially, this segment of duodenum is related to the common bile duct, the gastroduodenal artery, and the portal vein, the latter lying posterior to the bile duct and the artery.

The **second (longest) segment** of the duodenum is 10–12 cm long and is known as the **descending duodenum.** As it descends from the gallbladder fossa (fossa vesicae felleae), its lies ventral to the hilum of the right kidney, the right renal vessels, the right renal pelvis, and the superior portion of the right ureter. It drops from the level of vertebra L1 to the level of the interspace between L3 and L4. It is covered by peritoneum only on its anterior aspect. The covering peritoneum is reflected laterally onto the fatty tissues overlying the right kidney and then onto the right lateral abdominal parietes. The descending duodenum is fixed tightly to the posterior abdominal wall by fusion of its posterior surface to the posterior abdominal parietes. This segment of the duodenum is crossed anteriorly in its midsection by the transverse colon, to which it is attached by loose areolar tissue. This places its terminal half deep to that structure, which hides it.

▶ *Surgery on the supramesocolic segment of the descending duodenum. The surgeon can work with relative ease on the supramesocolic portion of the descending duodenum. Fortunately, the common bile duct and the major pancreatic duct empty into this segment, so that the surgical approach to their emptying papillae calls for only upper lateral duodenal mobilization followed by a posterolateral opening into the mobilized bowel. In contrast, it is difficult to see and approach the inframesocolic portion of the descending duodenum without first mobilizing the hepatic flexure. Disease in the inferior half of the descending duodenum causes signs and symptoms referable to the inframesocolic compartment of the abdomen.*

▶ *Injury to the second segment in genitourinary surgery. In procedures undertaken to mobilize the second segment of the duodenum, one must take care not to injure the renal or perirenal structures. Conversely, when one approaches the right kidney or upper ureter through a dorsal flank incision, care must be taken not to injure the duodenum.*

Anteriorly and superiorly, the descending duodenum is related to the free peritoneal cavity, the visceral surface of the right lobe of the liver, and the structures in the gallbladder fossa. Halfway along its course, the ventral surface of the descending duodenum is crossed by the transverse colon, whose dorsal surface at this point usually does not have a mesentery. The crossing posterior colonic surface is attached to the mid descending duodenum by loose areolar tissue.

Laterally, the descending duodenum is related to the right lumbar gutter, the right colic flexure, and the right kidney. Medial to the descending duodenum lie the head of the pancreas and the terminal branches of the superior and inferior pancreaticoduodenal vessels.

The common bile duct and the major pancreatic duct usually enter the left or medial posterior surface of the descending duodenum about 3 cm above the level of the transverse colon. However, the common bile duct may enter any portion of the descending duodenum or may even enter the proximal portion of the transverse duodenum. There are 3 ways in which the common bile duct and the major pancreatic duct may be anatomically related to each other and to the posteromedial descending duodenum: (1) The common bile duct may be joined by the major pancreatic duct (of Wirsung) within the substance of the head of the pancreas; then, via a common ductal channel, the structures thus joined may pierce the duodenal wall to empty via a single opening on the duodenal papilla. (2) The common bile duct may be joined by the major pancreatic duct within the medial duodenal wall, the secretions carried by the 2 ducts being emptied into the duodenum through a single opening on the duodenal papilla. (3) There may be no junction of the common bile duct and the major pancreatic duct; there are 2 separate ductal openings on the duodenal papilla.

The accessory pancreatic duct (of Santorini), if present, empties into the posterial medial wall of the descending duodenum via a small papilla about 2 cm above the major duodenal papilla.

The major duodenal papilla, which contains the opening or openings for the common bile duct and the major pancreatic duct, is a tubular projection that protrudes 3–4 mm into the posteromedial segment of the duodenal lumen. It is partially hooded by a semilunar fold of mucosa. One of the enlarged plicae circulares will often overhang this papilla, making it difficult to see the ductal openings.

The **third (transverse) segment** of the duodenum (horizontal portion) is 6–7 cm long and begins just to the right of the vertebral column at the level of the disk between L3 and L4. It runs transversely, terminating to the left of the vertebral column at the level of vertebra L2, where it lies anterior to the abdominal aorta. The transverse duodenum is posterior to the dorsal peritoneum of the inframesocolic compartment and is completely retroperitoneal. As it crosses the abdomen from right to left, the transverse duodenum passes in front of—and in this sequence—the right renal vessels, the right psoas muscle, the right ureter, the inferior vena cava, the vertebral column, and the abdominal aorta. Just to the right of its mid portion, the transverse duodenum is crossed ventrally by the superior mesenteric artery and veins as they enter or leave the root of the mesentery of the small bowel. The inferior mesenteric artery arises from the aorta just below the inferior edge of the transverse duodenum. Just before its termination, the transverse duodenum is crossed obliquely from left to right by the root of the mesentery of the small bowel. Just above the transverse duodenum is the inferior margin of the pancreas. In the groove between the pancreas and the transverse duodenum are the right and left terminal branches of the inferior pancreaticoduodenal artery, a branch of the superior vertebral artery.

➠ **The Whipple procedure.** *The third segment of the duodenum must be removed, either partially or completely, along with the pancreas and the pyloric antrum and the first and second segments of the duodenum, in the Whipple procedure for operable cancer of the pancreas, the lower common bile duct, or the descending duodenum.*

➠ **Injuries to the transverse duodenum.** *Despite its deep position, the retroperitoneal transverse portion of the duodenum is occasionally crushed against the vertebral column by severe anterior or posterior abdominal wall trauma. Rupture of the bowel and resultant spilling of duodenal contents may lead to retroperitoneal cellulitis and abscess formation or generalized peritonitis. Rupture is usually difficult to diagnose, often requiring mobilization of the hepatic flexure of the colon and of the ligament of Treitz to achieve adequate exposure of the transverse duodenum. Multiple small air bubbles ("ground glass" appearance) covering the upper right psoas muscle may be seen on abdominal x-rays. Rupture of the third portion of the duodenum is often accompanied by rupture of the body of the pancreas. In exploring the abdomen for trauma, the transverse duodenum must always be exposed and explored. Failure to do so may lead to fatal consequences.*

The **fourth (ascending) segment** is the shortest part of the duodenum and is about 2.5–3 cm long. It lies on the left crus of the diaphragm and runs superiorly and to the left along the left side of the vertebral column to L2. There it bends ventrally and downward to join the proximal jejunum at the duodenojejunal flexure (Fig 26–5). The ascending duodenum receives a fibromuscular band that runs from the left crus of the diaphragm to the final 1.25 cm of the antimesenteric border of the bowel. This is

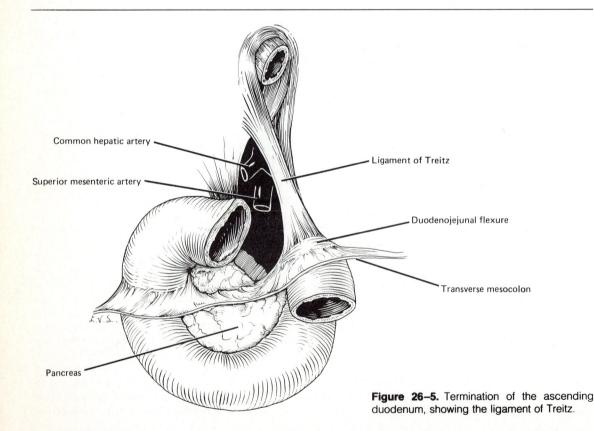

Common hepatic artery

Superior mesenteric artery

Pancreas

Ligament of Treitz

Duodenojejunal flexure

Transverse mesocolon

Figure 26–5. Termination of the ascending duodenum, showing the ligament of Treitz.

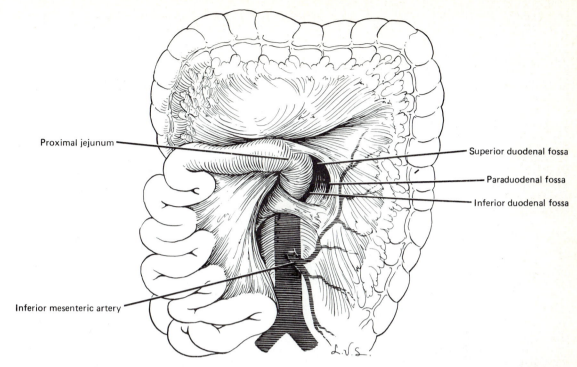

Proximal jejunum

Superior duodenal fossa

Paraduodenal fossa

Inferior duodenal fossa

Inferior mesenteric artery

Figure 26–6. The paraduodenal fossae.

the suspensory ligament of the duodenum (**ligament of Treitz**). If the transverse colon and the transverse mesocolon are lifted anteriorly and then superiorly, the ligament of Treitz is put on stretch and is relatively easy to locate as it runs to the duodenum. At the level of the suspensory ligament, the bowel leaves its retroperitoneal position and again becomes an intraperitoneal structure.

PARADUODENAL PERITONEAL FOSSAE (Fig 26–6)

Two or 3 inconstant peritoneal fossae are located about the duodenal jejunal flexure. The **superior duodenal fossa** lies dorsal to the superior duodenojejunal fold. This peritoneal fold runs to the left for about 2.5 cm after it leaves the duodenojejunal flexure. The fold's concave free border faces inferiorly and to the left. Occasionally, the inferior mesenteric artery runs in the free margin of the fold. The opening into the fossa, which is created by lifting of the fold, looks inferiorly and to the left, whereas its cavity passes upward and to the right toward the ventral surface of the pancreas. This fossa is present in about 50% of people.

The **inferior duodenal fossa** (of Jannesco) looks downward and to the right. Its ventral wall is formed by the inferior duodenojejunal fold that stretches to the left of the aorta and the vertebral column after

it branches off from the left side of the ascending duodenum. Its free edge is avascular. It is present in about 75% of people.

The **paraduodenal fossa** (of Lanzert) is the largest of the paraduodenal cul-de-sacs. It lies just to the left of the ascending segment. It results when a peritoneal fold is raised by the ascending branches of the left colic artery and the inferior mesenteric vein. Its opening looks medially, and its cul-de-sac looks laterally. Its lateral crescentic margin may unite the inferior and superior duodenal fossae. Its sac usually lies anterior to the left ureter. It is present in only about 25% of people.

➠ *Herniations into the paraduodenal fossa. The presence of the 3 paraduodenal fossae can result in internal hernias in the upper left abdominal quadrant. These internal hernias tend to incarcerate and strangulate. The presence and size of the fossae depend primarily on the method and degree of fixation of the terminal portion of the duodenum. If a loop of small bowel enters one of these fossae, it creates a peritoneal sac at the expense of the posterior parietal peritoneum. Strangulation of the bowel may occur as a result of impingement of one of the crescentic peritoneal borders of the fossa upon the bowel. In dividing the neck of the sac during procedures to correct these hernias, care must be taken not to injure the inferior mesenteric artery, the inferior mesenteric vein, or the ascending branches of the left colic artery.*

BLOOD VESSELS, LYMPHATICS, & NERVES

Arteries
(Fig 26–7)

The **first segment** of the duodenum receives its blood supply from the descending gastroduodenal artery via its duodenal branches. The branches run to the superior surface of the first portion of the duodenum.

The **descending duodenum** is supplied primarily by the 2 superior pancreaticoduodenal arteries, the right branch of the inferior pancreaticoduodenal artery, and a few small terminal branches of the gastroduodenal artery. The 2 superior pancreaticoduodenal arteries, which are paired in ventral-dorsal fashion, run in the groove between the head of the pancreas and the medial surface of the descending duodenum, sending branches to these structures. Little or no blood supply reaches the lateral border of the descending duodenum along its line of peritoneal reflection.

The **transverse** and **ascending** portions of the duodenum are supplied by the left major branch of the inferior pancreaticoduodenal artery, which runs in the groove between the inferior surface of the pancreas and the superior surface of the transverse duodenum. The main inferior pancreaticoduodenal artery, after leaving the superior mesenteric artery, divides into right and left branches on reaching the pancreaticoduodenal groove. The right branch of the artery anastomoses with the superior pancreaticoduodenal arteries, thus connecting the celiac artery and the superior mesenteric artery.

Veins

Venous return from the duodenum empties into the portal venous system via vessels that roughly parallel the branches of the superior and inferior pancreaticoduodenal arteries. These venous channels may drain directly into the portal vein, the splenic vein, or the terminal segment of the superior mesenteric vein before reaching the portal vein.

Lymphatics

Duodenal lymphatic drainage usually empties into (1) the celiac lymph nodes clustered about the celiac

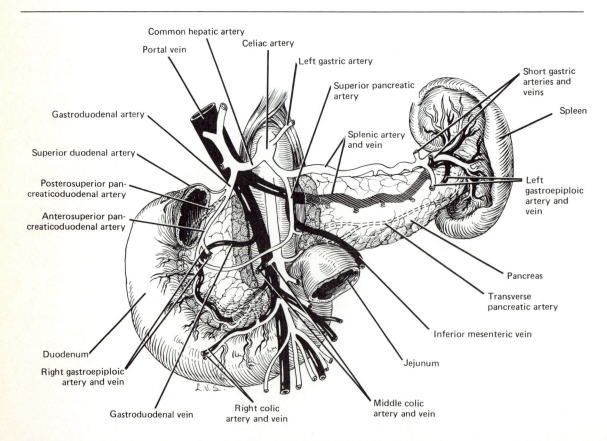

Figure 26–7. Arterial supply and venous return to the descending and transverse duodenum, pancreas, and spleen.

artery as it branches from the aorta; (2) the right aorticorenal nodes closely related to the right renal vessels; and (3) a group of nodes related to the tail of the pancreas and the hilum of the spleen (pancreaticosplenic nodes).

Nerves

The large hepatic branch of the **left vagus nerve** gives off a branch that accompanies the right gastric artery. This nerve gives small branches to the pylorus and the first segment of the duodenum.

A second branch from the hepatic branch of the left vagus runs with the gastroduodenal artery and the right gastroepiploic artery and supplies the remainder of the duodenum and the distal part of the greater gastric curvature.

The **posterior (right) vagus nerve** runs into the celiac plexus. Vagal fibers from secondary plexuses (postceliac) also reach the duodenum.

The small intestine is that portion of the gastrointestinal tract that begins at the pylorus and ends at the ileocecal junction. It is composed proximally of the duodenum and jejunum and distally of the ileum. Actually, the duodenum is the proximal segment of the small intestine but unlike the jejunoileum it is not mobile, most of it being fixed to the posterior abdominal wall.

EMBRYOLOGY
(See also Chapter 22.)

The prearterial loop of the midgut forms part of the duodenum, the jejunum, and most of the ileum.

Anomalies

Anomalies include stenosis and atresia, valve formation (rare), Meckel's diverticulum and associated vitellointestinal duct and vascular anomalies, other congenital small bowel diverticula (rare), and enterogenous cysts (reduplication of bowel). The small bowel may lie in the right lower abdomen, filling and joining the cecum from right to left. Reversed rotation of the midgut loop may also occur. (Figs 27–1 and 27–2.)

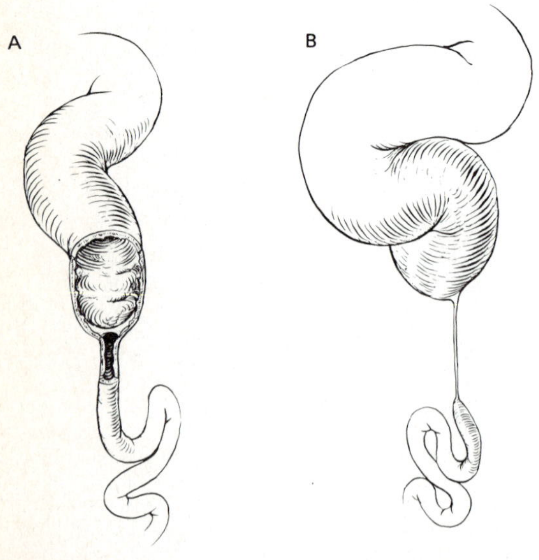

GROSS ANATOMY
(Fig 25–2)

The small bowel proper extends from the duodenojejunal flexure in the left upper abdominal quadrant to the ileocecal junction, usually in the right iliac fossa. Arbitrarily, the proximal two-fifths of the length of the small bowel is called the **jejunum** and the distal three-fifths the **ileum.** If it were fully extended, the small bowel would be 6–7 m long from the pylorus to the cecum. Its most proximal coils usually lie distal to the **ligament of Treitz** in the left upper abdominal quadrant. Its more distal coils tend to lie obliquely across the abdomen from the left upper quadrant to the right pelvis. The coils of mid ileum usually lie in the pelvis, whereas the terminal 30 cm of ileum usually rises from the pelvis to lie in close relationship to the cecum and the ascending colon.

The outer **serosal coat** of the small bowel is derived from the coelomic visceral peritoneum. It completely covers the gut except at its mesenteric border, where a small space, not covered by serosa, permits the entrance and egress of the blood vessels, lymphatics, and nerves of the bowel.

Deep to the small bowel serosa is the 2-layered **muscular coat** of the bowel. The outer layer is made up of longitudinal smooth muscle and is relatively thin. The inner layer is composed of circular smooth muscle and is thick and well-developed along the entire length of the small bowel. The inner circular smooth muscle is thicker in the jejunum than in the ileum.

The submucosal layer lies deep to the 2 layers of smooth muscle and is made up of fibroblastic and areolar tissue. It is very firm and is in the center of the circular mucosal folds, present only in the proximal jejunum and in the duodenum (plicae circulares). Within the submucosal layer are the nerves, lymphatics, and blood vessels that supply the small intestine. Single or small groupings of lymphatic follicles and

Figure 27–1. Types of intestinal atresia. **A:** A membranous web. **B:** Fibrous band connecting 2 blind ends. (Reproduced with permission, from Way LW [editor]: *Current Surgical Diagnosis & Treatment,* 7th ed. Lange, 1985.)

A — Membranous web

B — Fibrous band connecting 2 blind ends

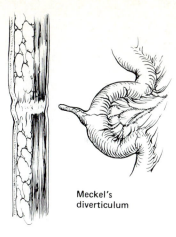

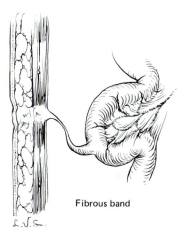

Figure 27–2. Omphalomesenteric duct anomalies arising from the primitive yolk. Remnants include Meckel's diverticulum, enterocystoma, or a fibrous band or fistulous tract between the ileum and the umbilicus. (Reproduced, with permission, from Way LW [editor]: *Current Surgical Diagnosis & Treatment,* 7th ed. Lange, 1985.)

➠ *Presence of small bowel in hernial sacs. Probably the most striking attribute of the small intestine is its great mobility; consequently, one may expect to find a single loop or coils of small bowel anywhere within the abdominal cavity. In addition, the small bowel may wander extra-abdominally as the sole occupant or as one structure present in the sacs of femoral, inguinal, umbilical, obturator, and diaphragmatic hernias.*

➠ *Intussusception. The small bowel may telescope into itself or into adjacent cecum and ascending colon. Occasionally, the small bowel will telescope upward through the opening of a gastrojejunostomy. In most cases of intussusception, the small bowel eventually becomes obstructed (Fig 27–3).*

➠ *Tears of small bowel close to a fixed area of bowel. Tears of the small bowel wall or of the small bowel mesentery are frequent sequelae of both penetrating and blunt abdominal trauma. Such tears nearly always occur close to an area of normal or abnormal fixation of a loop of bowel. A normal area of fixation would be the duodenojejunal flexure; an abnormal area of fixation would be one close to a pathologic kink or adhesion of the bowel in malignant, infectious, or congenital disease.*

nodules are present in the submucosa, mainly in the ileum. A thin layer of muscularis mucosae is interposed between the submucosa and the mucosa.

The mucous membrane of the small bowel is composed of a single layer of columnar epithelial cells. Protruding from the surface of the mucous membrane are multiple intestinal villi, larger and more numerous in the jejunum than in the ileum. Their presence causes the mucosal surface to appear velvety. Opening on the mucosal surface of the small bowel are the orifices of the intestinal glands, these openings being interspersed between the intestinal villi. The mucous membrane of the small bowel contains multiple lymphatic follicles (Peyer's patches) located between the intestinal villi and present in greatest numbers in the terminal ileum. These lymphatic follicles protrude from the neighboring submucosa, thus occupying both layers. As they protrude into the mucosa, they tend to flatten some of the intestinal villi.

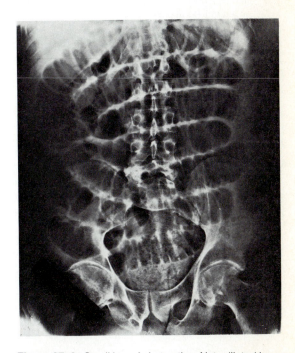

Figure 27–3. Small bowel obstruction. Note dilated loops of small bowel in a ladderlike pattern. Air-fluid levels are not obvious, because the patient is supine. (Reproduced, with permission from Way LW [editor]: *Current Surgical Diagnosis & Treatment,* 7th ed. Lange, 1985.)

➠ **Differences of appearance between the jejunum and ileum** (*of great importance to the operating surgeon*). *These include the following:*

(1) *The caliber of the small bowel diminishes, as does the thickness of its muscular wall, from proximal jejunum to distal ileum.*

(2) *The plicae circulares—circular folds in the duodenum and proximal jejunum—serve to thicken the walls of the small bowel. They are easily palpated through the proximal jejunal wall.*

(3) *Peyer's patches, small submucous lymphoid nodules, are visible and often palpable on the antimesenteric border of the ileum. They are only occasionally found in the jejunum but become quite numerous as the ileum approaches the ileocecal junction.*

(4) *The mesentery of the proximal small bowel is thinner, contains less fat between its leaves, and is more translucent than the mesentery of the distal small bowel, and its vascular pattern is simpler and more easily discernible than that of the distal small intestine.*

(5) *As one progresses distally along the small bowel, the lymphatics and lymph nodes present in its mesentery become larger and more numerous. The greatest number of lymphatic elements is present at the ileocecal-colic angle.*

(6) *There is a more marked tendency toward arborization and anastomosis of arterial and venous arcades in the mesentery of the distal ileum than in the mesentery of the proximal and mid jejunum (Fig 27–4).*

➠ **Identification of segments of small bowel.** *The operating surgeon often must be able to rapidly identify a segment of small bowel that must be handled. The gross differences listed above are of help in differentiating jejunum and ileum except in the presence of inflammation and distention. In such cases, the surgeon must manually trace the small bowel proximally or distally to its fixed points at the ligament of Treitz and the ileocecal junction to identify the position of a loop of bowel.*

➠ **Impaction of gallstones in small bowel.** *Since the small bowel becomes smaller in caliber as it descends from its origin at the ligament of Treitz, a fairly large gallstone passed from the gallbladder into the small bowel will frequently become lodged just distal to the jejunoileal junction. This junctional area usually marks the beginning of the narrower lumen of the ileum.*

➠ **Tube jejunostomy.** *Prior to the introduction of intravenous hyperalimentation, patients who could not tolerate food by mouth were nourished*

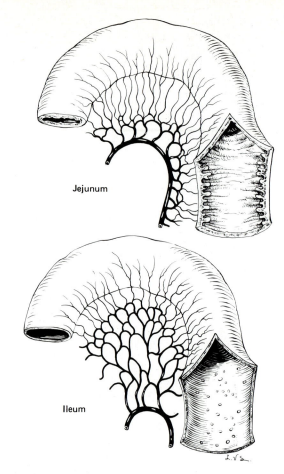

Figure 27–4. Variation in arterial supply to the small bowel. Note the more intricate arborization in the mesentery of the ileum. (Reproduced, with permission, from Way LW [editor]: *Current Surgical Diagnosis & Treatment,* 7th ed. Lange, 1985.)

by means of a tube jejunostomy. Tube ileostomy is still used occasionally.

➠ **Small bowel procedures in abdominal surgery.** *The small bowel—usually the proximal jejunum—is used as the segment of gut to which the esophagus, stomach, duodenum, pancreas, or extrahepatic biliary tract is anastomosed. Enteroenterostomy just distal to such an anastomosis is frequently done in order to ensure the proper emptying of the anastomotic loop and to prevent reflux. Enteroenterostomy may be performed to short-circuit small bowel flow around an area of unresectable obstruction, such as that resulting from cancer or chronic inflammation. Sections of proximal jejunum may be interposed between esophagus and duodenum as part of total gastric resection or partial gastroesophageal resection for stricture or cancer.*

⫸ ***Granulomatous disease of small bowel.*** *Intestinal tuberculosis and other granulomatous diseases of the small bowel cause hyperplasia of the lymphatic patches on the antimesenteric border of the terminal small bowel. This assists in the clinical recognition of such diseases when the abdomen is explored.*

⫸ ***Regional enteritis.*** *In regional enteritis (Crohn's disease), the mesenteric fat tends to climb the small bowel toward its antimesenteric border. This phenomenon may suggest the proper diagnosis. (Fig 27–5.)*

⫸ ***Ileostomy.*** *The terminal ileum may be brought to the surface of the anterolateral abdominal wall to serve as an end vent for the intestinal contents in cases where total colectomy has been required for ulcerative colitis, multiple polyposis, or multiple cancers of the colon.*

⫸ ***Ureteral implantation into closed ileal loop.*** *A short loop of ileum may be defunctionalized and separated from the intestinal stream to serve as a pouch into which one or both ureters may be implanted in cases in which the bladder has been removed because of cancer or tuberculous infection. The ureters are attached to the proximal end of the ileal loop; the distal end of the loop is exteriorized onto the skin of the anterior abdominal wall.*

THE MESENTERY OF THE SMALL BOWEL (Fig 27–6)

The mesentery of the jejunoileum is the means by which the entire small bowel is attached to the parietes of the posterior abdominal wall. The attachment of the "root" of the small bowel mesentery runs obliquely across the abdomen, starting just to the left of the second lumbar vertebra and ending near the right sacroiliac joint. The attachment of this mesentery to the posterior abdominal wall is normally about 15 cm long. As the root of the mesentery runs obliquely from left to right, it crosses, in order, the abdominal aorta, the vertebral column, and the transverse (third) portion of the duodenum. The superior mesenteric artery lies ventral to the third portion of the duodenum and crosses it to enter its base; the superior mesenteric vein leaves its base to pass superiorly across the transverse duodenum. The remainder of the root of the small bowel mesentery crosses, in order, the inferior vena cava, the right ureter, the right testicular or ovarian vessels, and the right iliac fossa.

The small bowel mesentery measures 14–30 cm from its root to the mesenteric border. The mid portion of the small bowel has the largest mesentery, whereas the segments of the small bowel closest to the cecum and the duodenojejunal flexure have the shortest mesentery. Failures of proper mesenteric root attachment and failure of proper mesenteric development (particularly failure of length) lead to various clinical syndromes. (See Chapter 22.)

⫸ ***Abnormally long small bowel mesentery leading to volvulus.*** *Occasionally, the mesentery of the small bowel just proximal to the cecum may be abnormally lax, conferring abnormal mobility on this segment of bowel. If, in addition, the cecum and the lower ascending colon and its mesentery are not well fixed to the posterior abdominal wall, there is a risk of ileocecalcolic volvulus. If the root of the small bowel mesentery is too short, there is a risk of volvulus of the entire small bowel about the shortened mesentery root.*

Within the leaves of the mesentery of the small bowel are the arteries, veins, lymphatics, and nerves supplying and draining the jejunoileum.

BLOOD VESSELS, LYMPHATICS, & NERVES

Arteries
(Fig 27–7)

The arterial supply to the entire small bowel is derived from the **superior mesenteric artery.** This

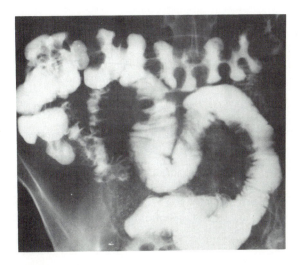

Figure 27–5. Barium x-ray showing spicules, edema, and ulcers in Crohn's disease. (Reproduced, with permission, from Way LW [editor]: *Current Surgical Diagnosis & Treatment,* 7th ed. Lange, 1985.)

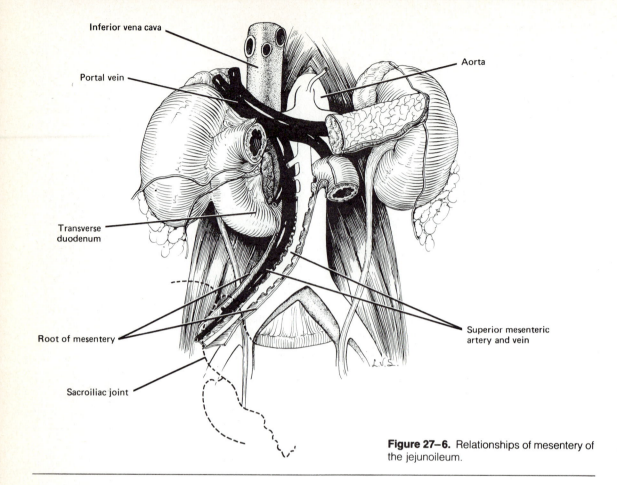

Inferior vena cava

Portal vein

Aorta

Transverse
duodenum

Root of mesentery

Superior mesenteric
artery and vein

Sacroiliac joint

Figure 27–6. Relationships of mesentery of
the jejunoileum.

branch of the abdominal aorta first appears visually
in the peritoneal cavity at the lower border of the
neck of the pancreas, ventral to its uncinate process.
It crosses the ventral surface of the third portion of
the duodenum and enters the root of the mesentery.
Within the small bowel mesentery, the artery forms
a long curve whose convexity faces the left side of
the abdomen. Most branches to the small intestine
are given off from the convex or left side of the
arterial curve; a few branches to the terminal ileum
are given off from the ileocolic artery.

➭ *Occlusion of superior mesenteric artery. Occlusion of the superior mesenteric artery or
of one of its distal branches may result in total
or segmental infarction of the midgut (the entire
small bowel, cecum, and appendix, the right
colon, and the right side of the transverse colon). Obviously, if the occlusion occurs near
the arterial takeoff from the abdominal aorta,
a large segment of small bowel and proximal
large bowel may become infarcted. The farther
distally the plugging of the artery occurs, the
smaller the segment of bowel infarcted. When*

*the terminal arterial arcades only are occluded,
usually only a relatively small area of bowel
will become gangrenous. If the occlusion occurs
slowly over many months, the involved bowel
is nourished by blood from the inferior mesenteric artery via the marginal artery (of Drummond). In such cases, the inferior mesenteric
artery almost doubles its caliber and length
and becomes markedly tortuous. This is easily
visible on inferior mesenteric arteriograms.*

➭ *Surgical treatment of superior mesenteric arterial occlusion. Arterial blockage may be relieved either by opening the affected vessel and
removing the blocking thrombus or plaque or
by using a bypass graft to the artery distal to
its point of obstruction. In many instances, such
surgery has prevented irreversible small bowel
gangrene.*

The **ileocolic artery** is the most distal segment
of the superior mesenteric artery. It is found in the
right lower abdominal quadrant, where it gives off
branches that supply the terminal ileum, the cecum

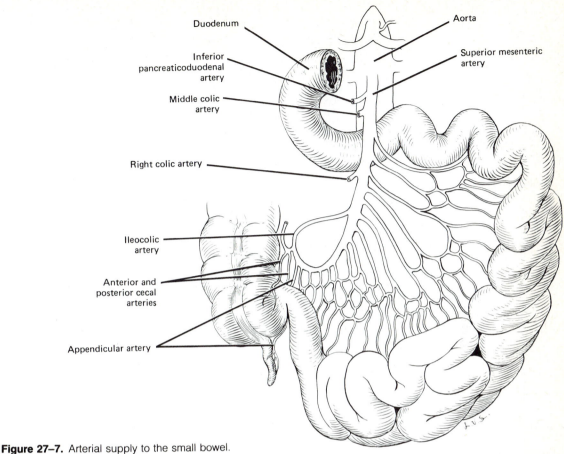

Figure 27–7. Arterial supply to the small bowel.

and appendix, and the proximal ascending colon. The inferior pancreaticoduodenal, middle colic, and right colic arteries (in that order) are all branches from the concave surface of the superior mesenteric artery.

There are usually 12–16 branches of the superior mesenteric artery running to the jejunum and ileum and entering the small bowel at its mesenteric border. There they penetrate the outer longitudinal smooth muscle of the bowel and then proceed to run within the circular muscle layer before reaching the antimesenteric border of the bowel.

➡ ***Arterial circulation to antimesenteric border of small bowel.*** *During resection and subsequent anastomosis of the small bowel to another loop of small bowel, to the esophagus or stomach, or to the colon or rectum, the surgeon must remember that the arterial circulation to the antimesenteric border of the small bowel is not as rich as that to the mesenteric border. Consequently, transection of small bowel before anastomosis should be done obliquely to leave a longer segment of bowel on the mesenteric border than on the antimesenteric border.*

Veins
(Fig 27–8)

Blood from the bowel capillaries funnels into venous channels, which are directed to the mesenteric border of the bowel, where they enter veins that parallel the branches of the superior mesenteric artery. These venous channels coalesce, and close to the root of the mesentery they form the **superior mesenteric vein.** Small bowel venous return joins with venous blood from the cecum and appendix, the ascending colon, and the right three-fourths of the transverse colon to form the superior mesenteric vein. The superior mesenteric vein (or 2–3 veins) leave the root of the small bowel mesentery, crossing the transverse duodenum and then lying on the uncinate process of the pancreas before dipping dorsal to the neck of the pancreas to join with the splenic vein to form the portal vein. Blood from the superior mesenteric vein ends mainly in the right side of the liver.

➡ ***Pylephlebitis.*** *Pylephlebitis of the veins of the superior mesenteric and portal system usually occurs after inflammation in the terminal ileum, cecum, appendix, or ascending colon. The in-*

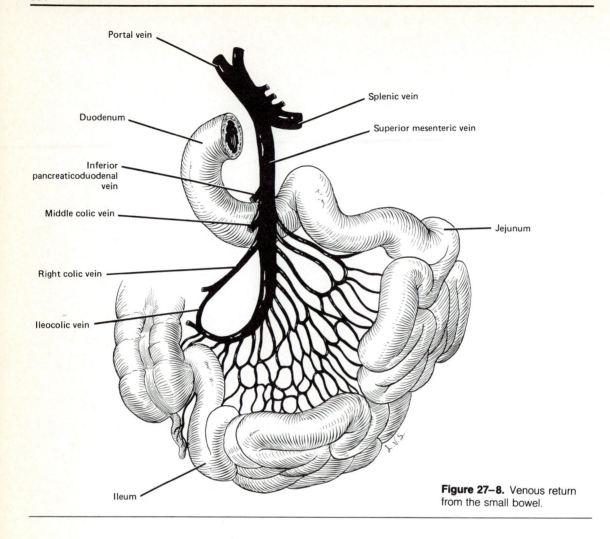

Figure 27–8. Venous return from the small bowel.

fected venous emboli will usually seed the right lobe of the liver, where multiple small pylephlebitic abscesses develop that may coalesce. Since the advent of antibiotics and the earlier diagnosis of gastrointestinal disease, this life-threatening clinical syndrome has become rare.

Lymphatics
(Fig 27–9)

The lymphatic system draining the jejunoileum includes the following: (1) lymphatic follicles within the small bowel wall, (2) lymph channels within the bowel wall, and (3) lymph nodes and lymph channels in the mesentery.

The mucosa and submucosa of the small bowel contain the deepest lymphatic elements of the jejunoileum. In addition, lymphatic follicles are present in the submucosa along the entire small bowel, becoming more numerous as the terminal ileum is approached. These follicles are located primarily in the submucosa but tend to protrude into the mucosal layer.

During small bowel disease, aggregated lymphatic follicles or Peyer's patches enlarge and move toward the serosa of the bowel. These patches hypertrophy in some diseases, tending to coalesce and increase in size near the ileocecal junction.

Individual small lymph channels that drain the small bowel begin in the submucosa and course through layers of smooth muscle to coalesce into larger lymphatic channels that accompany the venous drainage at the mesenteric border of the bowel. The large subserosal lymphatics drain into adjacent lymph nodes lying within the mesentery of the small bowel. The **cisterna chyli** is the dilated distal end of the lymph collection system, which eventually forms the thoracic duct.

Lymph nodes are few within the mesentery of the jejunum and proximal ileum. However, in the mesentery of the mid and terminal ileum they appear in large numbers, particularly at the ileocecal-colic angle. These distal mesenteric nodes plus the Peyer patches of the terminal ileum plus the lymphoid tissue aggregates of the appendix form a nearly complete

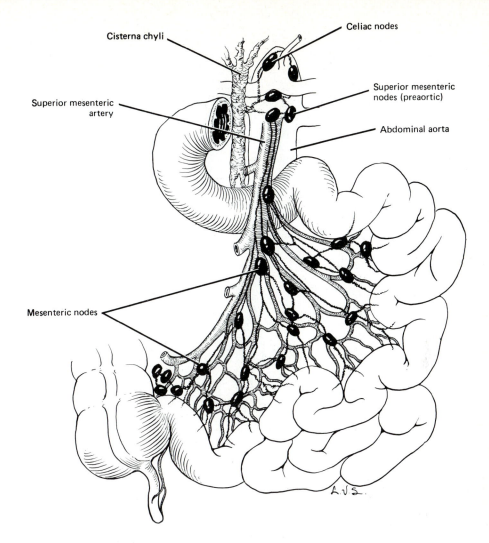

Figure 27–9. Lymphatic drainage from the small bowel.

circle of lymphatic tissue around the junction of the small and large bowel systems. This ring of lymphatic tissue serves as a filtration area and probably plays an important role in the immune response.

Ascending lymphatic drainage from the small bowel mesenteric nodes generally follows the pattern of the arterial circulation to the small bowel and runs to the root of the mesentery to empty into the preaortic nodes located at the celiac branch of the abdominal aorta.

⇒ *Lymphadenitis in mesentery of terminal ileum. The lymph nodes in the mesentery of the terminal ileum become enlarged and hyperplastic in a variety of gastrointestinal diseases, including regional enteritis, intestinal tuberculosis, and acute mesenteric lymphadenitis. Very rarely, these nodal enlargements will form a* *mass large enough to cause compression and obstruction of the terminal ileum.*

Nerves
(Fig 27–10)

The small intestine is served by nerves derived from the autonomic plexuses grouped around the take-off of the superior mesenteric artery from the aorta. These plexuses include the cranial preganglionic parasympathetics from the vagus as well as postganglionic sympathetic fibers from the celiac plexus. The 2 sets of fibers run to the myenteric plexuses in the bowel between the circular and longitudinal muscle fibers. Some branches from the myenteric plexus pierce the circular muscle fibers and form the submucosal plexus.

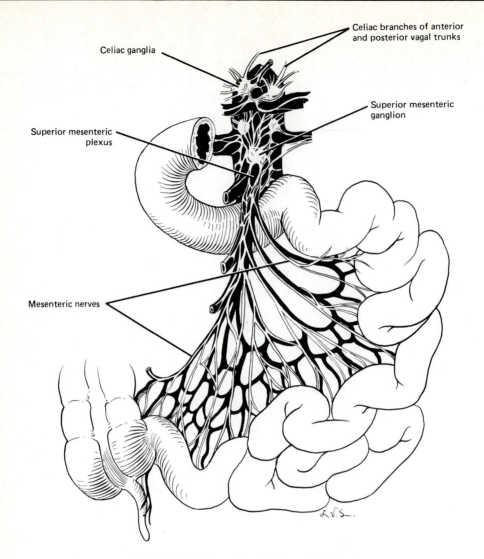

Celiac ganglia

Celiac branches of anterior and posterior vagal trunks

Superior mesenteric ganglion

Superior mesenteric plexus

Mesenteric nerves

Figure 27–10. Nerve supply to the small bowel.

➤ *Referred pain from the terminal ileum. The initial pain in acute appendicitis is usually felt in the periumbilical region. This is referred from the appendix itself or due to distention of the terminal ileum, which lies adjacent to the appendix. Pain in the terminal ileum is referred to the thoracic eighth, ninth, and tenth dermatomes.*

The submucosa of the small intestine contains the nerve plexus of Meissner. Between the longitudinal and circular muscle of the small bowel is the intramuscular myenteric (Auerbach's) plexus, consisting of nonmyelinated nerve fiber plus numerous ganglion cells.

The Large Bowel

28

The large bowel (Fig 28–1) can be divided into 5 sections for study purposes: (1) the cecum and vermiform appendix; (2) the ascending colon and the hepatic (right colic) flexure; (3) the transverse colon and mesocolon; (4) the splenic (left colic) flexure and the descending colon; and (5) the sigmoid colon.

EMBRYOLOGY
(See also Chapter 22.)

Right Portion of Large Bowel

The postarterial loop of the midgut develops into the terminal ileum, the cecum, the vermiform appendix, the ascending colon, the hepatic flexure, and the right three-fourths of the transverse colon. Anomalies: The cecum, appendix, and ascending colon may be found in the midline or in the left abdomen. The ascending colon may be absent, with a subhepatic cecum, or it may have an abnormally long mesentery.

Left Portion of Large Bowel

The hindgut develops into the left one-fourth of the transverse colon, the splenic flexure, the descending (left) colon, the sigmoid colon, and the rectum as far inferiorly as the anorectal line. Anomalies: The mesentery of the transverse or sigmoid colon may be abnormally long. There may be a single true congenital diverticulum, usually of the right colon or cecum, as well as congenital megacolon or congenital familial polyposis of the colon (Gardner's syndrome, Peutz-Jeghers syndrome).

Congenital stenosis or atresia and enteric cysts are rare anomalies.

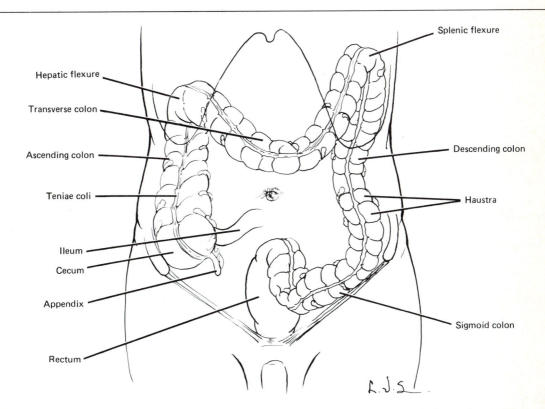

Figure 28–1. The colon. (Modified and reproduced, with permission, from Way LW [editor]: *Current Surgical Diagnosis & Treatment,* 7th ed. Lange, 1985.)

GROSS ANATOMY
(Fig 28–2)

The colon is about 1.4–1.7 m in length. Its diameter is greatest on the right side in the area of the cecum and ascending colon. The colon gradually narrows, so that the distal sigmoid colon is often no wider than a loop of terminal ileum—and is always narrower than a segment of the proximal jejunum. The cecum is about 7.5 cm wide and the ascending colon about 6 cm wide. The descending and sigmoid colon are 3.5–4 cm wide. The cecum is 6–7 cm long; the ascending colon varies from 8 to 20 cm in length; the transverse colon—the longest colonic segment—is 40–50 cm in length; the descending colon is 10–12 cm in length; the fixed sigmoid about 12 cm; and the mobile sigmoid about 38 cm in length. Just distal to the rectosigmoid junction, the large bowel once again dilates to form the wide ampulla of the rectum.

Similar to the remainder of the gastrointestinal tract, the large bowel is made up of 5 distinct layers: serosa, muscularis externa, submucosa, muscularis mucosae, and mucosa.

The outer **serous coat (tunica serosa coli)** is a component of the peritoneum. Normally it completely covers the cecum, the appendix, and the transverse and sigmoid colonic segments, except for a narrow slot along the mesenteric attachments of the bowel.

Since the ascending and descending segments of the colon are normally fused to the fascia covering the muscles of the abdominal wall, these portions of the colon are not covered with serosa along their areas of fusion.

The **muscularis externa (tunica muscularis coli)** of the large bowel is composed of a complete inner circular and an incomplete outer longitudinal layer of smooth muscle.

The **submucosa (tela submucosa)** is composed of areolar tissue and lies between the muscularis externa and the muscularis mucosae. It contains the terminations of the blood and lymphatic vessels supplying the bowel. It contains also lymphatic nodules, most abundantly in the proximal and distal colonic segments.

The thin **muscularis mucosae** is made up of circular and longitudinal smooth muscle.

The inner layer, the **mucosa (tunica mucosa coli)** is smooth and devoid of villi, consisting of a layer of simple columnar epithelium containing goblet cells. The straight tubular intestinal glands are wedged together and open onto the mucosal surface at small round apertures.

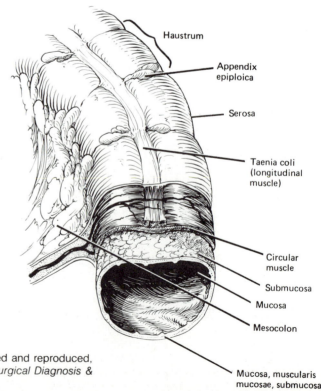

Haustrum

Appendix epiploica

Serosa

Taenia coli (longitudinal muscle)

Circular muscle

Submucosa

Mucosa

Mesocolon

Mucosa, muscularis mucosae, submucosa

Figure 28–2. Cross section of the colon. (Modified and reproduced, with permission, from Way LW [editor]: *Current Surgical Diagnosis & Treatment,* 7th ed. Lange, 1985).

The muscular coats of the colon are arranged differently from those of the stomach, small intestine, and rectum. Longitudinal smooth muscle covers the large bowel incompletely. The longitudinal fibers are arranged in 3 narrow but distinct bands called teniae coli. Between these 3 bands, the deeper circular muscle coat is visible. Contractions of the colon result in pouching or sacculation of the bowel between the longitudinal bands. The pouchings, or haustra, are randomly distributed; they are easily noted on gross examination and usually visible in roentgenograms.

On the cecum and the ascending colon, the teniae have a constant position relative to the bowel circumference, one band lying on the ventral surface of the colon while the other 2 lie medial and lateral to the ventral band. In the transverse colon, the teniae are less constant in position. Near the rectosigmoid junction, the teniae become quite indistinct, and the 3 bands merge into 2 aggregates of longitudinal muscle that widen and ultimately completely cover the rectosigmoid and rectum with longitudinal muscle fibers. Projecting from the antimesenteric border of the transverse, descending, and sigmoid segments are numerous lobules of fat, the appendices epiploicae, each enclosed within a complete peritoneal sac.

➡ *The teniae of the colon. The teniae of the colon are of clinical importance for the following reasons: (1) They hold sutures better than areas not covered with longitudinal muscle; (2) colotomy is nearly always performed by incising the colonic wall through one of the teniae; and (3) the teniae assist in anastomosis of one segment to another segment and help to line up corresponding areas of bowel circumference for suturing with maintenance of proper physiologic action.*

Diastatic rupture occurs most frequently in the cecum, alongside its anterior longitudinal band. This condition occasionally accompanies a distal large bowel obstruction.

➡ *Relationship of teniae to the base of the appendix. At the posteromedial side of the cecum, the 3 longitudinal bands converge to mark the base of the appendix. This anatomic landmark is indispensable to the surgeon in the search for a "wayward appendix."*

➡ *Infarction of the appendices epiploicae. The appendices epiploicae of the transverse and left colon may very rarely become acutely inflamed or infarcted and may give rise to a puzzling syndrome of intra-abdominal signs and symptoms. Diagnosis is seldom made before laparotomy. Following infarction, the fatty lobules may be cast off from the colonic surface and found lying free in the peritoneal cavity.*

Topographic Anatomy
(Fig 28–3)

The **cecum,** the most proximal segment of the large bowel, projects inferiorly from the ileocecal junction. It is usually in the right iliac fossa anterior to the iliacus muscle, but it may be at any level from the low pelvis to the subhepatic area.

The **ascending colon** lies on the right side of the abdomen and runs superiorly from the ileocecal junction to the hepatic or right colic flexure. Just above the ileocecal junction, the ascending colon lies on the right psoas major muscle and the iliacus and quadratus lumborum muscles. Near the hepatic flexure, the ascending colon lies ventral to the right kidney and the aponeurotic fibers of origin of the transverse abdominis muscle.

The **hepatic flexure** is the area where the ascending colon turns to become the proximal transverse colon. The hepatic flexure lies in apposition to the posteroinferior surface of the right lobe of the liver.

The **transverse colon** crosses the abdomen from right to left to the splenic flexure. Its mesentery is attached to the ventral surface of the head, neck, body, and tail of the pancreas and to the ventral surface of the mid portion of the descending duodenum.

The **splenic flexure,** which is 2 vertebrae higher than the hepatic flexure, lies adjacent to the tail of the pancreas and the inferior pole of the spleen. It is attached by a peritoneal fold, the phrenicocolic ligament, to the left lateral leaf of the diaphragm at the level of the tenth and 11th ribs.

The **fixed left** or **descending colon** passes almost vertically from the splenic flexure to the level of the iliac crest. It lies closer to the left abdominal parietes than the ascending colon does to the right parietes. The level at which the left colon acquires a mesentery marks the beginning of the sigmoid colon.

The **sigmoid colon** is a mobile loop of colon that takes off from the descending colon to merge in the true pelvis with the superior segment of the rectum. As it descends, it describes a broad S-shaped loop. Its junction with the upper rectum is just to the right of the midline at the level of S3.

CECUM & VERMIFORM APPENDIX

1. CECUM
(Figs 28–4, 28–5, & 28–6)

The cecum, the thinnest portion of the colon, is about 6 cm long and lies caudal to the entrance of the ileum into the colon. It normally lies on the right iliacus muscle with its midpoint near the anterosuperior iliac spine, but it may be higher or lower. The cecum presents 3 well-differentiated teniae that merge at its medial inferior border, where they always mark the base of the appendix (an indispensable surgical landmark). In the fetus and young child, the teniae join at the most dependent segment of the cecum,

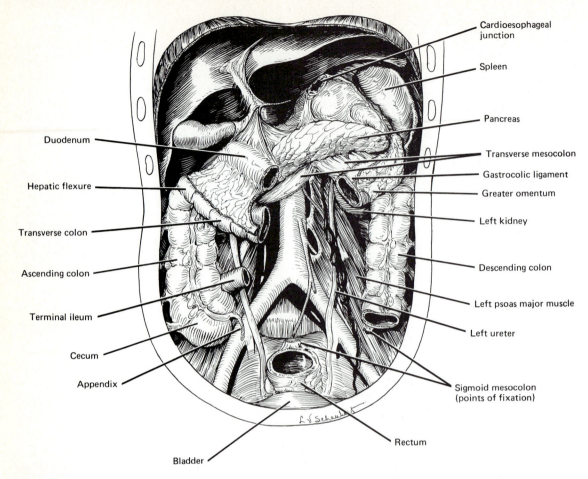

Cardioesophageal junction

Spleen

Pancreas

Transverse mesocolon

Gastrocolic ligament

Greater omentum

Left kidney

Descending colon

Left psoas major muscle

Left ureter

Sigmoid mesocolon (points of fixation)

Duodenum

Hepatic flexure

Transverse colon

Ascending colon

Terminal ileum

Cecum

Appendix

Rectum

Bladder

Figure 28–3. Relationships of the large bowel. The stomach and the mid portion of the transverse colon have been removed.

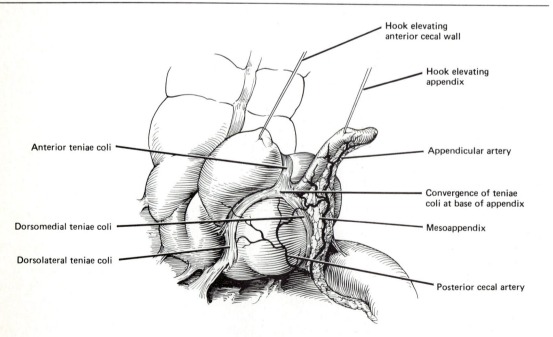

Hook elevating anterior cecal wall

Hook elevating appendix

Anterior teniae coli

Appendicular artery

Convergence of teniae coli at base of appendix

Mesoappendix

Dorsomedial teniae coli

Dorsolateral teniae coli

Posterior cecal artery

Figure 28–4. Convergence of the teniae coli on the posterior cecum.

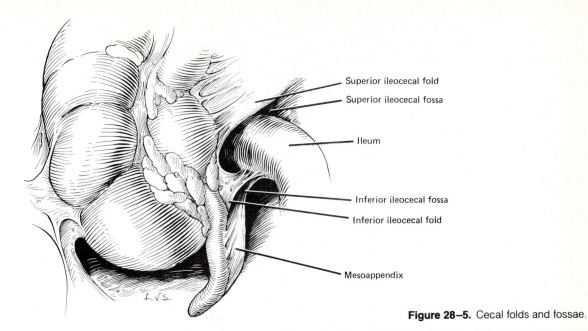

Superior ileocecal fold
Superior ileocecal fossa
Ileum
Inferior ileocecal fossa
Inferior ileocecal fold
Mesoappendix

Figure 28–5. Cecal folds and fossae.

the caput coli. Later, the portion of the cecum between the anterior and posterolateral teniae grows more rapidly than the remainder, pushing the inferior cecal segment with its attached appendix and its junction of the 3 teniae posteriorly and to the left. Consequently, after early childhood, the appendix normally opens into the cecum posteromedially.

Ileocecal colic angle. The ileocecal colic angle is the site of many pathologic entities.

Intestinal obstruction in the ileocolic area may be due to the following: (1) volvulus; (2) ileocolic intussusception; (3) hyperplastic tuberculosis of bowel and adjacent mesentery; (4) cicatrizing enteritis; (5) congenital or in-

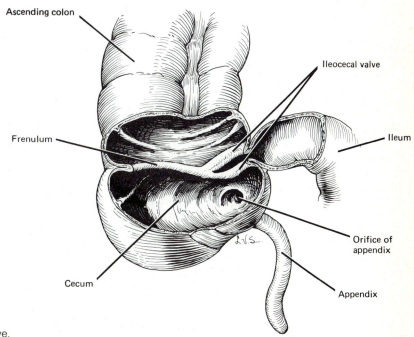

Ascending colon
Ileocecal valve
Frenulum
Ileum
Orifice of appendix
Cecum
Appendix

Figure 28–6. The ileocecal valve.

flammatory regional bands; (6) cancer of the terminal ileum, cecum, or ascending colon; (7) amebic granulomas of the cecum; (8) benign bowel tumors (fibromas, lipomas, myomas); (9) carcinoid tumors of the appendix or cecum; (10) congenital reduplications or absences of portions of bowel; (11) stenosis or atresia of bowel segments (rare in the ileocolic angle); (12) marked dilatation of the cecum and ascending colon with secondary diastatic rupture of the cecum due to distal large bowel obstruction in the presence of a competent ileocecal valve; and (13) right-sided sliding hernia, with cecum and, on occasion, lower ascending colon as the sliding component in the indirect hernial sac (Fig 28–7).

Vascular diseases involving the bowel in the ileocolic angle include pylephlebitis of the ileocolic veins and acute or chronic segmental infarction of bowel due to arterial or venous occlusion, or both.

*Acute, subacute, or chronic **ileocolitis**— both specific and nonspecific in origin—may occur.*

Other pathologic conditions that may occur in the area include tuberculosis, parasitic infection (amebiasis, ascariasis, etc), typhoid fever, mycotic infection, and nonspecific acute ulcerative colitis.

The cecum is normally mobile, and in over 90% of individuals it is completely covered with peritoneum and possesses no mesentery. In cases where the cecum becomes attached to the posterior abdominal wall, there is a fusion between the peritoneum of the dorsal wall of the cecum and the posterior parietal peritoneum covering the iliac fossa.

There are usually 3 folds of peritoneum arising from the area of the terminal ileum. The ''superior ileocecal fold'' extends from the mesentery of the terminal ileum to the lowest segment of the ascending colon and on to the adjacent segment of the cecum. It encloses the anterior cecal branch of the ileocolic artery and forms the overhanging crescentic margin of the superior ileocecal fossa. Two inferior ileocecal folds extend inferiorly from the left leaf of the mesentery of the terminal ileum, one running to the cecum and the other to the appendix. Between these 2 folds lies the triangular inferior ileocecal fossa. The shorter anterior fold is usually avascular; the longer, more posterior fold acts as a mesentery for the appendix and contains the appendicular artery, a branch of the ileocolic artery.

The terminal loop of ileum usually rises from the pelvis to join the cecum, approaching it either obliquely or directly from left to right at a 90-degree angle to the long axis of the cecum. The mesentery of the terminal ileal loop varies in length from rather short, tightly apposed to the bowel, to quite long, allowing marked mobility of the bowel. Both of these

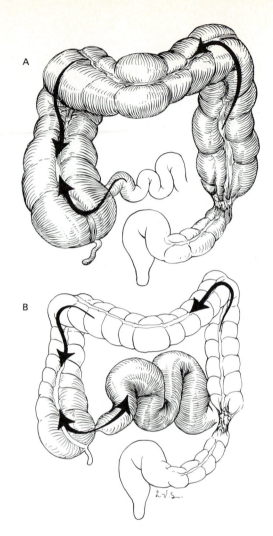

Figure 28–7. The role of the ileocecal valve in obstruction of the colon. The obstruction is in the upper sigmoid. **A:** The ileocecal valve is competent, creating a closed loop between the obstruction and the valve. Tension in the closed loop is increased further by emptying of gas and fluid from the ileum into the colon. **B:** The ileocecal valve is incompetent. Reflux into the ileum is permitted. The colon is relieved of some of its distention, and the small bowel has become distended. (Reproduced, with permission, from Way LW [editor]: *Current Surgical Diagnosis & Treatment,* 7th ed. Lange, 1985.)

extremes of terminal ileal mobility play an important role in the causation of both volvulus of the ileocecal colon and intussusception of the ileum into the cecum and ascending colon.

Penetration of the posteromedial wall of the cecum by the ileum forces mucosa, submucosa, and circular muscle of the terminal small bowel into the lumen of the cecum and forms the **ileocecal valve.** If the cecum is opened, this protrusion may be seen on the posteromedial surface as 2 transverse parallel folds. The superior and inferior lips of the valve fuse at its lateral borders to form 2 ridges that continue laterally, encircling the cecum. These ridges—the cecal frenula—probably act as a minor cecocolic sphincter. The surface of the lips of the ileocecal valve facing toward the ileum is covered with small bowel mucosa; the surface facing toward the large bowel is covered with large bowel mucosa.

The physiologic mechanism of the ileocecal valve is not fully understood. Most probably, intracecal tension tightens the 2 frenula of the valve, regulating valvular competence. A sphincterlike action of the circular muscle of the protruding ileum contributes to the efficiency of the valve. The primary function of the valve is to prevent rapid flow of ileal contents into the colon rather than to prevent reflux of colonic feces into the ileum.

➡️ *Competence of the ileocecal valve. Retrograde flow caused by incompetence of the ileocecal valve seems to be the rule rather than the exception. Consequently, regurgitation of liquid and gaseous colonic contents into the ileum nearly always occurs in colonic obstruction. Consequently, distal small bowel dilatation often follows large bowel obstruction. In contrast, failure of relaxation of the ileocecal sphincter mechanism in complete, prolonged large bowel obstruction results in cecal thinning and marked dilatation. It may lead to diastatic rupture of*

the thin-walled cecum if the obstruction is not relieved.

2. VERMIFORM APPENDIX (Fig 28–8)

The appendix is the remnant of the embryonic apex of the cecum. In postfetal life, overgrowth of that portion of cecum lying between the anterior and right lateral teniae rotates the original apical portion of the cecum into a posteromedial position. The 3 bands of longitudinal muscle on the surface of the right colon that originally joined at the most dependent portion of the cecum now join at its medially rotated apex. The junction of the bands marks the site of the appendiceal base even though the cecal apex has moved from its original dependent position.

Congenital absence, diverticula, and reduplication are rare appendiceal anomalies.

Histologically, the appendix consists of the same 5 layers as the remainder of the large bowel. The outer serous coat completely invests the organ save for a narrow strip along which the mesoappendix attaches. There are no teniae on the appendiceal surface. There is a well-delineated appendiceal submucosa with large aggregations of lymphoid tissue. These lymphoid aggregations cause the mucosal coat of the appendix to bulge into the appendiceal lumen. The mucosa of the appendix is lined by columnar

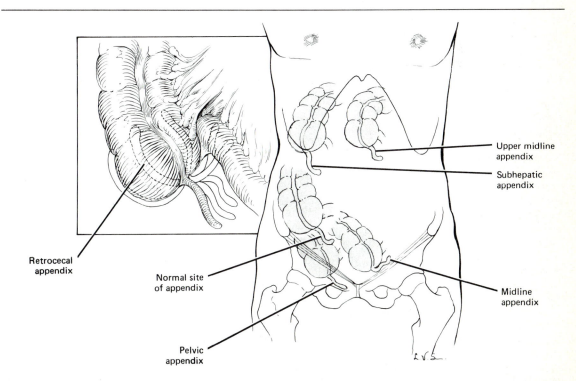

Figure 28–8. Positions of the appendix. (Modified and reproduced, with permission, from Way LW [editor]: *Current Surgical Diagnosis & Treatment,* 7th ed. Lange, 1985.)

epithelial cells similar to those in the large bowel. There are fewer intestinal glands in the appendiceal mucosa than in the mucosa of the large bowel.

The site of entrance of the appendix into the cecal lumen is marked by an inconstant, crescentic mucosal fold—the "apendiceal valve"—which, when present, limits the amount of fecal material that enters the appendix.

The appendix varies in length from 2 to 20 cm (average, 9 cm) and in width from 0.2 to 1 cm (average, 0.6 cm). In the great majority of individuals, the appendix is held in position by the posteroinferior ileocecal fold. This fold is roughly triangular and contains the appendiceal artery. The fold acts as the mesentery of the appendix and forms the posterior border of the shallow ileocecal fossa. In about 5% of cases, the mesentery of the appendix runs directly from the posterior peritoneum in the region of the ileocecal junction onto the mid portion of the appendix, at which point it is usually joined by the appendicular artery, a branch of the ileocolic artery.

The location of the body and tip of the appendix depends on (1) the length of the appendix and its mesentery, (2) the final positioning of the cecum during gut rotation and fixation, (3) the degree of fixation to the posterior abdominal wall of the cecum and lower ascending colon, and (4) pathologic processes at or in the vicinity of the ileocecal colic angle. In about 45% of individuals, the tip of the appendix floats free in the peritoneal cavity and points upward and medially. The appendix may be tightly attached to the ventral surface of the psoas muscle by a short mesentery. The distal segment of the appendix may lie in the pelvis if it is long and the tip points caudally or if it is short and develops from a low-lying cecum. The pelvic appendix may lie among the pelvic viscera or it may lie against the bladder in the female or against the seminal vesicles, prostate, or bladder in the male. A true retrocecal or retrocolic appendix is one held in position dorsal to the cecum and the proximal ascending colon. In such individuals, the tip of the appendix may rise posterior to the cecum and ascending colon to a subhepatic position if the appendix is abnormally long.

Several inconstant peritoneal bands and membranes may bind the appendix down to the cecum or to the lateral or posterior abdominal walls. The most common membrane—the pericolic membrane, or "Jackson's veil"—usually presents as a vascular structure extending from the posterior abdominal wall onto the anterolateral surface of the cecum (Fig 28–9). Because the blood vessels run transversely in a parallel pattern, it is usually easy to distinguish such a membrane from lateral adhesion of the cecum secondary to inflammation.

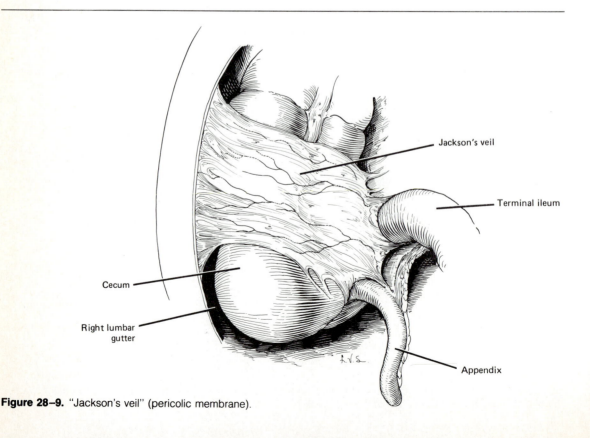

Figure 28–9. "Jackson's veil" (pericolic membrane).

3. BLOOD VESSELS, LYMPHATICS, & NERVES

Arteries
(Fig 28–10)

The terminal 14 cm of ileum, the cecum, and the appendix plus the adjoining ascending colon are supplied by the **ileocolic artery,** the terminal segment of the **superior mesenteric artery.** The ileocolic artery runs obliquely from left to right in the mesentery of the small bowel, terminating in the right lower quadrant. It ends just proximal to the ileocecal junction, dividing into 4 major branches. The most superior of these, the **colic artery,** passes to the ascending colon, anastomosing with the descending branches of the right colic artery—or of the middle colic artery if the right colic artery is not present. This anastomosis lies close to the mesenteric border of the beginning of the ascending colon and initiates the right colic segment of the marginal artery of Drummond, the vessel that is essential in maintenance of circulation during colonic surgery.

The second branch of the ileocolic artery is the **cecal artery,** which leaves the ileocolic artery just below the takeoff of the colic branch. The cecal artery divides almost immediately into 2 branches, the anterior and posterior cecal arteries, which encircle the mid cecum.

The **appendicular artery** arises either as a branch of the posterior cecal artery or directly from the main ileocolic trunk. On rare occasions it may arise from the ileal branch of the ileocolic artery. Regardless of its site of origin, the appendicular artery will pass dorsal to the most distal segment of the terminal ileum before it enters the mesoappendix.

The **ileal artery** supplies the terminal 12–14 cm of the ileum. This vessel is practically an end artery, since there is little or no anastomotic flow between it and the other major branches.

➠ *Psoas extension test in acute appendicitis. The appendix is on occasion attached by a short mesentery to the posterior peritoneum covering the ventral surface of the right psoas major muscle. If such an appendix becomes inflamed, forced extension of the right thigh causes increased pain in the right lower quadrant, a positive right psoas extension test. The test is also positive if an acutely inflamed appendix rests directly on the psoas muscle.*

➠ *Pelvic appendicitis. A pelvic appendix may lie against any of the pelvic viscera (uterus, adnexa, bladder, seminal vesicles, etc). Dysuria or pyuria may be caused by an inflamed appendix lying against the bladder. A pelvic appendix is often responsible for female pelvic adnexal tenderness, suggesting a diagnosis of pelvic inflammatory disease. A true pelvic appendix is difficult to diagnose, particularly in infants and in the aged, and appendicitis is associated with high morbidity and mortality rates in these age groups.*

➠ *Obturator test. A long appendix pointing caudally or a normal-sized appendix arising from a cecum low in the pelvis may lie against the obturator internus muscle. If such an appendix becomes inflamed, the obturator test will be*

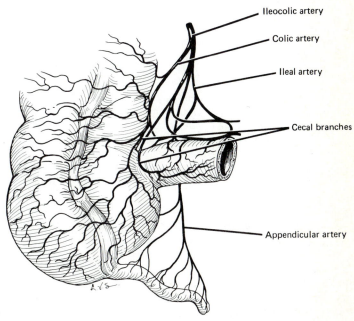

Ileocolic artery

Colic artery

Ileal artery

Cecal branches

Appendicular artery

Figure 28–10. Arterial supply to the cecum.

positive, ie, flexion and lateral rotation of the right thigh on the lower abdomen will cause increased lower abdominal pain and spasm.

⇒ ***Retrocecal appendicitis.*** *A true retrocecal appendix is held down to the posterior abdominal wall, dorsal to the cecum and ascending colon, as a result of embryonic serous layer fusion, or an inflammatory adhesion may hold the appendix in a retrocecal position. When a true retrocecal appendix held by serous layer fusion is approached surgically, the cecum must be freed from the posterior abdominal wall by sharp dissection along the line of its fusion plane, the dissection beginning laterally where the cecum impinges on the right lumbar gutter. When the appendix is bound in a retrocecal position by an inflammatory process, it may be freed by careful blunt dissection. A retrocecal appendix may lie behind the cecum and the ascending colon or behind the peritoneum of the right lumbar gutter. The appendiceal tip may be as high as the gallbladder fossa.*

⇒ ***Paracecal membranes.*** *The presence of inconstant peritoneal membranes, related to the cecum, terminal ileum, and appendix, may result in small bowel obstruction, the small bowel twisting on or being compressed by one or more of the membranes. If such membranes are present when the abdomen is explored for an acutely inflamed appendix, they may tend to obscure the appendix.*

⇒ ***Diseases of the appendix.*** *Common diseases of the appendix include (1) acute suppurative appendicitis, with or without rupture; (2) cancer; (3) carcinoid tumors; and (4) mucocele.*

⇒ ***Blood supply to terminal ileum.*** *In resection of the cecum and ascending colon for malignant or inflammatory disease, it is necessary to resect the distal 6–8 cm of the terminal ileum. Resection of the terminal segment of ileum is necessary because it is supplied directly by the ileal branch of the ileocolic artery, as an end artery. Such resection endangers the arterial supply, and the ileotransverse colostomy may be at risk as a result of the lack of circulation to the terminal ileal segment.*

Veins
(Fig 28–11)

The venous return from the ileocecal colic segment is through veins that parallel the arterial blood supply. The veins eventually form one or 2 major ileocolic trunks that join the superior mesenteric vein. The junction is below the point where the superior mesenteric vein disappears behind the neck of the pancreas, just above the root of the mesentery of the small bowel.

⇒ ***Pylephlebitis.*** *The main ileocolic vein and its distal tributaries play an important role in venous spread of infection and cancer cells, primarily toward the right lobe of the liver via the portal vein. This occurs in phylephlebitis secondary to suppurative processes in the ileocolic angle.*

Lymphatics
(Fig 28–12)

Lymphatic drainage from the ileocecal colic segment passes via lymphatic channels that closely parallel the arterial supply to the area (ileocolic artery). Clustered around the ileocolic artery are 2 groups of nodes: the inferior and superior ileocolic nodes. Most of the lymph from the ileocolic nodes eventually drains into lymphatics that run deep to the pancreas to empty into the lumbar aortic chain of nodes. About 5% of ileocolic lymph passes ventral to the pancreas to empty into the subpyloric gastric group of nodes. The collection of ileocecal colic mesenteric lymph nodes with their multiple anastomosing lymphatic channels, the large amount of lymphatic tissue in the submucosa of the appendix, and the numerous terminal ileal lymphatic patches together make this area a prime lymphatic filtration center.

⇒ ***Ileocolic lymphatics and arteries.*** *Generally, lymphatic flow from the ileocecal colic angle is via channels in close apposition to the arteries supplying the area. Consequently, ligation of these arteries close to their origins is probably the best method of handling lymphatic spread from the area.*

Nerves
(Fig 28–13)

The nerve supply to the ileocecal colic segment is derived from nerve trunks that closely follow the arterial pathway to the bowel. The nerves are branchings from the celiac and mesenteric autonomic plexuses. Both the right and left vagi give off branches to the celiac and mesenteric plexuses, so that branches to the bowel from this plexus carry parasympathetic fibers as well as sympathetic ones. The postganglionic cell bodies of the sympathetic fibers to the bowel lie within the celiac plexus. The afferent fibers are concerned with pain from either the ileocecal colic mesentery or from the bowel. Neither vagotomy nor sympathectomy seems to have any marked effect on colonic activity in the ileocolic area.

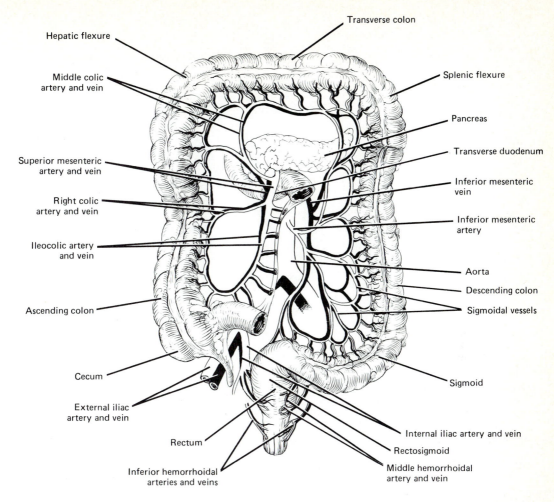

Figure 28–11. Arteries and veins of the colon. (Modified and reproduced, with permission, from Way LW [editor]: *Current Surgical Diagnosis & treatment,* 7th ed. Lange, 1985.)

ASCENDING COLON & HEPATIC (RIGHT COLIC) FLEXURE

1. ASCENDING COLON

The ascending colon occupies most of the right side of the abdominal cavity and extends from the cecum to the hepatic flexure. Its length and the degree of fixation vary greatly. Normally, the inferior limits of the ascending colon are at the level of the iliac crest, while the superior segment reaches to about the level at which the right tenth rib crosses the midaxillary line.

The posterior surface of the ascending colon is usually fused to the peritoneum of the posterior abdominal wall, so that the bowel surface is covered only anteriorly and laterally by peritoneum. In 8–10% of patients, part or all of the ascending colon and cecum may be mobile and may swing on a mesentery. Conversely, the entire cecum and ascending colon may be tightly fixed to the posterior abdominal wall.

The superior segment of the ascending colon is related anteriorly to the visceral undersurface of the right lobe of the liver and to the structures that lie in the fossa of the gallbladder. Posteriorly, the ascending colon is usually related by its fusion fascia to the underlying iliacus, psoas major, and quadratus lumborum muscles. The superior third of the ascending colon is related posteriorly to the lower pole of the right kidney and the branchings of the right renal vessels. The mid portion of the ascending colon is related posteriorly to the right testicular and ovarian arteries and the abdominal portion of the ureter. Medially, on a more posterior plane, is the distal half of the descending duodenum. Laterally, the ascending colon is related to the right lumbar gutter that separates it from the right lateral abdominal parietes. This wide gutter connects the right supra- and inframesocolic compartments of the abdomen. Occasionally, the

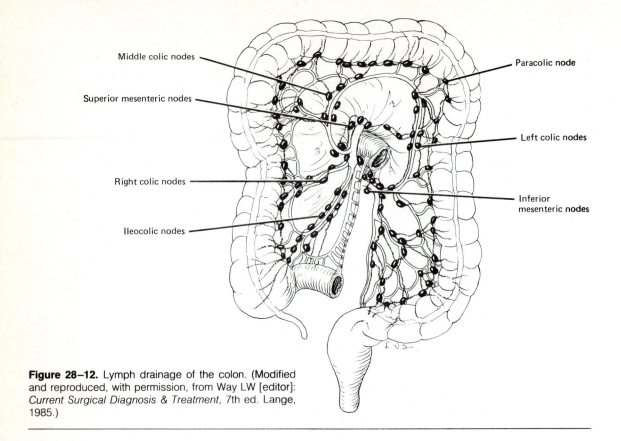

Figure 28–12. Lymph drainage of the colon. (Modified and reproduced, with permission, from Way LW [editor]: *Current Surgical Diagnosis & Treatment,* 7th ed. Lange, 1985.)

greater omentum fuses to the anteromedial surface of the ascending colon. When this occurs, the most proximal segment of the transverse colon is close to the medial superior border of the ascending colon, creating a double-barreled relationship. Normally, the dorsal leaf of the mesentery of the ascending colon is fused to the posterior peritoneum of the abdominal cavity. When the right colon is mobilized by incising the lateral peritoneal fusion fascia along its antimesenteric border, a fusion fascial plane can be developed between the mesentery and the posterior peritoneum anteriorly and the retroperitoneum posteriorly, making it relatively easy to preserve the right ureter and gonadal vessels.

➠ **Right sliding hernia.** *When the dorsal fusion fascia of the ascending colon, which fixes the bowel to the posterior abdominal parietes, becomes attenuated by advancing age or long-standing debilitating disease, it allows the ascending colon to slide down on the posterior abdominal parietes toward the true pelvis. This often places the cecum and the lower ascending colon close to the internal inguinal ring, with the risk of a right-sided sliding hernia.*

➠ **Right retrocolic and paraduodenal hernias.** *If the mesocolon to the ascending colon persists as part of the mesenteric complex of the small bowel and the superior mesenteric artery, it is possible for either a right retrocolic hernia or a right paraduodenal hernia of the mesoparietal type to develop. In both conditions, loops of small bowel become trapped dorsal to the mobile unfixed mesocolon of the right colon.*

➠ **Mobilization of right colon.** *Resection of the cecum and ascending colon is done for cure of infections or malignant disease. The right colon is mobilized by incising the lateral peritoneal fusion area along the antimesenteric border of the bowel. The colon can easily be drawn medially along with its supplying vessels, nerves, and lymphatics. Great care must be taken during dissection and elevation of the colon to preserve the underlying renal and ureteral structures as well as the testicular or ovarian arteries.*

➠ **Diverticulosis.** *Diverticula of the cecum or ascending colon are usually single and on the mesenteric border. They are seldom part of a generalized diverticulosis. A single diverticulum of the right colon is prone to acute inflammation and possible rupture.*

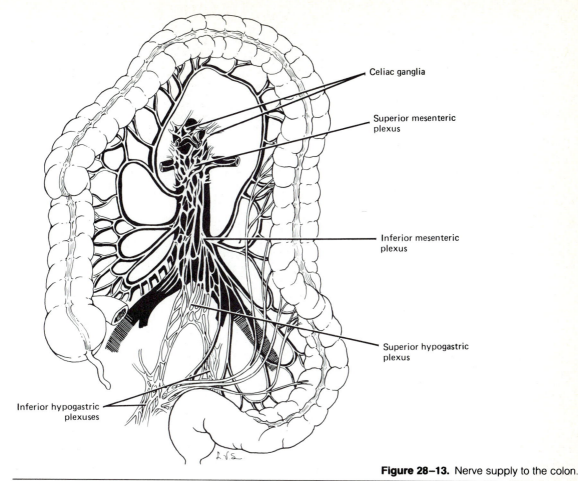

Figure 28–13. Nerve supply to the colon.

Celiac ganglia

Superior mesenteric plexus

Inferior mesenteric plexus

Superior hypogastric plexus

Inferior hypogastric plexuses

▥▶ *Upper ascending colon and gallbladder fossa. The proximity of the upper ascending colon, the hepatic flexure, and the right quarter of the transverse colon to the structures in the gallbladder fossa makes it possible for gallstones to pass into these segments of the colon through a cholecystocolic fistula.*

2. HEPATIC (RIGHT COLIC) FLEXURE

The hepatic flexure is the junction of the ascending and the transverse colon. It usually lies at the level of the right ninth or tenth rib in the midaxillary line. While the angle of the transverse to the ascending colon may vary, it is usually less acute than the angle formed at the splenic flexure. The angle at the hepatic flexure may be influenced by 2 fibrous bands: the **hepatoduodenocolic ligament,** which runs from the right lobe of the liver to the hepatic flexure of the colon; and the **cholecystocolic ligament,** which runs from the gallbladder to the hepatic flexure of the colon. Ptosis of the midsection of the transverse colon makes the angle at the hepatic flexure more acute.

The hepatic flexure usually lies between the right lobe of the liver and the ventral surface of the lower pole of the right kidney. Posterior to the hepatic flexure is the lower segment of the right kidney. The inferior half of the descending duodenum is dorsal and just medial to the flexure. Lateral to the hepatic flexure are the upper reaches of the right lumbar gutter. The hepatic flexure is covered with peritoneum except on its dorsal surface, where it adheres to the external layer of the perirenal fascia. The proximity of the hepatic flexure and the gallbladder fossa explains why adhesions occur between the flexure and the gallbladder in biliary tract disease.

▥▶ *Surgical mobilization. Mobilization of the hepatic flexure is often required. Incision of the fascia just lateral and superior to the flexure is a relatively bloodless procedure. When combined with the Kocher procedure for mobilization of the descending duodenum, it provides excellent exposure of the inferior half of the descending duodenum. It also allows good exposure of the superior half of the portal vein and the adjacent inferior vena cava, which is needed when a portocaval shunt is to be performed.*

3. BLOOD VESSELS, LYMPHATICS, & NERVES

Arteries
(Fig 28–11)

The ascending colon and the hepatic flexure are supplied by the superior mesenteric artery via (1) colic branches of the ileocolic artery, (2) the right colic artery, and (3) the right-sided branches of the middle colic artery. Each of these vessels, upon reaching the mesenteric border of the bowel, divides into 2 branches, one running distally and the other proximally along the bowel's mesenteric border, thus preserving the integrity of the marginal artery of Drummond. The colic branches of the ileocolic artery are described in the section on the cecum. The right colic artery is the most variable artery supplying the colon and is completely absent in 5–7% of people. It usually arises from the superior mesenteric artery, but it may be a branch of either the middle colic artery or the ileocolic artery. It runs toward the ascending colon between the 2 leaves of the right celiac mesentery. It lies ventral to the right ureter and right gonadal vessels. At the mesenteric border of the ascending colon, it divides into ascending and descending branches, each contributing to the marginal artery of Drummond. Generally, the right colic artery supplies the superior three-fourths of the ascending colon and the right 5 cm of the transverse colon. Since the vessels to the ascending colon run in the fused mesentery of that segment of bowel, they may be dissected free from the underlying peritoneum and retroperitoneal tissues when the peritoneum along the lateral border of the ascending colon is incised and the right colon is mobilized. The middle colic artery also supplies the hepatic flexure and the upper segment of the ascending colon via the marginal artery of Drummond.

Veins
(Fig 28–11)

Venous return from the ascending colon and the hepatic flexure is via vessels that closely parallel the arteries to this segment of bowel. The veins drain into the superior mesenteric system and thence into the portal venous systems.

➠ *Ligation of ileocolic venous channels. In operations for cancer of the terminal ileum, appendix, or proximal colon, the main ileocolic should be tied off as high as possible and as early as possible. It also should be ligated in the event of early pylephlebitis.*

Lymphatics
(Fig 28–12)

Lymphatic return from the ascending colon and the hepatic flexure is via vessels that closely parallel the arteries to these segments of bowel. The lymphatics drain, as do those of the cecum and terminal ileum, into nodes lying close to the origin of the superior mesenteric artery.

Nerves
(Fig 28–13)

The nerve supply to the ascending colon and hepatic flexure is derived from the celiac and mesenteric autonomic plexuses.

TRANSVERSE COLON & MESOCOLON

1. TRANSVERSE COLON

The transverse colon begins at the hepatic flexure and runs transversely to terminate at the splenic flexure. Dorsally, from right to left, the transverse colon is related to the inferior half of the descending duodenum, the surface of the pancreas, and the lower pole of the spleen. Ventrally, the right one-fourth of the transverse colon is related to the fossa of the gallbladder and to the right lobe of the liver. Lying just anterior to the transverse colon and attached to it is the greater omentum. Superiorly, the transverse colon is related to the greater curvature of the stomach and connected to it by the 2 anterior layers of the greater omentum (gastrocolic ligament). Superior to the transverse colon is the inferior recess of the lesser omental bursa (lesser sac). The central segment of the transverse colon sags inferiorly. The superoposterior surface of the transverse colon is related to the lesser sac, while its inferoposterior surface is related to the greater peritoneal cavity.

➠ *The transverse colon and mesocolon. The transverse colon and transverse mesocolon act as a barrier between the superior and inferior peritoneal cavities, keeping fluid accumulations in the supramesocolic compartment from descending into the lower abdomen. The fluids are retained superiorly for 4–48 hours. The anatomic route of egress from the supramesocolic compartment is nearly always via the right lumbar gutter.*

➠ *Position of transverse colon. The ventral surface of the mid portion of the transverse colon is closely related to the anterior abdominal wall. This makes exposure of this segment of the colon simple and aids in rapid performance of transverse colostomy if the transverse mesocolon is not too short.*

2. TRANSVERSE MESOCOLON

The transverse colon is completely invested by peritoneum except for a narrow area on its dorsal surface, where its mesentery, the transverse mesocolon, splits to envelop it. The transverse mesocolon connects the transverse colon dorsally to the ventral surface of the pancreas. In about 10–15% of individuals, it also connects the right edge of the transverse colon to the ventral surface of the descending duodenum.

The transverse mesocolon varies markedly in length: It may be as short as 3–4 cm or as long as 10–12 cm. Running in the mesocolon are the vessels supplying and draining the transverse colon. In addition, the mesocolon contains lymph nodes.

➠ *Middle colic artery. The segment of transverse mesocolon that contains the main trunk of the middle colic artery is frequently attached by a fusion fascia to the subpyloric region of the stomach. During gastric and gastroduodenal procedures, the surgeon must detach this adhesion, so as not to injure the vessel while freeing the right side of the greater curvature of the stomach. Failure to do so can result in infarction of the mid transverse colon.*

➠ *Vascular pattern in transverse mesocolon. To the left of the middle colic artery, the transverse mesocolon contains a relatively avascular space through which bloodless entry may be made into the lesser omental sac. Such an entry is made for drainage of the lesser sac, exploration of the body and tail of the pancreas, or construction of a posterior gastrojejunal anastomosis.*

➠ *Intussusception. Intussusception of colon into colon occurs occasionally in both the transverse and the left colon. The process is often initiated and led by a tumor in the bowel.*

➠ *Injury to transverse colon. Because of their relatively superficial positions, the transverse and the sigmoid colon may be injured by penetrating abdominal trauma. The first step in treatment is usually a diverting proximal colostomy. However, if the case is seen early and fecal contamination is minimal, primary closure may be done.*

3. BLOOD VESSELS, LYMPHATICS, & NERVES

Arteries
(Fig 28–11)

The extreme right side of the transverse colon receives blood from the **right colic artery;** the extreme left side receives blood from the ascending branch of the **left colic artery.** The major supplier of blood is the **middle colic artery,** a branch of the superior mesenteric artery. It enters the transverse mesocolon near the neck of the pancreas and supplies blood to the entire middle section of the transverse colon, anastomosing via the marginal artery of Drummond with both right and left colic arteries. Its arterial arcades in the transverse mesocolon are less complex to the left than to the right of the midline, providing a relatively avascular space that makes left-sided mesocolic incisions less troublesome.

Just inferior to the pyloric region of the stomach, the transverse mesocolon is usually attached by a fusion fascia to the gastrocolic ligament.

Veins
(Fig 28–11)

Venous return from the transverse colon is complex. Some veins from the right side of the transverse colon join with the right gastroepiploic veins to form the gastrocolic trunk, which empties directly into the portal vein. Most of the venous return from the right three-fourths of the transverse colon, however, joins with the superior mesenteric vein through its tributaries. Blood from the left one-fourth of the transverse colon usually joins venous channels that empty into the inferior mesenteric vein to join the portal venous flow via the splenic vein.

Lymphatics
(Fig 28–12)

Lymphatic flow from the right two-thirds of the transverse colon is into vessels roughly paralleling the right and middle colic arteries. These channels run to the nodal area near the origin of the superior mesenteric artery. From these nodes, the lymph flows into the para-aortic nodes that lie close to the origin of the superior mesenteric artery. From there, drainage from the entire right side of the transverse colon connects with small bowel lymphatic drainage to form the intestinal lymphatic trunk.

Lymphatics from the left side of the transverse colon run into nodes along the left colic artery and then along the inferior mesenteric artery to a group of lumbar nodes. Lymph from the lumbar nodes joins the aortic system of nodes eventually, but not via the intestinal trunk.

Nerves
(Fig 28–13)

The transverse colon receives the same autonomic nerve supply as does the right colon. Vagal fibers probably extend all the way to the splenic flexure of the colon, being supplied by fibers from the celiac and superior mesenteric plexuses.

SPLENIC (LEFT COLIC) FLEXURE & DESCENDING COLON

1. SPLENIC FLEXURE

The splenic flexure marks the end of the transverse colon and the beginning of the left or descending colon. It is higher than the hepatic flexure, usually at the level of the eighth interspace in the left midaxillary line. Anteriorly, the splenic flexure is well protected by the overhang of the left costal margin. Anterior to the splenic flexure is the greater curvature of the stomach. Posterior to the splenic flexure are the left kidney, the left suprarenal gland, and the left leaf of the diaphragm.

➠ *Palpation and mobilization of splenic flexure. The following anatomic factors make attempts to palpate the splenic flexure difficult: (1) deep posterior placement of the flexure, (2) marked overhang of the left costal margin, and (3) overhang of the flexure by the greater curvature of the stomach or by an enlarged spleen. These relationships make it difficult to diagnose disease in and around the splenic flexure or to mobilize the splenic flexure at exploration. After making certain that the inferior pole of the spleen, the greater curvature of the stomach, and the tail of the pancreas are not adherent to the phrenicocolic ligament—a bloodless peritoneal fold—the ligament may be cut to facilitate mobilization and exposure of the splenic flexure.*

The splenic flexure lies on the left leaf of the diaphragm and on the tendinous origin of the transversus abdominis muscle. Just superior to the flexure is the tail of the pancreas and the inferior surface of the spleen. The splenic flexure is covered with peritoneum anteriorly and laterally, but its posterior surface is fixed by a fusion fascia to the posterior abdominal parietes. In rare cases, the entire splenic flexure is covered with peritoneum and is attached by the transverse mesocolon to the tail of the pancreas. The splenic flexure may receive an attachment from the left free border of the greater omentum. Running from the splenic flexure to the surface of the left leaf of the diaphragm is a thickening of peritoneum called the phrenicocolic ligament. This ligament is normally at the level of the tenth rib in the midaxillary line, and the inferior pole of the spleen rests on it. It holds the splenic flexure tightly against the left lateral abdominal parietes and marks the superior end of the left lumbar gutter. The phrenicocolic ligament is the left lateral limit of the greater omentum.

➠ *Thoracoabdominal injuries. Because of its proximity to the left leaf of the diaphragm,* the splenic flexure is often involved in penetrating left thoracoabdominal injuries.

➠ *Malignant neoplastic disease. Because of the close relationship of the splenic flexure to the tail of the pancreas, the lower pole of the spleen, the left leaf of the diaphragm, and the underlying left kidney and suprarenal gland, direct tumor spread from the flexure may involve any and all of these structures.*

2. DESCENDING (LEFT) COLON

This segment is about 10 cm long and runs from the splenic flexure to the level of the left iliac crest. It lies at first lateral to and then curves around the lower pole of the left kidney, from lateral to medial. Posterior to the left colon is the quadratus lumborum muscle; posteromedially from above downward lie the left suprarenal gland, the left kidney, the left ureter, the left gonadal vessels, and the iliohypogastric and ilioinguinal nerves. Lateral to the descending colon is the left lumbar gutter. The descending colon seldom possesses a mesocolon. It is covered only ventrally and laterally by peritoneum.

➠ *Mobilization of fixed left colon. The left colon may be mobilized by incising its fusion fascia along the medial border of the narrow left lumbar gutter. Care must be taken not to injure the underlying kidney and left ureter.*

3. BLOOD VESSELS, LYMPHATICS, & NERVES

Arteries
(Fig 28–11)

The descending colon is supplied by the ascending branch of the **left colic artery.** This artery participates in formation of the marginal artery of Drummond along the mesenteric border.

Arterial supply to the splenic flexure is via the ascending branch of the left colic artery and the left branch of the **middle colic artery,** the 2 vessels anastomosing just proximal to the splenic flexure.

Veins
(Fig 28–11)

The left colon and the splenic flexure are drained by veins that empty into the inferior mesenteric vein. Occasionally, there may be minor venous drainage from the splenic flexure into vessels that empty into either the superior mesenteric or splenic veins.

➠ *Pylephlebitis. Venous flow from the left colon, sigmoid colon, and rectum via the inferior mes-*

enteric venous system is the source of septic emboli in cases of left-sided pylephlebitis. The emboli are usually from infected thrombosed internal hermorrhoids or diverticulitis with rupture and abscess formation. In such cases, the left lobe of the liver develops abscesses.

Lymphatics
(Fig 28–12)

Lymphatics that drain the left colon run primarily to nodes near the origin of the inferior mesenteric artery from the aorta. Eventually, the lymph passes upward to nodes near the origin of the superior mesenteric artery and occasionally into the pancreaticosplenic group of nodes.

Lymphatic drainage from the splenic flexure passes primarily into the pancreaticosplenic nodes and into nodes that lie along the left side of the gastrocolic ligament.

Nerves
(Fig 28–13)

The nerves to the descending colon are both sympathetic and parasympathetic and are branches from the inferior mesenteric and hypogastric plexuses. These branches continue into the left colic and sigmoid plexuses before reaching the decending colon. The preganglionic parasympathetic cell bodies lie in the spinal cord at S2–4.

➠ *Diseases of the descending colon. The descending colon is frequently the site of a stenosing, encircling type of carcinoma that, because of the small caliber of this segment, leads to early colonic obstruction with dilatation of the large bowel proximal to the area of obstruction (Fig 28–14). The descending colon is frequently involved in generalized left colonic diverticulosis or diverticulitis and may be involved in generalized ulcerative colitis or segmental granulomatous colitis.*

SIGMOID COLON

The sigmoid colon, so called because it frequently has an S shape, is divided into a fixed superior or iliac portion and a mobile inferior or pelvic portion. The fixed portion of the sigmoid colon begins at the level of the iliac crest. It runs inferiorly to the level of the anterosuperior iliac spine, where it begins to parallel the inguinal ligament. It continues to the brim of the true pelvis, crossing the left psoas muscle from left to right. Most of the superior portion of the sigmoid colon is tightly fixed to the fascia covering the iliacus muscle. It does not possess a mesentery. At the point where the sigmoid colon becomes mobile, it lies directly anterior to the external iliac artery.

The fixed portion of the sigmoid colon separates

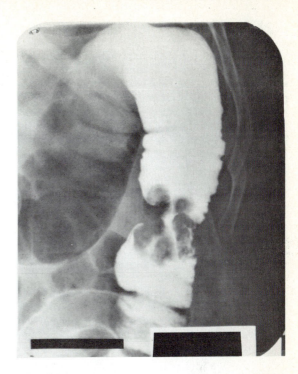

Figure 28–14. Barium enema roentgenogram of an encircling carcinoma of the descending colon presenting an "apple core" appearance. Note the loss of mucosal pattern, the "hooks" at the margins of the lesion owing to undermining by the growth, the relatively short (6 cm) length of the lesion, and its abrupt ends. (Reproduced, with permission, from Way LW [editor]: *Current Surgical Diagnosis & Treatment,* 7th ed. Lange, 1985.)

the left inframesocolic compartment of the abdominal cavity from the left paracolic gutter. Since the fixed portion of the sigmoid lies close to the anterior abdominal parietes, one may (in a thin person) palpate a tumor within the colonic lumen, pressing against the unyielding iliacus muscle.

The pelvic (mobile) portion of the sigmoid colon begins at the medial border of the left psoas major muscle and terminates at the rectosigmoid junction. Its length, the location of its loops, the degree of its convolutions, its relationships, and its mobility all vary markedly.

Normally, the proximal sigmoid colon lies in the false pelvis and the distal loops in the true pelvis. In case of an abnormally long mesentery, some sigmoid loops may be found in the right lower quadrant, close to the cecum. The more distal sigmoid loops are close to the bladder in the male. In the female, the distal sigmoid loops are related ventrally to the uterus and the upper vagina. As it lies in the true pelvis, the sigmoid colon in both the male and the female is related dorsally to the upper sacrum, the sacral plexus of nerves, and the left piriformis muscle. In the male, the distal sigmoid may be related to the upper rectum. This occasionally allows the diagnosis of a low sigmoid tumor by digital examination of the rectum.

Normally, the mobile segment of the sigmoid colon is attached to the dorsal abdominal wall by a mesentery of variable length. The line of the mesenteric attachment resembles an inverted V. The left limb of the inverted V starts at the medial border of the left psoas major muscle and climbs along the external iliac artery to the origin of the internal iliac artery from the common iliac artery. From there, the right limb of the inverted V descends almost vertically across the promontory of the sacrum to near the midline of the third sacral vertebra. The left limb of the mesenteric attachment crosses the left ureter.

⟫ *Intersigmoid mesenteric recess. The intersigmoid mesenteric recess, lying at the apex of the inverted V of the sigmoid mesocolon, is a site for internal herniation of the mesoparietal type. It can also serve as a guide to the location of the left ureter, since a finger placed into the recess can usually roll the left ureter onto the underlying common iliac artery.*

⟫ *Sigmoid volvulus. (Figs 28–15 and 28–16.) Volvulus of the sigmoid colon is the commonest*

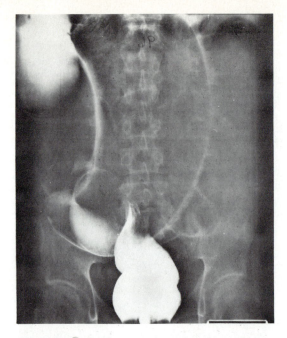

Figure 28–16. Volvulus of the sigmoid colon. Roentgenogram with barium enema taken with the patient in the supine position. The barium column resembles a "bird's beak" or "ace of spades" because of the way in which the lumen tapers toward the volvulus. (Reproduced, with permission, from Way LW [editor]: *Current Surgical Diagnosis & Treatment,* 7th ed. Lange, 1985.)

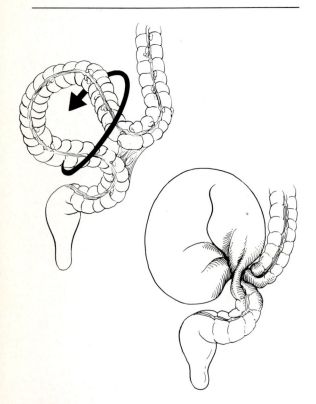

Figure 28–15. Volvulus of the sigmoid colon. The twist is counterclockwise in most cases of sigmoid vovulus. (Reproduced, with permission, from Way LW [editor]: *Current Surgical Diagnosis & Treatment,* 7th ed. Lange, 1985.)

adult form of bowel twist. The volvulus occurs about the apex of the short, inverted V-shaped attachment of the mesentery. It is more common in elderly and debilitated patients, in those with abnormally close sigmoid mesenteric attachments, and in those with abnormally long sigmoid colons. The passage of a sigmoidoscope helps to make the diagnosis (along with the radiographs) and often serves to untwist the volvulus. Sigmoid volvulus is frequently transient and tends to remit and recur spontaneously. For permanent cure, a portion of an abnormally long sigmoid colon should be resected.

1. BLOOD VESSELS, LYMPHATICS, & NERVES

Arteries
(Fig 28–11)

The **inferior mesenteric artery** is the major vessel to the terminal transverse colon, the splenic flexure, the left colon, the sigmoid colon, and the rectum. It arises from the left lateral surface of the abdominal aorta about 3.5 cm above the bifurcation and runs retroperitoneally for about 2.5 cm before giving off its first branch.

The **left colic artery** is the first branch of the inferior mesenteric artery, arising about 2.5 cm distal to its origin. It runs in the direction of the superior half of the descending colon. It divides into ascending and descending branches at a point about 5 cm proximal to the mesenteric border of the mid descending colon.

The **ascending branch** usually divides into 2 major divisions. The first runs superiorly, paralleling the left colon and contributing to the marginal artery of Drummond. The second branch climbs toward the terminal left one-fourth of the transverse colon and the splenic flexure, close to the superior mesenteric vein. It anastomoses with the left transverse branch of the middle colic artery.

The **descending branch** of the left colic artery parallels the inferior segment of the descending colon and the fixed (iliac) segment of the sigmoid colon. It anastomoses with the highest of the sigmoid arteries.

The **sigmoid arteries,** the second branches of the inferior mesenteric artery, are usually 2–5 in number (may be 1–9). Occasionally, the highest sigmoid artery may be a branch of the left colic artery and the lowest sigmoid artery a branch of the superior rectal artery. Generally, the sigmoid arteries run behind the posterior peritoneum ventral to the left psoas major muscle, the gonadal vessels, and the left ureter. The arteries then enter the sigmoid mesocolon to run to the mesenteric border of the mobile sigmoid loop. They anastomose freely with one another via an intricate series of arcades, and at the mesenteric border of the sigmoid colon they join the sigmoid portion of the marginal artery of Drummond. They supply the lower portion of the descending colon, the sigmoid colon, and a small segment of the upper rectum.

The superior rectal artery is the continuation of the inferior mesenteric artery. It supplies the area of the rectosigmoid junction and the upper and mid rectum. It becomes the superior rectal artery when it enters the sigmoid mesocolon. It continues inferiorly, crossing the left common iliac vessels, and it divides high on the surface of the rectum into its right and left terminal branches, which eventually anastomose with the middle and inferior rectal arteries.

➠ *Marginal artery of Drummond. The sigmoid marginal artery is usually adequate to ensure viability of the proximal sigmoid stump despite ligation of the lower sigmoid arteries. There is excellent circulation to the proximal sigmoid stump, even where the inferior mesenteric artery has been ligated close to its origin. This results from the anastomosis of the main superior rectal artery with the descending superior rectal arteries. It is good clinical practice always to check for arterial pulsations in the marginal artery of Drummond at the level of the proximal sigmoid stump, and to check also*

the briskness of bleeding of the stump at the time of its transection.

Veins
(Fig 28–11)

Venous return from the sigmoid colon is via the inferior mesenteric vein. It begins on the surface of the rectum as the superior rectal vein and proceeds superiorly at the mesenteric borders of the sigmoid colon and descending colon. It may join the splenic vein or the superior mesenteric vein, or it may empty directly into the portal vein.

➠ *Transection of inferior mesenteric vein. The inferior mesenteric vein should usually be transected as high as possible early in resection for malignant disease of the left colon, sigmoid colon, and rectum. This helps to prevent venous malignant emboli.*

➠ *Anatomic portacaval shunt. The inferior mesenteric venous system, into which the superior rectal veins empty, anastomoses with the middle rectal veins and the inferior rectal veins at about the level of the anorectal junction, establishing an anatomic portacaval venous shunt. The shunt exists because the middle and inferior rectal veins empty into the inferior caval system, whereas the inferior mesenteric vein terminates in the portal venous system.*

Lymphatics
(Fig 28–12)

Lymphatics draining the descending colon and the fixed portion of the sigmoid colon join together to run into lymph channels that drain into nodes along the left colic artery. Additional drainage from the left colic area is into nodes that lie close to the origin of the inferior mesenteric artery. This lymph flows either into the left lumbar nodes or into nodes lying to the left side of the abdominal aorta near the inferior mesenteric artery. Some lymphatic flow from the splenic flexure and the upper descending colon follows the inferior mesenteric vein to finally empty into nodes close to the base of the mesentery of the small bowel. Lymphatics from the sigmoid colon run directly to the lumbar or para-aortic nodes near the inferior mesenteric artery.

➠ *Lymphatic drainage of sigmoid colon. Wide sigmoid bowel resection and a deep sigmoid mesenteric resection are called for in carcinoma of the sigmoid colon. Lymphatics draining the sigmoid area converge toward the aortic and lumbar nodes and nodes lying close to the marginal artery of Drummond both above and below the level of the lesion being resected.*

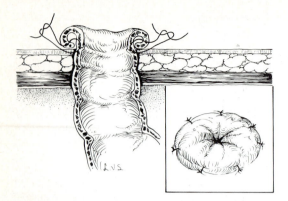

Figure 28–17. Single-barreled end colostomy. The margins of the stoma are fixed to the skin with sutures. (Reproduced, with permission, from Way LW [editor]: *Current Surgical Diagnosis & Treatment,* 7th ed. Lange, 1985.)

➡ Terminal sigmoid colostomy. *Sigmoid colostomy may be terminal or double-barreled. There is a trend toward performing more terminal colostomies as a primary diversionary step in resection for obstructing carcinoma and di-*

verticulitis of the left colon. However, with the ability to prepare the bowel properly before surgery, more one-stage procedures are being performed (primary anastomosis).

➡ Sigmoid and left colon colotomy. *(Fig 28–17.) Colotomy with polyp removal, or localized colonic resection with end-to-end anastomosis of bowel, may be used for polyps of the left colon and sigmoid colon. However, the best procedure for removal of most colonic polyps is to use the flexible fiberoptic colonoscope if the polyp is amenable to such a procedure.*

➡ Operations on the lower sigmoid colon. *Combined abdominoperineal resection has been the usual procedure in the past for removal of carcinoma of the rectum and lower sigmoid. Where an adequate inferior margin of normal bowel tissue can be obtained, anterior resection of the upper and mid rectum with end-to-end bowel anastomosis is now the procedure of choice.*

➡ Left colon and sigmoid colitis. *The sigmoid colon and left colon are frequently the site of ulcerative and granulomatous colitis. The rec-*

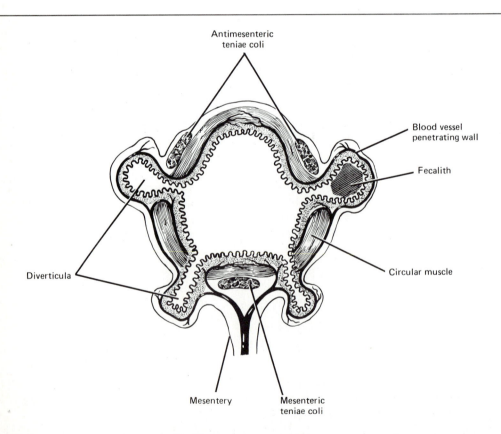

Figure 28–18. Cross section of the colon showing diverticula. (Modified and reproduced, with permission, from Way LW [editor]: *Current Surgical Diagnosis & Treatment,* 7th ed. Lange, 1985.)

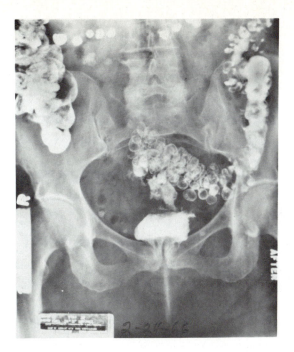

Figure 28–19. Barium enema roentgenogram showing multiple diverticula of the colon.

tum and sigmoid are the areas most commonly involved.

➠ ***Diverticula.*** *(Figs 28–18 and 28–19.) The sigmoid colon is the most common site for colonic diverticula; about 60% of such lesions occur in this area. Left colon and sigmoid colon diverticula typically show absence of the muscular coats of the bowel, are usually multiple, and occur most frequently in middle-aged and elderly people. They usually arise between the mesenteric border of the bowel and the lateral border teniae. They tend to pierce the muscular coats of the bowel with nutrient vessels to the colon and then proceed with the colonic vessels in the direction of the mesentery. Their presence is probably due to muscular dyskinesia of the bowel. Diverticulosis without inflammation may result in massive bleeding and is frequently difficult to localize. Left colon and sigmoid colon diverticulitis are common gastrointestinal diseases of civilized populations. Obstruction, perforation, hemorrhage, fistula formation, and tumorlike diverticuloma formation frequently call for operative management. It may be impossible to distinguish a diverticular inflammatory mass from invasion of the colon by a malignant tumor.*

Nerves
(Fig 28–13)

The sigmoid colon is supplied by sympathetic and sacral parasympathetic fibers via the hypogastric and inferior mesenteric plexuses.

EMBRYOLOGY
(See also Chapter 22.)

The epithelium of the rectosigmoid is derived from entoderm. Anomalies of this part include congenital megacolon.

Rectum

The rectum and the superior portion of the anal canal derive from the entodermal cloaca into which opens the allantois ventrally and the tailgut dorsally. The latter disappears by the eighth fetal week. **Anomalies** of the urorectal septum, which divides the cloaca, are usually associated with complete or partial imperforate anus and high-lying rectum and include persistence of the primitive cloaca; in females, rectouterine, rectocervical, or rectovaginal fistula; in males, rectovesical or rectourethral fistula; and rectoperineal fistula in both sexes (Fig 29–1).

Anal Canal

The epithelium of the inferior anal canal develops from ectoderm and cranially comes into contact with the entoderm of the hindgut to form the anal membrane. The latter breaks down by about the eighth fetal week. The invaginated perianal ectoderm is called the anal pit, or proctodeum. **Anomalies** of the anorectum include anorectal stenosis and imperforate anus with or without atresia of most of the distal hindgut segment. *Note:* Sixty percent of anal anomalies are associated with anomalies of urorectal septum and complicated by anorectal fistula (see above).

GROSS ANATOMY

1. THE RECTOSIGMOID
(Fig 29–2)

The precise position of the rectosigmoid junction, where the sigmoid ends and the rectum begins, varies with the criteria used. Operationally, there are only small differences when different criteria are applied.

Because of the gradual transition of sigmoid into rectum, it is better to think of the rectosigmoid as an area rather than a point of junction—especially if one regards the level of the peritoneal reflection from the anterior surface of the bowel as the major factor in designation of the rectosigmoid area.

⇒ *Endoscopy. The rectosigmoid area can only be properly viewed by passage of a sigmoidoscope or colonoscope. It is frequently a "blind area" in barium enema x-rays of the bowel.*

⇒ *Rectosigmoid disease. Carcinoma, benign and malignant polyps, diverticulitis, specific and nonspecific colonic mucosal ulcerations, bowel perforations, and sigmoid colonic volvulus all are among the many pathologic conditions occurring in or near the rectosigmoid.*

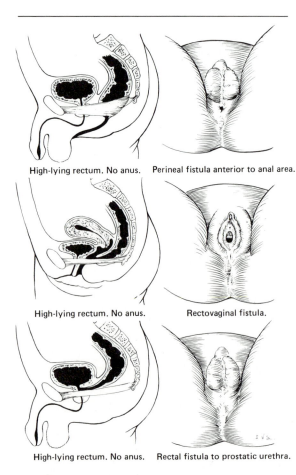

High-lying rectum. No anus.   Perineal fistula anterior to anal area.

High-lying rectum. No anus.   Rectovaginal fistula.

High-lying rectum. No anus.   Rectal fistula to prostatic urethra.

Figure 29–1. Anomalies of the rectum. (Modified and reproduced, with permission, from Way LW [editor]: *Current Surgical Diagnosis & Treatment,* 7th ed. Lange, 1985.)

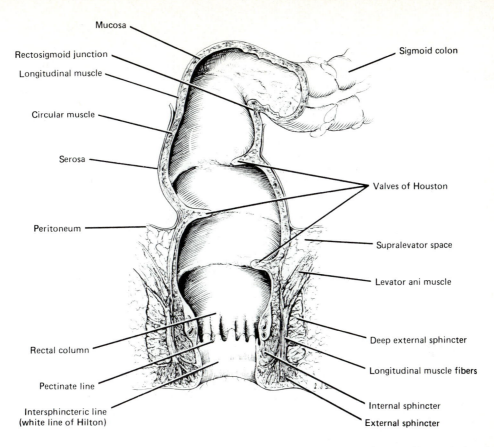

Figure 29–2. Anatomy of the rectosigmoid rectum and anus. (Modified and reproduced, with permission, from Way LW [editor]: *Current Surgical Diagnosis & Treatment,* 7th ed. Lange, 1985.)

2. THE RECTUM

Location & Peritoneal Covering (Fig 29–3)

The rectum is that portion of the large bowel interposed between the terminal portion of the sigmoid colon and the anal canal. It lies within the concavity formed by the posterior bowing of the anterior surfaces of the sacrum and coccyx. It possesses no appendices epiploicae, haustra, or teniae. Only its upper segment is related to the peritoneum, anteriorly and laterally. The mid and inferior segments of the rectum lie below the peritoneum of the posterior portion of the pelvic floor.

The superior third of the rectum is covered ventrally and laterally by peritoneum. The middle third of the rectum is invested only ventrally by a peritoneal layer. Below this level, the rectum has no peritoneal covering.

In the male, at the junction of the upper and middle thirds of the rectum, the ventral covering of peritoneum is reflected onto the upper third of the seminal vesicles and then onto the posterosuperior surface of the bladder, the vesicorectal peritoneal pouch being created by the reflection. Depending upon the level of the peritoneal reflection, the pouch may on occasion reach a level higher than the summits of the seminal vesicles. If the peritoneum is reflected from the anterior surface of the rectum at an abnormally low level, it may completely cover the seminal vesicles; if it is reflected at an even lower level, it may—in addition to covering the vesicles—cover the superior surface of the posterior lobe of the prostate. In such cases, the lower limit of the rectovesical pouch is palpable digitally through the ventral wall of the rectum.

In the female, the serous coat of the upper and mid rectum is reflected onto the posterior vaginal wall, forming the rectovaginal pouch (pouch of Douglas), and then onto the posterior surface of the uterus.

⤷ *Peritoneal pelvic pouch. In both males and females, a finger in the rectum may palpate collections of pus, blood, or ascitic fluid in the rectouterine or rectovesical pouch. It is easier to palpate fluid in the rectouterine pouch because of the lower level of the female peritoneal cul-de-sac and the ability to reach it via the posterior vaginal vault as well as via the rectum.*

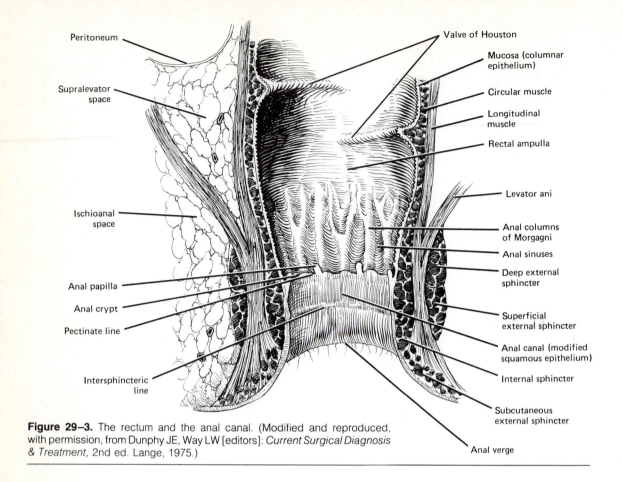

Figure 29–3. The rectum and the anal canal. (Modified and reproduced, with permission, from Dunphy JE, Way LW [editors]: *Current Surgical Diagnosis & Treatment,* 2nd ed. Lange, 1975.)

⇒ *Drainage of collections. In the male, fluid collections in the rectovesical pouch may drain spontaneously into—or be drained operatively through—the rectum. In the female, such collections are usually drained through the posterior vaginal vault.*

The rectum leaves the pelvic cavity by perforating the levator ani muscular diaphragm, the distal rectal segment thus becoming a perineal structure. The rectum is 14–18 cm long and quite variable in diameter. Its upper and lower levels are relatively constricted, whereas its mid portion, the **rectal ampulla,** is 2–3 times the diameter of its proximal and distal segments.

Rectal & Anal Curves

Together, the rectum and anus exhibit a series of curvatures. Two of these are in the sagittal plane, the upper one following the curve of the sacrum, its concavity facing anteriorly; the lower curvature, the perineal flexure, begins at the junction of the rectum and anus, and its concavity faces posteriorly. There are 3 lateral rectal curvatures, 2 with their convexities facing toward the left and one with its convexity facing toward the right. The lateral rectal curvatures form the plicae transversales recti (valves of Houston). The rectal valves are simple exaggerated folds of rectal mucosa, submucosa, and a small amount of circular muscle that project into the lumen of the rectum.

Because of the constant contraction of the sphincteric muscular system of the rectum, the lowest segment of the rectal mucosa is gathered into a group of vertical pleats, or folds, each about 1 cm long, the **columns of Morgagni.** The upper part of each column is covered with columnar epithelium, but toward the base the epithelium becomes the stratified type found in the anal canal. The grooves between the anal columns are known as anal sinuses. Transversely placed at the inferior margin of each anal sinus are semilunar cups, the anal valves. Each anal valve is open superiorly; at the base of each valve is a crypt 3–5 mm deep.

RELATIONSHIPS OF THE RECTUM (Fig 29–4)

From superior to inferior, the rectum is related posteriorly to the bifurcation of the superior rectal

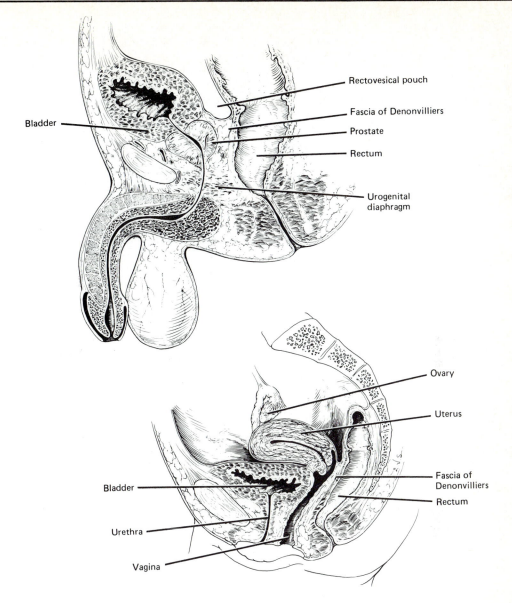

Figure 29–4. Relationships of the rectum and anus to genitalia. (Modified and reproduced, with permission, from Smith DR: *General Urology,* 11th ed. Lange, 1984.)

vessels, the left piriformis muscle, the sacral plexus of nerves, the anterior covering fascia of the bony sacrum and coccyx, and the most posterior fibers of the levator ani muscle. Anteriorly, the rectal relationships differ in the male and female. In the male, the rectum is related anteriorly to the lowest loops of bowel, the base of the bladder, the seminal vesicles, the ductus deferens, the posterior surface of the prostate, and the base of the urogenital diaphragm.

In the female, the rectum is related anteriorly to the lowest loops of the bowel, the posteroinferior surface of the uterus, and the upper and middle thirds of the posterior vaginal wall.

➠ *Digital rectal examination. The examining finger placed in the rectum aids in the diagnosis of genitourinary disease in the male. The prostate and seminal vesicles lie just anterior to the examining finger, separated from it only by the thickness of the rectal wall and by the rectovesical fascia (Denonvilliers' fascia). Many rectal cancers can be reached by the examining finger. A finger placed in the rectum may also palpate cystic or solid tumors in the retrorectal (presacral) space.*

In the female, a finger placed in the rectum can usually palpate the uterine cervix and a retroflexed posterior uterus. Ovaries and uterine tubes prolapsed into the rectouterine pouch of Douglas may also be palpated rectally.

Separating the enveloping fascia of the rectum from the more anteriorly related structures of the urogenital pelvis in both the male and female is a frontally placed fibrous septum, the rectovesical or rectovaginal fascia (Denonvilliers' fascia), which extends downward from the end of the pelvic peritoneal pouch to a point just above the upper segment of the **central tendinous point of the perineum.**

⇒ *Denonvilliers' fascia in surgery. Since Denonvilliers' fusion fascia is not as well developed in the female as in the male, it is not as clinically significant in females. In males requiring radical prostate surgery or with an anterior infiltrating rectal carcinoma, this fascia must be clearly identified, since it is the line of separation between the anorectal and urogenital pelves.*

THE POSTERIOR & LATERAL RECTAL LIGAMENTS

Below the level of the peritoneal reflection from the anterolateral surface of the rectum and extending as far caudally as the superior surface of the levator ani muscles, the rectum is enclosed within a strong outer fibrous sheath that is derived from the true pelvic lining fascia. This fascia is a branching of the great lining fascia of the peritoneal cavity. The external enclosing fascial sheath of the lower and mid rectum consists of an inner cellular and an outer fibrous layer. At about the midpoint of the ampulla of the rectum, these 2 layers fuse to form the so-called posterior rectal ligaments (stalks), which are attached to the anterior surface of the sacral fascia at the level of S3–4. There are also 2 lateral rectal ligaments that run from the lateral pelvic walls to the rectal walls. These lateral rectal ligaments are formed by the thickening of the fasciae that accompany the middle rectal arteries and the rectal nerves from the pelvic retroperitoneal tissues to the lateral surfaces of the rectum.

⇒ *Surgical mobilization of rectal ligaments. In order to mobilize the mid and inferior thirds of the rectum for removal or anastomosis, the posterior and the lateral rectal ligaments must be located, isolated, and transected. The transection allows the pelvic dissection of the rectum to proceed to the posterior surface of the prostate in the male and to the posterior vaginal fornix in the female.*

Structure of the Wall

The walls of the rectum are composed of 4 distinct layers.

An outer **serous layer** surrounds the deeper muscular, submucosal, and mucosal coats. The peritoneal or serous outer coat, however, is found only on the superior half of the rectum.

The **muscular coat** of the rectum consists of an outer longitudinal and an inner circular layer of smooth muscle fibers. The outer longitudinal layer arises from fusion of 3 longitudinal muscular bands—teniae—present on the colon from the cecum to the rectosigmoid junctional area. The 3 bands merge at the rectosigmoid area to form a complete longitudinal muscular coat around the rectum down the anorectal junction. Just above the level of the anorectal junction, the levator ani fibers encircle the rectum to meet the longitudinal smooth muscle fibers of the rectum and blend with the levator ani fibers.

The circular muscle of the rectum is not well defined, particularly over the upper and mid rectum. However, it thickens markedly as it encircles the lower third of the rectum at the level of the ring of external sphincter ani fibers, to form the **internal anal sphincter.**

The **submucosal layer** is loosely attached to the underlying mucosa, allowing the mucosa to glide easily upon it. It is composed of a thick layer of connective tissue within which the terminal ramifications of the arterial, venous, and lymphatic vessels are found.

The **mucosal coat** of the rectum is extremely vascular, thick, and reddish. It is lined with simple columnar epithelium which, at the level of the inferior margins of the anal columns of Morgagni, becomes stratified squamous epithelium. The loose rectal mucosa presents 3 obliquely transverse folds, the valves of Houston, which pouch into the rectal lumen as a result of the 3 lateral curvatures of the rectum. Two of the 3 transverse folds usually lie on the left and one on the right.

Deep to the submucosa lies a thin muscularis mucosae made of longitudinal and circular smooth muscle.

BLOOD VESSELS, LYMPHATICS, & NERVES

Arteries
(Figs 29–5 and 29–6)

The **superior rectal artery** is the continuation of the rectosigmoid branch of the inferior mesenteric artery. The superior rectal artery divides into right and left rectal branches high on the dorsal surface of the rectum at about the level of S3. When the branches reach the levator ani muscles, they anastomose with the branches of the middle and inferior rectal arteries.

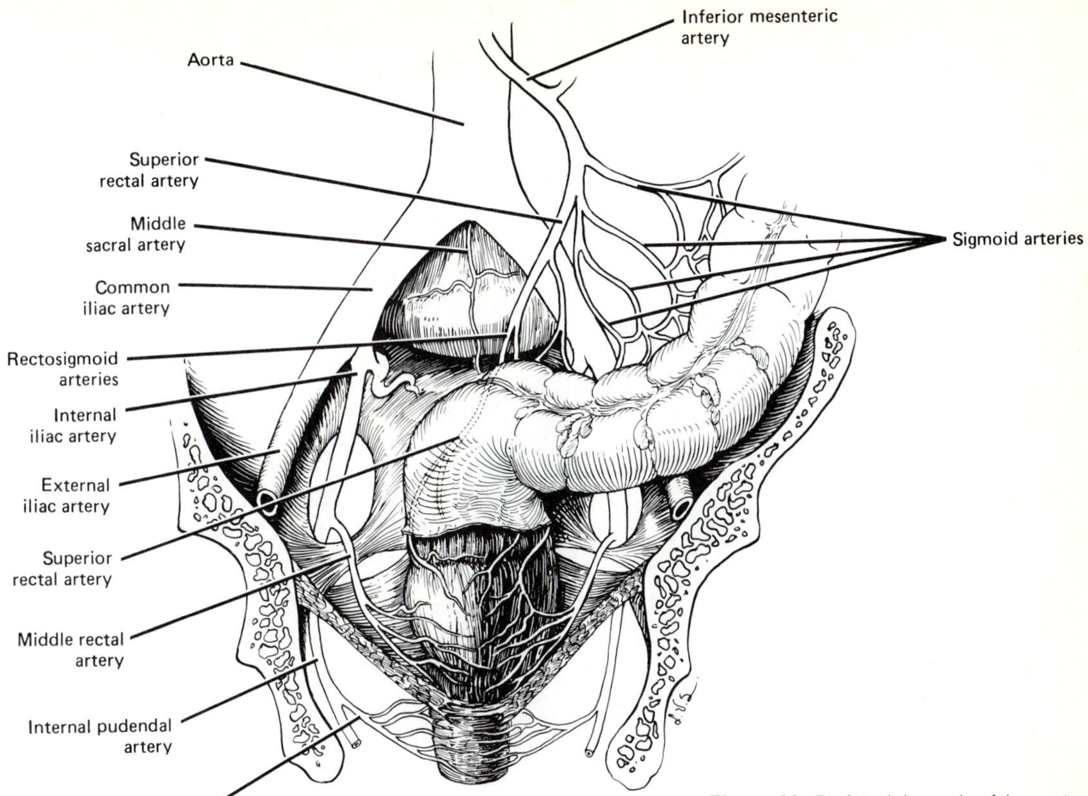

Figure 29–5. Arterial supply of the rectosigmoid and rectum (anterior view).

The **middle rectal artery** is a branch of the anterior division of the internal iliac artery. It runs along the superior surface of the levator ani muscle. This places the artery in the superior pelvirectal space. At the level of insertion of the levator ani fibers into the rectum, the middle rectal artery anastomoses with the 3 other arteries supplying the rectum (superior rectal, inferior rectal, and median sacral).

▸ *Ligation of middle rectal artery. The middle rectal artery, as it runs on the superior surface of the levator ani muscle, must be searched for, isolated, and ligated during the later stages of pelvic rectal dissection in an abdominoperineal rectal removal. Failure to do so may lead to serious operative or postoperative pelvic hemhorrhage.*

The **inferior rectal artery** is a branch of the internal pudendal artery, derived from the internal iliac artery. The internal pudendal artery leaves the pelvis through the greater sciatic foramen to enter the anorectal perineum through the lesser sciatic foramen by winding anteriorly around the ischial spine. In the perineum, it lies in a fascial envelope on the inner surface of the obturator muscle (pudendal [Alcock's] canal). The inferior rectal branch of the internal pudendal artery, after piercing the medial fascia of the pudendal canal, crosses the base of the ischiorectal fossa from lateral to medial, just deep to the skin and subcutaneous tissues of the anorectal perineum. Its terminal branches lie below the levator ani muscles and supply the internal and external sphincters of the rectum and the anal canal. The artery has a rich anastomosis with branches of the middle and superior rectal arteries, at about the level of the anorectal junction.

The **median sacral artery** is the centrally placed terminal branch of the abdominal aorta. It runs inferiorly in the retrorectal space, dorsal to the rectum and just deep to the fascia on the ventral surface of sacrum and coccyx. It sends minor branches to the dorsal rectal wall, the branches anastomosing with branches of the other 3 arteries supplying the rectum.

Veins
(Fig 29–7)

Just superior to the anorectal junction, a large submucosal venous plexus called the internal hemorrhoidal plexus drains the mucosa of the lower rectum. The plexus empties into large venous channels that run upward in the submucosa of the rectum. These channels eventually penetrate the muscular layers of the rectum and coalesce on the posterior rectal surface

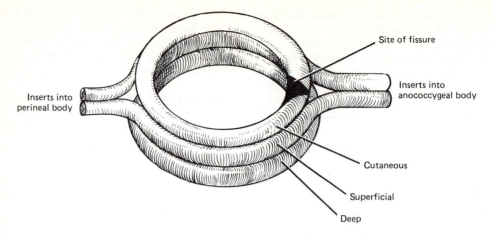

Figure 29–11. Model of the external sphincter ani, showing its three components and site of fissure. (Modified and reproduced, with permission, from Dunphy JE, Way LW: *Current Surgical Diagnosis & Treatment.* Lange, 1973.)

on the anorectum, the anorectal perineum, the pelvis, the levator ani complex, the external sphincter ani, and the internal sphincter ani.

⫸ *Examining the anorectum. The examining finger, the proctoscope, and the sigmoidoscope are the keys to diagnosis and treatment of the many diseases of the anorectum. Knowledge of the curvatures of the anorectum is necessary for proper passage of the finger or the endoscope. This can avoid pain and trauma to the bowel. Knowledge of the presence and angulation of the transverse rectal folds, the valves of Houston, aids in the painless passage of both the proctoscope and the sigmoidoscope. With the endoscope in place, tumors may be seen, and internal fistulous openings and ulcerative lower bowel disease may be examined. Cultures, smears, and biopsies of visualized lesions may be carried out through the endoscope.*

⫸ *Valves of Houston. As the sigmoidoscope is advanced through the rectum, the 3 transverse mucosal valvular projections indicate levels of lateral rectal curvature that must be negotiated by the endoscopist. Occasionally, an ulcer, polyp, or malignant tumor on the superior surface of one of the rectal valves may be hidden from the endoscopist. Accordingly, the rectal valves must be flattened against the rectal wall by the sigmoidoscope so that their superior surfaces can be inspected.*

⫸ *Anorectal prolapse. Anorectal prolapse, common in children and the elderly, presents at the anal orifice. In children, conservative treatment by simple reduction is often successful. In adults, treatment consists of resection of*

redundant colon and fixation of the rectosigmoid to the sacral prominence.

⫸ *Anorectal trauma. Anorectal trauma from a variety of causes is fairly common. It may result from perineal wounds or from perforation of the rectum or anus by a foreign body that either passed along the gastrointestinal tract (eg, a chicken bone) or was inserted into the anorectum. It may result from diagnostic endoscopy, particularly if the rectum is diseased. It may be a sequela of penetrating injury when the wound of entrance is through the perineum. It is important to determine if the rupture is intraperitoneal, extraperitoneal, or both. Frequently, the only way to diagnose the relationship of the site of rupture to the peritoneal cavity is by exploratory laparotomy. There are often associated gynecologic, anal, and urinary tract injuries. A diverting colostomy at the low sigmoid level is the preliminary step in treatment of the severely traumatized or perforated rectosigmoid, rectum, or anus.*

⫸ *Common anal lesions. Fig 29–12 shows fistulas, Fig 29–13 common lesions of the anal canal, and Fig 29–14 anorectal abscesses.*

BLOOD VESSELS, LYMPHATICS, & NERVES

Arteries & Veins

The anal canal is supplied by the **inferior rectal artery,** a branch of the internal pudendal artery. The inferior rectal artery is given off in the pudendal canal and crosses the base of the ischiorectal fossa to reach the anus. The **inferior rectal veins** draining the anus carry blood transversely across the ischiorectal fossa to the **internal** pudendal veins that empty into the

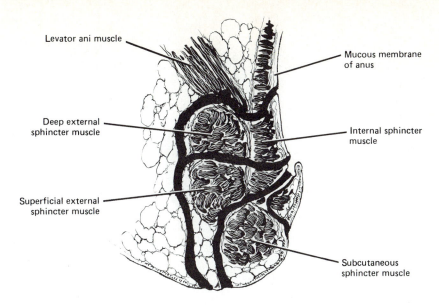

Figure 29–12. Cross section of the muscles of the anal wall, showing the usual paths of anal fistulas. (Modified and reproduced, with permission, from Wilson JL: *Handbook of Surgery,* 5th ed. Lange, 1973.)

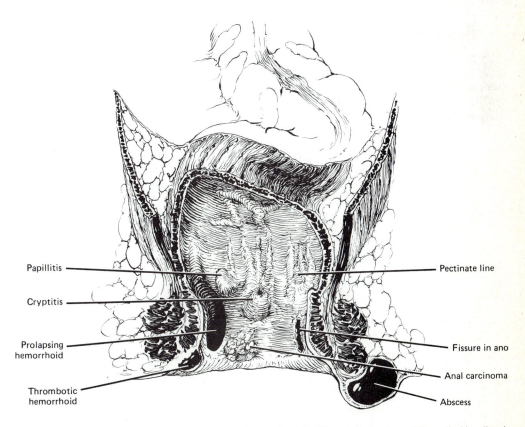

Figure 29–13. Common lesions of the anal canal. (Modified and reproduced, with permission, from Wilson JL: *Handbook of Surgery,* 5th ed. Lange, 1973.)

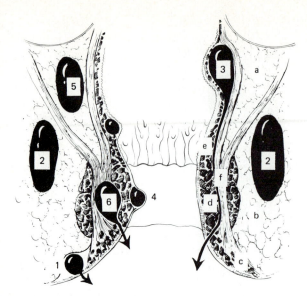

ANORECTAL ABSCESSES

1. Perianal
2. Primary ischiorectal
3. Submucous
4. Marginal
5. Pelvirectal
6. Intermuscular
   Retrorectal (not
   visualized)

ANATOMIC SPACES

a. Pelvirectal
b. Ischiorectal
c. Perianal
d. Marginal
e. Submucous
f. Intermuscular

Figure 29–14. Composite diagram of acute anorectal abscesses and spaces. (Modified and reproduced, with permission, from Way LW [editor]: *Current Surgical Diagnosis & Treatment,* 7th ed. Lange, 1985.)

internal iliac veins, the blood finally reaching the inferior vena cava.

Lymphatics

There is a large lymphatic plexus deep to the mucosa of the anal canal. From the anus, lymph is carried either to the inguinal lymph nodes or to the iliac nodes in the retroperitoneum of the pelvis. The submucosal perianal ring of lymphatics connects with the lymphatics of the rectum and may empty into them if the normal ischiorectal pathway is blocked.

Nerves

The anal canal and perianal skin are innervated by the somatic or cerebrospinal nervous system. The anal canal below the level of the anal valves is supplied by the inferior rectal nerve (third or fourth sacral nerve). This nerve is a branch of the pudendal nerve and crosses the ischiorectal fossa along with the inferior rectal artery and vein. The skin posterior to the anus is supplied by the anococcygeal nerves that are branches of the coccygeal plexus (coccygeal nerve with branches from S4 and S5).

The Greater Omentum

EMBRYOLOGY

The part of the foregut that forms the stomach is attached to the posterior abdominal wall by the dorsal mesogastrium. As the stomach rotates through 90 degrees around its long axis, the dorsal mesogastrium bulges sinistrally and inferiorly from the greater curvature as the greater omentum. Within the greater omentum initially is an extension of the lesser sac, but it is usually obliterated in later fetal life. Fat accumulates within the greater omentum, and it extends for a variable distance anterior to the transverse colon and the small intestine. The peritoneum of the posterior surface of the greater omentum generally fuses with the mesentery of the transverse colon.

Anomalies of development lead to congenital omental cysts; abnormal openings, or too long or too short a greater omentum; or failure of fusion of the anterior and posterior omental layers, leaving a cavity that connects with the lesser omental sac.

GROSS ANATOMY
(Figs 30–1, 30–2, & 30–3)

The greater omentum consists of a double sheet of peritoneum that hangs from the greater curvature of the stomach and folds back upon itself to become a 4-layered serous structure. The 2 anterior layers of the greater omentum are a direct continuation of the 2 layers of the gastrohepatic omentum that have descended from the porta hepatis and have split at the level of the lesser curvature of the stomach to envelop the stomach as its serous coat. The 2 gastric covering layers join again just below the greater curvature of the stomach. As they descend, they lie ventral to the transverse colon and mesocolon and the coils of small intestine. Between the greater curvature of the stomach and the transverse colon, the 2 descending serous layers are called the **gastrocolic ligament.** It may or may not have a relatively avascular fusion with the surface of the transverse colon.

The further descent of the greater omental layers varies. In some individuals, they reach down to the true pelvis; in others they reach only a few centimeters below the transverse colon. This is the usual case in infants and children. From the lowest level, the 2 anterior omental layers turn dorsally upon themselves and form the 2 posterior serous layers of the omental apron. All 4 omental layers eventually ascend to the transverse colon.

From the inferior border of the greater omentum to the inferior margin of the gastrocolic ligament, the few omental layers are normally fused tightly together. As a result, the cavity of the lesser sac, which in fetal life extends inferiorly between the 2 anterior and the 2 posterior greater omental layers, is obliterated and normally does not exist below the transverse colon.

At the antimesenteric border of the transverse colon, the 2 posterior layers of the greater omentum pass superior to the colon. They fuse with the peritoneum of the transverse colon and with the mesentery of the transverse colon, and thus become part of the transverse mesocolon.

The right free border of the greater omentum extends to the right to the first segment of the duodenum; the left free border becomes continuous with the gastrosplenic ligament, a poorly defined structure that runs from the fundus of the stomach to the left leaf of the diaphragm. The greater omentum contains varying amounts of fat between its thin serous layers; in adults, the greater omentum is longer and more mobile and contains more fat than in children.

⠿➡ *Function of the greater omentum. The greater omentum acts as a plug or shield in most cases of acute abdominal inflammation. An old surgical rule is to "follow the omentum to the site of inflammation." This rule is particularly appropriate in appendicitis, gallbladder disease, pelvic inflammatory disease, and diverticular disease. In children, the greater omentum is poorly developed and short, and as a consequence its plugging and directional characteristics are usually missing in patients under age 12.*

⠿➡ *Omental infarction. Omental infarction, either segmental or complete, presents as an occasional intra-abdominal emergency. It may occur as a result of omental twisting, iatrogenic interruption of the vascular supply to the omentum—particularly in the aged—or as a result of arteriosclerotic plugging of the omental vessels.*

The porta hepatis is attached to the lesser curvature of the stomach by the double-layered gastrohepatic ligament and to the pyloric portion of the duodenum by the hepatoduodenal ligament. The liver is thought to be held in position by positive intra-abdominal pressure exerted superiorly and by pressure upon its visceral surface by multiple adjacent organs. It may be held against the posterior abdominal wall by the areolar tissue that lies posteriorly.

Falciform Ligament

The falciform ligament consists of 2 closely applied layers of peritoneum. It has a scythelike shape. The right surface of the ligament faces forward and is in contact with the peritoneum of the anterior abdominal wall inferiorly and the undersurface of the diaphragm superiorly. Its left surface faces posteriorly and is in contact with the left lobe of the liver. As the falciform ligament passes over the dome of the liver, it divides into 2 leaflets, the right leaflet becoming part of the coronary ligament and the left leaflet becoming the left triangular ligament. The attachment of the falciform ligament to the liver extends from the umbilical notch on the superior surface of the liver onto its inferior surface to the porta hepatis. The 2 layers of peritoneum that comprise the falciform ligament merge at its base. The base of the falciform ligament contains the ligamentum teres hepatis (round ligament) and the paraumbilical veins.

➠ *Falciform ligament and abdominal incisions. In obese individuals, the falciform ligament of the liver becomes a nuisance when abdominal incisions are made in the mid or right upper abdomen. The surgeon must usually divide the ligament to gain adequate exposure of the upper abdominal areas. Division of the ligament is complicated by the frequent presence of large amounts of fat between its 2 peritoneal layers.*

Left Triangular Ligament
(Fig 31–6)

The left triangular ligament becomes prominent when the left lobe of the liver is drawn away from the undersurface of the diaphragm. The ligament is a peritoneal fold that connects the superior surface of the left lobe of the liver to the undersurface of the diaphragm. The ligament has 3 borders: The first is attached to the posterosuperior surface of the left lobe of the liver and is a continuation of the left layer of the falciform ligament. The second border is attached to the central tendon of the diaphragm. The third border is a free edge directed toward the left upper abdominal parietes. The left inferior phrenic vessels run near the lateral free border of the left triangular ligament.

➠ *Section of the left triangular ligament. In order to inspect the proximal portion of the lesser gastric curvature, the abdominal esophagus, the vagus nerves, the left suprarenal gland, and the decussation of the crura of the diaphragm, the surgeon often must mobilize and medially retract the left lobe of the liver. This may be done either by incising the free border of the left triangular ligament or by manual retraction medially and anteriorly of the left liver lobe. If the left triangular ligament is severed, care must be taken to avoid the left inferior phrenic vein that runs close to the posterior surface of the ligament.*

Coronary Ligament

The coronary ligament lies on the superior surface of the right lobe of the liver and consists of superior and inferior layers. The superior layer can be palpated by passing the fingers of the right hand posteriorly over the surface of the liver. The fingers will eventu-

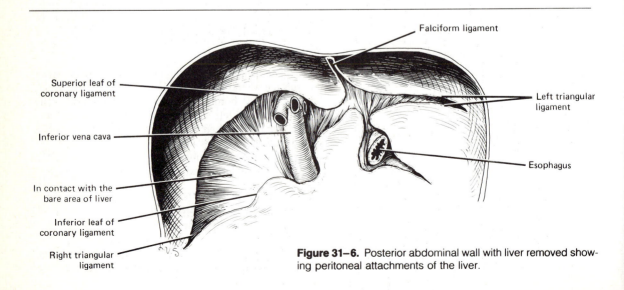

Figure 31–6. Posterior abdominal wall with liver removed showing peritoneal attachments of the liver.

Falciform ligament

Left triangular ligament

Esophagus

Superior leaf of coronary ligament

Inferior vena cava

In contact with the bare area of liver

Inferior leaf of coronary ligament

Right triangular ligament

ally be blocked by a layer of peritoneum, the upper layer of the coronary ligament. This layer is reflected from the superior surface of the liver onto the inferior surface of the diaphragm. As one pushes the fingers of the left hand upward along the superior reaches of the right lumbar gutter, dorsal to the right lobe of the liver, they will be stopped by the lower layer of the coronary ligament. This layer is reflected from the posterior surface of the right lobe of the liver onto the right kidney, the right suprarenal gland, and the inferior vena cava. The inferior leaf of the coronary ligament is often called the hepatorenal ligament and is the upper boundary of the right lumbar gutter. Between the upper and lower layers of the coronary ligament there is a large triangular area on the posterosuperior surface of the right lobe of the liver which is devoid of peritoneal covering and is therefore called the **bare area of the liver.** The retroperitoneal tissues lying posterior to the bare area of the liver are joined to the liver substance by areolar tissue and the small veins of Retzius. These veins are a minor area of anatomic portacaval anastomosis.

Right Triangular Ligament

The right triangular ligament begins at the extreme right of the bare area of the liver where the converging upper and lower layers of the coronary ligament fuse. It attaches the liver to the undersurface of the right leaf of the diaphragm.

Round Ligament

The round ligament is a fibrous cord that ascends within the base of the falciform ligament from the umbilicus to the umbilical notch on the inferior surface of the left lobe of the liver. From the umbilical notch it runs in its own fossa on the visceral surface of the liver to the porta hepatis. There, the round ligament becomes continuous with the ligamentum venosum.

LIVER FISSURES & FOSSAE
(Fig 31–2)

Longitudinal Fissure

The longitudinal fissure is a deep trench on the visceral surface of the liver running in an anterior-to-posterior direction. Inferiorly, the porta hepatis divides the fissure into anterior and posterior segments. The anterior segment is the fissure for the ligamentum teres hepatis and the posterior segment the fissure for the ligamentum venosum. The longitudinal fissure forms the right lateral border of the quadrate lobe.

Transverse Fissure

At the porta hepatis, the major hepatic blood vessels and nerves enter and the biliary ducts and liver lymphatics exit. The fissure lies on the visceral surface and presents as a narrow transverse slit not covered by peritoneum. It is bounded by the ventral and dorsal layers of the gastrohepatic ligament. The porta hepatis forms the crossbar of the H formed on the visceral surface of the liver by the fissures and fossae. The left anterior upright of the H is the ligamentum teres hepatis; the left posterior upright is the ligamentum venosum. The right posterior upright is the fossa for the inferior vena cava, the right anterior upright is the gallbladder and its fossa. The posterior uprights of the H enclose the caudate lobe; the anterior uprights enclose the quadrate lobe. The transverse fissure separates the anterior quadrate lobe from the posterior caudate lobe.

Gallbladder Fossa

The gallbladder fossa lies anteriorly on the visceral surface of the right lobe of the liver parallel to and to the right of the fissure for the ligamentum teres hepatis. It is quite shallow and extends posteriorly as far as the right free border of the porta hepatis. It is not covered by peritoneum.

Fossa for the Inferior Vena Cava

The fossa for the inferior vena cava is an almost completely enclosed tunnel sunk deeply into the liver. It lies on the posterior liver surface between the bare area of the liver and the caudate lobe. It is separated from the posterior termination of the gallbladder fossa by the porta hepatis. A line drawn from the anterior margin of the gallbladder fossa to the fossa for the inferior vena cava marks the true anatomic division between the right and left lobes.

THE INTRAHEPATIC & BILIARY DUCTS

Each of the 4 major portions of the liver—the right anterior and posterior segments and the left medial and lateral segments—is drained by a major segmental biliary duct. The right posterior segmental duct usually joins with the right anterior segmental duct to form the right major intrahepatic biliary duct. In about 25% of people, the anterior and posterior segmental ducts join the common hepatic duct separately. The medial segmental duct from the left lobe joins with the lateral segmental duct from the same lobe to form the left hepatic duct. Bile leaving the caudate lobe empties into both the right and left lobe biliary radicles, whereas bile leaving the quadrate lobe (ie, the medial segment of the left lobe) empties only into left biliary ducts.

THE SUBPHRENIC OR PERIHEPATIC SPACES
(Fig 31–7)

The subphrenic space is the region inferior to the diaphragm and superior to the transverse colon and mesocolon. The liver divides the subphrenic area into

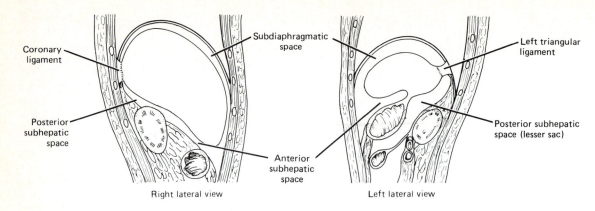

Figure 31–7. Subphrenic spaces.

(1) a suprahepatic area, bounded above by the diaphragm and below by the superior surface of the liver; and (2) an infrahepatic area, bounded above by the visceral surface of the liver and below by the transverse colon and transverse mesocolon.

The Suprahepatic Spaces

The suprahepatic space is divided into right and left segments by the falciform ligament, which runs from the superior surface of the liver to the diaphragm. The **right suprahepatic space** extends from the anterior margin of the right lobe to the upper margin of the triangular ligament. It thus spans the entire undersurface of the right diaphragm.

The **left suprahepatic space** is bounded above by the diaphragm, below by the upper surface of the left lobe of the liver, and medially by the falciform ligament. The left triangular ligament, which runs along the superior border of the left lobe of the liver, forms the posterior boundary of the space. The tip of the left lobe of the liver lies in the midclavicular line. To the left of this point, the subdiaphragmatic space houses the spleen.

The Infrahepatic Space

The infrahepatic space is divided into right and left segments by the combined round and falciform ligaments. The **right infrahepatic space** is bounded superiorly by the visceral surface of the right lobe of the liver and below by the transverse colon and mesocolon. Medially, it extends to the round ligament, and laterally, it merges with the upper end of the right lumbar gutter. The space contains the gallbladder, the cystic duct and the extrahepatic biliary ducts, the pylorus of the stomach, the first and second portions of the duodenum, and the lateral portion of the head of the pancreas.

The **left anterior infrahepatic space** (epigastric space) lies ventral to the stomach and to the left of the round ligament. It lies below the left lobe of the liver and above the left half of the transverse colon and mesocolon. The **left posterior infrahepatic space** (or lesser peritoneal sac) is bounded above by the inferior surface of the left lobe of the liver, below by the transverse colon and mesocolon, anteriorly by the stomach and the gastrohepatic omentum, and posteriorly by the parietal peritoneum covering the body and the tail of the pancreas.

Perihepatic spaces. The supra- and infrahepatic spaces are of clinical significance because (1) they are favored areas for the collection of free pus, blood, and gas; (2) they lie close to organs vulnerable to traumatic or pathologic perforation (gallbladder, common bile duct, stomach, duodenum, pancreas); and (3) pathways from the mid and lower abdomen lead to these spaces, allowing blood, pus, and gas to pool within them.

The right infrahepatic space is the space most frequently involved by disease in adjacent organs. The posterior recess of the right suprahepatic space is continuous with the right lumbar gutter, which runs between the lower and the upper abdomen. Fluid or air in the perihepatic spaces may be manifested by fever, leukocytosis, splinting of the diaphragm, elevation of the diaphragm, fluid in the pleural cavity, pain on respiration, and subcostal tenderness. Sonography and CT body scans help in the diagnosis of perihepatic collections.

Surgical approaches. (Fig 31–8.) Most subphrenic abscesses can be adequately drained by a catheter inserted with CT or ultrasound guidance. If surgical drainage is required, abscesses in the right perihepatic spaces and the left suprahepatic space may be drained through an abdominal incision. Posterior right subhepatic abscess may occasionally be drained through a posterior incision through the bed of the resected 12th rib (Ochsner approach). The lesser sac is usually drained through either the gastrocolic ligament or the transverse mesocolon.

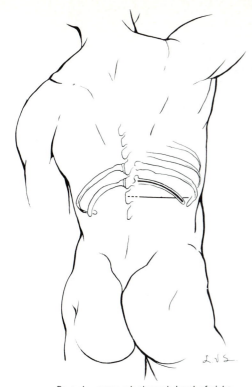

Posterior approach through head of right twelfth rib (Ochsner) reaches posterior superior space and upper end of right lumbar gutter.

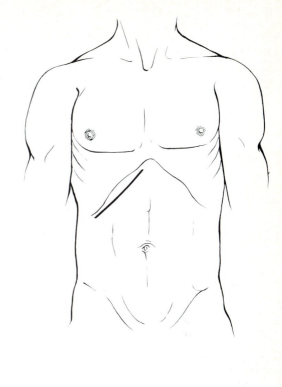

Paracostal incision gives a transperitoneal anterior approach to the anterior superior and visceral surfaces of the liver.

Figure 31–8. Surgical incisions for approach to liver.

LIVER STRUCTURE
(Fig 31–9)

The liver is composed of a vast number of polygonal lobules held together in a fine meshwork of connective tissue. The cellular columns of the liver lobule are grouped around a central vein that is the most peripheral part of the hepatic venous system.

Branches of the portal vein and the hepatic artery and small peripheral bile ducts traverse the liver along the portal canal. The 3 structures are held together by intrahepatic extensions of Glisson's fibrous capsule. Portal canals are associated with each liver lobule and are placed peripherally at angles of the lobular polygon.

Between the columns of hepatic cells that make up the individual liver lobules run the liver sinusoids (modified capillaries) and the small bile canaliculi. The sinusoids connect with branches of the portal vein and the hepatic artery at the periphery of the lobules. They then pass from the periphery to empty into the central hepatic veins. The sinusoidal walls contain elements of the reticuloendothelial system (macrophages or Kupffer cells).

The most peripheral portions of the biliary system begin as tiny channels (bile canaliculi) between the liver cells. These channels are always separated from the vascular capillaries by the thickness of a liver cell. The intercellular bile canaliculi run to the periphery of the liver lobule and empty into the interlobular biliary ducts. These ducts are close to the peripheral radicles of the portal vein and the hepatic artery.

BLOOD SUPPLY, LYMPHATICS, & NERVES
(Fig 31–10)

Arteries

The liver receives its blood supply from 2 sources: the **hepatic artery** and the **portal vein.**

Arterial blood reaches the liver through the **hepatic artery,** normally a branch of the celiac artery. The hepatic artery runs transversely behind the posterior peritoneum of the lesser sac, dividing into its 2 major branches at the border of the hepatoduodenal ligament. The ascending hepatic artery runs upward in the right free border of the hepatoduodenal ligament

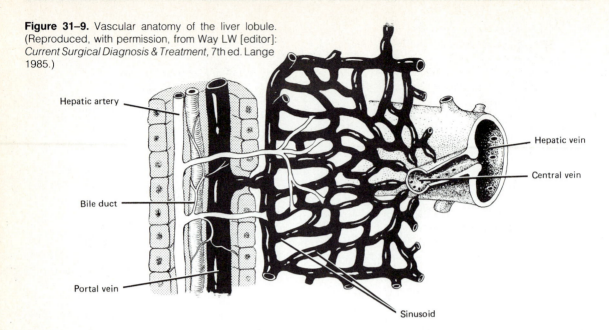

Figure 31–9. Vascular anatomy of the liver lobule. (Reproduced, with permission, from Way LW [editor]: *Current Surgical Diagnosis & Treatment,* 7th ed. Lange 1985.)

on the same plane as the common bile duct but medial to it. The common bile duct and the hepatic artery both lie ventral to the portal vein. Superior to the entrance of the cystic duct into the common bile duct, the hepatic artery divides into right and left branches that enter the liver at the porta hepatis. The hepatic artery and its terminal branches are variable in their sites of division and their relationships to structures in the hepatoduodenal ligament, the gallbladder fossa, and the porta hepatis. On occasion, the hepatic artery originates from the superior mesenteric artery, from the gastroduodenal artery, or directly from the aorta.

In 5% of cases, a branch of the **left gastric artery** runs to the left liver lobe in the left free border of the gastrohepatic omentum.

The **right terminal branch** of the ascending he-

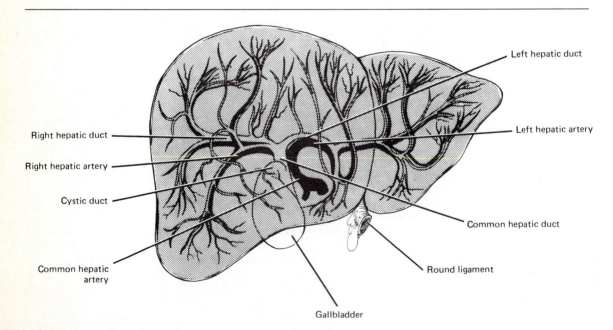

Figure 31–10. Bile ducts and hepatic arterial branches. Bile ducts are represented by lighter vessels, arteries by darker vessels.

patic artery usually passes from left to right behind the common bile duct. Entering the porta hepatis, this branch divides into right anterior and posterior segmental branches. The anterior segmental branch parallels the major biliary duct serving the anterior segment of the right lobe. The right hepatic artery eventually divides into an inferior and a superior vessel for the right anterior segment. The left hepatic artery usually divides within the liver into medial and lateral segmental branches. The medial segmental artery supplies the quadrate lobe.

A branch from the right hepatic artery supplies the right portion of the caudate lobe; a branch of the left hepatic artery supplies the left half of the lobe. Branches of the left hepatic artery supply portions of the liver immediately to the right of the falciform ligament. The major intrahepatic branches of

the hepatic artery follow the lines of the major liver fissures, making it relatively easy to identify the vessels in segmental hepatic resections.

Veins
(Figs 31–11 and 31–13)

The **portal vein** is normally formed posterior to the junction of the head and neck of the pancreas by the union of the splenic vein and the superior mesenteric vein. The portal vein then runs in the right free border of the hepatoduodenal ligament posterior to both the common bile duct and the hepatic artery. At the porta hepatis, the portal vein divides into right and left branches.

The right branch divides into anterior and posterior segmental branches that accompany the segmental branches of the right hepatic duct and the right hepatic

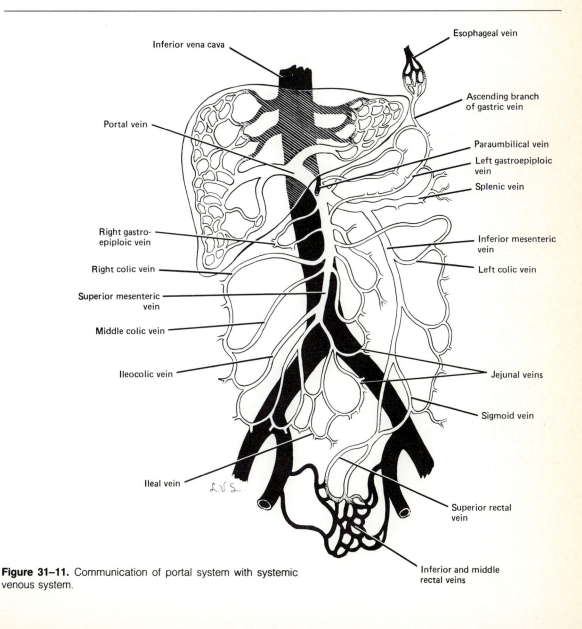

Figure 31–11. Communication of portal system with systemic venous system.

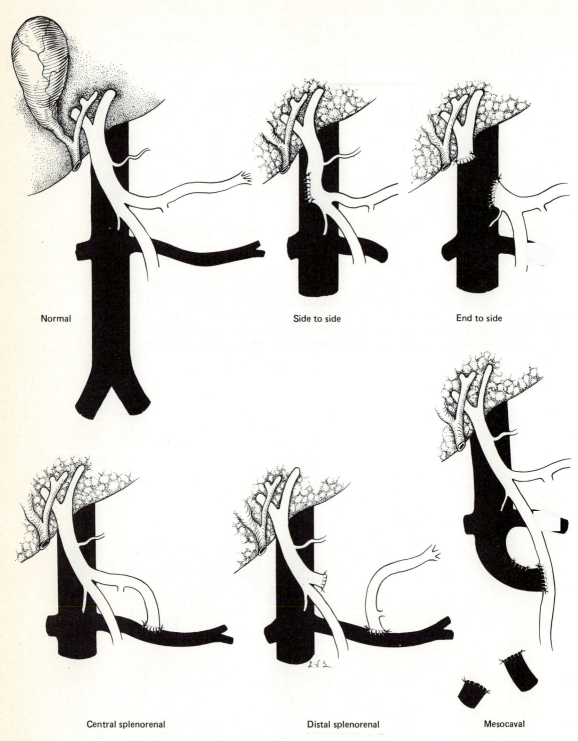

Normal

Side to side

End to side

Central splenorenal

Distal splenorenal

Mesocaval

Figure 31–12. Types of portacaval anastomoses.

artery. All 3 structures—venous, arterial, and ductal—terminate as superior and inferior segmental branches.

The left branch of the portal vein divides into 2 trunks. The transverse trunk runs to the left in the porta hepatis; the umbilical trunk descends to the umbilical fossa.

The medial and lateral segmental branches of the left portal vein run from the umbilical fossa to the medial and lateral subsegments of the left lobe. The portal venous supply to the caudate lobe arises from both the right and left portal venous trunks.

➠ ***Portacaval shunting.*** *(Fig 31–12.) In cirrhosis of the liver, the high pressure in the portal system can be relieved by anastomotic connections with vessels in the lower-pressure systemic venous system. Portal hypertension may be of intrahepatic or extrahepatic origin. The commonest cause of intrahepatic portal hypertension is cirrhosis; portal vein thrombosis and pressure of diseased or malignant structures on the portal vein are the commonest causes of extrahepatic portal hypertension. Shunting of portal blood into the caval system by surgical portacaval anastomosis has been used to avoid the sequelae of portal hypertension. The shunting is most often done just below the transverse fissure of the liver, where the portal vein and the inferior vena cava are in close proximity for anastomosis. Portal vein pressure should always be checked by direct manometry: Pressure greater than 300 mm of water indicates portal hypertension.*

The principal indication for portacaval shunting is one or more episodes of bleeding from esophageal varices.

Other surgical procedures for relief of portal hypertension are (1) shunting of the splenic vein to the left renal vein, and (2) shunting of the superior mesenteric vein to the inferior vena cava.

Normally, there are 3 major **hepatic veins:** right, middle, and left. They form within the liver and empty into the inferior vena cava. The 3 major hepatic veins each lie in one of the 3 major liver fissures and drain adjacent liver segments. The middle hepatic vein lies in the major lobar fissure and drains the left middle and right anterior segments. The right hepatic vein lies in the right segmental fissure and drains the right posterior and the anterior right lobar segment. The left hepatic vein lies in the left segmental fissure and drains the left lateral and the left medial segment. As a rule, the left and middle hepatic veins join to

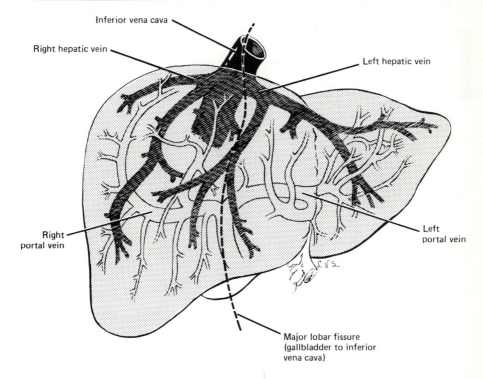

Inferior vena cava

Right hepatic vein

Left hepatic vein

Right portal vein

Left portal vein

Major lobar fissure (gallbladder to inferior vena cava)

Figure 31–13. Veins of the liver. The major lobar fissure is represented by the dashed line. Branches of the hepatic artery and biliary ducts follow those of the portal vein. The darker vessels represent the hepatic veins and vena cava; the lighter system represents the portal vein and its branches. (Reproduced, with permission, from Way LW [editor]: *Current Surgical Diagnosis & Treatment,* 7th ed. Lange, 1985.)

form a single trunk to empty into the inferior vena cava. The right hepatic vein usually joins the vena cava independently. Frequently, 3–6 smaller venous channels issuing from the liver also empty directly into the vena cava. There are no valves in the major hepatic veins.

➠ *Liver resection. The 3 major hepatic veins in the 3 major hepatic fissures serve as anatomic landmarks in segmental resection of the liver.*

➠ *Liver trauma. When liver trauma causes tearing of hepatic veins near their entrance into the inferior vena cava, a serious bleeding problem exists. The tears are usually not discovered until late in the course of surgical exploration, because the bulk of the liver tends to tamponade bleeding from these veins. Hepatic vein tears carry a very high mortality rate.*

➠ *Contrast x-rays. Since there are no valves in the major hepatic veins, they are easily visualized by means of x-rays taken after injection of opaque media into the adjacent inferior vena cava.*

Lymphatics
(Fig 31–14)

The lymphatics of the liver are divided into deep and superficial groups. One group of deep liver lymphatics begins near the small terminals of the portal vein and accompanies these portal venous radicles to the liver hilum. These lymphatic vessels terminate in the hepatic nodes around the superior termination of the ascending hepatic artery. Other deep lymphatic radicles follow the course of the hepatic veins to terminate near the caval opening in the diaphragm. These lymphatics then drain into the middle phrenic nodes, which lie in the posteroinferior mediastinum.

The superficial lymph channels lie in the subperitoneal connective tissue that covers the entire surface of the liver. The channels from the diaphragmatic surface drain into the lower phrenic nodes. Some upper subperitoneal channels drain through the caval foramen to the middle phrenic nodes. There is some (slight) drainage from superficial tissues of the upper surface of the liver toward the esophageal hiatus. Most lymphatics from the subperitoneal areas of the visceral surface of the liver drain directly into the celiac nodes, while some drain first into the nodes grouped about the porta hepatis and then into the celiac nodes.

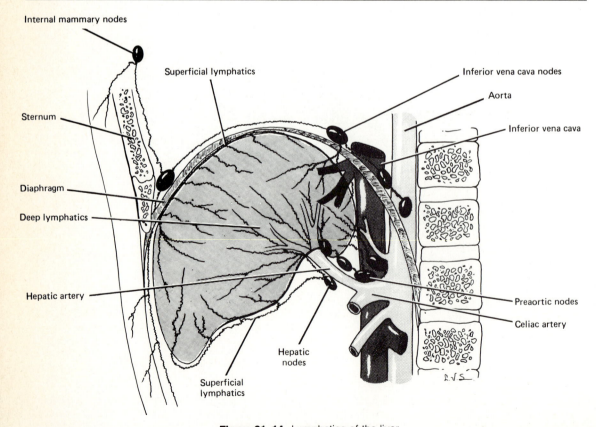

Figure 31–14. Lymphatics of the liver.

Nerves

The hepatic nerve supply is derived from the left vagus and from the abdominal sympathetic nerves, particularly those from the celiac plexus. Both groups of nerves enter the liver at the porta hepatis and accompany the liver vessels and ducts toward their hepatic terminations. The specific mechanism of these nerves is still in doubt, since most of the functions of the liver are probably under endocrine control. For example, secretion of bile is probably not under nervous control. Many pain fibers accompany the smaller biliary ducts into the liver.

➠ *Liver transplantation. Experimental and clinical investigations are being carried out on liver transplantation, particularly in patients with congenital biliary duct atresia. Liver transplants give promise of becoming useful therapy in selected cases.*

➠ *Surgical approaches. Most procedures on the liver can best be carried out via an anterior transperitoneal approach. On occasion, an abdominothoracic approach may give the best exposure. The posterior (Ochsner) approach gives good exposure of the bare area of the liver and leads the surgeon into the posterior suprahepatic space. For this approach, the 12th rib is resected, and care must be taken not to enter the pleural cavity when an incision is made through the bed of this rib.*

➠ *Drainage of abscesses. Only large, confluent liver abscesses are amenable to surgical therapy. They may be approached through the transabdominal, abdominothoracic (diaphragmatic sinus), or lumbar pathways, but more commonly are drained by percutaneous aspiration.*

32

Extrahepatic Biliary System

EMBRYOLOGY
(Fig 32–1)

The inferior knob of the liver diverticulum (see Chapter 31) develops into the gallbladder and the cystic duct. The latter opens into the common bile duct which, as a result of duodenal rotation and differential growth, comes to open into the left side of the second part of the duodenum.

Anomalies. Anomalous development results in a great variety of defects: congenital absence or anomalies of position of the gallbladder, double gallbladder, diverticulum of the gallbladder, complete or partial gallbladder mesentery, intrahepatic gallbladder, ab-

normalities of the gallbladder lumen, aberrant valves of Heister in the cystic duct, supernumerary right or left extrahepatic duct, congenital cyst of the common bile duct, and congenital absence, atresia, or stenosis of the extrahepatic biliary duct (Figs 32–2 and 32–3).

GROSS ANATOMY

1. THE GALLBLADDER
(Fig 32–4)

The gallbladder is a pear-shaped organ that lies in a depression ("bed") on the visceral surface of

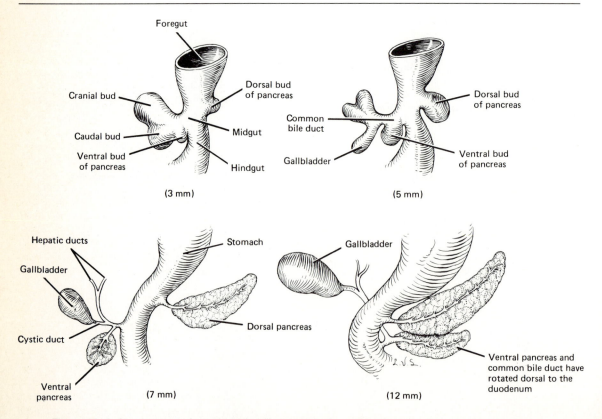

Figure 32–1. Development of extrahepatic biliary tract in the embryo from the 3-mm to the 12-mm stage.

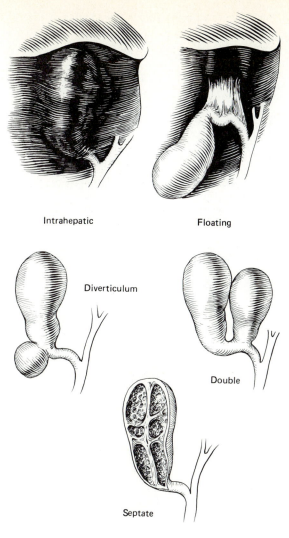

Intrahepatic

Floating

Diverticulum

Double

Septate

Figure 32–2. Anomalies of the gallbladder.

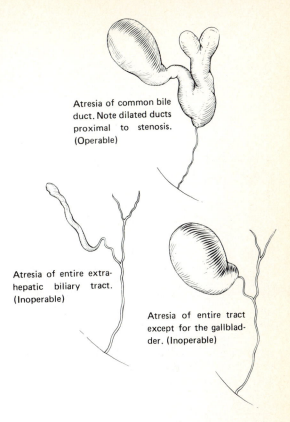

Atresia of common bile duct. Note dilated ducts proximal to stenosis. (Operable)

Atresia of entire extra-hepatic biliary tract. (Inoperable)

Atresia of entire tract except for the gallblad-der. (Inoperable)

Figure 32–3. Atresia of the extrahepatic biliary tract.

the right lobe of the liver. It is attached to its bed in the liver by areolar connective tissue that contains many small lymphatics and veins. These lymphatics and veins connect the venous and lymphatic systems of the gallbladder with those of the liver.

➠ *Inflammation of the liver secondary to gall-bladder disease. Since the gallbladder body is tightly attached to its bed in the liver and since the liver bed is not covered by peritoneum, gallbladder inflammation often spreads directly to the liver bed. The acutely inflamed gallblad-der may cause a neighboring hepatic cellulitis, or the gallbladder may rupture directly against its unprotected liver bed.*

Only that portion of the gallbladder circumference which is not adherent to the gallbladder bed of the liver is covered with peritoneum. However, some gallbladders possess a mesentery and consequently are almost completely covered with peritoneum. The amount of the gallbladder surface in direct contact with the liver and the degree with which the gallblad-der surface is covered with peritoneum vary markedly with the shape of the gallbladder. Since the fundus of the gallbladder normally protrudes a short distance below the margin of the liver, the fundus is nearly always completely covered with peritoneum.

The fundus of the gallbladder usually lies at the point where the lateral border of the rectus abdominis muscle intersects the right ninth costal cartilage. How-ever, the positions of these structures may vary mark-edly. In hepatic and biliary tract disease, the relation-ship of the gallbladder to the anterior abdominal peri-toneum will change markedly depending on whether the organ swells or shrinks.

➠ *Importance of relationship of fundus of gall-bladder to anterior abdominal wall. The fact that the tip of the fundus of the gallbladder lies against the parietal peritoneum of the right upper quadrant accounts for the ease with which a distended gallbladder can be palpated and for the early signs of peritoneal irritation when the gallbladder is inflamed.*

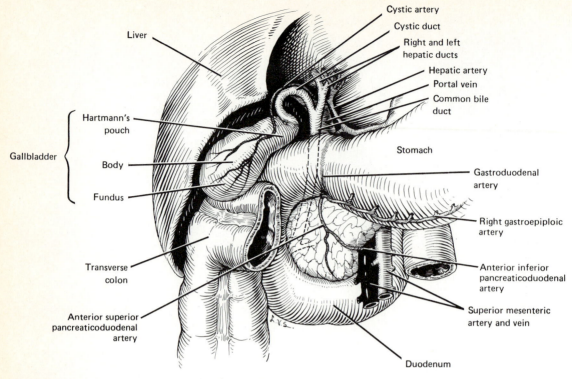

Figure 32–4. Relationships of the gallbladder.

DIVISIONS OF THE GALLBLADDER

The gallbladder is usually divided into a fundus, body, infundibulum, and neck.

Fundus

The fundus, the rounded blind end of the gallbladder, usually projects 0.5–1 cm beyond the free edge of the inferior border of the right lobe of the liver. The tip of the fundus usually lies in the angle formed by the lateral border of the right rectus abdominis muscle and the ninth costal cartilage. There, the fundus is in contact with the peritoneum of the abdominal wall.

The fundus is palpable in the right upper quadrant when the gallbladder is distended. Occasionally, the fundus of the gallbladder is kinked on itself, with a resulting so-called phrygian cap deformity.

➡ *Phrygian cap deformity on cholecystograms. The phrygian cap anomaly of the gallbladder fundus may be confused during gallbladder visualization with the presence of gallstones or mucosal polyps within the fundus.*

The gallbladder fundus passes without transition into the gallbladder body. Unless a mesentery is pres-

ent, the entire superior surface of the gallbladder body is attached to the visceral surface of the liver.

➡ *Complications from close coaptation of the gallbladder to the visceral surface of the liver. Close coaptation of the gallbladder to its liver bed allows for early spread of carcinoma of the gallbladder into the liver bed. On occasion, rupture of a gallbladder containing stones will allow the stones to fall between the body of the gallbladder and the liver bed surface.*

Body

The free surface of the body and the infundibulum of the gallbladder lie close to both the first and the second portion of the duodenum.

➡ *Clinical import of relationship of gallbladder to duodenum. In diseases involving both the duodenum and the biliary tract, adhesions frequently form between the proximal portions of the duodenum and the gallbladder. Such adhesions favor fistula formation with the possibility of passage of gallstones into the upper small bowel.*

The body and infundibulum of the gallbladder are also close to the hepatic flexure of the colon and the right third of the transverse colon. The serosal surfaces of the gallbladder may also come into close contact with loops of small bowel in the right hypochondrium. In cases of a high-lying cecum and appendix, in which these structures retain their embryonic subhepatic position, they too may come into close contact with the gallbladder body. The prepyloric and pyloric areas of the stomach are also close to the gallbladder.

➠ *Clinical import of relationship of gallbladder to right colon and hepatic flexure. Adhesions between the gallbladder, the hepatic flexure, and the right side of the transverse colon are common. Biliary stones can pass directly from the gallbladder into the large bowel.*

Infundibulum

The infundibulum of the gallbladder is the tapering transitional area between the gallbladder body and the neck. It usually lies close to the undersurface of the cystic duct and may completely hide the cystic duct from view. The infundibulum is attached to the first part of the duodenum by a relatively avascular double-layered peritoneal fold derived from the right free border of the hepatoduodenal ligament. This fold, the **cholecystoduodenal ligament,** is of great importance in the operative search for major vascular and ductal structures in the biliary fossa.

Hartmann's pouch is a bulging of the inferior surface of the normally shallow gallbladder infundibulum. The bulge lies close to the neck of the gallbladder. The surgeon usually uses the pouch for traction toward the fundus in order to better visualize the neck and cystic duct of the gallbladder, which the pouch overhangs.

➠ *Surgical importance of Hartmann's pouch. Hartmann's pouch may, as a result of inflammation, adhere so closely to the cystic duct that mobilization of the cystic duct cannot be carried out until the pouch has been dissected free. Hartmann's pouch may also adhere to the common bile duct, predisposing to injury of the extrahepatic biliary tree close to the entrance of the cystic duct into the common bile duct.*

Neck

The infundibulum of the gallbladder rapidly tapers into the neck, which is narrow and curves upon itself in the form of the letter "S." The neck of the gallbladder is usually 5–7 mm long. It is constricted at its junction with the cystic duct. The transition between the neck and the cystic duct can be abrupt or gradual. The neck occupies the deepest part of the so-called "cystic fossa," close to the free border of the hepatoduodenal ligament.

BLOOD VESSELS, LYMPHATICS, & NERVES

Arteries

Arterial supply to the gallbladder is usually from a single **cystic artery.** In about 12–13% of cases, a double cystic artery is present. Normally, the cystic artery arises from the right hepatic artery and soon divides into 2 branches, one related to the peritoneal surface of the gallbladder and the other between the body of the gallbladder and its liver bed. The artery usually lies superior to the cystic duct, but it may lie anterior or dorsal to it.

The site of origin of the cystic artery or arteries varies. It may originate from the right hepatic artery, the left hepatic artery, the common hepatic artery, or a branch of the celiac artery. It rarely arises from the superior mesenteric artery.

After it leaves the right hepatic artery, the cystic artery may parallel the parent artery for some distance in the direction of the liver. In such cases, it may easily be confused with the right hepatic artery. In 7–10% of cases, the cystic artery does not leave the right hepatic artery until just before that vessel enters the right lobe of the liver. In such cases, the cystic artery is only a few millimeters long and close to the visceral surface of the liver. It reaches the gallbladder at the superior surface of its neck. The cystic artery usually branches close to the neck of the gallbladder. If only one branch is found there, one must suspect the possibility of a double cystic artery.

Veins

Venous return from the gallbladder is by many small veins that run either from its hepatic surface directly into the liver bed or toward the cystic duct, where they join with venous radicles from the common bile duct before entering the portal venous system. There is no single major cystic vein.

Lymphatics

Lymph may run directly into the gallbladder bed of the liver through many small lymphatic channels that accompany the small venules. This is the main pathway for hepatic cellulitis in the area of the liver immediately adjacent to the gallbladder. From the subserous levels, lymph drainage may run toward the cystic duct and into nodes overlying the cystic duct just before it empties into the common bile duct. From these so-called cystic nodes, lymph may pass either through the hepatoduodenal ligament, to reach nodes close to the hilum of the liver, or into nodes lying about the celiac axis of the aorta.

Nerves

The gallbladder receives nerve fibers from both the sympathetic and parasympathetic nervous systems. The nerve supply to the gallbladder is via the hepatic plexus, which begins within the celiac plexus and then extends toward the gallbladder, along the hepatic artery and the portal vein. The hepatic plexus contains afferent, sympathetic, and vagal (parasympathetic) fibers. It is joined just below the liver by branches from the left (anterior) trunk of the vagus. The afferent fibers in the hepatic plexus include some pain fibers. Consequently, pain from the extrahepatic biliary tree is usually referred to the epigastric or the right hypochondrial areas, or to the right scapular region. Conduction of pain from the biliary tract is entirely through fibers that run with the sympathetic rather than with the parasympathetic nerves. The nerves supplying the gallbladder and the sphincter of Oddi are not essential for emptying of the organ. There is hormonal control over the contractions of the gallbladder; the presence of fats in the small intestine brings about the release of secretin and cholecystokinin, with resulting gallbladder contraction.

FUNCTIONS OF THE GALLBLADDER

The main function of the gallbladder is to store bile and to reabsorb water from the stored bile, thereby concentrating it. This process is dependent on an active sodium- and chloride-transporting mechanism in the gallbladder epithelium. Water reabsorption is probably by osmosis as a result of the sodium pump. Studies of its epithelial layer suggest that the sodium, chloride, and water cross the membrane of the cell apex, then move to the intercellular spaces and from these spaces to the blood vessels of the lamina propria of the organ.

⟐ *Surgical procedures involving the gallbladder. Cholecystostomy* (*gallbladder drainage*) *is reserved for cases of acute gallbladder disease in which it is felt that an elderly or debilitated patient would be unable to withstand more radical procedures (cholecystectomy, choledochostomy). It may be used in cases where the pathologic process (acute or subacute) has so obliterated the normal anatomic relationships in the gallbladder fossa as to make the more definitive procedure of cholecystectomy a risky one. Cholecystostomy is best done under general anesthesia, although local field block may be used. It is usually done through a subcostal incision. The gallbladder is drained through a lateral stab wound inferior to the major incision. Care must be taken not to displace a stone from the gallbladder or the cystic duct into the common bile duct during the procedure. Many patients subjected to cholecystostomy need later definitive gallbladder or common bile duct surgery.*

In **cholecystectomy,** *the gallbladder is usually removed by beginning dissection at the cystic duct level and working toward the gallbladder fundus. Removal must not be started until all of the structures in the gallbladder fossa have been visualized and identified. One can also remove the gallbladder in retrograde fashion, beginning dissection at the fundus and continuing down to the level of the cystic duct. This procedure is the bloodier of the 2 methods but is frequently the procedure of choice in acute empyema of the gallbladder, where the junction of the cystic and common bile ducts is so inflamed and edematous that specific anatomic structures at the junctional area cannot readily be identified.*

Mobilization of the liver aids greatly in the performance of biliary tract surgery. This is done by placing the hand over the anterosuperior liver surface and allowing air to enter the space between the liver and the diaphragm. This maneuver involves a risk of spreading infection into the perihepatic space. A pack placed above the liver will aid in moving a small high liver down into the operative field. Traction on the falciform and round ligaments of the liver will also help to bring the liver down into the surgeon's view. Before biliary tract surgery, a nasogastric tube should be passed to empty the stomach and thus provide better surgical access to the right upper abdomen. All mobile structures in the right upper quadrant of the abdomen—such as loops of small bowel and the hepatic flexure—are packed away from the operative field. The stomach is packed to the left. A pack placed in the upper end of the hepatorenal pouch of Morison will push the small bowel and the hepatic flexure caudally. The first portion of the duodenum and the pyloric end of the stomach are packed caudally and held there by the first assistant's left hand. Caudal displacement of the duodenum puts the hepatoduodenal ligament, the common bile duct, and the hepatic artery on stretch, leading to easier identification of the gallbladder fossa structures. Clamps placed on the fundus of the gallbladder and subsequently on Hartmann's pouch will pull the cystic duct to join with the common bile duct at a right angle and put the cholecystoduodenal ligament on stretch. Entering the space between the 2 leaves of the cholecystoduodenal ligament usually leads the surgeon directly to the junction of the cystic and common bile ducts. **Cholecystoduodenostomy** *and* **cholecystojejunostomy** *are used for short-circuiting of bile into the intestine in cases in which permanent blockage of the distal common duct exists.*

2. THE RIGHT & LEFT HEPATIC DUCTS; THE COMMON HEPATIC DUCT

The right and left hepatic ducts initiate the delivery of bile from the liver into the gastrointestinal tract. The ducts are formed within the substance of their respective hepatic lobes, and 1–3 cm of each duct may lie within the liver tissue. Generally, the intrahepatic segment of the left hepatic duct is easier to delineate than that of the right. This is because a stretch of terminal intrahepatic left hepatic duct is left without branching. This is of considerable importance in operations in which an additional length of biliary duct is needed for plastic repair or anastomosis.

The right and left hepatic ducts usually unite in an extrahepatic junction just inferior to the porta hepatis. In only about 5% of cases is their union intrahepatic. The usual extrahepatic length of the 2 hepatic ducts varies from 0.5 to 1.5 cm. This length of duct only becomes apparent when the pylorus, the duodenum, and the hepatoduodenal ligament are put on stretch inferiorly. If this maneuver is not performed, the ducts are difficult to locate and appear shorter than they are.

Usually the 2 ducts unite at an acute angle about 1 cm below the porta hepatis to form the common hepatic duct. Rarely, the 2 hepatic ducts continue as separate ducts to a level just above the junction of the cystic duct with the common hepatic duct. Occasionally, the 2 hepatic ducts join after the cystic duct has joined the right hepatic duct. In such cases, there is no common hepatic duct.

The common hepatic duct varies in length from 2 to 6.5 cm. Its course is inferior and slightly to the right.

As soon as the hepatic ducts leave the porta hepatis, they lie between 2 serous layers of the hepatoduodenal ligament, as does also the common hepatic duct. When the 2 hepatic ducts exit from the porta hepatis, they are separated from the adjacent right and left hepatic arteries and the portal vein and its branches by a well-marked areolar tissue sheath (Fig 32–5). This sheath normally encloses all structures in the upper portion of the hepatoduodenal ligament down to the junction of the cystic duct with the common hepatic duct. The condensation of fibrous areolar tissue around the upper biliary ductal system begins intrahepatically. When the right and left hepatic ducts leave the liver, the fibrous sheath accompanies them. As a result, the 2 hepatic ducts and their junction are partially obscured by the fibrous tissue sheath. This strong sheath of fibrous tissue binds the hepatic ducts to the adjacent vascular structures.

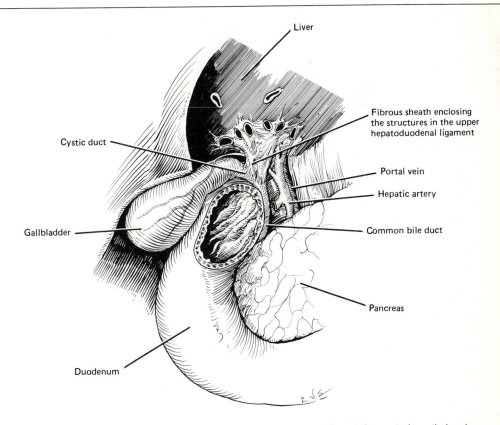

Figure 32–5. Fibrous sheath binding the biliary structures together at the porta hepatis level.

➡️ *Importance of fibrous tissue sheath about upper end of hepatoduodenal ligament.* *Because of the presence of the strong sheath of fibrous tissue that binds the structures in the superior segment of the hepatoduodenal ligament to the hilum of the liver, previous dissection, trauma, or infection usually does not affect ductal and vascular relationships.*

The relationship of the right hepatic duct and the common hepatic duct to the right hepatic artery is extremely variable. Usually the artery crosses from left to right, dorsal to the right hepatic duct and just superior to the junction of the right and left hepatic ducts forming the common hepatic duct. However, the artery frequently passes ventral to the right hepatic duct. The right hepatic artery frequently crosses the common hepatic duct either ventrally or dorsally just above the transverse course of the cystic artery. In such cases, it is difficult to distinguish it from the cystic artery. Finally, the right hepatic artery may not cross the right hepatic duct until just before the duct disappears into the porta hepatis.

➡️ *Right hepatic artery trauma in biliary tract surgery.* *It is usually the right hepatic artery that is in the danger area in biliary tract surgery. A diligent search must be made for it and its usual arterial branching before the cystic artery is ligated.*

In almost 80% of people, the left hepatic artery lies ventral to the main trunk of the portal vein. In the remainder, it lies slightly to the left of the portal vein. In almost 90% of people, the left hepatic artery lies to the left of the common hepatic duct and the common bile duct, but when there is a particularly low union of the left and right hepatic ducts, it can run superiorly between the 2 ducts.

The common hepatic duct is crossed by the right hepatic or the cystic artery in about 30% of cases. In about 90% of cases, the right hepatic duct is related closely to the right hepatic artery.

The hepatic ducts receive their nerve supply from the anterior and posterior divisions of the hepatic plexus.

➡️ *Presence of gallstones in the hepatic ducts.* *Gallstones often lodge in the hepatic ducts. Whenever the common bile duct is opened and explored, exploration of the hepatic ducts should be carried out manually, by endoscope, and by an operative cholangiogram so that stones in these ducts will not be missed.*

➡️ *Noninvasive techniques for locating stones in the hepatic ducts.* *Diagnostic ultrasound and* CT scan of the upper abdomen are good noninvasive techniques for evaluating the gallbladder and the intra- and extrahepatic ducts for enlargements, distortions, or biliary stones.

The hepatic ducts and the common bile duct are lined by a mucous membrane of columnar epithelium. The lamina propria of the cells is thin and surrounded by a thin layer of smooth muscle. As the common bile duct nears the duodenum, its muscular layer becomes thicker, and it is thickest in the pancreatic and intramural portions of the duct. There is a fibrous coat external to the thin muscular layer of the ducts. The internal mucous coat of the common bile duct contains numerous mucous glands that are markedly lobulated and open through minute orifices.

3. THE CYSTIC DUCT
(Fig 32–6)

The cystic duct normally connects the neck of the gallbladder to the common hepatic duct to form the common bile duct, though occasionally it connects with the right hepatic duct. The cystic duct is about 5 cm long (range, 0.5–8 cm). The caliber of the duct varies from 3 to 12 mm. Ducts of large caliber can pass gallbladder stones into the common bile duct with relative ease. In the rare instances of congenital absence of the cystic duct, the gallbladder is interposed between the hepatic and common bile ducts.

With the hepatoduodenal ligament placed on stretch, the cystic duct usually runs dorsally, to the left, and inferiorly to join with the common hepatic duct. On occasion, its course may be quite tortuous. The junction of the cystic duct with the main biliary stream can vary. The cystic duct may (1) join the common hepatic duct at a right angle; (2) parallel the common hepatic duct before joining its right lateral side; (3) run dorsal to the common hepatic duct and enter its dorsal surface; (4) run dorsal to the common hepatic duct and join it from its left lateral surface; (5) enter the right hepatic duct; (6) join the common hepatic duct after passing behind the first portion of the duodenum; and (7) (rarely) join the common hepatic duct just before it pierces the duodenal wall.

There are 3 modes of entrance of the cystic duct into the common hepatic duct: angular, parallel, and spiral. The angular position is the most common, occurring in over 70% of people. The angle of junction varies from 90 to 10 degrees. In the parallel type of junction, the 2 ducts run alongside for 1.5–6 cm and adhere closely to each other. In the spiral type of junction, the cystic duct may pass ventrally or dorsally to the common hepatic duct before joining it. On occasion, the spiraling duct empties into the common hepatic duct.

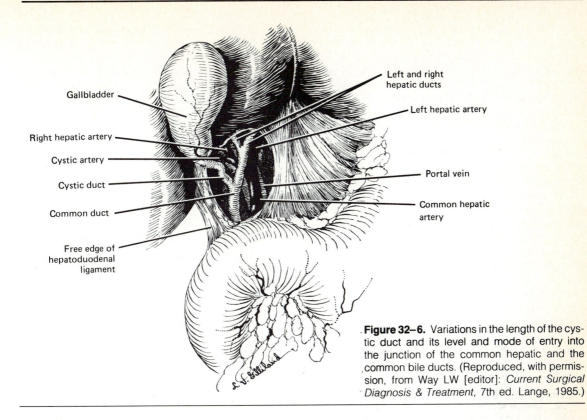

Gallbladder

Right hepatic artery

Cystic artery

Cystic duct

Common duct

Free edge of
hepatoduodenal
ligament

Left and right
hepatic ducts

Left hepatic artery

Portal vein

Common hepatic
artery

Figure 32–6. Variations in the length of the cystic duct and its level and mode of entry into the junction of the common hepatic and the common bile ducts. (Reproduced, with permission, from Way LW [editor]: *Current Surgical Diagnosis & Treatment,* 7th ed. Lange, 1985.)

⮕ ***Importance of recognition of angle of entrance of cystic duct.*** *Variations in the anatomy of the formation of the common bile duct by the joining of the cystic duct and hepatic ducts call for meticulous dissection of the biliary tree to prevent injury to the common bile duct when the cystic duct is ligated. Care must be taken not to leave a long stump of cystic duct attached to the common bile duct, since the stump may later become inflamed or serve as a nidus for formation of "postcholecystectomy stones." However, no effort should be made to remove the stump if it is tightly adherent.*

The mucous membrane that lines the interior of the cystic duct and the neck of the gallbladder shows crescentic folds. The folds persist in spiral fashion the entire length of the cystic duct and are known as the plicae spirales. With distention of the cystic duct, the intervals between valves widen and cause the lumen of the duct to appear twisted upon itself. The spiral valves of the gallbladder neck and the cystic duct tend to impede the passage of a gallstone through the cystic duct into the common bile duct.

⮕ ***Use of stump of cystic duct for cholangiographic studies.*** *The stump of the cystic duct is normally used for the introduction of opaque media for visualization of the biliary tree.*

The distal end of the cystic duct usually lies within the right free border of the hepatoduodenal ligament. Running from the undersurface of the cystic duct is the cholecystoduodenal ligament—the landmark in the operative search for the cystic duct and the cystic artery.

If the cystic artery is given off from the right hepatic artery in a relatively low angular position, close to the cystic duct, the artery usually runs transversely just superior to the cystic duct; but it may lie dorsal to the duct or run inferior to the cystic duct. If the cystic artery is given off from the right hepatic artery in a high position, just below the porta hepatis, the cystic artery usually passes down to the neck or body of the gallbladder, lacking a relationship with the cystic duct.

The right hepatic artery usually lies to the left of the cystic duct, but in 7–10% of cases it passes behind the cystic duct, and rarely it passes ventral to the cystic duct. The portal vein lies just dorsal and to the left of the cystic duct. The cystic duct and the cystic artery usually lie superior to the epiploic foramen, the entrance into the lesser peritoneal sac. Bleeding from the right hepatic or cystic artery can be stopped by inserting one or 2 fingers into the epiploic foramen and exerting pressure ventrally against the hepatoduodenal ligament.

The Common Bile Duct

Short descriptions of the hepatoduodenal ligament, the ascending branch of the common hepatic artery, the portal vein, and the epiploic foramen (of Winslow) are necessary to set the stage for an anatomic description of the common bile duct. This is because the intimate relationship of the long supraduodenal portion of the common bile duct with these structures must always be considered during operations on the duct.

The **hepatoduodenal ligament** is the right free border of the hepatogastric ligament, or lesser omentum. The hepatogastric ligament consists of 2 layers of peritoneum that run from the porta hepatis to the lesser curvature of the stomach, where they form the ventral and dorsal serosal coats of the stomach. Dorsal to the hepatogastric ligament lies the lesser peritoneal sac. The hepatoduodenal ligament therefore forms the right ventral border of the lesser peritoneal sac. Between the 2 leaves of the hepatoduodenal ligament lie the common bile duct, the common hepatic duct, the right and left hepatic ducts, the ascending hepatic artery and its extrahepatic branches, and the portal vein and its terminal branches, lymphatics, and nerves. The inferior vena cava lies dorsal to the hepatoduodenal ligament and is separated from it by entrance into the lesser peritoneal sac and by the peritoneum of the posterior abdominal wall.

The **common hepatic artery** normally arises from the celiac artery dorsal to the posterior peritoneal wall of the lesser sac and proceeds toward the right upper border of the head of the pancreas. It then turns ventrally and superiorly near the first part of the duodenum and enters the hepatoduodenal ligament close to the foramen of Winslow. There, the artery gives off its right gastric branch, which runs on the right segment of the lesser curvature of the stomach; and its gastroduodenal branch, which runs inferiorly, dorsal to and closely attached to the first portion of the duodenum. The course of the ascending hepatic artery in the hepatoduodenal ligament is variable. Normally, the artery runs to the left of the common bile duct and the common hepatic duct.

⇒ *Relationship of the hepatic artery to the foramen of Winslow. Just after it enters the hepatoduodenal ligament, the common hepatic artery runs ventral to the foramen of Winslow. This relationship allows a surgeon's fingers, placed in the foramen, to palpate the arterial flow and to occlude the vessel at this level.*

The common hepatic artery lies ventral to the portal vein and the inferior vena cava. An aberrant common hepatic artery on occasion arises from the superior mesenteric artery, directly from the abdominal aorta, and, rarely, from a common celiac and superior mesenteric artery.

The **portal vein** is formed dorsal to the neck of the pancreas by the junction of the splenic vein with the superior mesenteric vein at a right angle. The portal vein rises above the superior border of the

neck of the pancreas and turns ventrally to enter the hepatoduodenal ligament. There it receives blood from the coronary vein, the superior pancreaticoduodenal vein, the pyloric vein, and, on occasion, the cystic vein. The portal vein lies dorsal to the common bile duct and the ascending hepatic artery.

⇒ *Recognition of the portal vein. The portal vein should seldom be confused with the common bile duct. A small-gauge needle placed in the vein will clarify the identification.*

The **epiploic foramen** is the connection between the greater and lesser peritoneal cavities. It lies just superior to the first portion of the duodenum and is bounded ventrally, by the hepatoduodenal ligament; dorsally, by the peritoneum of the posterior abdominal wall, which covers the inferior vena cava; superiorly, by the coronary ligament of the liver; and inferiorly, by the first portion of the duodenum.

The common bile duct is formed by the junction of the common hepatic duct with the cystic duct. The length of the duct varies between 5 and 17 cm. It varies in caliber from 0.4 to 1.5 cm (range usually 9–11 mm).

With the exception of atresia and stenosis of the duct or a choledochal cyst, anomalies of the common bile duct are rare. The site of the opening of the common bile duct into the duodenum in 13–16% of cases is not at its usual termination in the midposterior descending duodenum. Doubling of the lower third of the common duct can occur. Rarely, the common bile duct is doubled along its entire length, one of the ducts draining the right lobe of the liver and the other draining the left. In most cases of double common bile duct, the 2 ducts open separately into the duodenum. The common bile duct has an outer fibrous coat of fibroareolar tissue that contains scant amounts of smooth muscle fibers, usually arranged in circular fashion about the duct. The mucosal layer of the duct is continuous with the lining of the gallbladder and the other extrahepatic ducts. It is also continuous with the mucous membrane lining the duodenum. The epithelium is of the columnar type and contains mucous glands which are lobulated and open into the ductal lumen by minute orifices.

4. DIVISIONS OF THE COMMON BILE DUCT

For purposes of gross description, the common bile duct is divided into 4 segments: supraduodenal, retroduodenal, pancreatic, and intraduodenal.

Supraduodenal Segment

The supraduodenal (first) segment of the common bile duct is usually the longest, averaging 2.5–5 cm. This segment is usually inspected for biliary tract disease and opened for exploration or drainage of the tract. It lies within the inferior half of the right free border of the hepatoduodenal ligament, between its 2 serosal surfaces. The ascending hepatic artery lies on the same plane as the duct and slightly to the left of it. The portal vein lies dorsal to the duct, separated by loose areolar tissue. Just above the first portion of the duodenum, the common bile duct lies ventral to the epiploic foramen, separated by areolar tissue, the portal vein, and the posterior peritoneal layer of the hepatoduodenal ligament.

⟹ *Importance of relationships of the common duct to the epiploic foramen. This allows the index finger of the left hand to be inserted into the foramen and the supraduodenal portion of the duct then to be palpated between the left forefinger and the thumb. The maneuver also allows a stone to be milked superiorly from the lower segment of the supraduodenal portion of the duct.*

Many lymph nodes are related to the superior portion of the common bile duct, and when enlarged they may be mistaken for gallstones or may compress the underlying common duct. The full length of the supraduodenal portion of the common bile duct becomes evident only when caudal pressure is exerted against the first portion of the duodenum, the pylorus, and the head of the pancreas.

⟹ *Fistulization between the common bile duct and the duodenum. In ulcerative disease of the duodenum or the pyloric end of the stomach and in acute cholecystitis, the gallbladder may closely adhere to these structures. A fistulous tract is occasionally formed, allowing the passage of gallstones into the upper gastrointestinal tract. Such a tract may also form between the infundibulum of the gallbladder and the common bile duct in cases where the infundibulum overhangs and adheres to the common bile duct.*

⟹ *Anastomoses of the supraduodenal segment of the common bile duct. Use of the lower portion of the supraduodenal segment of the common duct for anastomosis either to the adjacent duodenum or the proximal jejunum has become popular as a bypass procedure for either malignant, calculous, or inflammatory obstructions of the common duct. The anastomosis may be by the end-to-side, side-to-side, or Roux-en-Y method.*

Retroduodenal Segment

The retroduodenal (second) segment of the common bile duct is 2.5–4.5 cm long and lies dorsal to the first portion of the duodenum, slanting obliquely from right to left. Just to the left of the retroduodenal portion of the duct lies the descending gastroduodenal branch of the hepatic artery. The artery slants gradually to the right, placing the common bile duct closer to the artery at the lower margin of the duodenum than at the upper margin.

⟹ *Involvement of the retroduodenal segment of the common bile duct in duodenal disease. The common bile duct is frequently involved in edema and inflammation secondary to a posterior duodenal ulcer. Furthermore, in transecting the proximal part of the first portion of the duodenum during a Billroth I or II procedure for duodenal ulceration, care must be taken not to sever the common bile duct and not to involve it in suture closure of the duodenum or in the edema that always follows operation. If there is difficulty in locating the retroduodenal portion of the common bile duct, a catheter or sound should be passed down the duct from an opening in its supraduodenal portion; the retroduodenal portion of the duct will then become palpable and much easier to avoid during the procedure.*

The superior 1–1.5 cm of the retroduodenal segment of the common duct is loosely attached, by areolar tissue, to the posterior surface of the duodenum.

⟹ *Use of the Kocher procedure to visualize the distal common bile duct. (Fig 32–7.) The superior 1.5 cm of the retroduodenal segment of the common bile duct may be exposed by incising the ventral layer of the hepatoduodenal ligament, just above the upper border of the duodenum, and then pulling the duodenum inferiorly. To expose the entire retroduodenal segment of the common bile duct, one must mobilize the upper half of the descending duodenum, making use of the Kocher procedure. The avascular peritoneum on the left margin of the upper descending duodenum is incised and the duodenum bluntly dissected from the underlying tissues and rolled to the left.*

The retroduodenal segment of the common bile duct is closely associated with the middle colic artery. The artery is given off the superior mesenteric artery, just below the pylorus and the first portion of the duodenum. The artery often lies in a fold of the transverse mesocolon. During any mobilization of the retroduodenal segment of the common bile duct, the fold containing the middle colic artery must be searched for, mobilized, and allowed to drop away

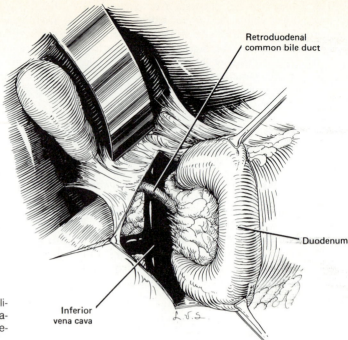

Figure 32–7. The Kocher maneuver for mobilization of descending duodenum and visualization of lateral pancreatic head and retroduodenal portion of common bile duct.

from the pylorus. As the retroduodenal segment of the common bile duct passes posterior to the superior surface of the duodenum, it may be crossed by the variable supraduodenal artery ventral to the duct. Farther inferiorly, the common bile duct is crossed ventrally by the posterosuperior pancreaticoduodenal artery. This relatively large vessel must always be dealt with in mobilizations of the retroduodenal segment of the common bile duct.

Pancreatic Segment

The pancreatic (third) segment of the common bile duct is 2–3 cm long, but when the duct empties distal to its normal point of entrance into the duodenum, it can be up to 6 cm long. The pancreatic segment of the duct may be entirely retropancreatic, or it may lie within the substance of the pancreatic head. The pancreatic segment of the common bile duct at first descends close to the left border of the descending duodenum. To the left side of the duct lies the vertebral column. About halfway along its pancreatic course, the third segment of the common bile duct curves rather sharply to the right to enter the posteromedial surface of the descending duodenum. The inferior vena cava lies just dorsal to the pancreatic segment of the duct. As the portal vein runs obliquely, it is unrelated to this segment of the duct. Related to the upper half of the third segment of the common bile duct is the gastroduodenal artery, which lies just to the left of it. The superior pancreaticoduodenal branch of the gastroduodenal artery crosses the third segment of the common bile duct either ventrally or dorsally. The many duodenal and pancreatic branches make

exposure of the third ductal segment hazardous. The large pancreaticoduodenal vein on the posterior surface of the pancreatic head is related to the pancreatic segment of the duct just before the vein joins the portal vein. The vein is easily torn during surgery on the duct or on the duodenum and pancreatic head.

Intraduodenal Segment
(Fig 32–8)

The intraduodenal (terminal) segment of the common bile duct lies dorsal to the major pancreatic duct where the common bile duct passes through the duodenal wall in an oblique fashion. Its course through the duodenal wall is almost 2 cm long. It passes first through the smooth muscle layers and then lies in the submucosa. The site of perforation of the duodenum by the common bile duct is the posteromedial wall just above the crossing by the transverse mesocolon. This site is generally about 7 cm distal to the pylorus of the stomach.

The major pancreatic duct also empties into the duodenum via the major duodenal papilla. The terminal segment of the common bile duct is related to the terminal segment of the major pancreatic duct in one of 3 ways: (1) There frequently is an extraduodenal junction of the 2 ducts just external to the duodenal wall. In such instances, the 2 ducts run parallel for 2–10 mm, or the lumens of the 2 ducts may join. (2) During passage of the bile duct and pancreatic duct through the duodenal wall, the internal septum between their lumens is lost, and together they form a true common duct that opens through a single ostium on the major duodenal papilla. (3) In

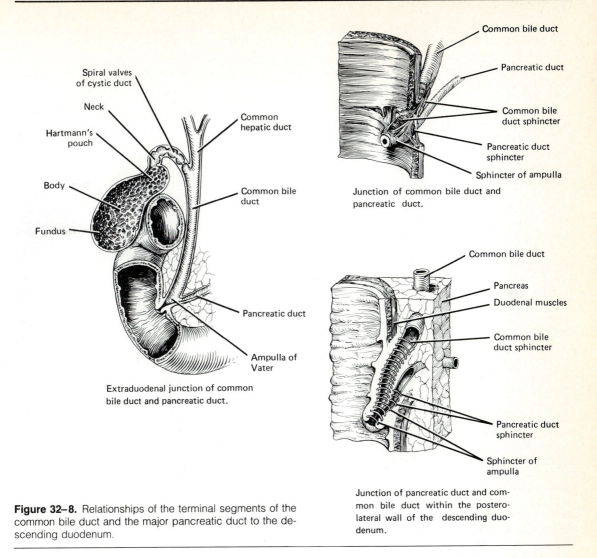

Figure 32–8. Relationships of the terminal segments of the common bile duct and the major pancreatic duct to the descending duodenum.

about 20% of cases, the septum between the lumens of the 2 ducts persists during the passage of the ducts through the duodenal wall, and the 2 ducts empty on the duodenal papilla by separate ostia.

As the common bile duct proceeds through the duodenal wall, it narrows markedly, from an extra-duodenal 10 mm to an average diameter of 6 mm. The narrowing is so pronounced that it forms a ridge between the wide extraduodenal segment of the duct and the narrow intraduodenal segment. This fact is of great importance in common duct exploration, because unless care is taken in the probing of this junctional area, a false passage may easily be formed.

The **ampulla of Vater** is formed when there is a junction of the lumens of the common bile duct and the major pancreatic duct. The length of the ampulla of Vater will vary. It can be as long as 14 mm and as short as 3 mm. If there is no ductal junction, there is no true ampulla of Vater. The ampulla reaches from the confluence of the 2 ducts to just proximal to their exit through a single opening on the duodenal

papilla. In over 50% of cases, the common bile duct narrows just before it empties into the ampulla, and in all cases its exit from the ampulla narrows just before the duodenal papilla. The 2 intraduodenal ductal areas of narrowing of the common bile duct become favorite places for stone impaction in calculous disease of the biliary tract. Blockage of the ampulla of Vater by a stone has been looked upon as the most frequent cause of pancreatitis (common channel theory), the blockage allowing for reflux of bile into the pancreatic duct. Although 60% of cases of acute pancreatitis are due to the passage of bile into the pancreatic duct, only 10% are due to blocking of the ampulla by a gallstone. The other 90% of cases of pancreatitis, caused by biliary reflux, may result from spasm of the sphincter of Oddi or are due to edema of the biliary papilla.

▅⇒ *Impaction of stone within the ampulla of Vater. The ampulla of Vater is a common site of impacted of biliary calculi. The smooth muscle fibers of the lower biliary tract sphincter apparatus frequently show an imbalance (dyssynergia) in many liver, gallbladder, and common duct diseases.*

Muscular Apparatus at Terminal End of Common Bile Duct (Sphincter of Oddi) (Fig 32–8)

The intraduodenal segment of the common bile duct, including the terminal area of the ampulla of Vater, is surrounded by a sheath of smooth muscle fibers. This entire sphincteric system is referred to as the sphincter of Oddi. The smooth musculature of the sphincter is both circular and longitudinal in character. The term ''sphincter'' of Oddi is thus an extremely loose one and should perhaps not be used.

The sphincter develops much later in fetal life than the duodenal muscle. The biliary tract sphincter operates separately from the action of the duodenal musculature, and spasms of the biliary duct sphincter result in pain quite similar to that of biliary colic.

The arrangement of smooth muscles surrounding the intraduodenal segments of the common bile duct is extremely complex. The biliary and pancreatic ducts enter the duodenum through an elliptical slit in the circular muscle of the bowel. At their points of entrance, some smooth muscle fibers reach to the angles of the duodenal opening to prevent its extension by splitting; other fibers connect the margins of the opening in the longitudinal and circular muscles of the duodenum with the major duodenal papilla. These connecting fibers erect the papillae and anchor the ducts to the apertures in the duodenal musculature. The common bile duct is wrapped in a sheath of circular muscle, the sphincter choledochus (of Boyden). This sphincter is responsible for filling of the gallbladder during periods of fasting between meals. When the common bile duct and the major pancreatic duct lie side by side within the duodenal wall, the choledochal sphincter usually interlaces with an inconstant sphincter pancreaticus in a figure-8 pattern.

Disturbances of physiologic function of the sphincter choledochus, with resultant hyper- or hypotonicity of the duct, are thought to be responsible for (1) pancreatic reflux of bile, (2) the presence of pancreatic juice in bile, and (3) reflux of duodenal contents into the biliary tract.

⇒ *Exploration of the common bile duct. The surgeon must be prepared to explore the common bile duct and hepatic duct as part of any operation on the biliary tract. The indications for common duct exploration are (1) a recent history of jaundice; (2) the presence of many small stones in the gallbladder, with obvious disproportion between the stones and the cystic duct (small stones, wide cystic duct); (3) a dilated*

or thickened common duct; (4) a thickening of the head of the pancreas or the presence of a palpable mass of the pancreatic head; (5) the presence of dark bile or biliary sludge in the common duct aspirate; (6) palpable or visible evidence of stone in the common duct; and (7) evidence of a possible stone or stones in the common duct at the time of operative cholangiograms.

The supraduodenal segment of the common duct is usually opened just below the entrance into it of the cystic duct. The common duct is opened for about 1 cm in a longitudinal direction. A soft rubber catheter is passed both superiorly and inferiorly within the lumen of the common duct to check its patency. It is usually easier to palpate a stone against a catheter within the ductal lumen than simply against the duct wall. If obstruction or stones are present, the duct is first irrigated with normal saline solution. Bougies, dilators, and stone forceps may be used to clear the duct. A transduodenal approach to the duodenal papilla may be an adjunctive procedure in difficult cases.

All common bile duct procedures should be preceded by an operative cholangiogram, preferably through the stump of the cystic duct, and followed by final operative cholangiograms with the T-drainage tube in place. Most surgeons feel that any common bile duct that is opened should be drained. A T-tube that passes up into the common hepatic duct and down the common bile duct for a short distance is used for drainage. The drainage tube is usually brought out to the skin surface through a stab wound in the right flank. Before the T-tube is withdrawn from the common duct (usually 7–10 days after surgery), a final postoperative cholangiogram should be taken through it. Retained common duct stones may be removed 6–8 weeks after surgery by the nonoperative instrumental method of Burhenne.

BLOOD VESSELS, LYMPHATICS, & NERVES

Arteries (Fig 32–6)

The great variation in distribution of the arterial supply to the common bile duct and the inconstant anastomotic patterns probably account for a high percentage of the postoperative ischemic sequelae that occur when long segments of the duct are stripped in order to mobilize it.

Generally, the arterial twigs supplying the common bile duct are small and inconstant and easily disrupted.

The major arterial branches to the duct usually arise from either the **cystic artery** or the **posterosuperior pancreaticoduodenal artery.** The supraduodenal segment of the duct is usually nourished by small branches from the cystic artery. These vessels also supply the common hepatic duct and the lower part of the right hepatic duct. Sometimes the cystic artery or the **right hepatic artery** will send off one or 2 descending branches to the common bile duct.

The retroduodenal (second) segment of the common bile duct is usually supplied by 4–6 branches from the posterosuperior pancreaticoduodenal artery as this vessel loops around this segment of the duct. On occasion, one of the branches will become an accessory cystic artery. The supraduodenal branch of the gastroduodenal artery will occasionally send a twig to the retroduodenal portion of the duct. This branch is usually ablated by the surgeon when the first part of the duodenum is mobilized. The third and fourth segments of the common duct are supplied by the anterior and posterosuperior pancreaticoduodenal arteries, and these segments of the duct have a better anastomotic arterial pattern than the 2 superior ductal segments.

Veins
(Fig 32–6)

The superior portion of the common bile duct sends its venous drainage along the surfaces of the common duct and the hepatic and cystic ducts. The drainage enters the liver directly rather than by joining branches of the portal vein. The venous drainage from the inferior half of the common bile duct is into small venous radicles that enter the portal vein. The supraduodenal segment of the common bile duct is divided by the presence of a most constant ascending vein. This vessel can become a nuisance during common duct surgery if it is not ligated above and below the site of opening of the common duct.

Lymphatics

Lymphatic drainage from the common bile duct is first into nodes along the entire course of the duct and finally into a group of 6–10 nodes closely related to the structures at the porta hepatis. The nodes that lie along the common duct are on occasion mistaken for stones within the duct. The nodes that lie about the porta hepatis, when enlarged as a result of infection or tumor invasion, often compress the biliary ducts, thereby causing obstructive jaundice. Some lymphatic drainage from the common bile duct reaches the deep

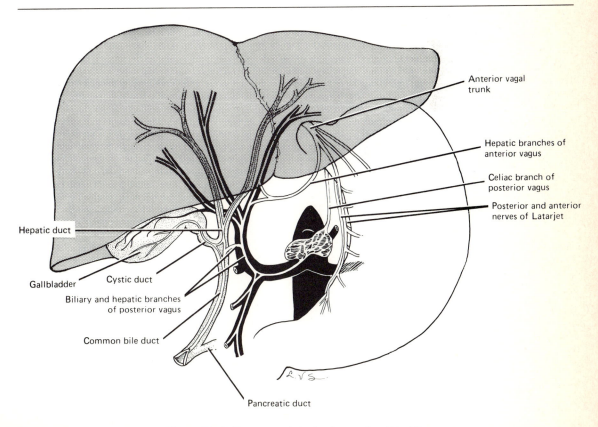

Figure 32–9. Nerve supply to the liver and gallbladder.

Anomalies
(Fig 33–1)

Anomalous development of these structures leads to heterotopic pancreatic tissue (usually found in gastric or duodenal mucosa or in Meckel's diverticulum); divided pancreas, from failure of fusion of the 2 buds; and annular pancreas, which probably occurs when the ventral pancreatic bud extends around the ventral and dorsal aspects of the duodenum before fusing with the dorsal pancreatic bud.

GROSS ANATOMY
(Figs 33–2 and 33–3)

The pancreas is a solid viscus that lies transversely across the posterior abdominal wall at the level of

L1 and L2. It measures close to 15 cm in transverse diameter. It lies deep within the epigastrium in a retroperitoneal position. The pancreas is quite firmly fixed in position, with only slight superior and inferior range of movement. Because the mid portion of the body of the pancreas overlies the abdominal aorta, aortic pulsations may be transmitted to the gland.

➡ *Position of pancreas in abdomen. The deep (retroperitoneal) position of the pancreas protects it from blunt trauma. The flare of the costal arch and the thick skeletal and muscular structure of the posterior abdominal wall also shield against trauma. Even so, the pancreas may be injured in the following manner: (1) By penetrating wounds through the abdominal walls. (2) By combined abdominothoracic wounds, nearly always left-sided. (Such wounds frequently injure the spleen and splenic flexure of the colon as well as the pancreas.) (3) By*

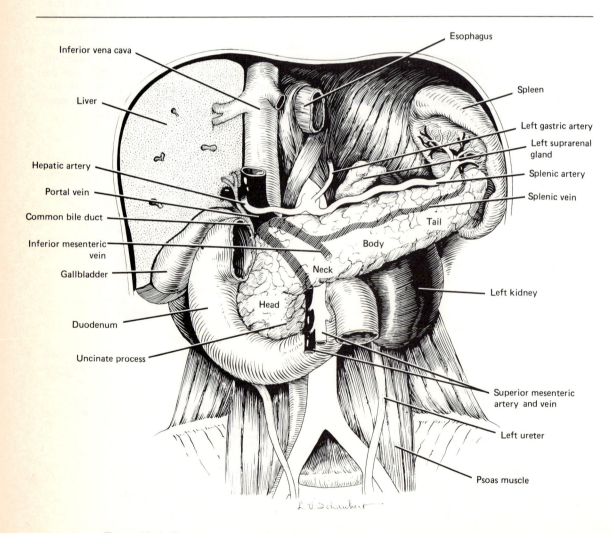

Figure 33–2. The pancreas, showing relations of the major vessels and venous drainage.

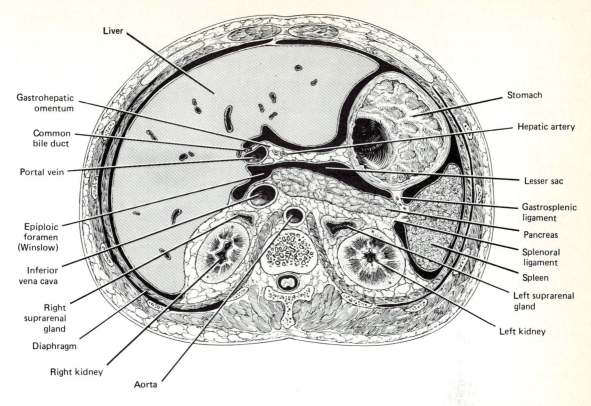

Figure 33–3. Cross section of the abdomen at approximately T12, showing the relationship of the pancreas to the stomach lesser sac, and retroperitoneal structures.

nonpenetrating trauma to the upper anterior abdominal wall. (*These are often minor, and the pancreatic injury is frequently overlooked.*) *(4) By nonpenetrating wounds of the posterior abdominal wall. (These may involve the transverse duodenum and the upper abdominal aorta as well as the pancreas and are usually secondary to forcible flexion of these 3 structures over the bony spinal column.)*

Pancreatic pseudocyst. *Injury to the pancreas usually results in liberation of pancreatic enzymes, and hemorrhage may occur within the pancreatic tissue. Blood and enzymes may be confined by the pancreatic capsule or, if the capsule is torn, may be released into the peritoneal cavity. If confined by the capsule, pancreatic pseudocyst may result. The cysts may attain great size and most frequently present to the left of the abdominal midline, pushing ventrally either the gastrohepatic omentum, the stomach, the gastrocolic ligament, or the transverse mesocolon. They may be approached through any of the 3 mesenteric structures and treated by (1) external drainage; (2) marsupialization; or (3) anastomosis of the cyst, either directly to the ventrally related stomach or to*

adjacent small bowel via a side-to-side or Roux-en-Y procedure.

Diagnosis of pancreatic disease. *The deep location of the pancreas makes its disorders difficult to diagnose and surgical procedures technically difficult to perform. Increased blood and urine amylase and lipase concentrations are of great diagnostic value. Endoscopic retrograde cholecystopancreatography (ERCP) may outline the hepatic and pancreatic ducts and reveal the diagnosis.*

Pancreatic tumors. *Occasionally, a large pancreatic tumor in the left upper abdomen can be seen or felt to move on deep inspiration.*

Relationship of the pancreas to the lesser sac and retroperitoneum. *The surgical anatomy of the pancreas is closely allied to that of the lesser omental sac and the retroperitoneal tissues dorsal to the pancreas. Consequently, pancreatic disease frequently spreads to these 2 spatially related areas.*

DIVISIONS OF THE PANCREAS

The pancreas is composed of a head and uncinate process, a neck, a body, and a tail.

Head & Uncinate Process of the Pancreas

The head of the pancreas, the largest segment of the gland, fits into the concavity of the C curve formed by the first, second, and third portions of the duodenum. A small segment of the pancreatic head is overlapped by the first portion of the duodenum, a frequent site of posterior penetrating duodenal ulcer, which can erode into this pancreatic tissue. The caudal portion of the pancreatic head may overlap the third segment of the duodenum. The inferior surface of the pancreatic head is cleaved by the superior mesenteric artery and vein near where the 2 vessels cross the transverse duodenum. Just dorsal to the vessels lies a small flap of the pancreatic head—the uncinate process. The head of the pancreas is divided into supra- and inframesocolic segments by the attachment of the root of the transverse mesocolon to its ventral surface.

Relationships of the Head of the Pancreas

Ventrally, the head of the pancreas is related to the transverse colon and mesocolon, the gastrocolic ligament, and the greater omentum. Ventrally and medially, it is related to the posterior parietal peritoneum, which forms the dorsal wall of the lesser sac.

Dorsally, the pancreatic head is related to the following structures: (1) the superior mesenteric vein is dorsal to the pancreatic head but ventral to its uncinate process; (2) the superior mesenteric artery runs dorsal to the pancreatic head but ventral to the uncinate process; (3) the portal vein, related only to the superior portion of the dorsum of the head; (4) the third (pancreatic) portion of the common bile duct, which may lie dorsal to the head or enclosed within its tissues; (5) the right edge of the abdominal aorta; (6) the inferior vena cava; (7) the right crus of the diaphragm; (8) vertebrae L1 and L2; (9) the right and left renal veins; (10) the right renal artery; and (11) the ascending gastroduodenal vein.

Laterally, the head of the pancreas is related to the descending duodenum, the dorsal and ventral superior pancreaticoduodenal arteries, and the ascending branch of the inferior pancreaticoduodenal artery.

Superiorly, the head of the pancreas is related to the first portion of the duodenum and to the undersurface of the pylorus. It is related to the retroduodenal portion of the common bile duct and to the gastroduodenal, the right gastroepiploic, and the superior pancreaticoduodenal arteries.

Inferiorly, the head of the pancreas is related to the third portion of the duodenum and to the right branch of the inferior pancreaticoduodenal artery, which runs in the groove between the pancreas and the transverse duodenum.

Medially, the head of the pancreas blends into the pancreatic neck.

Neck & Body of the Pancreas

The neck of the pancreas extends medially from the pancreatic head as a thick bit of tissue 2.5 cm long. It connects the head to the body of the organ. The neck is related superiorly to the inferior surface of the pylorus and to the gastroduodenal artery. Dorsally, the neck is related to the junction of the splenic and superior mesenteric veins to form the portal vein. Its other relationships are similar to those of the left side of the head of the pancreas.

The body of the pancreas lies in a transverse plane as it crosses the abdomen at the level of L1–2. The left half of the body lies about one vertebra higher than the right. On cross section, the body of the pancreas is roughly triangular in shape. The base of the transverse mesocolon is attached to the apex of the anterior surface of the gland, dividing it into a larger superior surface lying in the supramesocolic and a smaller inferior surface related to the inframesocolic compartment. As a consequence, diseases affecting the 2 portions of the anterior surface of the pancreas will have differing manifestations, and the surgical approaches to reach or drain these surfaces will vary. The anterosuperior pancreatic surface is directly related to the lesser peritoneal sac, while the anteroinferior surface is related to the greater peritoneal cavity.

➤ *Cancer of the pancreas. Carcinoma may involve any portion of the pancreas, the pancreatic head and body being the commonest sites. It may be treated by partial or total pancreatectomy, but the cure rate is low, and cholecysto- or choledochoenterostomy is frequently the palliative procedure of choice if the common bile duct is blocked by the disease. If the disease is in the pancreatic head, it will eventually block the common bile duct, leading to jaundice, and—if the tumor is a large one—will serve to widen the duodenal loop.*

B cell (beta cell) adenomas of the pancreas, with their insulin-producing effect, are occasional pancreatic tumors. They are capable of producing a profound hypoglycemia.

Non-B cell adenomas of the pancreas, with their ability to initiate and sustain peptic ulceration of the Zollinger-Ellison type, may occur singly or may multiply in the pancreas, often in association with pituitary, parathyroid, and duodenal wall adenomas.

Relationships of the Body of the Pancreas

The body of the pancreas has the following posterior relationships from right to left: (1) the great vessels of the dorsal abdomen make a dorsal approach to the pancreas hazardous; (2) vertebrae L1 and L2;

(3) the left crus of the diaphragm; (4) the left psoas muscle; (5) the upper segment of the left lumbar sympathetic chain with ganglion L1; (6) the left kidney and suprarenal gland; and (7) retroperitoneal areolar tissue, the site of neighborhood cellulitis secondary to pancreatic infection.

⇢ ***Surgical approaches to the pancreas.*** *(Fig 33–4.) The pancreas may be approached surgically via either the retroperitoneal or lumbar route.*

The organ may be approached transperitoneally in the following ways: (1) By incising the gastrohepatic omentum. This gives poor exposure of the pancreatic body and tail and leaves little room for manipulation; furthermore, it is hard to secure drainage, since the liver and stomach interfere. It is occasionally used for lesions along the upper border of the pancreas. (2) Through the left half of the gastrocolic ligament. This gives the best exposure of the dorsal surface of the stomach and of the entire body and tail of the pancreas, spleen, and splenic vessels. There is good dependent drainage. (3) Through a relatively avascular area in the transverse mesocolon. This gives the best exposure of the mid portion of the body of the pancreas and provides good dependent drainage of the lesser peritoneal sac.

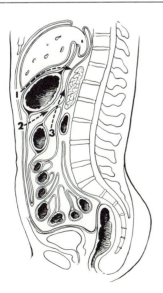

Figure 33–4. Surgical approaches to the lesser sac and pancreas via (1) the gastrohepatic omentum, (2) the gastrocolic ligament, and (3) the left side of the transverse mesocolon.

The retroperitoneal approach (seldom used) is technically difficult owing to the thickness of the posterior abdominal wall and the presence of major blood vessels.

The splenic artery grooves the posterior surface of the body of the pancreas on its tortuous course to the spleen. The splenic vein runs transversely just inferior to the splenic artery. This large vein is frequently diseased in hepatic, pancreatic, and splenic syndromes.

Ventrally, the superior two-thirds of the body of the pancreas is intimately related to the peritoneum of the dorsal surface of the lesser sac and the dorsal surfaces of the stomach and to the gastrocolic ligament containing the epiploic vessels. The transverse mesocolon attaches to the ventral surface of the pancreas as it runs across the abdomen. The inferior third of the ventral surface is related to the greater peritoneal cavity.

⇢ ***X-ray in diagnosis of pancreatic lesions.*** *If a pancreatic or lesser sac mass is suspected, a lateral view of the stomach filled with barium can reveal the mass pushing the stomach ventrally. Sonography may provide diagnostic information. CT scans or MRI can be used to examine the mass.*

Tail of the Pancreas

The tail of the pancreas continues from the pancreatic body, toward the left side of the abdomen, and terminates against the spleen in the region of the splenic hilum. On occasion, it may lie against the phrenicocolic ligament, where it is in contact with the left colic flexure and at risk of injury during operations on this portion of the bowel. The length of the pancreatic tail varies markedly. A short tail may not reach the gastric surface of the spleen, while a long one may cradle the greater curvature of the stomach as it lies in the concavity of the splenic hilum.

⇢ ***Surgical visualization of the pancreatic tail.*** *When splenectomy is performed—especially for a traumatized spleen, where bleeding is likely to be brisk, obscuring anatomic landmarks— the surgeon must be extremely careful in ligation of the splenic pedicle not to traumatize the tail of the pancreas. It is important to carefully locate and preserve the tail of the pancreas in high and total gastric resections and in resections of the splenic flexure.*

⇢ ***Total pancreatectomy.*** *In operative procedures involving a badly diseased or damaged pancreas, total pancreatectomy has been under-*

taken. The spleen is removed along with the pancreas. This leaves the patient with a relatively low requirement for insulin—an average of only 5–15 units of insulin daily to control blood sugar.

➡ **Etiology of acute pancreatitis.** *For the surgeon, acute pancreatitis is somewhat of a paradox, since it is frequently discovered at operation but seldom calls for operative treatment. The process may be secondary to (1) infection by mumps virus; (2) obstruction of the terminal common duct, with reflux of bile or duodenal contents into the pancreatic ducts; (3) acute alcoholism; (4) blood- or lymph-borne infected emboli; or (5) an operation in the area of the pancreas (duodenal stump syndrome; pancreatic tail syndrome following splenectomy).*

Pancreatitis must always be considered in the differential diagnosis of acute, painful upper abdominal disease. Elevations of blood and urinary lipase and amylase and of serum glutamic-oxaloacetic transaminase are important in diagnosis. Treatment consists of continuous nasogastric suction; analgesics; anti-cholinergic drugs; restoration of fluid and electrolyte balance and replacement of blood loss, which may be substantial; careful attention to calcium and potassium levels, which may drop as a consequence of saponification of fats; and broad-spectrum antibiotic therapy. Operation is contraindicated unless rapidly worsening jaundice suggests common bile duct obstruction, in which case the common bile duct should be explored and drained.

Chronic pancreatitis is a frequent sequela of acute pancreatitis. It consists of a sclerosing, scarring lesion which grossly resembles carcinoma and can only be differentiated from carcinoma by biopsy. It may be localized or diffuse and most frequently involves the head and body, secondarily obstructing the biliary and pancreatic ducts and causing pancreatic insufficiency. It may be treated by (1) sphincterotomy of the sphincter of Oddi; (2) pancreaticoduodenectomy (Whipple procedure); (3) partial or total pancreatectomy; (4) pancreaticojejunostomy (Puestow filleting procedure); or (5) medical management solely. Pancreatic pseudocysts often are present in chronic pancreatitis.

DUCTAL SYSTEM OF THE PANCREAS (Figs 33–5 and 33–6)

The major pancreatic duct (of Wirsung) runs in the body of the pancreas, closer to the dorsal than to the ventral surface. At the junction of the body and neck, the major pancreatic duct turns first inferiorly, then dorsally, and finally to the right where it joins with the common bile duct and enters the duodenum. (See common bile duct.) The accessory pancreatic duct (of Santorini), when present, drains the head of the pancreas. It occasionally joins with the major pancreatic duct. It empties into the duodenum about 2 cm superior to the main pancreatic duct on the posteromedial duodenal wall. It is occasionally possible to palpate the main pancreatic duct through the covering glandular tissue when it is dilated as a result of obstruction in the pancreatic head. Normally the major pancreatic duct is 3–4 mm in diameter. In elderly individuals, it is up to 6 mm wide. The tributaries to the major pancreatic duct join it at right angles along its central course.

➡ **Dilatation of major pancreatic duct.** *In operative procedures upon the pancreas, in those cases in which the major pancreatic duct is*

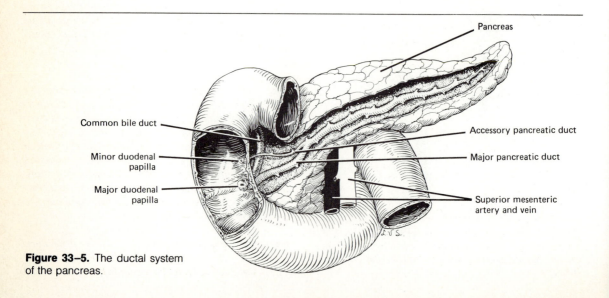

Figure 33–5. The ductal system of the pancreas.

Pancreas

Common bile duct

Minor duodenal papilla

Major duodenal papilla

Accessory pancreatic duct

Major pancreatic duct

Superior mesenteric artery and vein

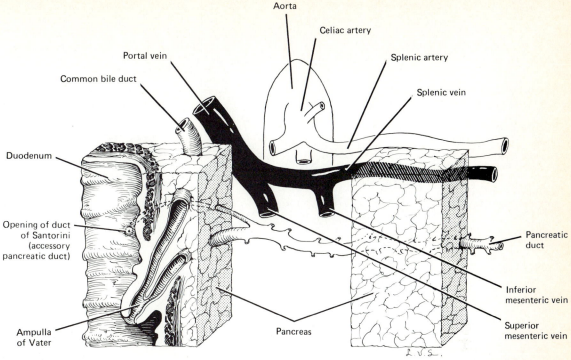

Figure 33–6. Diagram of blocks of the pancreas and the descending duodenum to illustrate the common bile and pancreatic ducts, the splenic vein, the portal vein, and the course of the splenic artery.

markedly dilated as a result of long-standing ductal obstruction, the widened duct can often be directly anastomosed to the small bowel in end-to-end fashion. If one is not able to use a dilated pancreatic duct for anastomosis, the cut end of the pancreas may be anastomosed to the small bowel in end-to-side fashion or via a Roux-en-Y type of anastomosis.

BLOOD VESSELS, LYMPHATICS, & NERVES
(Figs 33–7 to 33–9)

Arteries (Fig 33–7)

The arterial supply to the pancreas is quite constant. Anterior and posterior arterial arcades are formed by branches from the **gastroduodenal** (superior pancreaticoduodenal) and **superior mesenteric** (inferior pancreaticoduodenal) **vessels.** In addition, the **splenic artery** sends branches to the body and tail of the pancreas. The tail of the pancreas receives some arterial blood from the short gastric branches of the splenic artery and from the left gastroepiploic artery.

Veins (Fig 33–7)

Venous drainage from the pancreas is mainly via the splenic vein and its radicles. The gastroduodenal vein, paralleling the dorsal branch of the superior pancreaticoduodenal artery, drains the head of the pancreas. It empties directly into the portal vein, enlarges in cirrhosis of the liver, and is easily torn in the course of mobilization of the duodenum and the pancreatic head. The junction of the right gastroepiploic, anterosuperior pancreaticoduodenal, and middle colic veins forms the gastrocolic venous trunk. This empties into the superior mesenteric vein at the inferior border of the neck of the pancreas. Some small veins draining the head and neck of the pancreas empty directly into the portal vein.

Lymphatics (Fig 33–8)

Lymphatic drainage from the tail of the pancreas is to nodes at the hilum of the spleen, the pancreaticosplenic nodes. The head of the pancreas drains into the pancreaticoduodenal nodes, which lie between the pancreatic head and the descending duodenum. Lymph from the head of the pancreas also drains into the subpyloric nodes. Drainage from the body of the pancreas is into periaortic nodes, along the aorta near the celiac axis.

Nerves (Fig 33–9)

The pancreas is supplied by sympathetic nerve fibers that branch from the greater, lesser, and least

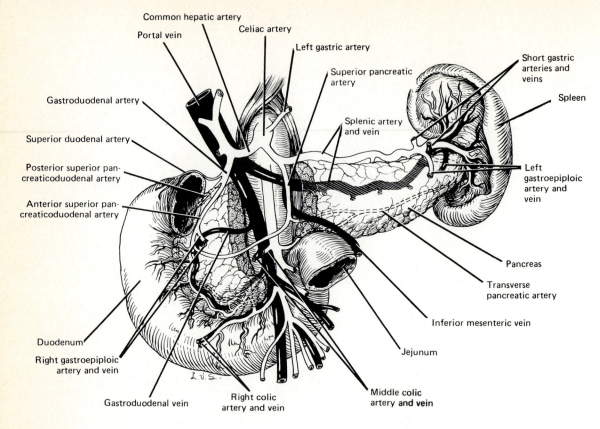

Figure 33–7. Arterial supply and venous return of the descending and transverse duodenum, pancreas, and spleen.

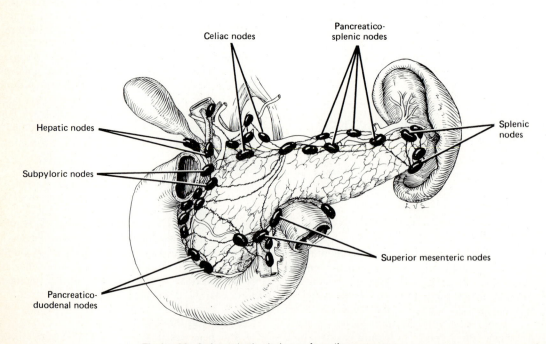

Figure 33–8. Lymphatic drainage from the pancreas.

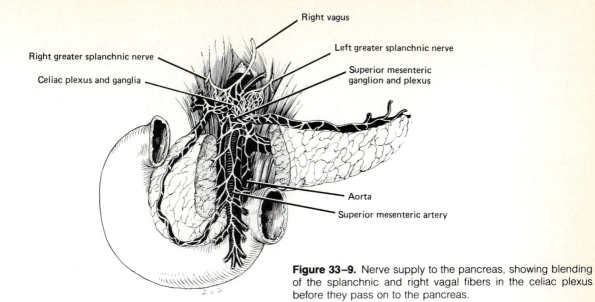

Right vagus

Left greater splanchnic nerve

Superior mesenteric ganglion and plexus

Right greater splanchnic nerve

Celiac plexus and ganglia

Aorta

Superior mesenteric artery

Figure 33–9. Nerve supply to the pancreas, showing blending of the splanchnic and right vagal fibers in the celiac plexus before they pass on to the pancreas.

splanchnic nerves and reach the gland via the celiac plexus. These sympathetic fibers intermingle with branches of the right vagus, forming the celiac plexus, the major nerve supply to the pancreas. The parasympathetic nerve supply to the pancreas comes from branches of the right vagus, and these vagal fibers can be spared if selective vagotomy is undertaken during gastric surgery.

➤ *Role of sympathetic system in pancreatic pain.* *The sympathetic impulses delivered to the pan-* *creas by the splanchnic nerves via the celiac ganglion may be obliterated by a lower thoracic sympathetic block. If the block alleviates pancreatic pain, longer-acting results may be achieved by a dorsal splanchnicectomy (since the sensory fibers pass to the spinal cord alongside the sympathetic fibers), or possibly by total pancreatectomy. In chronic pancreatitis with calculus formation, the severe, narcotic-demanding pain may be relieved by one of these measures, but only if it is performed relatively early.*

34

The Spleen

EMBRYOLOGY

Between the fourth and fifth fetal weeks, the primitive spleen first appears as a condensation of mesodermal tissue in the dorsal mesogastrium near the tail of the developing pancreas. As the stomach rotates 90 degrees to the right, the spleen moves to the left into a position dorsal to the stomach, close to the anterior surface of the left kidney. The portion of the dorsal mesogastrium between the spleen and the greater curvature of the stomach becomes the gastrosplenic ligament, while that between the spleen and the left kidney becomes the lienorenal (splenorenal) ligament.

Anomalies

There are marked variations in the size and shape of the spleen, its position in the abdominal cavity, and the distribution of the arterial and venous blood supply. The spleen is on the right side in complete dextrocardia. Accessory spleens (Fig 34–1) may be found in or near the splenic hilum, the gastrosplenic ligament, or the left side of the greater omentum (lienorenal ligament, tail of pancreas, small bowel mesentery, region of the left tube and ovary), or adjacent to the left testis in the scrotum. Congenital cysts of the spleen may occur.

HISTOLOGY
(Fig 34–2)

The spleen is enclosed within 2 capsular layers. The outer serous coat, derived from the peritoneum, is reflected off the spleen as the splenorenal, phrenicosplenic, and gastrosplenic ligaments. Deep to the external serous layer is an inner fibroelastic layer, which accompanies the large splenic vessels as they enter the spleen at its hilum. As they pass into the organ, this layer forms the splenic trabeculae and the fibrous framework of the organ. The presence of the enclosing fibroelastic layer gives to the spleen an elasticity that allows for variations in splenic size in response to physiologic stimuli.

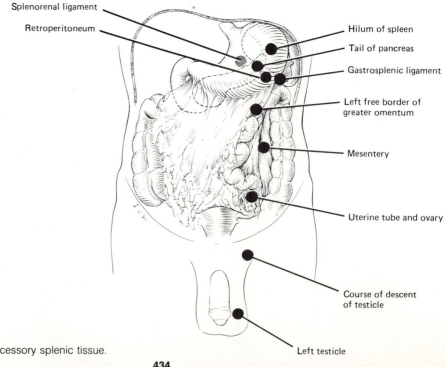

Splenorenal ligament

Retroperitoneum

Hilum of spleen

Tail of pancreas

Gastrosplenic ligament

Left free border of greater omentum

Mesentery

Uterine tube and ovary

Course of descent of testicle

Left testicle

Figure 34–1. Sites of accessory splenic tissue.

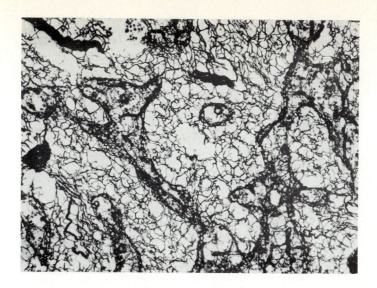

Figure 34–2. Photomicrograph of a silver-stained section of spleen to show general architecture. (×200.) (Reproduced, with permission, from Junqueira LC, Carneiro J: *Basic Histology,* 5th ed. Lange, 1986.)

GROSS ANATOMY
(Figs 34–3 and 34–4)

The spleen is a soft, roughly rectangular, purplish organ, between the fundus of the stomach and the left lateral leaf of the diaphragm (Fig 34–3). The average weight of the spleen is 100–250 g.

The spleen lies under cover of the left ninth, tenth, and 11th ribs in the midaxillary line and is closely related to the left pleural cavity, the lower lobe of the left lung, and the left costophrenic recess. It is separated from these structures only by the thickness of the left leaf of the diaphragm. Since the spleen

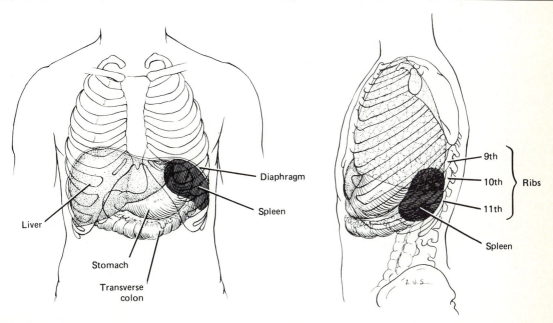

Figure 34–3. Anatomic locations of the spleen, with reference to the anterior and anterolateral abdominal and thoracic parietes. (Modified and reproduced, with permission, from Dunphy JE, Way LW: *Current Surgical Diagnosis & Treatment.* Lange, 1973.)

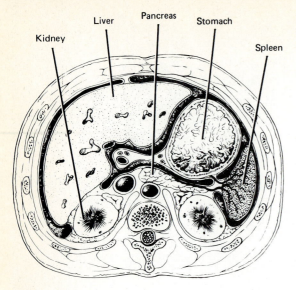

Kidney Liver Pancreas Stomach Spleen

Figure 34–4. Normal anatomic relations of the spleen. (Reproduced, with permission, from Way LW: *Current Surgical Diagnosis & Treatment,* 8th ed. Appleton & Lange, 1988.)

is normally hidden beneath the left costal border, it is not palpable. If it enlarges, it becomes palpable as it moves inferiorly and to the right across the upper abdomen. This pattern of splenic descent is governed by the oblique slant of the phrenicocolic ligament. The ligament prevents the enlarged spleen from descending into the left lumbar gutter.

⇒ *Injuries to the spleen. Fractures of the lower left ribs and fractures of the left upper lumbar vertebral transverse processes should always*

suggest the possibility of splenic rupture. The absence of early signs should not allay suspicion, since delayed splenic rupture commonly follows primary subcapsular rupture. A spleen enlarged by disease is more liable to rupture than a normal one.

The spleen—along with the splenic flexure of the colon, the tail of the pancreas, the fundus of the stomach, and the left kidney—is frequently injured in association with left thoracoabdominal injuries, particularly when the wound of entrance is close to the left midaxillary line.

Surfaces of the Spleen
(Fig 34–5)

The **diaphragmatic (phrenic) surface** is convex and smooth and lies against the undersurface of the left leaf of the diaphragm, which separates it from the left side of the thoracic cavity. The phrenic surface of the spleen faces superiorly, dorsally, and to the left.

The **visceral surface** of the spleen is divided by a centrally placed ridge into an anterior (gastric) surface and a posterior (renal) surface. The gastric surface is broad and concave. It lies against the posterior wall of the fundus of the stomach superiorly and against the tail of the pancreas inferiorly. The gastric surface of the spleen is fissured near its posterior border by the splenic hilum. The hilar area is perforated by apertures for the arteries, veins, and lymphatics.

⇒ *The pancreatic tail during splenectomy. In performing splenectomy, one must avoid the tail of the pancreas, which usually lies against the*

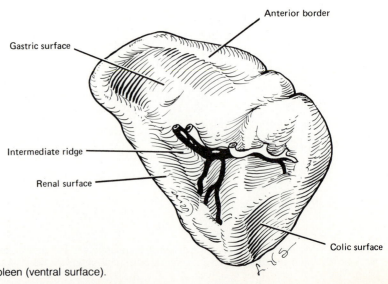

Anterior border

Gastric surface

Intermediate ridge

Renal surface

Colic surface

Figure 34–5. General shape of the spleen (ventral surface).

splenic hilum. This is accomplished by carrying out clean dissection of the splenic vessels and by avoiding mass ligation.

The renal surface of the spleen is flattened and narrower than the gastric surface. It is related to the upper pole of the left kidney and to the left suprarenal gland. It makes up the posterior third of the splenic visceral surface.

Splenic Extremities

The superior tip of the spleen inclines slightly posteriorly at the level of T11 and superiorly toward the undersurface of the diaphragm.

The inferior extremity of the spleen is roughly triangular and rests upon the phrenicocolic ligament. It usually lies just below the area of splenic contact with the tail of the pancreas.

Borders of the Spleen

The thin, free anterior border of the spleen separates its phrenic surface from the gastric surface. This border is frequently notched over its lower third. When the spleen is enlarged, the palpable presence of these notches helps to distinguish the spleen from other left upper quadrant organs or tumors.

The posterior border of the spleen is blunt, rounded, and separates the renal surface from the phrenic surface.

The inferior border of the spleen separates the diaphragmatic surface from the colic surface.

Fixation of the Spleen
(Fig 34–6)

The spleen is fixed in the left upper abdominal quadrant by 3 ligaments.

The **gastrosplenic ligament** connects the fundus and the superior edge of the greater curvature of the stomach to the spleen. Between its 2 layers are the short gastric and left gastroepiploic arteries and veins. The short gastric arteries arising from the splenic artery, just proximal to the splenic hilum, are covered ventrally by peritoneum derived from the gastrohepatic omentum. They are covered dorsally by peritoneum derived from the lateral abdominal parietes.

The **splenorenal ligament** connects the spleen to the lateral abdominal parietes and contains the splenic artery and vein. The splenic artery runs laterally and to the left behind the posterior wall of the lesser sac (the peritoneum of the posterior abdominal wall). Just before the artery reaches the spleen, it adheres to the layer of peritoneum that lies dorsal to it. The splenic artery picks up a ventral covering of peritoneum from the posterior wall of the lesser sac. Thus, the splenorenal ligament is composed of lesser sac posterior peritoneum ventrally and greater sac parietal peritoneum dorsally. The splenic artery runs to the spleen between these 2 serous layers.

The **phrenicocolic ligament** is a fold of the left lateral parietal peritoneum that runs from the splenic flexure of the colon to the left leaf of the diaphragm at the level of the tenth rib. It serves to support the lower pole of the spleen and to close off the upper reaches of the left lumbar gutter.

➠ *Mobilization of splenic ligaments during splenectomy. Skillful splenectomy requires proper anatomic exposure of the organ and proper mobilization of the splenic ligaments, particularly the splenorenal ligament, since this mobilization delivers the spleen up into the abdominal wound and allows the surgeon to inspect the splenic vessels through only one layer of peritoneum.*

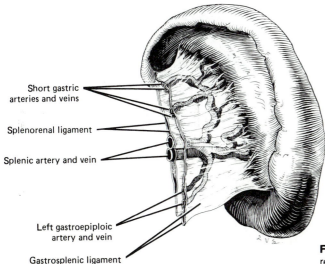

Short gastric arteries and veins

Splenorenal ligament

Splenic artery and vein

Left gastroepiploic artery and vein

Gastrosplenic ligament

Figure 34–6. Ligaments of the spleen and their relationships to the splenic vessels.

Other factors that tend to keep the spleen in position are (1) pressure of the stomach, the tail of the pancreas, and the left kidney against the spleen; (2) the shortness of the splenic vascular pedicle; and (3) intraabdominal pressure exerted superiorly.

BLOOD VESSELS, LYMPHATICS, & NERVES
(Fig 34–7)

Arteries

The **splenic artery** is the largest, longest, and most convoluted branch of the celiac artery. It runs transversely to the left, behind the posterior peritoneal layer of the lesser sac, superior to the splenic vein, and in close proximity to the pancreas, to which it gives many short branches. The terminal branches of the splenic artery are given off in the following manner.

The **superior polar branch** is given off about 2 cm before the artery reaches the splenic hilum. It runs between the 2 layers of the splenorenal ligament and enters the spleen through the upper portion of the hilum. The short gastric arteries (vasa brevia) arise from the superior polar branch of the splenic artery just before it enters the splenic tissue and pass to the right between the 2 leaves of the gastrolienal ligament. They supply the fundus of the stomach (see Chapter 25).

The **inferior polar branch** enters the lower portion of the splenic hilum between the leaves of the sple-

norenal ligament. The left gastroepiploic artery arises from the inferior polar branch of the splenic artery just before that vessel enters the splenic hilum. It passes to the right between the 2 anterior layers of the greater omentum (gastrocolic ligament), 1–2 cm below the line of the greater curvature of the stomach.

The terminal **intrasplenic branches** of the superior and inferior splenic polar arteries arborize within the splenic pulp. Their ultimate peripheral branches are end arteries supplying a wedge-shaped area of splenic periphery.

➠ *Aneurysms of the splenic artery. The tortuous splenic artery is occasionally the site of aneurysmal dilatation and weakening. The diagnosis may be suspected if one hears a bruit over the course of the splenic artery or if a calcified, rounded swelling appears along the course of the artery in plain abdominal films. Since splenic artery aneurysms may rupture spontaneously, they are usually removed along with the spleen when they are diagnosed.*

➠ *Splenic aortography and sonography. Splenic selective angiography is of great value in the diagnosis of disease of the spleen and vessels leading to and from the pancreas and the spleen. Splenic sonography is of help also in cases of splenic enlargement. If sonography fails to provide diagnostic information, either CT scan or MRI can be used.*

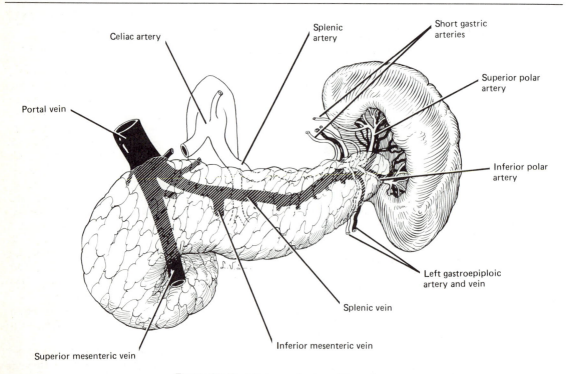

Figure 34–7. Arteries and veins of the spleen.

⇒ *Infarctions of splenic segments. Since the ultimate peripheral branches of the splenic artery are end arteries, an embolus wedged into one of these peripheral vessels will infarct a wedge-shaped area of splenic pulp, the base of the wedge always being located on the splenic periphery.*

Veins
(Fig 34–7)

The small peripheral splenic veins anastomose with one another to form large venous radicles that run toward the hilum along the supporting framework of fibrous trabeculae. Eventually, 5–7 large veins are formed that emerge individually from the splenic hilum. These individual veins usually unite rapidly to form a large single splenic vein between the splenic hilum and the pancreatic neck. Normally, the single **splenic vein** is formed as soon as the multiple issuing veins reach the body of the pancreas. Dorsal to the neck of the pancreas, splenic venous flow unites with the superior mesenteric venous flow to form the portal vein.

The splenic vein leaves the hilum of the spleen via the splenorenal ligament. As the splenic vein courses to the right, it runs behind the body of the pancreas below the splenic artery. Usually, the inferior mesenteric vein joins the splenic vein at about the mid portion of the body of the pancreas, but it may join directly with either the superior mesenteric vein or the portal vein. The splenic vein usually receives the left gastroepiploic vein and always receives short veins from the body, tail, and neck of the pancreas.

⇒ *Multiplicity of splenic veins makes splenorenal shunting difficult. Since the site of formation of a single large splenic vein from the many veins issuing from the splenic hilum is unpredictable, and since on occasion there are many splenic venous channels near the splenic hilum, it may be difficult or impossible to perform a proper splenorenal shunt for portal hypertension.*

⇒ *Splenoportography and splenic arteriography. Splenoportography consists of x-ray study following injection of radiopaque material into the spleen via percutaneous splenic puncture. It is of diagnostic usefulness in liver, portal vein, or splenic disease. In injecting the opaque medium, the operator must remember the presence of the costodiaphragmatic reflection of the parietal pleura (costophrenic recess), which in the left midaxillary line occurs at the level of the tenth rib. Splenic artery arteriography is probably a better method of investigating splenic and pancreatic disease.*

Lymphatics

The lymphatics draining the spleen are largely confined to the capsular and trabecular areas near the splenic hilum. Near the hilum, the major splenic lymphatics join with lymphatics draining the greater curvature of the stomach and the body and tail of the pancreas. The combined lymphatic flow empties into lymph nodes in the gastrosplenic ligament and also into nodes along the splenic vein (gastropancreaticosplenic nodes). The lymph from these nodes continues into the deep aortic nodes near the origin of the celiac artery.

Nerves

Splenic innervation is purely sympathetic. The sympathetic fibers reach the spleen from the celiac plexus via the splenic artery. Splanchnic stimulation causes splenic contraction.

⇒ *Incisions for removal of spleen. Many different kinds of incisions have been used for splenectomy. The organ may be removed through (1) a left rectus incision that can be extended by a transverse T to the left; (2) a left subcostal incision; (3) a left Hoag type of incision (see Chapter 23), with the patient placed on the right side and lying on a kidney rest; (4) a combined left thoracoabdominal incision; or (5) a pure thoracic approach. The choice depends on the patient's body habitus, the size of the spleen, the anticipated splenic disease, and the preferences of the surgeon.*

⇒ *Techniques of splenectomy. (Fig 34–8.) There are 2 approaches to the splenic pedicle.*

*(1) The **anterior approach,** by passage through the lesser sac, is used only in emergencies when brisk bleeding must be rapidly controlled. The lesser sac is entered via an incision through the left side of the gastrocolic ligament. The splenic artery is quickly palpated along the superior surface of the body of the pancreas, and the artery is then compressed either by the finger or by a bulldog arterial clamp. The artery should never be clamped too far medially, as pancreatic circulation may be compromised. The short gastric vessels are then visualized and ligated, care being taken not to include a portion of the gastric wall in the ligatures. Finally, vessels at the splenic hilum are identified and ligated, and the spleen is removed after the splenorenal ligament has been incised. This approach through the lesser peritoneal cavity means that 3 layers of peritoneum must be incised, ie, the 2 layers of the gastrosplenic ligament and the anterior layer of the splenorenal ligament.*

*(2) The **posterior approach** to the spleen is via the greater coelomic cavity. Following chronic or subacute inflammation, vascular ad-*

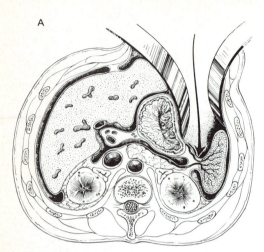 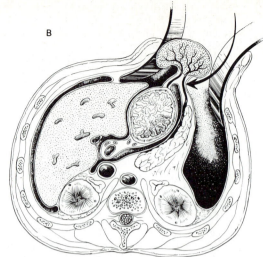

Figure 34–8. Surgical approaches to the spleen: **A:** Anterior approach to the splenic artery. **B:** Mobilization of the spleen with posterior exposure of the splenic artery. (Reproduced, with permission, from Way LW [editor]: *Current Surgical Diagnosis & Treatment,* 8th ed. Appleton & Lange, 1988.)

hesions may be found between the splenic surface and the diaphragm. These must first be isolated and the vessels in the adhesions ligated. A pack is then placed above the spleen to guide it inferiorly and to the right and to exert pressure upon any small bleeding diaphragmatic vessels. The first assistant retracts the stomach (always containing a nasogastric tube) to the right. An incision is made in the posterior leaf of the splenorenal ligament dorsal to the hilum. This releases the spleen from the posterolateral abdominal wall. The hilar vessels that appear after only one layer of peritoneum has been incised are ligated. The anterior leaf of the splenorenal ligament is incised, and the short gastric vessels in the gastrosplenic ligament are then ligated.

Splenectomy indications and contraindications. Indications for splenectomy have been grouped into 3 major classifications:

A. Absolute Indications:

1. Rupture or suspected rupture of the spleen.

2. Congenital hemolytic icterus (hereditary spherocytosis).

3. Many cases of acquired hemolytic anemia.

4. Many cases of idiopathic thrombocytopenic purpura.

5. Primary splenic neutropenia and pancytopenia.

B. Probable Indications: The spleen should probably be removed in—

1. Severe secondary hypersplenism due to hepatic cirrhosis or extrahepatic portal hypertension and congestive splenomegaly (Banti's disease), splenomegaly of sarcoid, rheumatoid arthritis, Gaucher's disease, and tuberculosis.

2. Severe hypersplenism, especially when associated with hemolytic anemia due to chronic lymphocytic leukemia; lymphosarcoma; Hodgkin's disease; or follicular lymphoblastoma.

3. When a greatly enlarged spleen causes disability due to weight or pressure, and in some cases of thalassemia and sickle cell anemia with splenomegaly and excessive hemolysis.

4. A few cases of marrow hypoplasia with critical thrombocytopenia.

C. Contraindications: The spleen should probably not be removed in—

1. Cytopenia with bone marrow hypoplasia.

2. Myelofibrosis with myeloid metaplasia of the spleen.

3. Acute symptomatic hemolytic anemias with hemoglobinemia.

4. Certain blood dyscrasias such as polycythemia vera, monocytic leukemia, and most cases of lymphocytic leukemia.

Preservation of traumatized spleen. There has been a tendency to preserve traumatized spleen, particularly in children and young adults. This is because such splenectomized individuals have decreased ability to combat some acute infections. Suturing of splenic lacerations, resection of portions of the spleen, and the use of hemostatic materials at the site of splenic rupture are the procedures of choice. Obviously, these patients must be carefully watched for further bleeding, and some of them eventually require splenectomy.

Kidneys, Ureters, & Suprarenal Glands

35

The kidneys, ureters, and suprarenal glands are the major viscera in the postfetal retroperitoneum. These organs lie ventral to the dorsal fascia lining the abdominal cavity and dorsal to the posterior peritoneum of the abdominal coelom. Although the initial development of the gonads (ovaries and testes) begins high in the retroperitoneum, the location of these structures is in the pelvis and scrotum, respectively. Therefore, the gonads are not included in this discussion of the abdominal retroperitoneum except for their relationship to the true retroperitoneal viscera during the embryonic period.

Many portions of the gastrointestinal tract are wholly or partially retroperitoneal in the adult (secondarily retroperitoneal): most of the duodenum, the cecum, the ascending and descending colon, and the pancreas. These structures are discussed in other chapters.

I. KIDNEYS

EMBRYOLOGY
(Fig 35–1)

The embryonic kidney develops from the intermediate mesoderm, as do the male and female genital systems. The intermediate mesoderm runs the entire length of the dorsal wall of the embryo from the future neck to the pelvis. The nephrogenic cord is the name given to the mesodermal mass positioned along each side of the fetal aorta in the lumbar region.

Pronephros

The pronephros is a temporary nonfunctional structure that appears in the fourth fetal week. It is composed of a group of tubules. From each pronephros a duct runs inferiorly and discharges into the cloaca. The structure rapidly degenerates, but the pronephric duct remains, to be utilized by the next, or mesonephric, stage of renal development.

Mesonephros

The mesonephros develops just caudal to the pronephros. It functions as an intermediate kidney until permanent renal function is established. Mesonephric

vesicles form within its mesenchyme, many becoming S-shaped and sending tubules to join the pronephric duct, now called the mesonephric, or wolffian, duct. Many of the vesicles are indented by capillaries to form glomeruli and Bowman capsules. Capsule plus glomerulus makes up the mesonephric corpuscle. The mesonephric tubule's medial segment elongates and becomes convoluted. The mesonephric ducts and a few tubules remain in postfetal life as the male genital ducts or as vestigial ducts in females.

Metanephros

The permanent kidneys start their development in the fifth week and begin excreting urine in the 11th week. The metanephros develops from 2 anlagen: the metanephric diverticulum (ureteric bud) and the metanephric mesoderm, or blastema, which is located in the terminal portion of the nephrogenic cord. The metanephric diverticulum arises from the mesonephric duct just before it enters the cloaca. It is the forerunner of the ureter, the renal pelvis and calices, and the collecting tubules. The diverticulum, proceeding dorsally and cranially, enters the nephrogenic cord and evokes the metanephros, or definitive kidney. The caudal portion of the diverticulum becomes the ureter, while its cranial widened end becomes the renal pelvis. From the renal pelvis develop the major and minor calices and the collecting tubules.

Vesicles and tubules form in the metanephros as in the mesonephros, but in much greater numbers. The distal end of each metanephric tubule joins with a collecting tubule. As a consequence, a uriniferous tubule is made up of 2 different embryologic segments: a nephron (renal corpuscle plus convoluted tubules) from the metanephric mesoderm and a collecting tubule from the metanephric diverticulum. As the metanephric tubule elongates, it forms the proximal convoluted tubule, the loop of Henle, and the distal convoluted tubule. The fetal kidneys are pelvic in position, but as a result of differential growth they come to lie in the abdomen. The kidney hilum at first faces ventrally, but after 90-degree rotation it faces ventromedially.

Anomalies
(Fig 35–2)

Renal anomalies include ectopy of the kidney, which may be simple (low position but on proper

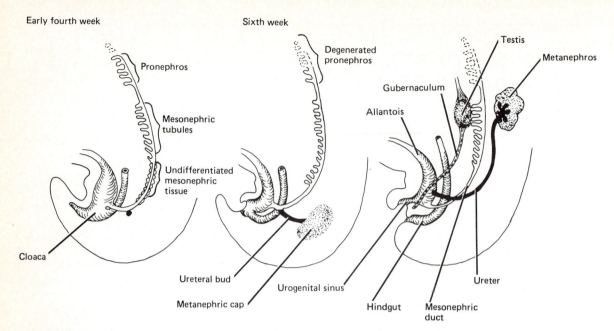

Figure 35–1. Schematic representation of the development of the nephric system. (Modified and reproduced, with permission, from Tanagho EA, McAninch JW [editors]: *Smith's General Urology,* 12th ed. Appleton & Lange, 1988.)

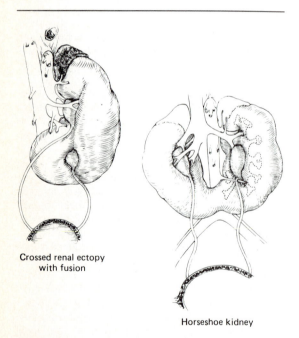

Crossed renal ectopy with fusion

Horseshoe kidney

Figure 35–2. Renal anomalies. **Left:** Crossed ectopy with fusion. The renal mass lies in the left flank. The right ureter must cross over the midline. **Right:** Horseshoe kidney. Pelves are anterior. Note the aberrant artery obstructing the left ureter and the low position of renal mass. (Reproduced, with permission, from Tanagho EA, McAninch JW [editors]: *Smith's General Urology,* 12th ed. Appleton & Lange, 1988.)

side), crossed (low position but on contralateral side), or crossed with fusion with opposite kidney (horseshoe kidney); malrotation of the kidney; congenital absence of a kidney (renal agenesis); supernumerary kidneys (rare); congenital polycystic kidneys; renal hypoplasia or hyperplasia; and multiple renal vessels.

Ureteral anomalies include bifid ureter, reduplication of the ureter; failure of development of the ureteral bud, leading to solitary kidney and hemitrigone of the bladder; congenital ureteropelvic and ureterovesical stenosis; and ectopic ureteral orifices.

GROSS ANATOMY
(Figs 35–3 and 35–4)

The kidneys are encased in 3 layers of fat and fascia and lie in the retroperitoneum on either side of the upper lumbar vertebral column. Although the exact position of the kidneys depends on many physiologic, pathologic, and embryologic factors, the upper pole of the kidney is generally near the level of vertebra T12 and the lower pole near L3. The right kidney is usually slightly lower than the left, owing to the presence of the liver on the right side of the abdomen. The long axis of each kidney is directed laterally and caudally. The normal adult kidney weighs about

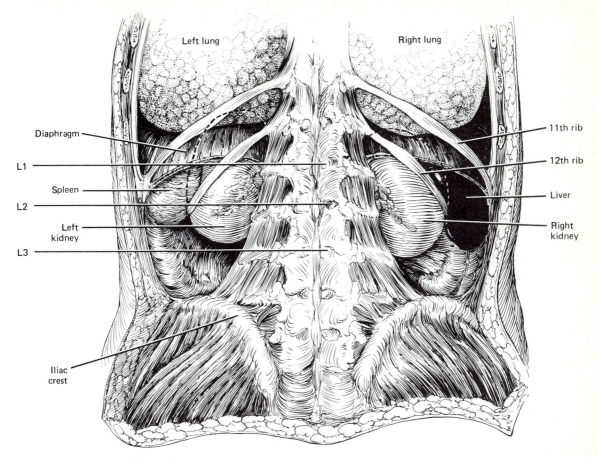

Figure 35–3. Relationship of the kidney to the dorsal abdominal wall. Dotted line represents the portion of the kidney obscured by overlying tissue. (Modified and reproduced, with permission, from Tanagho EA, McAninch JW [editors]: *Smith's General Urology,* 12th ed. Appleton & Lange, 1988.)

150 g in men and about 125 g in women. In infants, the kidney is about 3 times larger in proportion to the total body weight than it is in the adult.

Each kidney is bean-shaped, with its convexity facing laterally. The kidney and its supplying renal vessels are cradled in perirenal fat (adipose capsule). The fat enters the renal hilum and extends into the renal sinus. The kidneys usually move superiorly and inferiorly with diaphragmatic movement during respiration.

STRUCTURE OF THE KIDNEYS
(Fig 35–5)

On gross examination, the kidney is seen to consist of an outer granular zone, the **cortex,** and an inner striated zone, the **medulla.** The cortex derives its granular appearance from the many glomeruli contained within its boundaries. The medulla appears striated because of its many linear tubules and collecting ducts. However, tubules appear in the cortex, constituting the medullary rays. Cortical tissue ex-

tends centrally as far as the renal sinus, appearing as thin strips, the **renal columns,** which lie between the medullary pyramids. The **medullary pyramids** are pyramidal masses consisting of straight tubules and collecting ducts; the bases of the pyramids are directed peripherally and their apexes face centrally toward the renal sinus. The apexes of the pyramids terminate in papillae, which project into the lumen of the minor calices. The portion of the renal cortex that arches over the base of the medullary pyramid and connects the renal columns is called the cortical arch.

⭢ *Renal trauma. Because the kidneys lie partly under cover of the lower thoracic ribs, renal trauma should be suspected in all injuries associated with trauma to the posterior lower thorax or upper abdomen. Blunt trauma to the abdomen may also result in injury to the kidneys, and in contrecoup injury there may be excessive stretching of the renal vascular pedicle, causing it to rupture. (Fig 35–6.)*

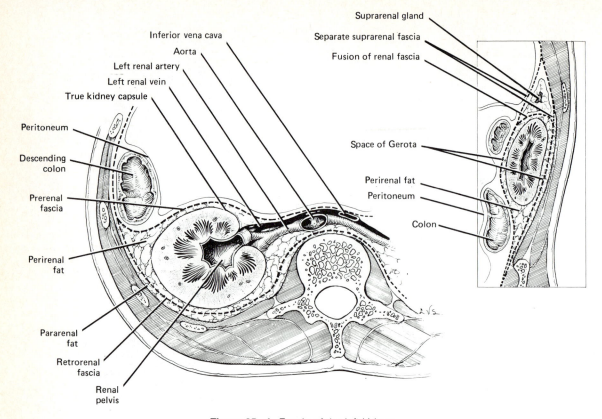

Figure 35–4. Fascia of the left kidney.

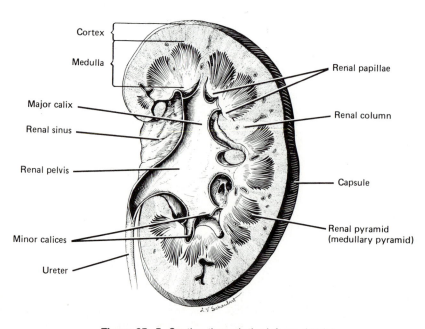

Figure 35–5. Section through the left renal pelvis.

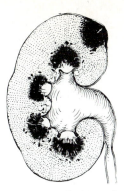

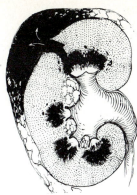

A. Renal contusion (ecchymosis) with small subcapsular hematoma.

B. Incomplete laceration of renal parenchyma and capsule with perirenal hematoma.

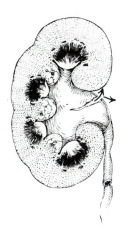

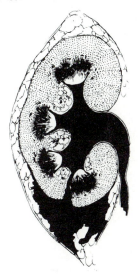

C. Laceration of renal pelvis or ureter; urinary extravasation occurs.

D. Complete laceration of kidney with gross hematuria; gross extravasation of blood and urine.

Figure 35–6. Renal injuries from blunt trauma. (Reproduced, with permission, from Tanagho EA, McAninch JW [editors]: *Smith's General Urology,* 12th ed. Appleton & Lange, 1988.)

➠ *Disorders of the perirenal fatty tissues. The perirenal fatty tissues may become the site of perinephric abscess formation, either from spread of infection from the kidney parenchyma or from blood-borne infection of nonrenal origin. Cutaneous furuncles are occasional causes of perinephric abscess, but antimicrobial therapy has reduced their incidence. Most perinephric abscesses are contained by the external layer of the perirenal fascia. With such an abscess, the diaphragm on the affected side is usually elevated and fixed; the ipsilateral psoas shadow may be obliterated on x-rays; and scoliosis of the lumbar spine with the concavity of the spinal curve facing the side of the abscess may also be seen. There is usually costovertebral angle tenderness.*

In about 5% of people, the perirenal fatty tissues of the right kidney may occasionally pouch superiorly into the mediastinum through an inconstant opening between the right lateral and medial lumbocostal arches. On x-rays, the herniated fat pad may resemble a tumor in the lower lobe of the right lung. Mediastinal tomograms must be obtained to rule out this possibility.

FASCIAL COVERINGS OF THE KIDNEYS (Fig 35–4)

The external renal fascia (Gerota's fascia or capsule, perirenal capsule) is a thickening of the abdominal subserous fascia that lies between the posterior lining of the abdominal fascia dorsally and the major subserous fascia ventrally. At the lateral border of each kidney, the subserous fascia of the lateral abdominal wall splits into sheaths that enclose the kidney and its covering of perirenal fat. In splitting into a ventral (prerenal) fascia and a dorsal (retrorenal) fascia, the subserous fascia delineates the space of Gerota, which lies between its 2 leaves. After surrounding the kidney and leaving its medial edge, the prerenal fascia is prolonged over the great vessels of the retroperitoneum and in the midline joins the prerenal fascia from the contralateral side. The retrorenal fascia also extends medially after covering the kidney dorsally; it blends with the fascia covering the ventral surfaces of the quadratus lumborum and psoas major muscles. At the midline, it covers the ventral surface of the vertebral column and joins with the retrorenal fascia from the contralateral side. In the midline of the retroperitoneum, the retrorenal fascia lies deep to the aorta. Both the prerenal and the retrorenal fasciae send off fibrous prolongations that pass through the perirenal fat (the fatty renal capsule) to attach to the true (fibrous) renal capsule. Dorsal to the external perirenal capsule is the so-called pararenal fat pad. This fatty tissue is not to be confused with the perirenal fatty capsule that lies deep to Gerota's fascia and superficial to the true renal capsule.

The 2 layers of perirenal fascia fuse at the superior pole of the kidney and thereby separate the kidney from the suprarenal (adrenal) gland, which is encased in a separate fascial envelope. The 2 layers of the perirenal fascia do not fuse at the lower pole of the kidney. Consequently, the kidney is able to move inferiorly between their layers.

In summary, the kidney has 3 capsules: an outer "perirenal" capsule derived from the subserous fascia; a fatty (adipose) capsule that cradles the organ and lies deep to the perirenal capsule; and an intrinsic (true) fibrous capsule that surrounds the kidney proper and is composed of relatively strong fibrous tissue, which in young and healthy patients strips easily from the underlying kidney parenchyma.

➠ *Fusion of the leaves of the perirenal fascia. Since the anterior and posterior leaves of the perirenal fascia fuse superior to the kidney and do not include the suprarenal gland, Gerota's space (perirenal fat) may be entered and the kidney surgically removed without injury to the suprarenal gland.*

RELATIONSHIPS OF THE KIDNEYS
(Fig 35–7)

Ventral Relationships
The right and left kidneys have different ventral relationships.

A. Right Kidney: Superiorly, the right kidney is related medially to the right suprarenal and laterally to the liver. Medially, the right kidney is related to the descending duodenum. Inferiorly, the right kidney is related to the hepatic flexure of the colon.

B. Left Kidney: Medially and superiorly, the left kidney is related to the left suprarenal gland. Laterally, the left kidney abuts the spleen. Medially, in descending order, the left kidney is related to the dorsal gastric surface, the pancreas, and the splenic flexure of the colon.

Dorsal Relationships
The dorsal surface of each kidney is not covered by peritoneum and is tightly adherent to fatty areolar tissue. Each kidney is related to the diaphragm and, from lateral to medial, to the tendon of the transversus abdominis, the quadratus lumborum, and the psoas major muscles.

Medial Relationships
The concave central segment of the kidneys is deeply fissured. Entering the fissure, the **kidney hilum,** are the arteries and nerves, and leaving it are the renal vein and the ureter. The hilum expands into an intrarenal space, the renal sinus, which contains the superior ureteral segment and the renal calices. The renal sinus usually contains much fat in which are buried the renal arteries, veins, and nerves.

BLOOD VESSELS, LYMPHATICS, & NERVES
(Fig 35–7)

Arteries
The renal arteries normally arise from the sides of the abdominal aorta near the level of L2. The arteries are large and pass laterally to the hilum of the kidney and in so doing cross the crura of the diaphragm and the psoas muscles. The right renal artery is longer and slightly lower in origin than the left artery; it passes dorsal to the inferior vena cava, the descending portion of the duodenum, and the head of the pancreas. The shorter left renal artery lies dorsal to the left renal vein, the body of the pancreas, and the splenic vein. At the hilum of the kidney each renal artery lies dorsal to the renal vein and ventral to the renal pelvis.

A branch of the renal artery runs in each renal column as it courses toward the periphery of the kidney from the renal pelvis. At the border between the cortex and the medulla, these interlobar arteries arborize into the arcuate arteries, branches of which become the afferent arterioles of the glomeruli. The efferent arterioles break up into small capillary networks surrounding the renal tubules.

Between the aorta and the hilum, each artery gives off ureteric and inferior suprarenal branches. Within the hilum, each artery splits into many branches that pass toward the renal periphery. Beyond the junction of the medulla and the cortex, the peripheral arterial

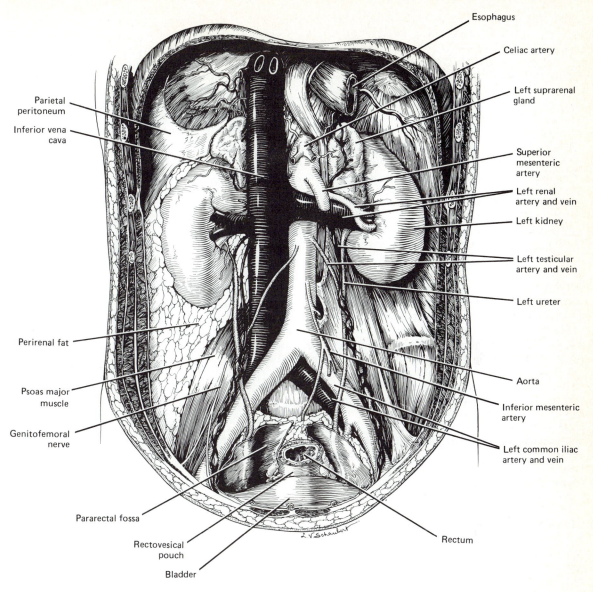

Figure 35–7. Vessels and organs of the retroperitoneum.

branches become true segmental arteries with no intercommunication.

Accessory renal arteries occur frequently, usually on the left side and below the major renal artery. They usually arise from the aorta or, rarely, from either the common or the external iliac arteries. For the most part, the accessory renal arteries are actually segmental arteries to the upper or lower renal poles that have been given off proximal to their usual site of branching within the renal sinus.

➠ *Segmental infarction of the kidney. At a variable distance between the abdominal aorta and the renal sinus, each renal artery branches into segmental (end) arteries. Because there*

is little or no communication between individual terminal renal arteries, segmental infarction of an area of kidney follows occlusion of one of these vessels. Infarction may follow infectious endocarditis, the propagation of atrial or ventricular cardiac thrombi, polyarteritis nodosa, or thrombosis of the renal artery following trauma.

➠ *Accessory renal arteries. When accessory renal arteries run to the lower pole of the kidney, they often exert pressure upon the upper ureteral segment just distal to the renal pelvis. Such compression may result in hydronephrosis.*

⟶ *Pathologic occlusion of the renal artery. Fibromuscular hyperplasia of the renal artery or the presence within a renal artery of arteriosclerotic plaques may lead to renal hypertension. If hypertension is severe, an aorticorenal bypass graft, renal endarterectomy, or renal artery prosthesis may be needed to maintain normotension.*

⟶ *Trauma to the kidney. Kidney trauma can follow a blow to the anterior abdomen, the flank, the lumbar region of the abdominal wall, or the perineum (contrecoup injury). Renal injury must be suspected in all cases of fracture of the lower posterior ribs or lumbar transverse processes and in all patients with marked costovertebral tenderness following trauma.*

Veins

Efferent blood flow from the kidneys is carried to the inferior vena cava by the renal vein. Each renal vein is formed within the renal sinus as a result of the junction of numerous smaller segmental renal venous branches. The major renal vein has a larger luminal diameter than the renal artery. It lies ventral to the renal artery. Both renal veins empty into the inferior vena cava at almost a right angle. Accessory renal veins are rare.

The left renal vein is longer than the right, since it must cross to the contralateral side of the abdomen to empty into the inferior vena cava. The left renal vein lies about 1 cm superior to the level of the right renal vein. As the left renal vein passes to the right, it lies ventral to the abdominal aorta just below the takeoff of the superior mesenteric artery. The left renal vein receives the upper left ureteric vein, the left testicular or ovarian vein, the left suprarenal vein, and the left inferior phrenic vein.

⟶ *Splenorenal shunting. The left renal vein is occasionally used for splenorenal shunting in patients with bleeding of esophageal varices due to portal hypertension. The splenic vein is mobilized and joined to the left renal vein in an end-to-side anastomosis. The left suprarenal vein, which empties into the left renal vein, usually must be ligated so that a splenorenal anastomosis can be constructed.*

The right renal vein is short. As it runs toward the inferior vena cava, it passes dorsal to the descending segment of the duodenum. The right renal vein has only one tributary, the right upper ureteric vein.

Lymphatics

Lymph drainage from the kidney is initiated at the renal hilum. Three major lymphatic plexuses are related to the kidney: one in the perirenal fat, one within the kidney parenchyma, and one just deep to the fibrous capsule of the organ. Three or 4 lymphatic pathways leave the kidney hilum and are joined by lymphatics that have drained the area just deep to the kidney's intrinsic fibrous capsule. These lymph channels follow the renal vein to the lumbar lymph nodes. Lymph from the perirenal fat flows directly into the lumbar nodes by an independent trunk.

Nerves

The kidneys are innervated by 12–16 nerves derived from the renal plexus. The renal plexus is made up of nerve fibers that reach the kidneys from the lesser and lowest thoracic splanchnic nerves, the celiac and aortic plexuses. Afferent nerves pass from the kidney to the spinal cord along the path followed by the sympathetics. The efferent nerve supply to the kidney is autonomic, with vasomotor fibers to both the afferent and efferent renal arterioles. The nerves from the kidneys connect with nerves from the testicular plexus. This association probably accounts for the testicular pain encountered in some kidney diseases.

II. URETERS

The ureters are tubes that run from the renal pelvis to the urinary bladder (Fig 35–8).

EMBRYOLOGY

Embryology and anomalies of the ureters are described under embryology of the kidneys, above.

⟶ *Urography before urologic surgery. It is important to determine whether the patient has a double ureter before pelvic surgery is performed, because the surgeon could inadvertently injure the second ureter once the first one has been recognized and isolated. Consequently, visualization of the kidneys and ureters by urography is often recommended prior to pelvic surgery.*

⟶ *Congenital ureteropelvic and ureterovesical stenosis. Congenital ureteropelvic stenosis results in hydronephrosis. Congenital ureterovesical stenosis results in hydroureteronephrosis. A stone lodged in the lower ureter can also produce hydroureteronephrosis (Fig 35–9).*

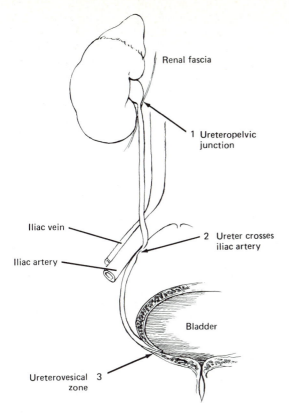

Figure 35–8. Points of ureteral narrowing. The ureter is narrow at 3 points: (1) at the ureteropelvic junction, (2) at the point where the ureter crosses over the iliac vessels, and (3) in the ureterovesical zone where the ureter joins the bladder. A stone that passes the ureteropelvic junction has an excellent chance, therefore, of continuing the whole distance. If it becomes arrested, it is usually in the lower 5 cm of the ureter. (Modified and reproduced, with permission, from Tanagho EA, McAninch JW [editors]: *Smith's General Urology,* 12th ed. Appleton & Lange, 1988.)

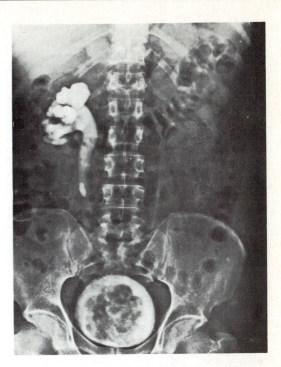

Figure 35–9. Excretory urogram showing right ureteral stone causing hydronephrosis. Large irregular filling defect from unsuspected vesical neoplasm. (Reproduced, with permission, from Tanagho EA, McAninch JW [editors]: *Smith's General Urology,* 12th ed. Appleton & Lange, 1988.)

GROSS ANATOMY

The 8–12 minor renal calices coalesce to form 3 or 4 major calices that in turn join to create a funnel-shaped dilated tube, the renal pelvis. The proximal portion of the renal pelvis normally lies within the renal sinus, whereas the distal portion is usually extrarenal. However, the renal pelvis may be completely intrarenal or completely extrarenal. It usually lies at the level of L1. The upper part of the adult ureter begins in the renal sinus as a continuation of the renal pelvis.

Each ureter is 26–34 cm long, and the right ureter is usually slightly shorter than the left. The lower end of the renal pelvis tapers to form a thick, narrow tube that varies in luminal diameter at different levels. The ureteropelvic junction is the first anatomic constriction of the ureter; the others occur (1) as the ureter crosses the pelvic brim and (2) as it enters the bladder wall (Fig 35–8). Below the ureteropelvic junction, the course of the ureter (for purposes of description) is divided into abdominal, pelvic, and intravesical segments.

⇒ *Ureteral trauma. Ureteral trauma may follow penetrating injuries to the dorsal or ventrolateral abdominal wall; may follow abdominal or pelvic surgery; and occasionally is secondary to perineal injury. Intravenous urography is helpful is diagnosing ureteral injury. The ureter can usually be repaired by an end-to-end anastomosis, but it may be necessary to anastomose the severed ureter to the contralateral ureter or directly to the bladder. Iatrogenic injury to the ureter can usually be avoided by the placement of ureteral catheters before difficult lower abdominal and pelvic surgery. (Fig 35–10.)*

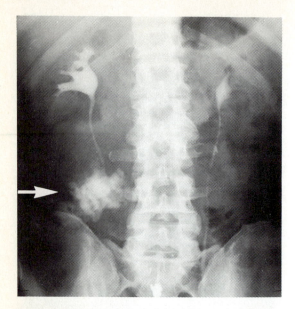

Figure 35–10. Stab wound of the right ureter shows extravasation of dye on intravenous urogram. (Reproduced, with permission, from Tanagho EA, McAninch JW [editors]: *Smith's General Urology,* 12th ed. Appleton & Lange, 1988.)

ABDOMINAL URETER

The abdominal ureter is essentially the same in males and females and is 18–20 cm long. The abdominal ureter runs inferiorly and slightly medially on the ventral surface of the psoas major muscle to the brim of the true pelvis. Superiorly, at the level of the inferior border of the renal pelvis, the ureter lies dorsal to the renal artery and vein; along its entire abdominal course, it is loosely embedded in the retroperitoneal areolar tissue from which it derives minor arterial circulation. The ureter lies ventral to the genitofemoral nerve and dorsal to the gonadal vessels that cross it obliquely.

The upper portion of the abdominal segment of the right ureter lies dorsal to the descending duodenum and just to the right of the inferior vena cava; it is crossed by the right colic and the ileocolic vessels as it lies dorsal to the fixed mesentery of the ascending colon. The left ureter lies to the right of the sigmoid colon; it is crossed by the left colic vessels.

➤ *Trauma to the abdominal segment of the ureter.* The extraperitoneal approach is usually used for surgery upon the abdominal segment of the ureter (eg, high ureterolithotomy). Because the abdominal ureteral segment is easy to locate, it is seldom injured during upper midabdominal surgical procedures. Surgeons often follow the abdominal ureter inferiorly, from the level of the pelvic brim, as a guide to its more vulnerable pelvic segment.

➤ *Vulnerability of the upper segment of the right ureter in surgery.* During surgery upon the descending duodenum, right lumbar sympathetic chain, or the upper segment of the inferior vena cava, the surgeon must consider the position of the upper segment of the right ureter. When the cecum, ascending colon, and terminal ileum are mobilized, the surgeon must always be careful not to injure the mid right ureter, since it lies in close dorsal relationship to these structures.

➤ *Stricture of the ureter.* Stricture of the ureter is common and may be due to congenital narrowing, infection, or trauma. Stricture may also be caused by nonureteral disease such as cancer of the colon, cancer of the genital tract in the female, cancer of the bladder, or retroperitoneal fibroplasia. Pressure on the ureter by an aberrant renal vessel is a frequent cause of upper ureteral stricture. Stricture is inevitably followed by urinary stasis and infection. Partial stricture may result when a stone lodges in the ureter.

➤ *Referral of pain in ureteral disease.* Pain secondary to ureteral disease in the male is often referred to the ipsilateral testicle, since the ureter crosses the genitofemoral nerve in its descent to the bladder. Pain from a stone in the kidney pelvis is referred to the ipsilateral flank. Pain from a stone in the mid ureter can be referred to the ipsilateral flank or right lower abdominal quadrant. Pain from a stone at the ureterovesical junction may be referred to the scrotum or vulva or to the right lower quadrant. (Fig 35–11.)

➤ *Vulnerability of the left ureter in resection of the sigmoid colon.* The left ureter lies well to the medial side of the descending colon and is crossed from right to left by the left colic vessels. However, inflammatory disease or cancer of the sigmoid colon tends to bind the left ureter closer to the colon, making it more vulnerable.

PELVIC URETER

The pelvic ureter begins at the superior border of the true pelvic cavity, where it crosses either the common iliac artery or the external iliac artery, just ventral to the sacroiliac joint. The pelvic ureter is 12–14 cm long. In the pelvic retroperitoneal tissues, it forms a mild convex curve that faces the lateral pelvic wall. It lies at first ventral and then inferior to the internal iliac artery and ventral to the obturator vessels and nerve.

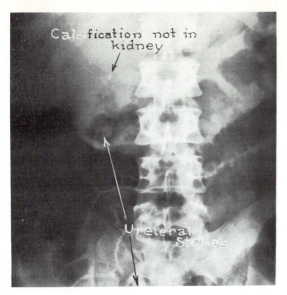

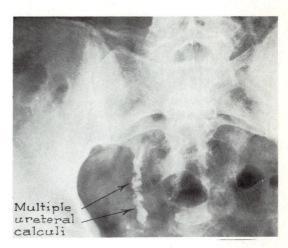

Figure 35–11. Plain films showing progress of stone down ureter. (Reproduced, with permission, from Tanagho EA, McAninch JW [editors]: *Smith's General Urology,* 12th ed. Appleton & Lange, 1988.)

> *Vulnerability of the ureters during midrectal resections. The ureters are particularly vulnerable to inadvertent injury during abdominoperineal or low anterior rectal resection.*

The superior half of the pelvic ureter is the same in both the male and the female. However, at the inferior depths of the pelvis, relationships obviously differ.

The pelvic ureter is anatomically constricted as it crosses the common or external iliac arteries.

> *Narrowing of the ureter in the pelvis. (Fig 35–8.) The 2 areas of anatomic constriction in the pelvic ureter are (1) where it passes over the common or external iliac arteries and (2) where it passes through the bladder wall. These are the most common sites for impaction of ureteral stones.*

> *Palpation of the left pelvic ureter. Since the most proximal segment of the pelvic ureter lies just ventral to the external iliac artery, it can usually be palpated by inserting a finger into the apex of the sigmoid mesentery and rolling the ureter upon the ventral surface of the underlying artery. This precaution serves to locate the left ureter and helps to prevent injury during pelvic surgery.*

Pelvic Ureter in the Male

In the male, after the ureter has descended below the bifurcation of the common iliac artery, it lies at first just deep to the peritoneum of the lateral pelvic wall along the anterior border of the greater sciatic notch. Each ureter then converges toward the contralateral ureter in a ventromedial curve. When the ureters reach the level of the ischial spine, they enter the sacrogenital fold and join with a group of vascular and nervous structures that are directed toward the urinary bladder. As it turns medially from the lateral pelvic wall, each ureter lies ventral to the apex of a seminal vesicle (Fig 35–7). The ductus deferens crosses over the ureter ventrally. As the pelvic ureter enters the sacrogenital fold, it is surrounded by veins of the vesical plexus. The ureter continues medially within the loose connective tissue that forms the lateral true bladder ligament and becomes closely related to the inferior hypogastric nerve plexus.

Pelvic Ureter in the Female

The female pelvic ureter lies at first deep to the parietal peritoneum of the lateral pelvic wall dorsal and inferior to the ovary. The ovarian vessels lie just lateral to the ureter in the ovarian fossa. The ureter then bends medially and comes to lie ventral to the internal iliac artery and medial to the obturator nerve and to the obturator, inferior vesical, and middle rectal branches of the internal iliac artery. It reaches the dorsal attachment of the uterosacral ligament, which it enters. In the ligament, it passes ventrally and medially toward the bladder and runs in the cardinal (lateral cervical) ligament at the base of the broad ligaments of the uterus. There the ureter is about 2 cm lateral to the uterine cervix and the lateral fornix of the vagina and is crossed superiorly by the uterine artery "water under the bridge." The ureter then enters the tissues of the true lateral bladder ligament, ventral to the vagina, and enters the posteroinferior surface of the bladder.

➠ **Vulnerability of the ureter in the ovarian fossa.** *The ureter, the ovarian vessels, and the suspensory ligament of the ovary (infundibulopelvic ligament) all lie in close proximity in the ovarian fossa on the lateral pelvic wall. Therefore, the ureter is vulnerable to injury during gynecologic surgery (eg, total hysterectomy), when it may be inadvertently clamped or ligated along with the vessels in the infundibulopelvic ligament.*

➠ **Relationship of the pelvic ureter to the uterine cervix.** *Because the ureters are closely related to the uterine cervix, they may be transected, ligated, or distorted during surgery involving the lower uterine segment. The gynecologic operative procedures most likely to cause injury to the ureters are total hysterectomy when the cervix is being removed and surgery upon the uterine tubes and ovaries at the point where the ovarian and tubal blood supply is ligated close to the lateral pelvic wall.*

INTRAVESICAL (TERMINAL) URETER

The intravesical (terminal) portion of the ureter in both males and females is about 2 cm long and runs obliquely through the bladder wall in a medial and caudal direction. The oblique path creates a valve-like effect that helps to prevent reflux of urine from the bladder into the ureters during bladder contraction and emptying. Urinary reflux is prevented by contraction of bladder muscle fibers surrounding the intravesical ureters; by compression of the ureters by the bladder as it fills with urine; and by the anatomic constriction of the ureters as they pass through the bladder wall. During its intravesical course, the smooth muscle of the ureter does not blend with the bladder musculature but fans out deep to the bladder trigone as a separate muscle layer that sends some fibers to the proximal urethra. The intravesical course of the ureter ends at the border of the bladder trigone.

➠ **Ureteral urinary reflux.** *Despite the sphincter-like action of the bladder musculature upon the intravesical ureter, urinary reflux during micturition is relatively common in some children who consequently suffer recurrent episodes of pyelonephritis.*

➠ **Relationship of retroperitoneal fibrosis to the ureters.** *Retroperitoneal fibrosis, a chronic in-flammatory process due to various causes including cancer, aortic aneurysm, and long-term use of methysergide, may involve the retroperitoneum in both the pelvis and abdomen. The resulting fibrotic tissue may completely obstruct the ureters or may cause their medial displacement, a factor in the x-ray diagnosis of the condition.*

➠ **Use of the ureters in bladder bypass procedures.** *The ureters may be used for urinary bypass procedures when malignant or granulomatous disease requires diversion of urine from the bladder. The ureters are usually anastomosed to an ileal conduit loop or occasionally to the sigmoid colon.*

BLOOD VESSELS, LYMPHATICS, & NERVES

Arteries

The various portions of the ureter are supplied almost in a segmental fashion, so that there is usually little arterial anastomosis between the vessels supplying the individual segments. The abdominal ureter receives its blood from the lowest branches of the renal artery. The pelvic ureter receives blood from the testicular or ovarian artery and occasionally from an inconstant ureteric branch of the common iliac or renal artery. The intravesical ureter receives blood from the uterine or inferior vesical artery and from the middle rectal artery. An occasionally significant amount of blood is supplied to the ureter by vessels in the areolar tissue in which it lies.

➠ **Ureteral rupture following radical hysterectomy with pelvic node dissection.** *Delayed rupture of the ureter may follow radical hysterectomy for cancer (Wertheim procedure) if a segment of ureter is deprived of its blood supply. The denuded ureteral segment becomes gangrenous and leaks or ruptures 7–10 days following surgery, often resulting in a urinary fistula.*

Veins

Venous return from the ureters drains into the inferior vena cava by means of veins that parallel the ureteral arterial supply.

Lymphatics

Lymphatic drainage from the ureters is into the regional lumbar and pelvic nodes.

Nerves

The nerves to the ureters are derived from inferior mesenteric, testicular or ovarian, and hypogastric plexuses.

III. SUPRARENAL (ADRENAL) GLANDS

The suprarenal (adrenal) glands are 2 brownish yellow organs that lie in the retroperitoneum in close relationship to the medial superior pole of each kidney. They are endocrine organs. The cortex produces steroid hormones, and the medulla produces epinephrine and norepinephrine. (Fig 35–12.)

EMBRYOLOGY

Cortex

The cortex of the gland is derived from mesoderm and appears during the sixth fetal week as a groove in the coelom near the superior end of the mesonephros. Cells at the base of the groove grow rapidly and move toward the aorta. Cortical tissue then divides into 2 zones: an outer zone of undifferentiated cells and an inner layer of well-differentiated cells. Soon after birth, the inner zone disappears and the outer zone divides into the 3 layers of the postfetal gland. The zona glomerulosa and the zona fasciculata are present at birth, whereas the zona reticularis does not form until early in the fourth year.

Medulla

The medulla of the gland develops from cells of the neural crest (neuroectoderm), which move ventrally along with the cells of the adjacent sympathetic ganglia. During the seventh fetal week, a group of neural cells grow into the cortical area and are encapsulated by the fetal cortex to form the medulla of the suprarenal gland. These cells are of sympathetic ganglion origin and are called the chromaffin cells of the suprarenal medulla.

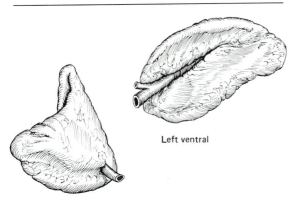

Left ventral

Right ventral

Figure 35–12. The suprarenal (adrenal) glands.

Anomalies

Hyperplasia of the fetal adrenal cortex can result in female pseudohermaphroditism. Congenital hypoplasia of the cortex may also occur. Accessory glands are found in the connective tissue adjacent to the gland or in paravertebral locations in the abdomen—and occasionally related to the testis or ovary.

➠ *Hyperplasia of the suprarenal cortex. The suprarenal cortex may be the site of hyperplasia that causes excessive adrenocortical secretion and leads to Cushing's syndrome. The disorder usually involves both suprarenal glands and is best treated by bilateral suprarenalectomy.*

➠ *Pheochromocytoma. Pheochromocytoma, a tumor of the suprarenal medullary tissue, causes severe hypertension plus diverse other symptoms resulting from excessive secretion of epinephrine. This can be alleviated by removal of the involved suprarenal gland. About 10% of such tumors are bilateral.*

GROSS ANATOMY (Fig 35–13)

The suprarenal glands are 3–5 cm long, 3 cm wide, and about 10 mm thick. Their concave deep surface fits snugly against the upper pole of the kidney. The right gland is roughly pyramidal; the left gland is usually larger and more superior and is crescent-shaped. The normal combined weight of the 2 glands is 7–20 g. The relationship of the right and left suprarenal glands to adjacent structures differs significantly.

The suprarenal glands are surrounded by fatty areolar tissue and are invested by tight fibrous capsules. The glands are separated from the kidneys by fusion of the leaves of the ventral and dorsal perirenal fascia at the upper poles of the kidneys.

Multiple small accessory suprarenal glands are often found in the areolar tissue surrounding the glands. Accessory cortical tissue is most often found close to the kidney and along the path taken by the gonads during their embryonic descent. Accessory medullary (chromaffin) tissue is most often located in the posterior portion of the abdominal cavity near the sympathetic ganglia or along the abdominal aorta.

➠ *Routes of surgical approach to the suprarenal glands. The suprarenal glands may be explored and removed by a posterolateral extraperitoneal or transperitoneal approach. The transperitoneal approach is preferred for the following reasons: (1) It allows exploration of both*

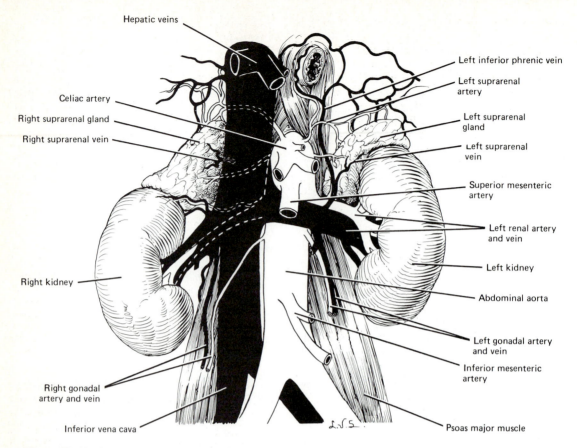

Figure 35–13. Anatomy of the kidney and the suprarenal glands, showing arterial supply and venous return.

suprarenal glands (12% of suprarenal gland tumors are bilateral); (2) it permits a more thorough search for possible ectopic suprarenal tissue (along the lumbar sympathetic trunks or in sympathetic nerve plexuses in the abdomen or in locations close to the testis or ovary); and (3) it provides better exposure for operating on a lateral tumor of the gland.

➠ **Suprarenal cortical and medullary tumors.** Tumors of the suprarenal cortex and medulla may be either secretory or nonsecretory. If they are large, they may displace the kidney inferiorly, and in rare cases the tumor itself may be palpable in the abdomen. Air injected into the retroperitoneal space formerly was used as a method of localization of these tumors, but angiography, ultrasonography, and CT scanning are now of much greater importance in diagnosis.

➠ **Bilateral suprarenalectomy for advanced carcinoma of the breast.** Bilateral adrenalectomy is occasionally performed for temporary palliation of carcinoma of the breast in both men and women. It is also used occasionally for

the purpose of slowing down tumor growth in men with advanced carcinoma of the prostate. In general, the best results after bilateral adrenalectomy are achieved in patients who have responded well to endocrine therapy, particularly castration.

➠ **Cysts of the suprarenal glands.** Suprarenal cysts may displace the kidney inferiorly and must be considered in the differential diagnosis of adrenal tumors. It is important to determine whether cysts are benign or malignant, since benign cysts do not require surgical excision unless they compress the gland. The cysts have no endocrinologic function. A thin line of calcification just deep to the capsule of the cyst is frequently seen on x-ray examination.

➠ **Suprarenal calcification as a diagnostic aid.** Punctate suprarenal calcification on a plain film of the abdomen suggests tuberculosis or a calcium-producing neuroblastoma. Suprarenal calcification may follow spontaneous hemorrhage into the gland and may be present in benign suprarenal cysts.

RIGHT SUPRARENAL GLAND

The right suprarenal gland is pyramidal in shape and lies dorsal to the inferior vena cava and the right lobe of the liver and ventral to the upper pole of the right kidney and to the right leaf of the diaphragm. A lateral segment of its ventral surface is in contact with the bare area of the liver. Just inferior to the apex of the ventral surface of the right suprarenal gland, the short right suprarenal vein emerges to run to the inferior vena cava. The superior segment of the dorsal surface is attached to and rests against the diaphragm; the inferior segments rest against the ventral surface of the right kidney.

➡ *Surgery involving the right suprarenal gland. The right suprarenal gland is usually more difficult to explore and remove than the left gland because of its close proximity to the right lobe of the liver. The adjoining inferior vena cava may be lacerated during removal of the right suprarenal gland because the short right suprarenal vein cannot be properly exposed until the gland itself has been mobilized. Likewise, the right suprarenal vein itself, only 6–8 mm long, may be accidentally torn during the procedure.*

LEFT SUPRARENAL GLAND

The left suprarenal gland is crescent-shaped; its concave surface is attached to the upper pole of the left kidney, and the gland extends almost to the renal hilum. The superior segment of the ventral surface is covered by the peritoneum of the omental bursa, which separates the left suprarenal gland from the cardia of the stomach and from the upper pole of the spleen. The inferior portion of the ventral surface is in contact with the pancreas and the splenic artery and is not covered with peritoneum. The relatively long left suprarenal vein emerges from the most inferior segment of the ventral surface of the gland. The dorsal surface of the left suprarenal gland rests medially upon the left crus of the diaphragm and laterally upon the left kidney.

BLOOD VESSELS, LYMPHATICS, & NERVES
(Fig 35–13)

Arteries

The suprarenal glands are supplied by at least 3 arteries of substantial size. The superior suprarenal artery is a branch of the inferior phrenic artery. The middle suprarenal artery branches directly from the abdominal aorta. The inferior suprarenal artery is derived from the renal artery. All 3 vessels usually divide into small branches before they enter the capsule of the suprarenal gland.

Veins

Only one major vein (the central suprarenal vein) issues from the hilum of the suprarenal gland. The right suprarenal vein runs a very short transverse course medially before emptying directly into the inferior vena cava. The left suprarenal vein is longer and courses across the surface of the gland before joining the left inferior phrenic vein, which empties into the left renal vein. Occasionally, the left suprarenal vein empties directly into the left renal vein.

Lymphatics

Lymph drainage from the suprarenal glands originates in 2 plexuses, one in the periphery of the cortex and the other lying within the suprarenal medulla. The efferent lymphatic flow from both areas is along the course of the suprarenal veins, which takes it to the highest nodes of the lumbar chain. These connect with the lowest posterior mediastinal nodes just above the diaphragm.

Nerves

The nerves that supply the suprarenal glands are mostly preganglionic sympathetic fibers. They are derived from all 3 of the splanchnic nerves that pass to the suprarenal glands from the celiac and aorticorenal ganglia.

The nerves pass through the cortex without innervating it and terminate in the medulla.

GROSS ANATOMY

The pelvis is the most inferior part of the abdominal cavity. It is angled about 10 degrees dorsally from the upper and mid portions of the abdominal cavity. The pelvis is enclosed by bony, ligamentous, and muscular walls that divide the area. The **false pelvis** is a direct continuation of the lower abdomen and is contained by the iliac fossae and the upper sacral vertebrae. The **true pelvis** lies below a boundary formed ventrally by the superior borders of the pubic bones and by the pectineal line of the pubis, laterally by the arcuate line of the ilium, and posteriorly by the sacral promontory. The true pelvis is separated from the perineum by the fasciomuscular, urogenital, and levator diaphragms.

The pelvis contains the urinary bladder, the terminal portions of the ureters, the pelvic male or female genital organs, the rectosigmoid, the upper and mid rectum, coils of small intestine, and the blood vessels, lymphatics, and nerves that supply and drain the pelvic and perineal muscles and viscera.

BONY & LIGAMENTOUS STRUCTURES OF THE TRUE PELVIS
(Figs 36−1, 36−2, & 36−3)

The true bony pelvis is bounded dorsally by the sacral and coccygeal vertebral column, laterally by the 2 innominate bones, and ventrally by the 2 pubic rami and the pubic symphysis. The outlet of the bony pelvis is bounded dorsally by the tip of the coccyx, laterally by the ischial tuberosities, and ventrolaterally by the inferior surfaces of the ischiopubic arch.

Dorsally, the space between the ischial tuberosities and the sacrum and the coccyx is partially filled by the sacrotuberous and sacrospinous ligaments. The sacrotuberous ligament passes from the posterosuperior iliac spine and the adjacent areas of the sacrum and coccyx and inserts into the ischial tuberosity. The sacrospinous ligament passes from the ventrolateral border of the lower sacrum and the coccyx and inserts into the ischial spine. The sacrospinous ligament lies medial and inferior to the sacrotuberous

ligament. These 2 ligaments, in their oblique course, almost completely fill the posterior bony notch of the pelvic outlet. They convert the sciatic notches into the greater and lesser sciatic foramens.

The greater sciatic foramen is bounded by the iliac bone laterally and by the sacrotuberous and sacrospinous ligaments medially and inferiorly. The **piriformis muscle** leaves the pelvis through the greater sciatic foramen. Superior to the piriformis muscle, the superior gluteal vessels and nerve leave the pelvis. Inferior to the piriformis muscle, the inferior gluteal vessels and nerve, the internal pudendal vessels and pudendal nerve, the sciatic nerve, the posterior femoral cutaneous nerve, and the nerves to the quadratus femoris and obturator internus muscles all issue from the pelvis.

The lesser sciatic foramen is enclosed by the ischial tuberosity and the ischial spine laterally and by the sacrospinous and sacrotuberous ligaments medially and inferiorly. Through it the obturator internus tendon and the nerve to the obturator internus leave the pelvis, while the internal pudendal vessels and the pudendal nerve, which have left the pelvis through the greater sciatic foramen, enter the perineum through the lesser sciatic foramen after winding around the ischial spine. The lesser sciatic foramen is about one-fifth as large as the greater sciatic foramen (Fig 36−2).

THE FEMALE PELVIS

The female pelvis differs from the male pelvis in that it is shallower and its bones generally more delicate. The greater lateral bony flare of the female hips is due to lateral projection of the ilium near the anterosuperior iliac spine. The entrance into the true pelvis is wider and more nearly circular in the female. The inferior (true) pelvic aperture in the female is wider, and the female coccyx is more loosely articulated. The ischial spines are smaller and protrude less toward the midline than in the male, thus creating a wider pelvic outlet. The ischial tuberosities and consequently the acetabula are farther apart in the female. The angle of the pubic arch is more obtuse and the intrapubic space more rounded than in the male. These anatomic features of the female pelvis facilitate parturition.

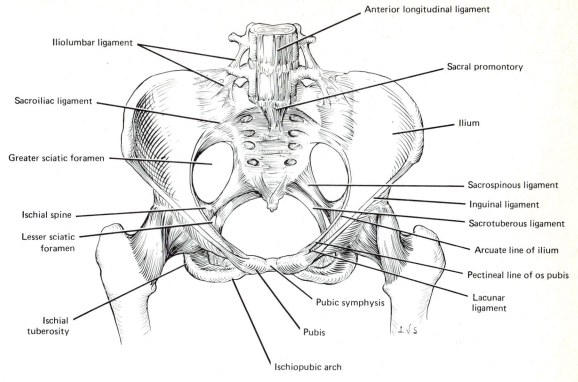

Figure 36–1. The bony pelvis (anterior view).

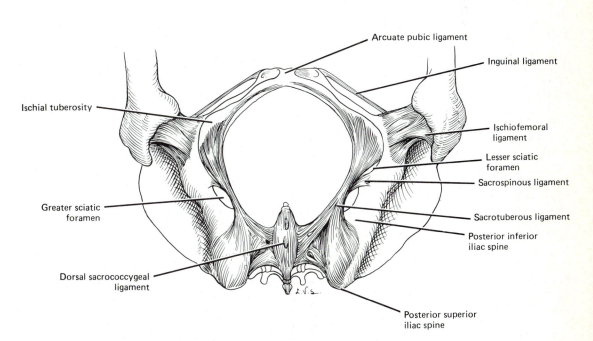

Figure 36–2. The bony pelvis (inferior view).

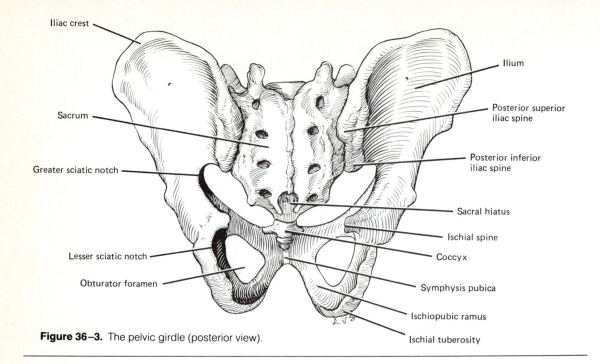

Figure 36–3. The pelvic girdle (posterior view).

Labels (clockwise from top left): Iliac crest, Ilium, Posterior superior iliac spine, Posterior inferior iliac spine, Sacral hiatus, Ischial spine, Coccyx, Symphysis pubica, Ischiopubic ramus, Ischial tuberosity, Obturator foramen, Lesser sciatic notch, Greater sciatic notch, Sacrum, Iliac crest.

THE HIP BONES
(Fig 36–4)

The bony pelvic ring, which marks the superior entrance into the true pelvis, is formed by the 2 large iliopubic bones, which join ventrally at the pubic symphysis and dorsally with the sacrum via the sacroiliac joints. The bony ring thus formed serves to transmit the weight of the body from the torso to the lower limbs. Each hip bone is the amalgamation of 3 separate bones: the ilium, the ischium, and the os pubis. The 3 bones unite laterally and inferiorly to form the acetabulum of the hip joint.

➤ *Fractures of the bony pelvic ring. Fractures of the bony pelvic ring may follow direct trauma to the pelvic bones or may be caused by forces transmitted to the pelvic bones from the lower extremities. The pelvic ring usually fractures at one of 2 areas: (1) close to the symphysis pubica or through the pubic rami; or (2) through the obturator foramen or the acetabulum. A fracture of the pelvic ring can result in concomitant dislocation of the sacroiliac joint. Pelvic fractures may be accompanied by severe pelvic soft tissue damage and hemorrhage and by injury to the intrapelvic organs.*

The Ilium

The ilium is the superior fan-shaped segment of the hip bone, the apex of the fan externally forming the superior arch of the acetabulum. The ilium is grossly divided into an inferior body and a superior ala, the division being marked externally by the acetabulum and internally by the arcuate line. The external surface of the body of the ilium contributes about two-fifths of the circumference of the acetabulum; its internal surface forms a portion of the lateral wall of the pelvis. The inner surface of the body is the site of origin of some of the fibers of the obturator internus muscle.

The ala of the ilium forms the superior portion of the bone. It slants obliquely, and its inner surface forms the internal lateral boundary of the false pelvis; the external surface is convex, and to it attach the 3 gluteal muscles. The internal surface of the ala presents a concavity, the iliac fossa, which is occupied by the iliacus muscle. The dorsomedial segment of the inner surface of the ilium presents a roughened area, which is covered anteriorly with cartilage and articulates with the lateral surface of the sacrum. The crest terminates anteriorly in the anterosuperior iliac spine (the upper anchor of the inguinal ligament) and dorsally at the posterosuperior iliac spine. The iliac crest is thinner centrally than at its anterior and posterior terminations; one can usually palpate the iliac crest along its entire length. The dorsal border of the ala presents a posterosuperior and a posteroinferior spinous process. Just below the latter lies the greater sciatic notch.

The Acetabulum

The acetabulum, the socket with which the ball-like head of the femur articulates, is the area of junction of the os pubis, ischium, and ilium. The acetabulum has a thick, uneven bony rim to which the acetabu-

Figure 36—4. The right hip bone (lateral view), showing the acetabulum.

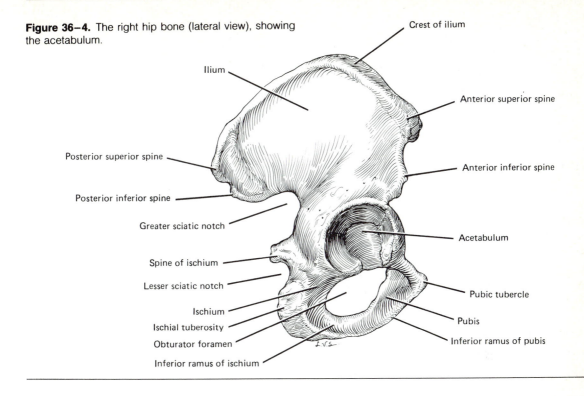

lar labrum is attached. The labrum serves to narrow the acetabular circumference and to deepen its articular surface. Inferiorly, the rim is deeply notched, has no covering of labrum, and is bridged by the transverse acetabular ligament. This creates a passageway deep to the ligament for the entrance of arteries and nerves. The ligamentum teres, attached to the fovea of the femoral head, articulates with the edges of the acetabular notch via 2 strong fibrous bands.

➧ *Fractures of the acetabulum. Fractures of the acetabulum with central dislocation of the head of the femur frequently cause disruption of the urinary bladder or urethra. A careful diagnostic bladder and urethral workup should always follow the diagnosis of such a fracture, so that urinary leakage can be promptly controlled.*

The Ischium

The ischium is roughly V-shaped, the blunt point of the V being the ischial tuberosity, which bears the weight of the body in the sitting position. The body of the ischium contributes to about two-fifths of the **acetabulum.** On the posteromedial surface of the ischial body is the ischial spine, to which attaches the sacrospinous ligament. From the inner surface of the ischial spine arise portions of the levatores ani and coccygeus muscles. At the pelvic outlet, the 2 ischial spines face each other; this is the narrowest space between the 2 ischial surfaces. Just superior to the ischial spine lies the greater sciatic foramen;

inferior to it lies the lesser sciatic foramen. The inner (pelvic) surface of the body of the ischium forms a portion of the bony wall of the true pelvis. This same segment of the ischium also forms the inferior border of the obturator foramen. The ramus of the ischium joins the inferior ramus of the os pubis, the combined rami forming the ischiopubic ramus. To the inner surface of the ischiopubic ramus attaches the most lateral expansion of the inferior fascia of the urogenital diaphragm (Colles). Farther dorsally on the ischiopubic ramus is the attachment of the superficial transverse perineal muscle. The crus of the penis in the male and the crus of the clitoris in the female attach to the inner surface of the ischiopubic ramus. Along the superior border of the ischial ramus is the attachment of the obturator membrane.

The Obturator Foramen (Fig 36—4)

The obturator foramen is a large, roughly circular lateral aperture situated between the ischium and the os pubis. The foramen is larger in males than in females. It is almost completely filled in by the obturator membrane, which is attached to the bony margins except superiorly, where there is an aperture through which the obturator vessels and nerves pass from pelvis to thigh.

The Os Pubis

The 2 pubic bones join ventrally in the midline via the symphysis pubica and form the pubic arch. The body of the pubic bone articulates medially at the symphysis pubica with the contralateral pubic body. The pelvic surface of the pubic body is smooth and in close approximation to the retropubic fat pad and the surface of the bladder. The lateral portion of the body of the os pubis forms the medial border of the obturator foramen. The superior portion of the body of the pubic bone is called the pubic crest, while its lateral boundary is marked by the pubic tubercle, into which the inguinal ligament inserts. The pubic tubercle is easily palpable in most males but difficult to palpate in females because of its smaller size and the presence of the fatty mons pubis. The superior ramus of the os pubis broadens to fuse with the ilium and the ischium to complete the acetabular cup. The pubic bone forms about one-fifth of the acetabulum. On the inner superior border of the superior pubic ramus is a sharp projecting edge called the pectineal line, which marks the anterolateral superior border of the true pelvis. The inferior pubic ramus joins the ischial ramus along the border of the obturator foramen; it is thinner than the superior ramus and is somewhat flattened.

The Sacrum
(Fig 36–5)

The sacrum is a massive triangular bone formed by the fusion of the 5 sacral vertebrae. Its superior base inclines ventrally; its mid segment projects dorsally. The bone forms the greater portion of the dorsal surface of the true pelvic cavity; it presents a smooth concave ventral surface and a roughened convex dorsal surface. The sacrum is widened laterally by the transverse processes and the costal appendages of the individual sacral vertebrae. The ventral surface presents 4 transverse ridges, each of which terminates laterally in a sacral foramen through which issue the ventral rami of the sacral nerves and the sacral vessels. The anterior surface of the first sacral vertebra, which resembles a lumbar vertebra, protrudes into the pelvic cavity at the true pelvic brim, considerably narrowing the true pelvic entrance. A midline dorsal projection— the middle sacral crest—is formed by the spinous processes of the upper 3 sacral vertebrae. S5 shows no fusion of its 2 laminae. Consequently, an opening—the sacral hiatus—leads into the sacral canal. Placed laterally on the dorsal sacral surface are 4 dorsal sacral foramens through which pass the dorsal divisions of the sacral nerves. The terminal end of the vertebral canal is lodged in the sacrum. The sacral hiatus sits at the end of the canal at about S5, and through its wide opening (no laminal fusion) caudal anesthesia is introduced.

➡ *Fractures of the sacrum. Fractures of the sacrum may occur as a result of direct violence. Sacral fractures often accompany fractures of the other pelvic bones. Most sacral fractures are linear and not displaced. Ventral displacement of sacral fractures may cause injury to the sacral nerve trunks; however, this complication is rare.*

The Coccyx
(Fig 36–5)

The coccyx consists of the 4 terminal spinal segments, which present either as articulated segments or as the fused caudal end of the bony spine. The coccyx is the lower dorsal border of the pelvis. The pelvic surface of the coccyx is concave, the dorsal surface convex. The coccyx articulates superiorly with the sacrum. To the ventral surface of its inferior 2 segments attaches the pubococcygeal portion of the levatores ani muscle diaphragm.

➡ *Fractures of the coccyx. Fractures of the coccyx usually follow a fall on the buttocks. Pain may be severe, and the disability may last many weeks. Only in the case of unusually slow healing or repeated painful fractures should coccygectomy be considered.*

PELVIC JOINTS
(Fig 36–6)

The bones of the bony pelvis articulate by means of the sacroiliac joint, the symphysis pubica, the lumbosacral joint, and the sacrococcygeal joint. These joints sacrifice mobility in order to preserve pelvic stability during transfer of body weight from the trunk to the pelvic girdle.

➡ *Pelvic joints are seldom dislocated. Because of the great strength of their surrounding ligaments and musculature, the pelvic joints can be dislocated only by a tremendous direct force. The bony portions of the adjacent pelvic rim, particularly the pubic rami, usually fracture instead.*

The Sacroiliac Joint

The sacroiliac joint connects the sacrum and the iliac bone. In children, the joint is a synchondrosis in which the articular surface of each bone is covered with thin cartilage and the surfaces are in close apposition. In later life, the joint usually remains a synchondrosis, but the 2 bones are occasionally separated by a space containing synovial fluid to form a gliding joint supported by the ventral and dorsal sacroiliac ligaments.

The Lumbosacral Joint

This articulation connects L5 with the sacrum. The joint is supported by (1) the anterior and posterior longitudinal ligaments of the vertebral column; (2) the intervertebral disk between L5 and S1; (2) the ligamentum flavum, which connects the lamina of L5 with the lamina of S1; (4) the capsules around the articular processes of the 2 vertebrae; and (5) the interspinal and supraspinal ligaments. The iliolum-

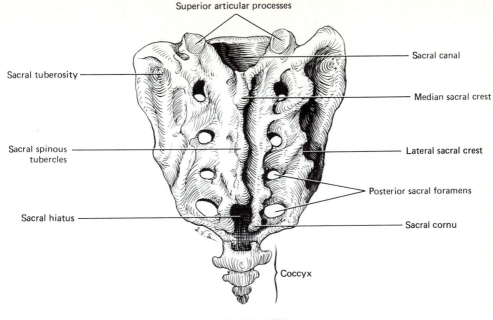

POSTERIOR VIEW

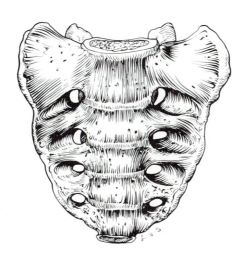

ANTERIOR VIEW

Figure 36–5. The sacrum (posterior and anterior views) and coccyx.

bar ligament between the transverse process of L5 and the pelvis helps to support the joint.

➡ ***Spondylolisthesis of L5.*** *Anterior movement (spondylolisthesis) of L5 upon S1 causes severe lower back pain that may require operation.*

The Pubic Symphysis

The symphysis pubica allows for only a slight degree of movement between the 2 oval articular surfaces of the bones. The joint is supported superiorly by the pubic ligament, which extends to connect the pubic tubercles, and inferiorly by a strong fibrous band, the arcuate pubic ligament, which forms the pubic arch. The inferior free border of the arcuate ligament does not reach the superior fascia of the urogenital diaphragm, leaving an aperture through which, in the male, the deep vein of the penis passes into the pelvis. The articular surfaces of the 2 pubic bones are separated by a fibrocartilaginous disk.

➡ ***Softening of symphysis pubica in pregnancy.*** *In females, the symphysis pubica, along with*

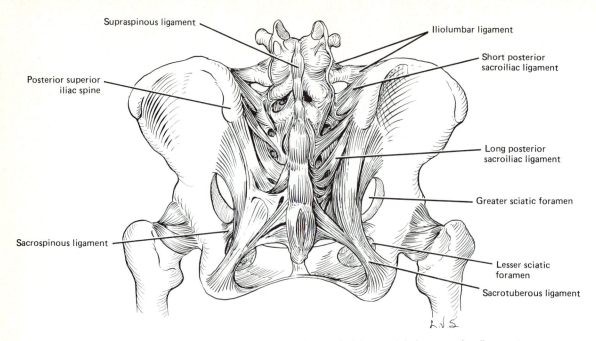

Figure 36–6. The bony pelvis, showing the posterior pelvic joints and their supporting ligaments.

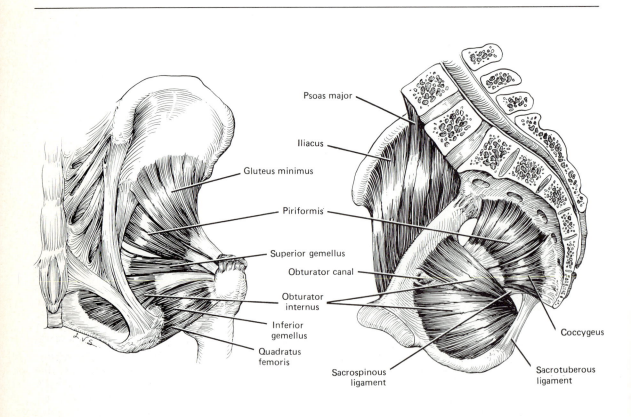

RIGHT POSTERIOR

RIGHT MEDIAL

Figure 36–7. The pelvic musculature.

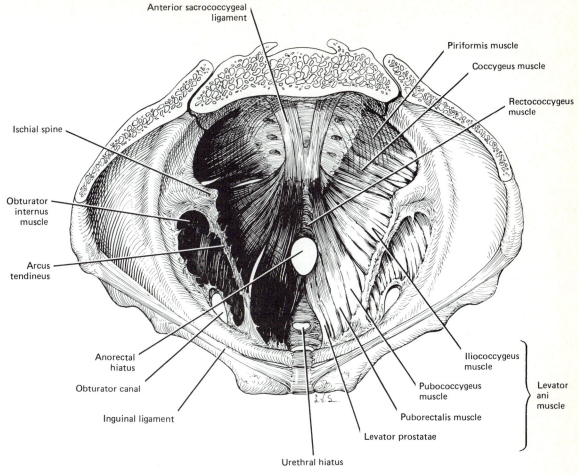

Figure 36–8. The male pelvic diaphragm (from above).

the sacroiliac joint and the sacrotuberous, sacrospinous, and inguinal ligaments, undergoes softening that tends to increase the pelvic diameters, making parturition easier.

MUSCULATURE OF THE PELVIS
(Figs 36–7 and 36–8)

The Iliacus Muscle & Psoas Major Muscle

The iliacus fills the entire cavity of the iliac fossa. It arises from the upper two-thirds of the fossa, from the iliac crest, and from the sacroiliac and iliolumbar ligaments. It joins with the tendon of the psoas major just before that muscle passes beneath the inguinal ligament to insert into the lesser trochanter of the femur. The iliacus and underlying iliac bone form most of the lateral wall of the false pelvis. The iliacus is innervated by branches from the femoral nerve (L2, 3). The muscle assists in flexing the thigh upon the abdomen and in medial rotation of the thigh.

The Obturator Internus Muscle & the Piriformis Muscle

The **obturator internus,** a fan-shaped muscle, arises from the pelvic surface of the superior and inferior pubic rami, the ramus of the ischium, and the pelvic surfaces of the obturator membrane and the obturator fascia. Its fibers pass dorsally to the lesser sciatic foramen and terminate in 5 tendinous bands. The bands turn at 90 degrees around the space between the ischial spine and the ischial tuberosity and leave the pelvis through the lesser sciatic foramen. The composite tendon of the muscle formed from the junction of the 5 bands passes across the capsule of the hip joint and inserts on the greater trochanter of the femur near the attachments of the 2 gemelli muscles. The obturator internus is supplied by the nerve to the obturator internus (L5, S1) from the sacral plexus (L4, 5). The muscle rotates the thigh laterally, and when the thigh is flexed, the obturator internus extends and abducts it.

The **piriformis** is a triangular muscle that arises from the ventrolateral surfaces of S2–4, passes laterally, and leaves the pelvis through the greater sciatic foramen. It inserts into the greater trochanter of the femur after traversing the dorsal surface of the hip joint. It externally rotates and abducts the thigh and is supplied by nerve branches from S1 and S2.

The Levatores Ani Muscles

The levatores ani and coccygeus are paired muscles which together form the pelvic diaphragm that separates the pelvis from the perineum. They give elasticity to most of the pelvic floor and support to the pelvic viscera. The levatores ani maintain the functionally correct anorectal angle and lift and contract the terminal rectum and anal canal during defecation. The 2 levatores ani muscles also assist in voluntary control of the anal sphincter apparatus and in completion of the act of defecation (Figs 36–8 and 36–9).

➡ *Disruptions of the pelvic diaphragm after pelvic fractures. Disruptions of the fascia and musculature of the urogenital and levatores ani pelvic diaphragms may accompany pelvic fractures.*

Each levator ani muscle arises ventrally from the superior ramus of the pubic bone. Laterally and dorsally, the 2 muscles arise from the pelvic surface of the obturator fascia. The origin of the obturator fascia is along a line that runs obliquely from the pubic ramus to the ischial spine. The most dorsal fibers of origin of the levatores ani arise from the ischial spine. Generally, the levatores ani muscle fibers pass dorsally, caudally, and medially to form the "pelvic hammock." The levatores ani may be morphologically divided into pubococcygeal and iliococcygeal fibers.

The **pubococcygeal fibers,** the most ventral fibers of origin of the levatores ani, are separated from the opposite fibers by the narrow genital hiatus (levator cleft) that allows the urethra and vagina in the female and the urethra in the male to pass from pelvis to perineum (Fig 36–8). The hiatus is filled by the muscles and fascia of the urogenital diaphragm. In the male, the pubococcygeal fibers insert into the periprostatic capsule (the puboprostatic levator fibers). Comparable fibers in the female encircle the vaginal walls and are called the sphincter vaginae levator fibers. Dorsal to the prostate in the male and the vagina in the female, the pubococcygeal levator ani fibers insert into a midline fibrous structure, the perineal body, where they interdigitate with fibers of the external sphincter ani and fibers of the superficial and deep transverse perineal muscles. Dorsal to the perineal body, the continuing pubococcygeal fibers encircle the walls of the anal canal at the level of the highest fibers of the external sphincter ani and interdigitate with these fibers. Finally, the most dorsal

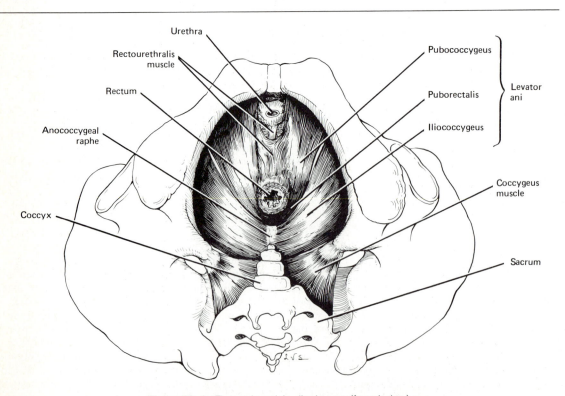

Figure 36–9. The male pelvic diaphragm (from below).

of the pubococcygeal fibers insert into the terminal 2 segments of the coccyx.

The levator ani fibers that originate from the oblique line on the obturator fascia and from the ischial spine are called the **iliococcygeal fibers.** They insert into the coccyx and unite in the midline to form the anococcygeal muscular raphe. As the iliococcygeal fibers pass around the lower rectum and anus, they blend with the longitudinal musculature of the rectal wall (Fig 36–9).

The Coccygeus Muscle

The fibers of the levatores ani muscles, which arise from the ischial spine, insert in the anococcygeal muscular raphe and into the coccyx and the terminal segment of the sacrum. These fibers constitute the paired coccygeal muscles.

The many sites of origin of the levatores ani muscles and the direction of their fibers as they run to the sites of insertion give to the levatores ani complex a hammocklike shape that is concave toward the pelvis and convex toward the perineum. The most ventral portion of the sling is open, and the gap is filled by the urogenital diaphragm. As the rectum passes through the levator diaphragm from pelvis to perineum, the levator fibers grasp the rectum tightly as a result of their attachment to the longitudinal rectal musculature. Some longitudinal smooth muscle fibers leave the rectal wall to run on the superior surfaces of the levatores ani. Dorsally, this strip of rectal longitudinal muscle fibers connects the rectum to the tip of the coccyx (rectococcygeal muscle). Ventrally, these fibers attach to the bulb of the urethra (rectourethralis muscle) in the male and to the lower posterior vaginal wall in the female. The rectourethralis muscle fibers maintain the 90-degree angle of the rectum as it passes through the levator diaphragm toward the anus.

➠ *Section of the rectourethralis fibers of the levatores ani muscles. In perineal prostatectomy or abdominoperineal resection of the rectum, the rectourethralis fibers running on the superior surfaces of the levatores ani muscles must be sectioned so that the rectum can be retracted dorsally, away from the vagina and urethra in the female and the prostate in the male— all of which lie in the urogenital perineum.*

The superior fascia of the levatores ani muscles is derived from the endopelvic fascia. This fascia lies just inferior to the extraperitoneal cellular tissue of the pelvis, which is rich in lymphatics, lymph nodes, and large venous plexuses. The inferior fascia of the levatores ani is derived from the parietal fascia of the perineum. Consequently, the muscle fibers of the levator complex and of the urogenital diaphragm serve as an anatomic division between pelvis and perineum (urogenital diaphragm, discussed in Chapter

38). The levatores ani are supplied by branches from the pudendal nerve plexus.

THE FASCIA & LIGAMENTS OF THE PELVIS (Fig 36–10)

Endopelvic Fascia

The endopelvic fascia is a segment of the great lining fascia of the abdominal cavity; it is continuous with the transversalis, lumbar, iliacus, and subdiaphragmatic fasciae. The fascia covering the iliopsoas muscle is called the iliopsoas of iliacus fascia. In the true pelvis, the endopelvic lining fascia is divided into the parietal fascia, the fascia of the outlet diaphragm, and the fascia of the pelvic viscera.

The **parietal fascia** (piriformis and obturator fascia) covers the piriformis and obturator internus muscles. It also attaches to the ligaments and bones of the pelvic outlet and is continuous superiorly with the iliopsoas fascia and the transversalis fascia.

The **fascia of the pelvic outlet diaphragm** covers the superior surfaces of the levatores ani and the coccygeus and the deep transverse perineal muscle and the sphincter of the membranous urethra (and sphincter vaginae in the female).

The **visceral fascia** is derived from the superior layer of the fascia of the levator and urogenital diaphragms and is reflected from the muscle complexes onto the various pelvic viscera, blending with their outer muscular coats and forming their muscular sheaths.

Ligaments

The ligaments of the pelvis are formed as a result of thickenings of the endopelvic fascia and the extraperitoneal fatty and areolar tissues, which, in conjunction with septa from the endopelvic fascia, form fibrous stalks that are reflected about the nerves and vessels running to the pelvic viscera.

➠ *Pelvic ligaments in surgery. Knowing the location of the pelvic ligaments is of great importance during mobilization of the pelvic organs in pelvic surgery.*

The **rectal stalks** pass from the posterolateral pelvic walls to the lateral rectal walls. (See Chapter 29.)

➠ *Lateral rectal stalks in rectal resection. The lateral rectal stalks must be identified and severed to properly mobilize the pelvic segment of the rectum during abdominoperineal or anterior resection of the rectum.*

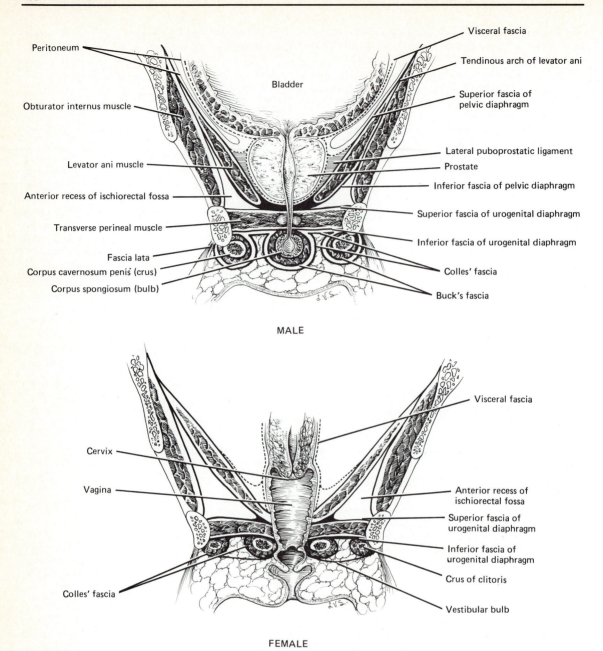

Figure 36–10. Fascia of the pelvis and urogenital region.

The **lateral bladder ligaments** pass from the pubic arches to the lateral bladder walls. They serve to hold the bladder firmly in place in the anterior pelvis.

The **lateral cervical ligaments**—Mackenrodt's ligaments—pass from the lateral pelvic walls to the uterine cervix and the lateral vaginal vaults. They help to maintain the cervix and the upper vagina in the midline of the lower pelvis.

➠ *Lateral cervical ligaments in the reconstruction of pelvic support after hysterectomy. Use*

of the lateral cervical ligaments is of prime importance in the reconstruction of pelvic support after total hysterectomy.

EXTRAPERITONEAL PELVIC SPACE

Pelvic extraperitoneal areolar tissue lies between the pelvic peritoneum and the endopelvic fascia. It contains the common, external, and internal iliac arteries and veins; the pelvic segments of the ureters; the nerves to the pelvic viscera; and the pelvic lymph nodes, both lumbar and iliac. The tissue is extremely vascular because it contains many large venous plexuses (vesical, uterine, prostatic).

⇥ *Cellulitis of the extraperitoneal pelvic areolar tissues. The areolar tissue of the extraperitoneal pelvis becomes the site of pelvic cellulitis, particularly following pelvic organ inflammatory disease in the female and in acute perforated sigmoid diverticulitis in both males and females.*

The Pelvic Peritoneum (Fig 36–11)

The ventral and dorsal layers of parietal peritoneum descend into the true pelvis but do not reach its most inferior limits. The 2 layers are separated from the pelvic outlet by the pelvic viscera, upon which they are reflected, and by the extraperitoneal cellular tissue and the endopelvic fascia. The pelvic viscera are not completely sheathed by peritoneum and lie largely inferior to it. Only portions of their superior and lateral surfaces are covered by the peritoneal layers.

Leaving the ventrolateral abdominal wall, the ventral layer of the parietal peritoneum forms a series of folds and fossae. The peritoneum is reflected from the abdominal wall onto the bladder and forms the so-called ventral and lateral false bladder folds. The ventral parietal peritoneum covers all of the bladder fundus and a small segment of the posterior superior bladder surface before being reflected dorsally onto the ventral and ventrolateral surfaces of the rectum in the male and the ventral surface of the uterus in the female.

The vesicorectal pouch in the male is a shallow depression lined with peritoneum, dorsal to the bladder and ventral to the rectum. Occasionally, the vesicorectal pouch is deeper, and its peritoneum may relate to the surfaces of the seminal vesicles and even to the superior surface of the prostate.

In the female, the peritoneal fossa between the rectum and the bladder divides into an anterior (vesicouterine) fossa and a posterior (uterorectal) fossa. The 2 fossae are formed by the interposition, between bladder and rectum, of the uterus and its supporting broad ligaments. The vesicouterine fossa is relatively shallow and descends only to the anterior surface of the uterine cervix; thus, it is usually not related to the ventral vaginal fornix.

⇥ *Vesicouterine disease. The examining finger placed in the vagina is seldom able to palpate lesions in the anterior or vesicouterine pelvic recess.*

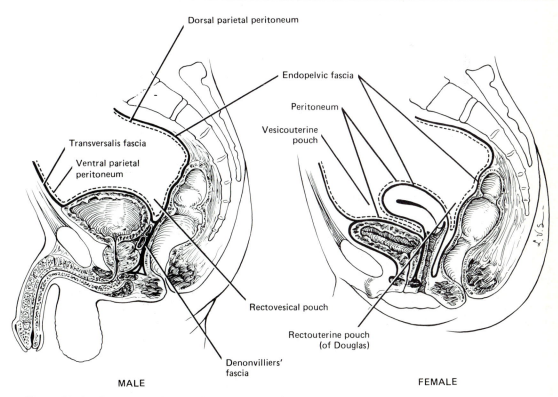

Figure 36–11. Peritoneal reflections in the male and female pelves. (Peritoneum indicated by dotted line.)

The pelvic peritoneum of the rectouterine pouch (pouch of Douglas) covers the posterior vaginal fornix. This relationship makes it easy to palpate structures in the posterior (uterorectal) pelvic recess with a finger inserted into the posterior vaginal fornix. Two thickened peritoneal folds extending from the posteroinferior surfaces of the uterus to the sacrum are called the uterosacral ligaments. The lower segment of the sigmoid colon and many loops of small bowel usually descend deep into the rectouterine space between these 2 ligaments.

➠ **Rectovesical pouch disease in the male.** *When the rectovesical peritoneal pouch descends lower than normal, thus covering the seminal vesicles and the prostate, the peritoneum of the lower reaches of the pouch may be irritated by acute disease of these organs (seminal vesiculitis, acute prostatitis). This may give rise to puzzling signs and symptoms referable to the peritoneal cavity that may be confused with disease of the cecum, appendix, and sigmoid colon.*

The depths of the rectouterine pouch and the rectovesical pouch differ markedly. In early fetal life, in both males and females, the pouches reach almost to the perineal floor. Later, the inferior reaches of each pouch are obliterated by fusion of their ventral and dorsal walls to form the retrovesical fascia. Normally, the rectouterine pouch extends considerably farther caudally than the rectovesical pouch in the male.

➠ **Rectouterine pouch disease.** *Since the rectouterine peritoneal pouch is intimately related to the posterior vaginal fornix, collections of pus, blood, etc, may be palpated and drained, if necessary, via the vagina. On occasion, such collections rupture spontaneously into the vagina or rectum.*

BLOOD VESSELS, LYMPHATICS, & NERVES

Arteries
(Fig 36–12)

At the level of L4, the abdominal aorta divides into the 2 **common iliac arteries.** Each vessel is 5–6 cm long, but the artery on the right side is a bit larger than its mate. Anterior to the sacroiliac joint, the common iliac arteries divide into the external and internal iliac arteries. There are normally no large branches of the common iliac arteries, but they occasionally give off small branches to the overlying peri-

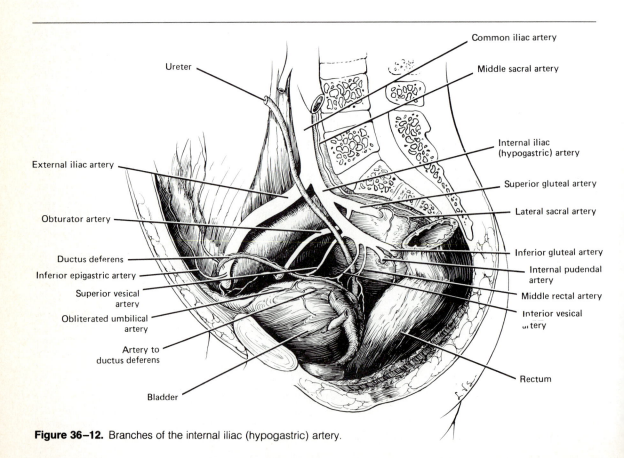

Figure 36–12. Branches of the internal iliac (hypogastric) artery.

toneum, the retroperitoneal areolar tissues, and the mid portions of the ureters.

On the right side of the pelvis, the **right common iliac artery** lies deep to the posterior peritoneum and to some branches of the pelvic sympathetic nerves. Close to its termination, it is crossed by the right ureter. Dorsal to the right common iliac artery is the junction of the 2 common iliac veins and the beginning of the inferior vena cava at the level of L5. These veins lie slightly lateral to the right common iliac artery close to the body of the psoas major muscle.

The ventral relationships of the **left common iliac artery** mirror those of the right common iliac artery. The left common iliac vein lies medial and dorsal to the left common iliac artery. The left common iliac artery is related laterally to the body of the left psoas major muscle.

➠ *Obliterative disease of the iliac arteries. The common, external, and internal iliac arteries and the abdominal aorta are on occasion the site of aneurysmal dilatation. Their lumens may also be completely or partially abolished by arteriosclerotic plaques. Such conditions call for aorticoliac grafts, bypass grafts, or endarterectomy.*

The **external iliac arteries** are usually thicker than the internal iliacs. They run from the point of bifurcation of the common iliac artery to beneath the midpoint of the inguinal ligament and issue onto the anterior surface of the thigh as the femoral arteries. Ventral to the external iliac artery in the pelvis lies the posterior parietal peritoneum, and the terminal ileum and the appendix lie superficial to the artery on the right. On the left, both the sigmoid colon and the ascending arm of its mesentery lie ventral to the artery. In the female, the artery is crossed by the ovarian vessels and occasionally by the ureter. In the male, the testicular vessels and the genital branch of the genitofemoral nerve lie ventral to the artery. The ductus deferens and the round ligament of the uterus are related to the medial surface of the artery. Dorsally, the artery is related to the psoas major muscle.

The 2 major branches of the external iliac artery are the inferior epigastric and the deep iliac circumflex arteries. The inferior epigastric artery arises from the external iliac artery just superior to the inguinal ligament; it runs between the peritoneum and the transversalis fascia to supply the lower anterior abdominal wall. The deep circumflex iliac artery arises from the external iliac artery just opposite the origin of the inferior epigastric artery; it runs to supply the internal oblique and transverse abdominal muscles below the anterosuperior iliac spine.

The **internal iliac artery** is the major vessel supplying the pelvic viscera and the walls of the pelvic cavity. The artery arises as a terminal branch of the common iliac artery just ventral to the sacroiliac joint and runs for 4 cm to terminate at the upper border of the greater sciatic foramen by dividing into ventral and dorsal branches. It lies dorsal to the pelvic ureter and just ventral to the internal iliac vein. The order and sites of takeoff of the branches of the internal iliac artery often vary.

The **posterior division** of the internal iliac artery normally supplies branches to the pelvic parietes. Its branches are (1) the iliolumbar artery, which supplies the iliacus muscle and the ilium; (2) the lateral sacral artery, which supplies the contents of the sacral canal, the piriformis muscle, and the muscles on the dorsal surface of the sacrum; and (3) the superior gluteal artery, which leaves the pelvis through the greater sciatic foramen, superior to the piriformis muscle, to supply all 3 gluteal muscles.

The **anterior division** of the internal iliac artery supplies not only the pelvic and perineal parietes but also the upper thigh and some pelvic viscera. Its branches are the obturator artery and the umbilical artery.

The **obturator artery** runs toward the obturator foramen. It passes through the superior quadrant of the foramen to appear on the anterosuperior thigh, where it divides into an anterior and a posterior branch, which supply the obturator (adductor) muscles. A small branch of the artery reaches the hip joint.

➠ *Fate of the distal segment of the umbilical artery. Following section of the umbilical cord, the distal segment of the umbilical artery running from the bladder to the umbilicus atrophies to become the medial umbilical ligament. The portion of the umbilical artery that persists as an active vessel is called the superior vesical artery. It supplies the superior portion of the bladder. In the male, it gives off a small branch, the artery to the ductus deferens.*

The **inferior vesical artery** arises either from the anterior division of the internal iliac artery or from the middle rectal artery. It runs on the superior surface of the urogenital diaphragm to reach the inferior surface of the bladder. It supplies the bladder's caudal surface and sends some blood to the prostate and seminal vesicles.

After leaving the internal iliac artery, the **uterine artery** runs medially along the superior surface of the levator ani diaphragm and enters the base of the broad ligament to reach the lateral uterine surface in the midcervical area.

The **middle rectal artery** runs medially on the superior surface of the levator ani muscle resting atop its puborectalis fibers, which converge toward the rectum. The vessel is intimately related to the superior fascia of the levator diaphragm; it has ascending and descending terminal branches that anastomose freely on the rectal wall with the superior and inferior rectal arteries.

The **internal pudendal artery** (see Chapter 38) leaves the pelvis and enters the perineum to supply the structures in the superficial perineal pouch and those between the 2 layers of the urogenital diaphragm.

⇒ *Importance of location of middle rectal arteries. Since the middle rectal arteries run on the superior surface of the levatores ani muscles, and since these muscles must be severed during deep pelvic surgery involving the rectum, the vessels must be identified and secured to prevent troublesome postoperative bleeding in the pelvis or perineum.*

The **vaginal artery** may arise either from the internal iliac artery or from the uterine artery. With descending branches of the uterine artery, the vaginal artery descends along the ventral and dorsal surfaces of the vagina, forming a rich arterial plexus.

⇒ *Descending vaginal arteries and surgery on the cervix. The descending vaginal arteries are branches of both the internal iliac and the uterine arteries, and they run on the ventral and dorsal surfaces of the cervix. In order to reduce the amount of bleeding associated with conization or reconstruction of the cervix, it is important to ligate these arteries beforehand.*

Veins
(Fig 36–13)

The **common iliac vein** is formed just ventral to the sacroiliac joint as a result of the junction of the internal and external iliac veins. From there, the common iliac veins run superiorly and at the level of L5 join at an acute angle to form the inferior vena cava. The right common iliac vein runs almost vertically and is shorter than the left vein. The right common iliac vein lies at first lateral and then dorsal to the right common iliac artery. The longer left common iliac vein runs obliquely superiorly and to the right. It lies medial to the left common iliac artery and then dorsal to the right common iliac artery. The

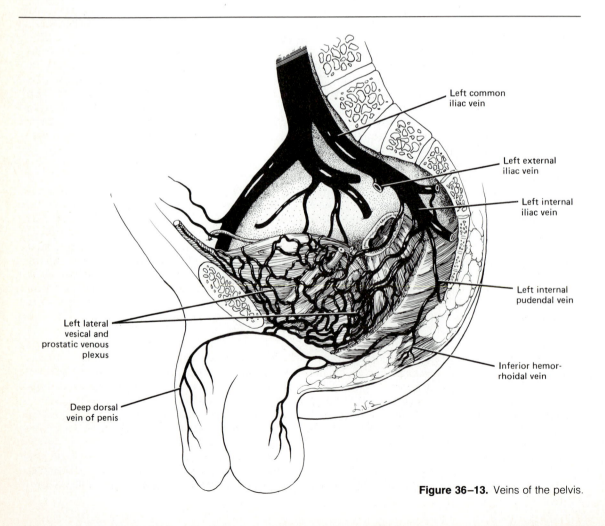

Left common iliac vein

Left external iliac vein

Left internal iliac vein

Left internal pudendal vein

Inferior hemorrhoidal vein

Left lateral vesical and prostatic venous plexus

Deep dorsal vein of penis

Figure 36–13. Veins of the pelvis.

lateral sacral and the iliolumbar veins join with the ipsilateral common iliac vein; the middle sacral vein joins only the left common iliac vein.

➡ *Injuries to common and internal iliac veins in plastic surgery for aneurysm. Because of their close relationship to the lower segment of the abdominal aorta, the common and internal iliac veins are occasionally injured during procedures for aortic aneurysm resection and anastomosis.*

The **internal iliac vein** is formed as a result of the junction of veins draining the areas supplied by the internal iliac artery. It is a wide, short vessel that begins at the upper border of the greater sciatic foramen and runs to the level of the sacroiliac joint. There the vein joins with the external iliac vein to form the common iliac vein. Each internal iliac vein lies medial and slightly dorsal to the internal iliac artery.

The tributaries of the internal iliac veins parallel the branches of the internal iliac artery. They are the superior and inferior gluteal veins, the internal pudendal vein, the obturator vein, the lateral and middle sacral veins, the middle rectal veins, the dorsal vein of the penis, and the vesical, uterine, and vaginal veins.

The **external iliac veins** return blood from the lower extremity and the lower ventrolateral abdominal wall. They begin just superior to the inguinal ligament and continue superiorly, joining the internal iliac vein to form the common iliac vein just ventral to the sacroiliac joint. The right external iliac vein lies first medial and then dorsal to the right external iliac artery. The left external iliac vein lies on the medial side of the left external iliac artery throughout its course. The external iliac veins are fed by the inferior epigastric, the deep circumflex iliac, and the pubic, scrotal, and bulbar veins.

The pelvic viscera are enveloped and supported by the dense endopelvic fascia. Between the layers of fascia and close to such pelvic viscera as the uterus, bladder, prostate, vagina, and rectum are aggregations of large fragile veins. These **venous plexuses of the pelvis** usually communicate with one another before emptying mainly into the internal iliac vein.

➡ *Role of pelvic venous plexuses in pelvic surgery. Because of the presence of the large venous plexuses, which lie close to the pelvic viscera, dissection of the tissues about these viscera may be a bloody procedure.*

➡ *Thrombophlebitis of pelvic venous plexuses. Thrombophlebitis of one or all of the pelvic venous plexuses may follow surgery upon the pelvic or perineal organs or upon the lower extremity. Infected emboli from the pelvic venous plexuses may complicate an existing pelvic disease process. Pelvic thrombophlebitis may be the source of ascending pylephlebitis or may cause an infected embolus to pass to the right heart and lungs via the inferior vena cava. On rare occasions, these emboli reach the liver if their ascending course is via the inferior mesenteric vein, which empties into the portal venous system. Such a route is taken by emboli that occur during infected internal hemorrhoids and diverticulitis of the sigmoid colon.*

Lymphatics
(Fig 36–14)

The external, common, and internal iliac lymph nodes receive most of their lymphatic drainage from the pelvic organs, except for lymph draining from the rectum. The rectal lymphatics proceed superiorly along superior rectal arteries and veins to reach the nodes in the base of the mesentery of the sigmoid colon. The 3 groups of iliac nodes lie in close approximation to the arteries from which they derive their names.

While most lymphatic drainage from pelvic viscera reaches the iliac lymph nodes, some also passes to nodes in the extraperitoneal cellular tissue of the pelvis. These nodes are usually close to the branches of the internal iliac artery. The nodes that drain the walls of the true pelvis are called the gluteal, obturator, sacral, etc, nodes. Lymphatic drainage from the internal and external iliac nodes is carried upward to nodes that lie in close relationship to the abdominal aorta. A small amount of pelvic and perineal lymph finds its way to the supra- and infrainguinal group of nodes.

➡ *Role of lymphatic drainage in surgery for pelvic cancer. Since lymphatic drainage from the pelvis usually reaches the internal and external iliac nodes in the extrapelvic cellular tissues close to the internal and external iliac arteries, any operation for cancer of the pelvic organs must completely strip the pelvic walls of areolar tissue and attempt to eradicate all of the involved iliac nodes. The Wertheim operation is such a procedure.*

Nerves
(Figs 36–15 and 36–16)

The major nerve trunks and plexuses of the pelvis lie close to its lateral and posterior walls and run to the pelvic viscera via the various stalks and ligaments raised from the pelvic peritoneum by the vascular supply to the pelvic organs.

The anterior rami of the **sacral and coccygeal nerves** form the sacral and pudendal plexuses. The anterior rami of S1–4 appear in the pelvis after emerg-

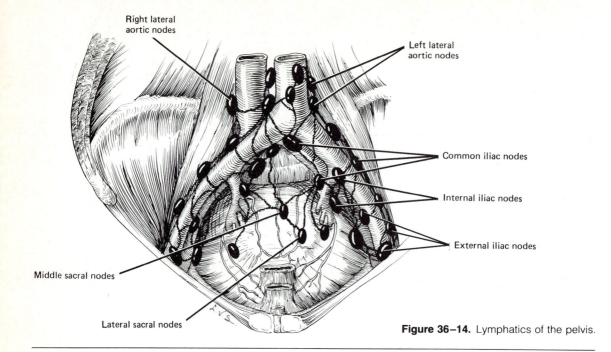

Right lateral
aortic nodes

Left lateral
aortic nodes

Common iliac nodes

Internal iliac nodes

External iliac nodes

Middle sacral nodes

Lateral sacral nodes

Figure 36–14. Lymphatics of the pelvis.

ing from anterior sacral foramens. S1 and S2 are large nerves; S3 and S4 are smaller; and S5 is very small.

The **sacral plexus** is made up of the descending lumbosacral trunk, derived from the lumbar plexus and the anterior rami of S1–3. The anterior ramus of S3 has a superior branch, which joins the sacral plexus, and an inferior branch, which aids in formation of the pudendal nerve. The nerves forming the sacral plexus converge and unite near the lower portion of the greater sciatic foramen to form the sciatic nerve.

➠ *The sacral plexus is seldom harmed in pelvic surgery. The deep position of the pelvic portion of the sacral plexus usually protects these pelvic nerves during pelvic surgery and from injury associated with penetrating wounds of the lower abdomen.*

➠ *Involvement of the sacral plexus by late malignant disease. The great number of pelvic nerve trunks that lie in close apposition to the pelvic viscera may be involved in the spread of cancer from a pelvic viscus to an adjacent nerve trunk. This spread is the major cause of severe, intractable pelvic pain in late pelvic cancer.*

➠ *Sacral anesthesia (caudal block). Sacral or caudal anesthesia is frequently used in genitourinary, gynecologic, and anorectal surgery. A needle is placed through the sacrococcygeal ligament so that it enters the sacral canal at*

the level of the hiatus between the terminal sacrum and the coccyx. The injected solution accumulates in the extradural space and anesthetizes the roots of the sacral nerves as they issue from the dense dural sheath that surrounds them.

The nerves comprising the sacral plexus lie on the pelvic surface of the piriformis muscle. Just ventral to the plexus lie the internal iliac artery and vein, the ureter, and (on the left) the sigmoid colon. As the superior gluteal vessels pass dorsally, they run between the lumbosacral trunk and S1. The inferior gluteal vessels pass dorsally between S2 and S3. All branches of the sacral plexus that emerge from the pelvis do so beneath the inferior border of the piriformis muscle—with the exception of the superior gluteal nerve, which emerges above the superior border of that muscle.

From the **ventral divisions** of the sacral plexus are derived (1) nerves to the quadratus femoris and gemellus inferior (L4, 5; S1); (2) nerves to the obturator internus and gemellus superior (L5; S1, 2); (3) the posterior femoral cutaneous nerve (S2, 3); and (4) the tibial branch of the sciatic nerve (L4, 5; S1–3). From the **dorsal divisions** of the nerves of the sacral plexus are derived (1) the nerve to the piriformis (S1, 2); (2) the superior gluteal nerve (L4, 5; S1); (3) the inferior gluteal nerve (L5; S2, 3); (4) the posterior femoral cutaneous nerve (S1, 2); and (5) the common peroneal branch of the sciatic nerve (L4, 5; S1, 2).

The **pudendal plexus** lies just ventral to the inferior edge of the piriformis muscle and is made up

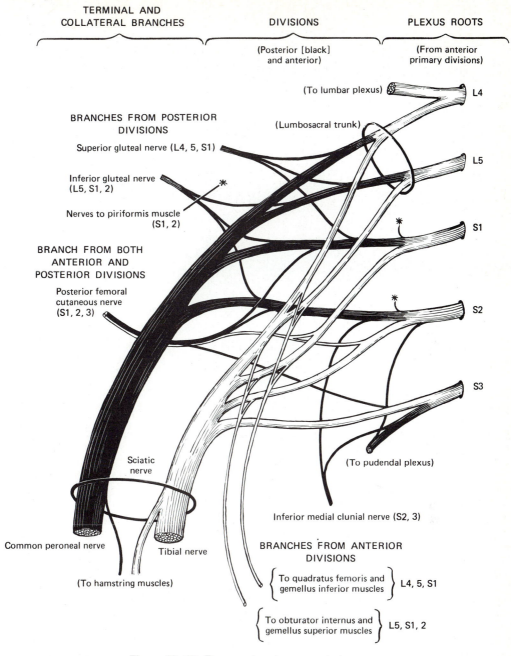

Figure 36–15. The sacral and coccygeal plexuses.

of the anterior branches of S2–4. It gives off pelvic visceral and muscular branches and the pudendal nerve. The pudendal nerve passes dorsally between the piriformis and coccygeus muscles to leave the pelvis through the greater sciatic foramen. It then runs across the ischial spine to enter the perineum via the lesser sciatic foramen. It continues ventrally in the perineum along with the internal pudendal vessels, encased in a sheath of the obturator internus fascia (Alcock's canal). It gives off the inferior hemorrhoidal nerve and ends by dividing into the perineal

nerve and the dorsal nerve of the penis or clitoris.

S4 and S5 join with the coccygeal nerve to form the coccygeal plexus. The anococcygeal nerves arise from this plexus and supply the skin about the coccyx.

The **obturator nerve** (L2–4) is a branch of the lumbar plexus and has a long intrapelvic course. However, none of its branches are distributed to pelvic viscera or muscles. The nerve enters the pelvis by running deep to the common iliac artery and vein. It then passes ventrally along the lateral pelvic wall, usually in a position lateral and deep to the pelvic

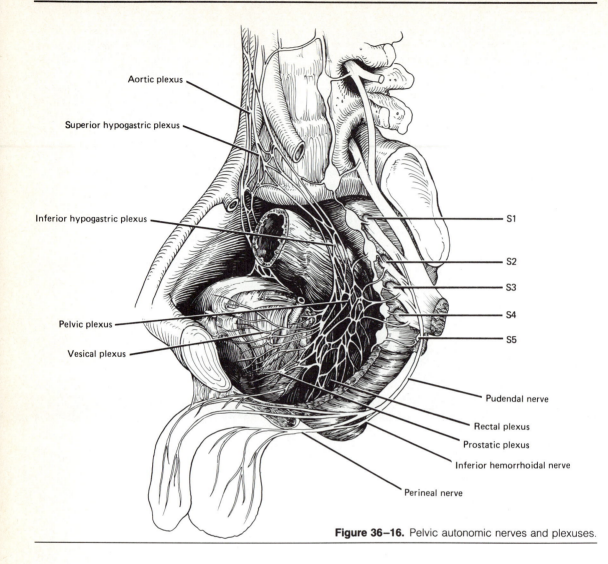

Aortic plexus

Superior hypogastric plexus

Inferior hypogastric plexus

Pelvic plexus

Vesical plexus

S1

S2

S3

S4

S5

Pudendal nerve

Rectal plexus

Prostatic plexus

Inferior hemorrhoidal nerve

Perineal nerve

Figure 36–16. Pelvic autonomic nerves and plexuses.

ureter and the internal iliac vessels. It crosses the obturator fascia and runs superior to the obturator artery and vein. It issues from the pelvis along with the obturator vessels by passing through the superior portion of the obturator foramen. An accessory obturator nerve, when present (10% of individuals), does not pass through the obturator foramen but leaves the pelvis by crossing over the superior surface of the pubic ramus, to be distributed—as is the primary obturator nerve—to the anterior thigh and to the hip joint.

▮▶ ***Obturator neurectomy.*** *Obturator neurectomy is on occasion performed for severe painful spasms of the adductor muscles of the thigh. The main trunk of the nerve is interrupted in an extraperitoneal but intrapelvic position. Intrapelvic interruption is done because once the obturator nerve appears on the thigh it has* *already given off its several branches to the thigh muscles.*

The nerves of the pelvic segment of the **abdominal autonomic trunk** are a continuation of the lumbar sympathetic trunk and consist of a nerve chain and 4–5 ganglia. The pelvic ganglia are the smallest ganglia of the entire autonomic chain. The chain and ganglia lie on the ventral surface of the sacrum just medial to the anterior sacral foramens. The right and left trunks are often connected across the midline by 2 or 3 fine nerve cords. The lowest (coccygeal) ganglion is frequently a single midline ganglion, resulting from fusion of the lowest ganglion on each side. From the sacral and coccygeal ganglia, branches are supplied to each of the sacral and coccygeal nerves as gray rami communicantes. Visceral branches from the pelvic trunk run to the hypogastric and pelvic nerve plexuses, and after passing through these plexuses are distributed to the pelvic blood vessels and organs.

The **pelvic autonomic plexuses** (Fig 36–15) result from the junction of the pelvic sympathetic and parasympathetic fibers. The result is the pelvic plexus, formed by the junction of the hypogastric plexus with rami from the sacral segment of the sympathetic chain and visceral branches from S2–4. The pelvic autonomic plexus, through its multiple secondary plexuses, sends nerves to all of the viscera in the pelvis. The nerves from the secondary plexuses are responsible for the formation of (1) the vesical plexus, (2) the middle rectal plexus, (3) the prostatic plexus, (4) the vaginal plexus, and (5) the uterine plexus.

⇒ *Surgery on the sacral autonomic plexus. Resection of the sacral autonomic plexus has been performed as treatment for a variety of gynecologic complaints (dysmenorrhea, etc) but has not proved effective. The plexus should never be resected in the male, as it will alter the sequence leading to ejaculation. The sacral parasympathetic nerves have a marked influence on penile and clitoral erection and are concerned with reflex emptying of the bladder and rectum and should ordinarily not be resected.*

The urinary bladder stores the urine excreted by the kidney and delivered via the ureters; this anterior pelvic reservoir eventually discharges urine to the exterior of the body under central nervous system control.

EMBRYOLOGY

The ventral portion of the cloaca—the terminal segment of the entodermal hindgut—known as the urogenital sinus is separated from the bowel dorsally by the growth of the urorectal septum. The descending mesonephric ducts terminate in the urogenital sinus. Projecting from the anterosuperior segment of the urogenital sinus is the urachal tube, which connects the sinus to the allantois in the umbilical stalk. The urogenital sinus is divided into 3 parts: a superior vesical portion connected to the allantois, a middle pelvic part into which the mesonephric ducts and the ureters (initially) open, and an inferior phallic part. The openings of the ureters gradually migrate from the mesonephric ducts to their definitive positions in the bladder wall. The muscle layers and the adventitia are derived from the splanchnic mesenchyme.

Anomalies

Failure of development of the transverse urorectal septum results in persistent cloaca and rectovesical, rectourethral, or rectovestibular fistulas. Failure of proper obliteration of the urachus results in patent urachus with umbilical urinary fistula and urachal cysts (single or multiple). Exstrophy of the bladder may also occur.

GROSS ANATOMY
(Figs 37–1 and 37–2)

The urinary bladder is a hollow muscular organ, which, when empty, lies anteriorly in the true pelvis. It is related ventrally to the dorsal surfaces of the pubic symphysis and the rami of the pubic bones, and dorsally to the rectovesical pouch of the peritoneum, the seminal vesicles, the vas deferens, the

ureters, and the rectum in the male, and the vesico-uterine pouch of peritoneum, the uterus, and the upper vagina in the female. The adult bladder normally can hold 400–500 mL of urine.

STRUCTURE OF THE BLADDER

The bladder is covered by an outer serous peritoneal coat only on its superior, posterior, and lateral surfaces.

The bladder wall consists of a maze of muscle fibers that run in many directions except near the internal orifice, where 3 definite muscular layers can be seen: the internal longitudinal, middle circular, and external longitudinal muscles. In the female, the external longitudinal layer extends the entire length of the urethra; in the male, it extends to the distal prostatic urethra. The middle circular layer—the so-called detrusor muscle—terminates at the internal bladder orifice as a well-defined circular band, the sphincter vesicae urinariae, whose fibers in the male are continuous with the prostatic muscle fibers. All 3 converging muscle layers make up the musculature of the vesical neck but do not function as a true bladder sphincter. Vesicoureteral reflux is usually due to attenuation of the trigone and of the intravesical ureteral musculature.

The voluntary external bladder sphincter is composed of striated muscle between the superior and inferior fasciae of the urogenital diaphragm. In the female, it is situated at about mid urethra, superior to the external layer of the urethral musculature. In the male, the striated fibers surround the distal prostate and the membranous urethra. The voluntary muscles of the pelvic floor also contribute to overall voluntary sphincter function.

The submucosa of the bladder is composed of areolar tissue that joins the muscular and mucous coats. The interior of the bladder is lined with a mucous membrane, which is loosely attached to the underlying submucosa.

In the midline of the posterior wall of the bladder is a triangular area, the **bladder trigone** (Fig 37–3). At the trigone, the bladder mucosa is tightly attached to the submucosa. The slitlike ureteral orifices form the lateral borders of the base of the bladder trigone. The ureteral orifices are about 2.5 cm apart in the empty bladder and 5 cm apart in the full bladder. Between the 2 ureteral orifices, a raised bar or ridge

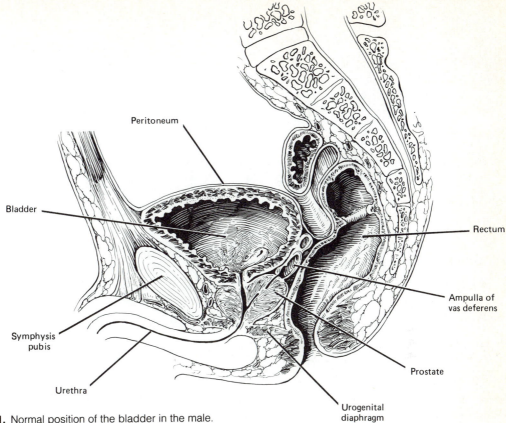

Figure 37–1. Normal position of the bladder in the male.

Labels: Peritoneum, Bladder, Symphysis pubis, Urethra, Rectum, Ampulla of vas deferens, Prostate, Urogenital diaphragm

of mucosa called the **plica interureterica,** is formed by underlying smooth muscle. The internal urethral aperture lies at the apex of the bladder trigone and occupies the most dependent portion of the bladder.

➠ *Fistulas between the bladder and adjacent structures. Fistulas between the bladder and the small or large bowel are fairly common complications of regional enteritis, deep x-ray therapy to the pelvic organs, diverticular disease of the distal colon, and cancer of the adjacent large bowel. Vesicovaginal fistula occurs from incision into the bladder during pelvic surgery, perforation of the bladder by invading neoplasms, or severe pelvic trauma during parturition.*

In the adult, as the bladder fills, it gradually rises from the pelvis into the abdominal cavity and elevates the parietal peritoneum superior to it from the deep surface of the ventrolateral abdominal wall. This brings the anterior surface of the bladder directly against the space of Retzius. In children under age 3, the pelvis is small and the bladder tends to be in an intra-abdominal position even when empty. In chil-

dren, when the bladder is empty, the bladder neck lies just superior to the pubic symphysis.

➠ *Partial and complete cystectomy. Partial cystectomy, with or without transplantation of the ureters into a retained bladder segment, the ileum, or the sigmoid is a treatment used for well-localized malignant bladder tumors, severe chronic benign bladder ulcerations resistant to treatment, large bladder diverticula, and as a step during the treatment of bladder fistulas into the colon, small bowel, or vagina. Complete cystectomy, always accompanied by ureteral transplantation (during diversion), is done for treatment of advanced bladder tuberculosis with a resultant constricted and very painful bladder. Total cystectomy with concurrent pelvic node dissection is often done for bladder cancer.*

➠ *Cystotomy and cystostomy. Cystotomy, the creation of a surgical opening into the urinary bladder, is done for the purpose of removing a bladder stone or other foreign body. The bladder is filled with fluid, so that it rises into the abdomen and becomes related to the space*

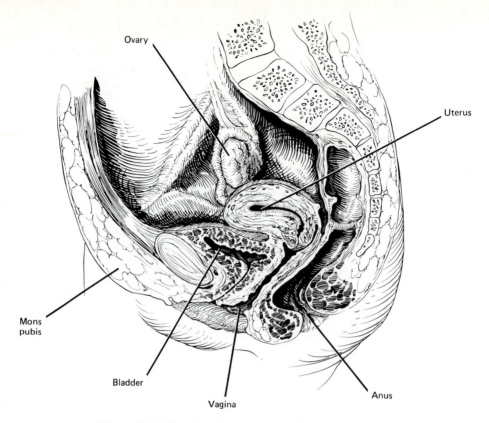

Figure 37–2. Normal position of the bladder in the female.

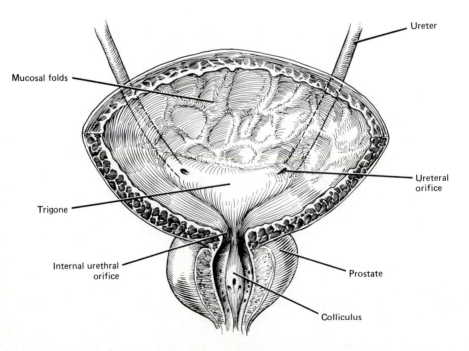

Figure 37–3. Bladder trigone (anterior portion of bladder removed).

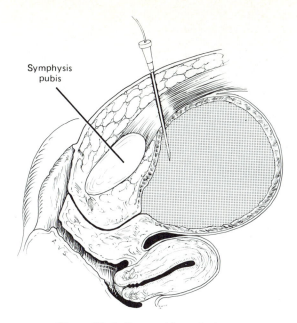

Symphysis
pubis

Figure 37–4. Suprapubic cystostomy.

of Retzius. An incision is made through this prevesical extraperitoneal space, and the ventral surface of the bladder is opened so that it can be explored. Cystotomy is performed also during removal of the prostate via the suprapubic or retropubic approach.

Cystostomy is used for bladder drainage when the normal urethral channel must be bypassed. (Fig 37–4.)

➠ *Insertion of catheter via cystotomy to re-establish urethral patency in the male. In the male, a cystotomy incision may be used for insertion of a urethral catheter via the bladder when partial or complete urethral transection distally precludes passage of the catheter into the bladder from below. The urethral and the cystotomy catheters can frequently be connected in the line of the urethra to establish urethral patency.*

➠ *Importance of emptying the bladder before intraperitoneal endoscopy. The bladder must always be emptied by catheter before abdominal or pelvic peritoneal endoscopy and before any lower abdominal intraperitoneal diagnostic tap is performed. Many women with cystocele and urethrocele and most elderly men with prostatic hypertrophy have difficulty, particularly under stress, in completely emptying the bladder. Consequently, the bladder containing high residual urine may be punctured by the entering instrument if it is not completely empty.*

➠ *Recognition of high-lying bladder in children and infants. In children under age 3, the blad-*

der is a lower abdominal viscus rather than a pelvic organ. This position must always be considered when lower abdominal incisions are made. Especially when performing hernia repair in infants, great care must be taken not to injure the high-lying bladder.

The superior surface of the empty bladder tends to be flat, and the empty organ thus appears to be roughly pyramidal in shape, with its apex facing inferiorly. When the bladder is filling, it rises superiorly and assumes a globular shape, its superior surface resembling a sphere. The superior, posterosuperior, and laterosuperior bladder surfaces are covered with peritoneum reflected from the adjacent ventrolateral and lateral abdominal and lateral pelvic walls. The bladder peritoneum is reflected off the upper posterior surfaces of the organ to form (posteriorly) the rectovesical pouch in the male and the uterovesical pouch in the female.

➠ *Relationships of peritoneal covering of bladder. Since the bladder is covered by peritoneum only superiorly, posterosuperiorly, and laterosuperiorly, the bladder must first be filled with fluid before an extraperitoneal incision can be made. The distended bladder then rises above the pubis, its anterior surface presenting against the abdominal wall in an extraperitoneal position.*

➠ *Urinary extravasation following injury to the bladder. Bladder lacerations may occur after pelvic bone fractures, abdominal trauma, or perineal injuries. The bladder is more apt to rupture as a result of trauma if it is distended. Extravasation of urine after bladder injury may be intra- or extraperitoneal, depending on the site of bladder laceration. (Fig 37–5.)*

POSITION OF THE BLADDER

In the male, the apex of the bladder is firmly attached to the base of the prostate and thus is fixed to the superior fascia of the urogenital diaphragm. In the female, the apex of the bladder rests ventrally on the superior surface of the urogenital diaphragm and dorsally on the superior fibers of the levator ani diaphragm. Ventrally, the bladder is separated from the os pubis and from the obturator internus muscle by the fat and loose areolar tissue that fills the prevesical fascial cleft, the space between the anterior levator ani fibers. Ventrally and laterally, the bladder is intimately related to the large perivesical venous plexuses. The superior surfaces of the bladder are related to the free peritoneal cavity, primarily to some coils of small bowel, a low-lying cecum, and the sigmoid colon. In the female, the anterior surface of the uterus lies atop and indents the posterosuperior bladder sur-

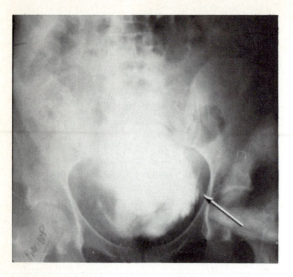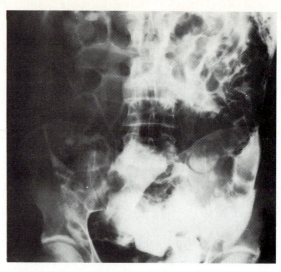

Figure 37–5. *Left:* Extraperitoneal bladder rupture. Extravasation (at arrow) seen outside the bladder in the pelvis on cystogram. ***Right:*** Intraperitoneal bladder rupture. Cystogram shows contrast surrounding loops of bowel.

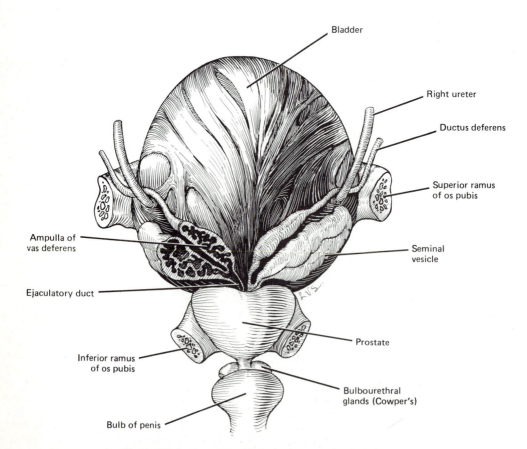

Figure 37–6. The dorsal aspect of the bladder in the male.

face. Dorsally, in the female, the bladder is related to the anterior fornix of the vagina, the cervix, and the lower uterine segment. In the male, the posterior bladder surface is closely related to the seminal vesicles, the terminal portion of the ductus deferens, and the vesicorectal peritoneal pouch. (Fig 37–6.)

FASCIA OF THE BLADDER & PELVIS

The bladder is fixed in position by condensations of the endopelvic fascia. Ventrally, in the female, the endopelvic fascia condenses to form the anterior and lateral pubovesical ligaments that attach the bladder to the os pubis. In the male, the medial and lateral puboprostatic ligaments, which run to the prostate from the os pubis and which are condensations of the endopelvic fascia, serve to fix the bladder anteriorly, since the prostate is tightly attached to the apex of the bladder. The lateral septa of the endopelvic fascia thicken about the neurovascular bundles running to the lateral bladder surface and form the true lateral bladder ligaments. The urachus runs from the superior bladder surface to the umbilicus. From the lateral superior bladder surfaces extend the paired lateral umbilical folds that were the 2 fetal umbilical arteries. Reflection of the bladder peritoneum laterally onto the side walls of the pelvis forms the so-called lateral false ligaments of the bladder.

➠ *Injury to the internal sphincter during prostatectomy. In the male, the sphincter is continuous with the muscular fibers of the prostate. It may be damaged during prostatectomy, but the injury does not usually result in incontinence. It is always weakened after prostatectomy. However, patients usually remain continent unless the injury extends distal to the verumontanum, destroying the distal smooth sphincteric mechanism. More distal injury will damage the external sphincter.*

➠ *Loss of urinary control from perineal hernia in females. Loss of urinary control in the female is often secondary to the presence of a large cystocele, urethrocele, or both. These perineal hernias are usually secondary to the trauma of parturition. In stress incontinence, the supportive structures about the bladder neck and the membranous urethra become lax—particularly the vesicouterine and pubovesical ligaments. Relaxation of these ligaments causes caudal and posterior movement of the urethra. The bladder sphincter in such cases becomes extremely lax, and sphincter control is markedly diminished. In order to correct the inferoposterior bladder displacement, normal anatomic relationships must be restored by a Marshall-Marchetti operation, in which sutures placed*

paraurethrally and to the posterior symphysis are used to lift the urethra and reduce the hernia.

BLOOD VESSELS, LYMPHATICS, & NERVES

Arteries

The bladder has a profuse and varied arterial blood supply, chiefly via the superior, middle, and inferior vesical arteries. All are branches of the anterior division of the internal iliac artery. In the female, the bladder receives additional arterial blood from the uterine and vaginal arteries. In both males and females, some arterial blood reaches the bladder from the inferior gluteal and obturator arteries.

Veins

The endopelvic areolar tissue surrounding the bladder contains a rich plexus of veins. The veins are most prominent in the endopelvic tissues close to the bladder neck. They extend to the entrance of the ureters into the bladder. A large venous plexus lies just ventral and lateral to the bladder dorsal to the pubic rami. The several venous plexuses coalesce into 4 or 5 large vesical veins on each side of the bladder. These veins eventually empty into the internal iliac veins.

➠ *Bleeding from the perivesical plexus of veins. The presence of the large venous plexuses that surround the bladder and adhere closely to it makes operation involving the paravesical tissues a bloody procedure.*

➠ *Perivesical hematomas following pelvic trauma. Pelvic trauma secondary to fractures of the bony pelvis and perineal trauma following severe straddle injuries and land mine explosions may result in massive hematomas about the bladder secondary to rupture of the large perivesical plexuses.*

Lymphatics

Lymphatics of the bladder arise in rich intra- and extramuscular plexuses. Lymphatics from the ventral surface of the bladder drain into the external iliac nodes after passing through anterior and lateral vesical nodes. The nodes on the dorsal surface of the bladder drain primarily into the external, internal, and common iliac nodes.

Nerves
(Fig 37–7)

Bladder control is mediated by a combination of sympathetic and parasympathetic nerves. The vesical plexus is mixed and is a continuation of the inferior

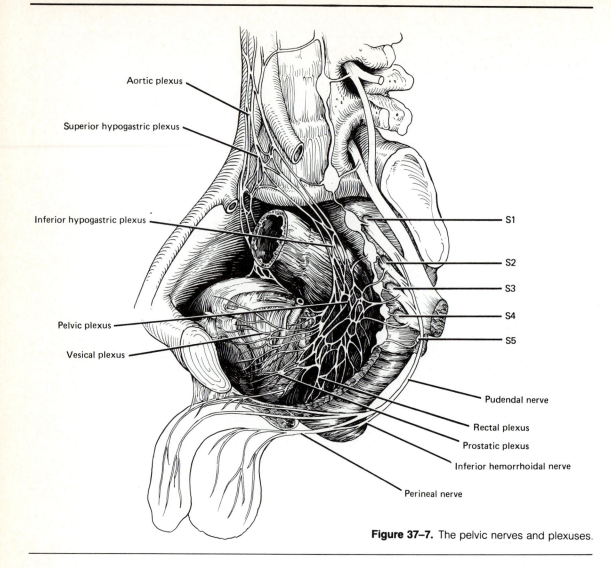

Aortic plexus

Superior hypogastric plexus

Inferior hypogastric plexus

Pelvic plexus

Vesical plexus

S1

S2

S3

S4

S5

Pudendal nerve

Rectal plexus

Prostatic plexus

Inferior hemorrhoidal nerve

Perineal nerve

Figure 37–7. The pelvic nerves and plexuses.

hypogastric plexus; it contains postganglionic sympathetic and preganglionic parasympathetic fibers. The parasympathetic fibers are derived from sacral nerves S2, S3, and S4. The vesical plexus surrounds the distal portion of the pelvic ureters. The parasympathetic nerves are responsible for the emptying reflex, which causes the bladder wall to contract. The sympathetic nerves are distributed to the trigonal muscle and to the blood vessels of the bladder. Afferent impulses of the reflex emptying arc are carried by nerve fibers running with the sympathetic and parasympathetic fibers.

The Perineum

38

The perineum is the outlet of the pelvis; it is separated from the pelvic cavity by the urogenital diaphragm ventrally and by the levator ani muscular complex laterally and dorsally. It is bounded ventrally by the pubic arch, the pubic symphysis, and the arcuate ligament; ventrolaterally by the inferior rami of the ischiopubic bones and by the ischial tuberosity; dorsolaterally by the sacrotuberous and sacrospinous ligaments, and dorsally by the tip of the coccyx.

If the patient stands erect with thighs adducted, the perineum consists merely of a narrow groove lying between the upper inner surfaces of the thighs. However, with the thighs flexed, abducted, and externally rotated (lithotomy position), the perineum opens to form a large diamond-shaped space (Fig 38–1).

Anteriorly, in the male, the perineum contains the roots of the scrotum and penis; in the female, it contains the clitoris and the openings of the vagina and urethra. The perineum may be divided into 2 triangles—ventral and dorsal—by drawing a line between the ischial tuberosities. The ventral triangle is called the urogenital perineum; the dorsal triangle is called the anorectal perineum.

ANORECTAL PERINEUM

SKIN

The skin covering the anorectal perineum is thin and attached to the superficial fascia. It covers a large plexus of subcutaneous perineal veins, particularly around the anal orifice. The skin is puckered around the anus by the underlying corrugator cutis ani muscle. In the midline is the anococcygeal raphe, a skin ridge running from the posterior anal verge to the coccyx.

➠ *Fistulous openings on the skin of the anorectal triangle. The skin of the anorectal perineum is often the site of openings of fistulous tracts that pass through the ischiorectal fossa after leaving the lower rectum or anus. Occasionally, fistulous tracts originating in the lower abdo-*

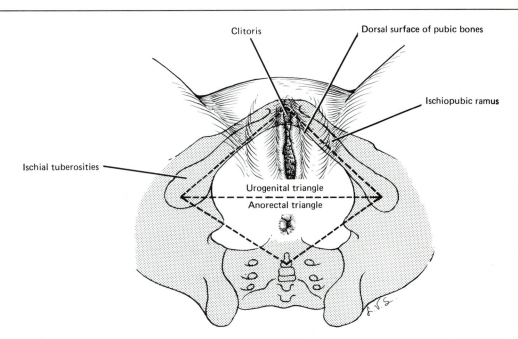

Figure 38–1. Urogenital and anorectal triangles. (Modified and reproduced, with permission, from Pernoll ML, Benson RC [editors]: *Current Obstetric & Gynecologic Diagnosis & Treatment,* 6th ed. Appleton & Lange, 1987.)

483

men or pelvis will open onto the perineum. Such fistulous tracts may be due to acute prostatitis or acute seminal vesiculitis or may be secondary to chronic enteritis, appendiceal abscesses, or abscesses from sigmoid diverticulitis or pelvic inflammatory disease. To be completely removed, these tracts must be dissected superiorly into the pelvis through the pelvic musculofascial diaphragms. On occasion, abdominal exploration must accompany the perineal procedure.

➠ ***Pruritus ani.*** *Acute or chronic pruritus ani may result in erythema, fissuring, maceration, lichenification, thickening, and fibrosis of the perianal skin. Chronic cases are difficult to treat and call for protracted proctologic care.*

➠ ***Thrombotic external hemorrhoids.*** *Thrombotic external hemorrhoids around the anal verge are swollen edematous skin tags. They present because of the rupture of subcutaneous veins into the subcutaneous connective tissue. The blood clots within the tags must be removed in order to relieve severe perianal pain.*

➠ ***Perianal skin cancer.*** *Basal cell epithelioma, perineal Bowen's disease, and extramammary Paget's disease of the anus are slowly growing cancers that occasionally occur around the anus.*

FASCIA

The superficial fascia of the anorectal perineum is continuous with the superficial fascia covering the buttocks and inner surfaces of the thighs. Alongside the anus, the superficial fascia contains large lobules of fat (perianal elastic pad). Where the anorectal su-

perficial fascia covers the ischial tuberosities, it is tough and stringy and separated from the underlying bony ischium by a bursa.

➠ ***Ischial bursitis (weaver's, tailor's, or lighterman's bottom).*** *The bursa that separates the bony ischial tuberosity from the underlying subcutaneous tissues may become inflamed and tender. The symptoms respond readily to direct injection of the bursa with a mixture of procaine and hydrocortisone.*

ANORECTAL MUSCULATURE
(Fig 38–2)

The anorectal musculature consists of the levator ani, the coccygeus muscle, and the external and internal anal sphincters. These muscles support the anorectum and are of great importance in maintenance of anorectal continence.

The 3 portions of the external anal sphincter, the muscles of the levator ani complex, and the posterior perineal muscles of the urogenital compartment of the perineum are all under conscious central control and under normal conditions constitute the effective sphincteric apparatus of the anorectum. They are supplied by a branch from S4 and by the inferior rectal and perineal branches of the pudendal nerve.

The levator ani complex is discussed in Chapters 28 and 29.

External Anal Sphincter

The external anal sphincter consists of 3 parts: deep, subcutaneous, and superficial.

The **deep portion** of the external anal sphincter is a circular bundle of voluntary muscle fibers surrounding the external longitudinal musculature of the terminal rectum and upper anus. It is closely related

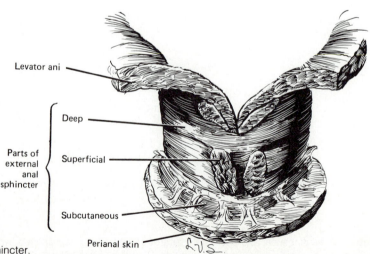

Figure 38–2. Musculature of the anal sphincter.

to the levator ani muscles just below the point where the levator ani inserts into the rectum, about 4.5 cm superior to the anal verge.

The **subcutaneous portion** of the external anal sphincter lies inferior to both the internal sphincter and the deep portion of the external sphincter. It is separated from the internal sphincter muscle by the intersphincteric groove.

The **superficial portion** of the external anal sphincter lies lateral and superior to the subcutaneous segment. It does not surround the rectum in tubelike fashion, like the other portions of the muscle, but runs from the coccyx to the central tendinous point of the perineum—and thus encircles the anus in a loose manner. Since its fibers decussate loosely in their relationship to the posterior subcutaneous quadrant of the anorectum, this area is less well supported than are the anterior and lateral anal quadrants.

The external anal sphincter receives its nerve supply via a branch from S4 and from the inferior rectal branch of the pudendal nerve.

⏵ *Fistulas and fissures associated with the external anal sphincter. The subcutaneous portion of the external anal sphincter is frequently involved in superficial anorectal fistulas. It is the portion of the external anal sphincter that is divided by the procedure of external sphincterotomy.*

⏵ *Subcutaneous sphincterotomy for anal fissures. Chronic anal fissures, which are usually in the posterior anal quadrants, become chronic because of associated spasticity of the denuded subcutaneous portion of the external anal sphincter that lies at the base of the fissure. This portion of the external sphincter apparatus must be incised to allow healing.*

Internal Anal Sphincter

The internal anal sphincter is circular and lies deep to the outer longitudinal layer. It thickens markedly just above the anorectal junction, is about 2.5 cm long, and has a free inferior border. It is easily seen on rectal dissection and felt on digital examination. The outer longitudinal muscle of the rectal wall separates the internal anal sphincter from the deep portion of the external anal sphincter. The lower border of the internal sphincter is separated from the subcutaneous portion of the external sphincter by the intersphincteric groove. The internal anal sphincter is not under central control and plays little or no part in conscious control of anal continence.

THE ISCHIORECTAL FOSSA (Fig 38–3)

The ischiorectal fossa is the roughly triangular space that lies in the posterior perineum on either side of the anorectum. The space is separated from

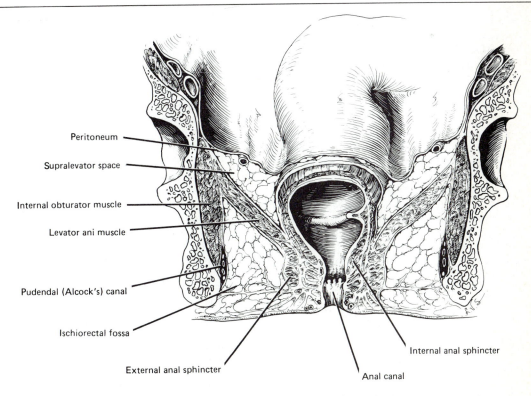

Peritoneum

Supralevator space

Internal obturator muscle

Levator ani muscle

Pudendal (Alcock's) canal

Ischiorectal fossa

External anal sphincter

Anal canal

Internal anal sphincter

Figure 38–3. The ischiorectal fossae and pelvic diaphragm.

the pelvis by the levator ani muscles and their fasciae. Because the levator ani muscles slope from a lateral superior to a medial inferior position, the lateral portions of the fossa rise higher than the medial portions. Laterally, the fossa is bounded by the obturator internus fascia and the ischial tuberosity; this boundary is essentially a vertical wall. The obturator internus fascia splits just above the level of the ischial tuberosity and forms the pudendal (Alcock's) canal, which is about 0.5 cm high and about 0.3 cm wide. The canal contains the internal pudendal artery and vein and the pudendal nerve. The ischiorectal fossa is bounded medially by the sloping surface of the levator ani muscle and by the walls of the terminal rectum and the anus, which are surrounded by the external anal sphincter; inferiorly by the subcutaneous tissues and the skin of the anorectal perineum; and anteriorly by the superficial and deep transverse perineal muscles.

The 2 ischiorectal fossae join posterior to the anal canal. Anteriorly, the fossae extend farther into the urogenital triangle above the level of the urogenital diaphragm. Dorsally, each ischiorectal fossa extends to the gluteus maximus muscle. The dorsal extension is called the posterior recess of the ischiorectal fossa.

Components of the Ischiorectal Fossa

The ischiorectal fossa is filled with coarse, stringy fat containing many fibrous strands that divide the area into lobules. The presence of fat about the anorectum allows for distention of the terminal bowel and the anorectum during defecation. Crossing the inferior portion of the ischiorectal fossa are the inferior rectal arteries and veins, a rich plexus of lymphatics leading from the anorectum to the obturator and inguinal lymph nodes, and branches of the pudendal nerve. All of these structures lie just deep to the skin and subcutaneous tissues of the anorectal perineum.

➧ *Ischiorectal and pararectal abscesses. Ischiorectal and pararectal abscesses are common and are usually drained via an incision into the ischiorectal fossa. Most ischiorectal abscesses probably begin as anorectal cryptitis. Since the 2 ischiorectal fossae join posterior to the anal canal, large, poorly defined posterior ischiorectal abscesses can develop. The ischiorectal fossae project superiorly and anteriorly into the urogenital triangle, and abscesses may tunnel into these anterosuperior recesses, where pus can be easily overlooked in perineal drainage.*

➧ *Penetrating wounds of the anorectal perineum. Penetrating wounds of the anorectal perineum (eg, from land mine injuries) frequently pass through the levator diaphragm to injure intrapelvic organs and vessels. Such wounds may call for abdominal as well as perineal*

exploration and, on occasion, for a diversionary colostomy.

THE UROGENITAL PERINEUM IN THE MALE (Fig 38–4)

The skin of the urogenital perineum in the male is relatively thin and is drawn tightly across the perianal area. A midline raphe runs from the scrotum to a line between the 2 ischial tuberosities. The superficial fascia of the urogenital perineum in the male is in 2 layers: superficial and deep. The superficial layer is fatty, ill-defined, and continuous with Camper's fascia of the abdomen and with the superficial fascia covering the anorectal area. In the male, this layer joins with the deep layer of the perineal superficial fascia (Colles' fascia) to form the tunica dartos of the scrotum; in the female, it makes up the bulk of the labium majus pudendi. The deep layer of the superficial perianal fascia is a tightly fitting membranelike structure over the entire urogenital triangle (Colles' fascia). It is attached anteriorly to the anterior lips of the inferior ischiopubic rami. Dorsally, it terminates along a line drawn between the 2 ischial tuberosities, at which point it tucks around the dorsal border of the 2 transverse perineal muscles to blend with the 2 layers of fascia that form the base of the urogenital diaphragm. Ventrally, Colles' fascia passes over the scrotum, penis, and spermatic cords (delivering a layer to each) and crosses the pubic bones and pubic symphysis to become Scarpa's fascia, the deep layer of the superficial fascia of the ventrolateral abdominal wall. Where Colles' fascia invests the scrotum, it contains little or no fat, but it does contain thin reddish involuntary muscle fibers (dartos muscle) that contract the scrotal skin into rugal folds.

➧ *Cutaneous fistulas in the male perineum. The urogenital perineum in the male is occasionally the site of fistulous openings, usually following perineal trauma or disease of the perineal portions of the urogenital tract. Such fistulas occur secondary to urethral stricture, instrumentation of the urinary tract, and blunt or penetrating perineal trauma. In the newborn, fistulas that may result from malformations of the anorectum usually are situated in the urogenital perineum.*

CONTENTS OF THE SUPERFICIAL PERINEAL POUCH

Colles' fascia in the urogenital perineum delineates a perineal fascial space, the superficial perineal pouch.

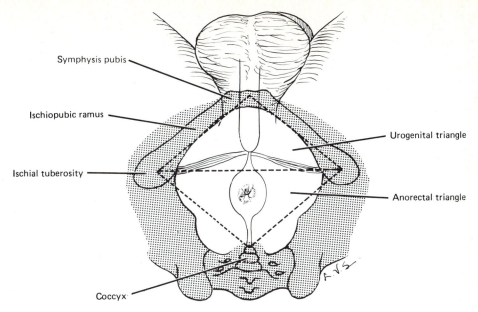

Figure 38–4. Area between the fascial layers of the urogenital diaphragm (male).

The pouch is bounded inferiorly by Colles' fascia, superiorly by the inferior fascia of the urogenital diaphragm, ventrally by the pubic bones and symphysis pubica, laterally by the ischiopubic arch, and dorsally by the union of Colles' fascia with the fused fascia of the urogenital diaphragm. Within the superficial perineal pouch lie the superficial transverse perineal muscles; the bulb of the urethra, covered by the bulbocavernosus muscle; the crura of the penis, with their overlying ischiocavernosus muscles; the fixed anterior urethra, covered by the bulbocavernosus muscle; and many important perineal vessels, nerves, and lymphatics. There may be a medial fascial septum. Colles' fascia is tightly fused to the inferior surfaces of the pubic bones and the ischiopubic arch, making the superficial perineal pouch a closed space, except ventrally, where the space joins the scrotum and penis.

⇒ *Urinary extravasation in the male perineum.*
(Fig 38–5.) Urinary extravasation into the superficial perineal pouch may follow trauma to the perineum that ruptures the portions of the urethra which lie below the urogenital diaphragm. The urine passes ventrally to the scrotum, penis, and spermatic cords and finally ascends to the lower abdomen, where it lies deep to Scarpa's fascia and superficial to the muscles of the abdomen. This leads to marked toxicity, particularly if the urine is infected.

The **superficial transverse perineal muscle** runs from the tuberosity of the ischium to the central perineal body into which it inserts, along with its contralateral muscle. Dorsally, in the midline, the muscle abuts the most ventral fibers of the external anal sphincter; ventrally, it is in contact with posterior fibers of the bulbocavernosus muscle.

⇒ *Role of the transverse perineal muscle in the perineal approach to the prostate. Radical prostatectomy through a perineal approach is occasionally required for treatment of prostatic cancer. The cutaneous incision is made in the posterior portion of the urogenital perineum and is developed superiorly, care being taken to stay anterior to the 2 layers of transverse perineal muscles. When the rectourethralis muscle is severed, the structures in the anorectal perineum fall away dorsally, and injury to the rectum is thus prevented.*

The 2 crura of the **corpora cavernosa penis** are spongy vascular bulbs containing large venous lakes. They arise from the inferior surfaces of the ischiopubic rami and run obliquely to the undersurfaces of the symphysis pubica, where they join to complete the formation of the dorsal aspect of the penis. They adhere to the inferior surface of the inferior fascia of the urogenital diaphragm.

The **ischiocavernosus muscles,** which are attached to the free inferior surfaces of the crura, serve to compress the crura against the pubic arch and thus obstruct venous return from the corpora cavernosa. The muscles arise from the undersurface of the ischial tuberosities and from the inner surface of the pubic rami; they insert into the inferior and lateral surfaces

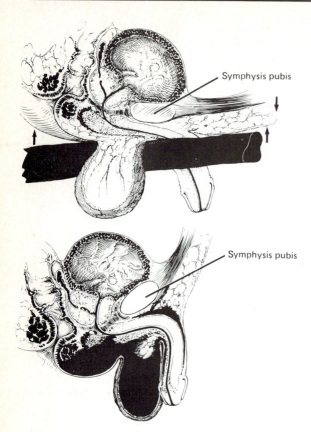

Symphysis pubis

Symphysis pubis

Figure 38–5. Injury to the bulbous urethra. **Top:** A perineal blow or a fall astride an object results in crushing of the urethra against the inferior edge of the pubic symphysis. **Bottom:** Extravasation of blood and urine enclosed within Colles' fascia. (Reproduced, with permission, from Tanagho EA, McAninch JW: *Smith's General Urology,* 12th ed. Appleton & Lange, 1988.)

of the crura where the crura join to form the dorsal surface of the penile body. The **bulb of the urethra** is the thinned, dilated dorsal portion of the fixed perineal urethra. It is in the superficial perineal pouch just anterior to the central tendinous point of the perineum. The bulb is firmly attached superiorly to the inferior fascia of the urogenital diaphragm and is the continuation of the membranous urethra.

The fixed anterior portion of the **perineal urethra** runs from the urethral bulb to the pubic arch. It is firmly attached to the inferior fascia of the urogenital diaphragm and thus is subject to injury from perineal trauma.

The **bulbocavernosus muscle** encloses the inferior and lateral surfaces of the urethral bulb and the inferior surface of the fixed anterior urethra. It arises from the perineal body, from the median raphe on the perineal surface of the bulb of the urethra, and from the dorsal portion of the fixed anterior urethra. Its fibers insert into the inferior fascia of the urogenital diaphragm, into the corpus spongiosum penis, and into the fascia of the dorsum of the penis. The muscle

has 2 halves joined by a midline fibrous raphe. The sphincter action of the muscle empties the urethral bulb by squeezing it and by pressing it against the undersurface of the urogenital diaphragm.

The superficial perineal pouch also contains branches of the perineal divisions of the **pudendal arteries, nerves,** and **veins.** All muscles in the superficial perineal pouch are supplied by the perineal branch of the pudendal nerve (S2–4).

THE UROGENITAL DIAPHRAGM (Fig 38–1)

The urogenital diaphragm is a triangular musculomembranous partition that stretches across the ventral segment of the pelvic outlet. The levator ani complex and the urogenital diaphragm together separate the pelvis from the perineum. The urogenital diaphragm separates the structures of the urogenital perineum from the organs of the anterior true pelvis (bladder, prostate, and seminal vesicles in the male; bladder, uterus, cervix, and vagina in the female).

The urogenital diaphragm is composed of 2 muscles: the sphincter of the membranous urethra ventrally and the deep transverse perineal muscle dorsally. They are enclosed within a superior and an inferior fascial sheath. The 2 fascial sheaths enclose the deep perineal pouch. The superior and inferior fascial sheaths blend just inferior to the pubic arch to form the transverse perineal ligament of the pelvis; they blend dorsally to form the triangular ligament, which is the posterior edge of the urogenital diaphragm. Between the transverse perineal ligament and the arcuate ligament of the symphysis pubica is a space through which passes the dorsal vein of the penis in the male and of the clitoris in the female. The superior and inferior fascial sheaths are fused laterally to the inferior margins of the pubic arch.

CONTENTS OF THE DEEP PERINEAL POUCH

The sphincter of the membranous urethra encircles that structure, which is the most dorsal portion of the urogenital diaphragm in the male. A central tendinous raphe is in the midline between the 2 membranous urethra sphincter muscles. The 2 deep transverse perineal muscles are actually the posterior transverse fibers of the sphincter of the membranous urethra. These muscles, acting in unison, compress the membranous urethra. In the male, the deep perineal pouch contains the membranous urethra; the bulbourethral glands of Cowper, the superior terminal branches of the internal pudendal vessels, and the dorsal nerve to the penis.

In males, in the upright position, the inferior fascia of the urogenital diaphragm faces toward the anterior perineum, while the superior fascia of the diaphragm faces toward the posterior pelvic cavity. The 2 muscles that occupy the deep perineal pouch lie in the same plane and are fused so tightly that they are difficult to separate. The sphincter of the membranous urethra, arises from the inferior surface of the pubic rami, and its fibers encircle the membranous urethra. The deep transverse perineal muscles comprising the greater muscular portion of the urogenital diaphragm arise from the ischial tuberosity and insert in the midline into the central tendinous segment of the perineum. Both muscles are supplied by the perineal branch of the pudendal nerve.

The inferior fascia of the urogenital diaphragm is pierced in the male by the membranous urethra, the internal pudendal artery, the dorsal nerve to the penis, the arteries to the urethral bulb, and the ducts of the bulbourethral glands that empty into the urethral bulb below the inferior fascia of the diaphragm. The superior fascia of the urogenital diaphragm is a derivative of the parietal layer of the endopelvic fascia. In contrast, the inferior fascia lies in the same plane as the bony wall of the pelvic outlet and the obturator membrane and is not related to the endopelvic fascia. The superior fascia is pierced by the membranous urethra. In the male, the apex of the prostate (surrounding the prostatic urethra) is anchored to the superior fascia. Since the neck of the bladder is surrounded by the prostate, this attachment holds the bladder tightly against the superior surface of the urogenital diaphragm.

BLOOD VESSELS, LYMPHATICS, & NERVES OF THE MALE PERINEUM

Arteries

The **internal pudendal artery** supplies both the superficial and the deep perineal structures that lie inferior to the urogenital and levator ani diaphragms. It is a branch of the anterior division of the internal iliac artery. After leaving the posterior pelvis, it enters the perineum and Alcock's canal, the split in the inferior margin of the obturator internus fascia. Within the canal, the artery lies lateral to the pudendal nerve. It gives off its inferior rectal branch to the anorectal perineum and then continues to run in Alcock's (pudendal) canal to the dorsal border of the urogenital diaphragm. At this point, it divides into 2 major terminal branches: the perineal artery and the artery to the penis.

The **perineal artery** supplies the skin of the perineum, the scrotum, the perineal body, and the superficial transverse perineal muscles. The **artery to the penis** perforates the inferior fascia of the urogenital diaphragm and runs forward between its 2 fascial layers. It gives off a branch to the urethral bulb and several branches to the fixed anterior urethra. The branch of the artery that supplies the penis leaves the deep perineal pouch, and within the superficial perineal pouch it supplies the crura of the penis and

the ischiocavernosus and bulbocavernosus muscles. The main trunk of the artery to the penis leaves the deep perineal pouch and, at the undersurface of the symphysis pubica, it divides into its 2 terminal branches: the dorsal and the deep arteries of the penis.

Veins

The major venous drainage from the male perineum is into veins that parallel the 2 major perineal branches of the internal pudendal artery. Thus, the internal pudendal vein receives tributaries from the penis and from all of the structures of the anterior and posterior perineum. This profuse venous drainage is carried into the pelvis via the single internal pudendal vein, which accompanies the internal pudendal artery in Alcock's canal. It exits the perineum through the lesser sciatic foramen and, after entering the pelvis via the greater sciatic foramen, joins the internal iliac vein to reach the inferior vena cava.

Lymphatics

Lymphatic drainage from the male perineum moves mainly into the superficial inguinal nodes. Some drainage from the penis goes directly to the deep inguinal nodes, and a few penile lymphatics parallel the course of the major pudendal vein to end in the pelvic nodal chains.

Nerves
(Fig 38–6)

The pudendal nerve is made up of fibers from S2–4 and is the major nerve to the perineal area. It first runs in Alcock's canal along with the internal pudendal artery and vein. The pudendal nerve leaves the pelvis via the greater sciatic foramen and reenters the perineum through the lesser sciatic foramen. Its 3 major branches, which are given off within Alcock's canal, are the inferior rectal nerve, the dorsal nerve to the penis or clitoris, and the perineal nerve.

The **inferior rectal nerve,** after leaving Alcock's canal, runs transversely across the base of the ischiorectal fossa to the lower rectum and the anus. It supplies the sphincter ani externus and the perineal skin.

The **dorsal nerve to the penis** runs forward with the dorsal penile artery, then leaves the deep perineal pouch by perforating its inferior fascia and supplies the corpus cavernosum penis. It then runs forward on the dorsum of the penis to the glans penis.

The **perineal nerve** is the largest branch of the pudendal nerve. It runs forward with the perineal artery and divides into 2 terminal branches—the posterior scrotal nerve, which supplies the scrotal skin; and the muscular branch of the perineal nerve, which supplies the muscles of the superficial and deep perineal pouch areas.

Small direct branches from S4 help to supply the levator ani, the coccygeus, and the external anal sphincter muscles. The greater and lesser cavernous nerves, branches of the sacral plexus, also help to supply the penis and corpora cavernosa.

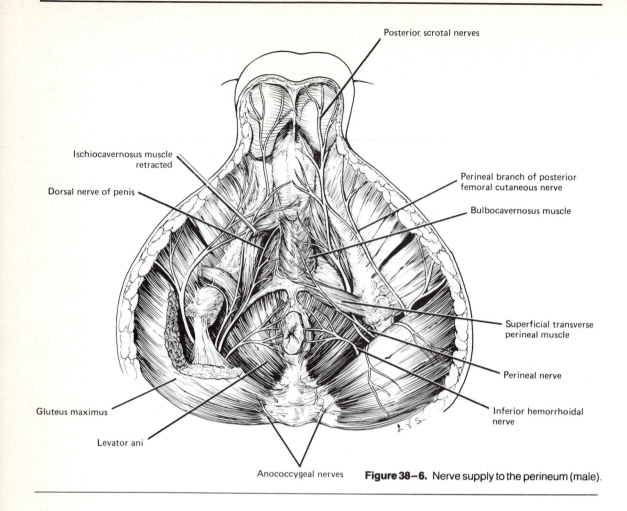

Posterior scrotal nerves

Ischiocavernosus muscle
retracted

Dorsal nerve of penis

Perineal branch of posterior
femoral cutaneous nerve

Bulbocavernosus muscle

Superficial transverse
perineal muscle

Perineal nerve

Inferior hemorrhoidal
nerve

Gluteus maximus

Levator ani

Anococcygeal nerves

Figure 38–6. Nerve supply to the perineum (male).

THE UROGENITAL PERINEUM IN THE FEMALE (Fig 38–7)

The **mons pubis** is a subcutaneous fat pad that in the female covers the abdominal area just ventral to the pubis. In adults, it is covered with hair. It is not part of the female external genitalia but is really a segment of the lower abdominal wall.

The vulva is the area of the perineum containing the labia majora, labia minora, clitoris, and perineal vestibule—the space between the spread labia minora that contains the urethral and vaginal orifices.

The **labia majora** are 2 cutaneous folds (each the homolog of half of the male scrotum) between the upper inner surfaces of the thighs. The outer surface of each fold of the labia majora is hairy and contains varying amounts of pigment; the inner surface of the fold is smooth and contains sebaceous follicles. The 2 labia majora unite anteriorly to form the anterior labial commissure and posteriorly to form

the posterior labial commissure. The labia majora form the lateral borders of the pudendal pouch.

With the labia majora spread laterally, the **labia minora** appear as 2 cutaneous folds extending from the clitoris ventrally to the fourchette dorsally. The fourchette is formed by the junction of the labia minora in the midline. The anterior segments of the labia minora join just ventral to the clitoris to form the prepuce of the clitoris. The dorsal segments of the labia become attached to the inferior surface of the glans of the clitoris to form its frenulum. Between the ventral margin of the fourchette and the posterior margin of the vaginal orifice is the shallow fossa navicularis of the vulva.

The **vestibule** of the vulva is the space between the labia minora when they are spread laterally. The urethral orifice opens into the vestibule ventrally, and the vaginal orifice dorsally. On either side of the vestibule are the openings of the ducts of Bartholin's glands, or greater vestibular glands.

The **clitoris** is the homolog of the male penis and lies just anterior to the urethral orifice in the vestibule. It is usually hidden by the labia and mons pubis. It is an erectile structure. The 2 crura of the

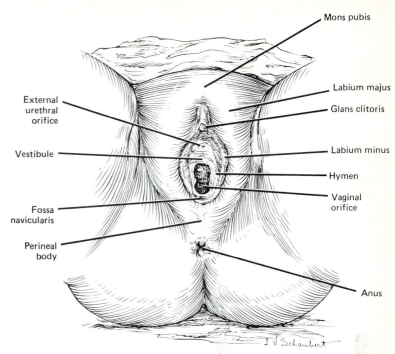

External
urethral
orifice

Vestibule

Fossa
navicularis

Perineal
body

Mons pubis

Labium majus

Glans clitoris

Labium minus

Hymen

Vaginal
orifice

Anus

Figure 38–7. External genitalia of the adult female (parous). Note labium minus spread laterally. (Reproduced, with permission, from Pernoll ML, Benson RC [editors]: *Current Obstetric & Gynecologic Diagnosis & Treatment*, 6th ed. Appleton & Lange, 1987.)

clitoris arise from the undersurface of the ischiopubic rami in the superficial perineal pouch. The 2 crura join on the vulval surface of the perineum to form the body of the clitoris, which is embedded in the vulval tissues and surmounted by a cap of erectile tissue, the glans clitoridis.

The **urethral orifice** is a small opening 4–6 mm in diameter situated about 2.5 cm dorsal to the clitoris. Many tiny glands—the paraurethral glands of Skene—surround the urethra near its orifice. These glands are the homologs of the prostate in the male. The paraurethral glands open via a pair of ducts situated laterally in the submucous coat of the urethra just above the urethral orifice.

➡ ***Infection of Skene's glands.*** *Chronic inflammation of Skene's glands may follow gonorrheal infection. Smears of the terminal can help to identify the etiologic agent.*

➡ ***Urethral caruncles.*** *Vascular urethral caruncles at the urethral orifice often become inflamed and painful and require surgical removal. The lesions are usually reddened, tender, and friable. They nearly always occupy the posterior lip of the urethral meatus and are more common in postmenopausal women.*

The **vaginal orifice** occupies the posterior two-thirds of the vestibule and in precoital females may be closed completely or partially by a fold of mucous membrane called the **hymen.**

The deep layer of the **superficial perineal fascia** (Colles' fascia) is much less well defined in the female than in the male. Furthermore, it does not have the same clinical significance as in the male, since perineal urinary extravasation is rare in women. Colles' fascia contains a moderate amount of fat within its fibrous meshes and invests and gives shape to the labia majora. It forms the superficial boundary of the superficial perineal pouch (as it does in the male). Within the pouch lie the crura of the clitoris (with their covering ischiocavernosus muscles), the bulb of the vestibule, the greater vestibular (Bartholin) glands, the superficial transverse perineal muscles, the bulbospongiosus muscles, and branches of the perineal vessels, nerves, and lymphatics. The muscles in the superficial perineal pouch of the female are usually poorly developed and hard to define surgically or by dissection.

CONTENTS OF THE SUPERFICIAL PERINEAL CLEFT (Fig 38–8)

The **superficial transverse perineal muscle** runs from the ischial tuberosity to the perineal body. The **ischiocavernosus muscle** arises from the medial surface of the ischial tuberosity, covers the crus of the clitoris, and inserts into the pubic arch, into the crus of the clitoris, or into the clitoris itself. The **bulbocavernosus muscle** in the female is also called the bulbospongiosus muscle or the sphincter vaginae (Fig 38–8). It is a paired muscle that arises from the perineal body dorsally. Ventrally, each bulbocavernosus mus-

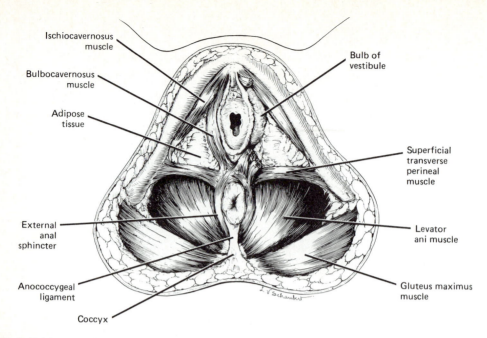

Figure 38–8. Pelvic musculature in the female (inferior view). (Reproduced, with permission, from Pernoll ML, Benson RC [editors]: *Current Obstetric & Gynecologic Diagnosis & Treatment,* 6th ed. Appleton & Lange, 1987.)

cle divides into 2 segments, the medial one inserting into the dorsum of the clitoris and the lateral one into the fascia of the urogenital diaphragm. All muscles in the superficial perineal pouch are supplied by the perineal branch of the pudendal nerve.

The vestibular bulbs are masses of extremely vascular connective tissue lying on either side of the vestibule deep to the bulbocavernosus muscles. They are the homologs of the erectile tissue of the bulb of the urethra and the corpus spongiosum penis of the male.

⇢ *Hemorrhage into the vestibular bulbs. The extremely vascular vestibular bulbs, lying on either side of the vagina, bear the brunt of the pressure exerted by the presenting part of the fetus during parturition. The bulbar tissues are occasionally torn as a result of fetal pressure or secondary to obstetric manipulations. As a consequence, considerable bleeding into the superficial perineal pouch may occur. The presence of the bulbar tissue about the vaginal orifice makes any surgical procedure in the female superficial perineal pouch quite bloody.*

The **greater vestibular (Bartholin) glands** are present on either side of the dorsal margins of the vagina, usually under the vestibular bulbs. They are drained by a long thin duct that empties into the vestibule just lateral to the vaginal orifice. The homo-

logs of these glands in the male, the bulbourethral glands, lie within the deep perineal pouch rather than in the superficial pouch.

⇢ *Inflammation of Bartholin's glands. The ducts of the vestibular glands are frequently the site of acute or chronic inflammation and often undergo abscess formation. Carcinoma seldom develops in these glands.*

THE PERINEAL BODY

The perineal body is the most important structure in the female perineum. It acts as the dorsal anchor of the vagina as well as the ventral anchor of the rectum. It is a fibromuscular nodule lying on a line drawn between the ischial tuberosities. Inserting into it are the superficial and deep transverse perineal muscles, the bulbocavernosus muscle, the external anal sphincter, the rectourethralis muscle, and some anterior fibers of the levator ani muscle. The perineal body is pyramid-shaped, with its apex pointing toward the pelvic cavity. It is about 0.5–1 cm high as it reaches superiorly from the perineal floor.

⇢ *Repair of the perineal body. Following parturition and also during operative procedures in the perineal area, care must be taken to properly rebuild the perineal body so that it will regain its proper anatomic and physiologic*

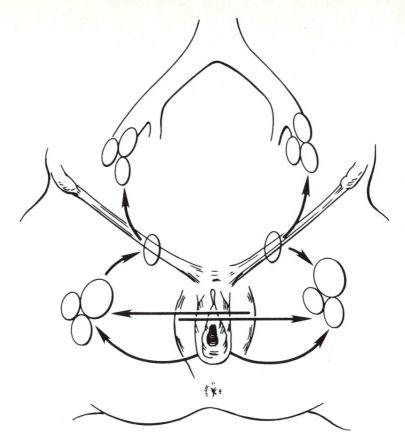

Figure 38–9. Diagram of lymphatic drainage of vulva, showing capacity for bilateral node involvement. (Reproduced, with permission, from Way S: Carcinoma of the vulva. In: *Progress in Gynecology*. Meigs JV, Sturgis SS [editors]. Vol 3. Grune & Stratton, 1957.)

functions of support and aid to muscular contraction.

THE UROGENITAL DIAPHRAGM

The urogenital diaphragm in the female separates the ventral portion of the female pelvis and its contained organs from the perineum. It is a triangular sheet of muscle with a superior and an inferior fascia. It is attached to the inferior rami of the os pubis and to the ischiopubic rami. Its 2 fascial layers fuse ventrally to form the transverse perineal ligament and dorsally to form the base of the urogenital diaphragm. In the female, the inferior fascia of the urogenital diaphragm is better-defined than the superior fascia, but the muscles lying between the fasciae of the diaphragm are thin and poorly defined. They have little or no sphincteric action on the membranous urethra. These muscles are the sphincter of the membranous urethra anteriorly and the deep transverse perineal muscle posteriorly. The vagina divides the deep perineal pouch—the space between the 2 fasciae of the urogenital diaphragm—and also the superficial perineal pouch into equal halves.

BLOOD VESSELS, LYMPHATICS, & NERVES OF THE FEMALE PERINEUM

Arteries

The **internal pudendal artery** is usually smaller in the female than in the male. Its branches in the female perineum are analogous to those in the male. Its perineal branch supplies the labia majora and minora; its bulbar branch supplies the vestibular bulbs and the vaginal erectile tissue; its deep clitoral branch supplies the corpus cavernosum clitoridis; and the dorsal artery of the clitoris supplies the dorsum of the clitoris as well as its glans and prepuce.

Veins

Venous drainage from the female perineum is via veins that parallel the perineal arterial branches. The flow is into the pudendal vein and thence via the internal iliac vein into the inferior vena cava. The vaginal venous plexuses lie on either side of the vagina and are drained by the vaginal veins that run directly into the internal iliac vein.

Figure 38–10. Arteries and nerves of the perineum (female). (Reproduced, with permission, from Pernoll ML, Benson RC [editors]: *Current Obstetric & Gynecologic Diagnosis & Treatment,* 6th ed. Appleton & Lange, 1987.)

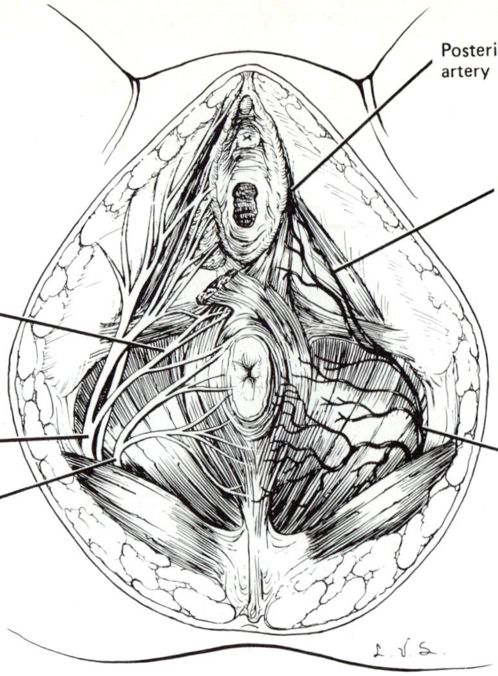

Posterior labial artery

Dorsal artery of the clitoris

Perineal nerve

Pudendal nerve

Inferior hemorrhoidal nerve

Internal pudendal artery

Lymphatics
(Fig 38–9)

Vulval lymphatic drainage is to the superficial inguinal lymph nodes via lymphatics that follow the course of the superficial external pudendal vessels.

Most of the lymph flow from the clitoris ends in the same nodes, although a small amount runs directly to the deep inguinal nodes. Occasionally, some clitoral drainage moves into the internal iliac pelvic nodes. The lower vagina and the adjacent labia drain into both the superficial and the deep inguinal nodes, with occasionally a small amount of drainage into the pelvic nodes.

Nerves
(Figs 38–10 and 38–11)

The female perineum is supplied by the pudendal nerve and its branches and also by direct branches from S4. Autonomic nerves are brought to the lower vagina, to the erectile tissue of the vestibule, and to the clitoris by fibers from the inferior portion of the pelvic plexus, which is a continuation of the hypogastric plexus. Some sacral fibers from S2, S3, and S4 and some fibers from the upper 2 sacral ganglia also supply the female perineum.

➠ *Perineal anesthesia in the female. Perineal anesthesia may be obtained by injecting the pudendal nerve as it lies in Alcock's canal. The ischial spine serves as the anatomic landmark. This procedure was a fairly common, simply performed obstetric practice. It has been superseded by epidural block anesthesia, an effective method for anesthetizing the perineum and relieving the pain of uterine contractions in the first stage of labor.*

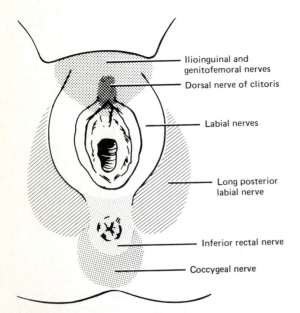

Ilioinguinal and genitofemoral nerves

Dorsal nerve of clitoris

Labial nerves

Long posterior labial nerve

Inferior rectal nerve

Coccygeal nerve

Figure 38–11. Cutaneous distribution of innervation in the female.

The Male Genital System

The male genital system is divided into extrapelvic and intrapelvic segments. The extrapelvic segment comprises the penis, scrotum, and testes. The intrapelvic segment consists of the ductus deferens, the seminal vesicles, the ejaculatory ducts, and the prostate.

I. EXTRAPELVIC SEGMENT

THE PENIS & URETHRA

EMBRYOLOGY
(Fig 39–1)

Sex differentiation of the male external genitalia begins during the eighth week of fetal life. By the end of the 12th week, one can distinguish the male from the female embryo by noting differences in the developing external genitalia. Three small elevations on the external cloacal membrane are the earliest evidence of sex differentiation in the male fetus. This central elevation is the genital tubercle, and on either side of it are the genital swellings. By the seventh week of fetal life, the urogenital membrane has broken down, and the primitive urogenital sinus opens on the undersurface of the genital tubercle. The opening of the urogenital sinus, which is on the ventral surface of the genital tubercle, is called the urethral groove. The urogenital sinus and the urethral groove are bounded by urethral folds. The genital tubercle elongates and eventually becomes the phallus.

By the seventh week, the corpora cavernosa are first noted as paired cellular rods of mesenchymal origin lying within the penile shaft. By the tenth week, the urethral folds begin to fuse, starting at the orifice of the urogenital sinus and continuing outward to the end of the phallic tip. The fusion is completed by the 14th week, and the penile urethra is thus formed. The corpus spongiosum results from differentiation of the mesenchymal mass around the formed penile urethra.

The penile glans develops after the circular coronary sulcus appears at the end of the phallus. The urethral groove and fusing urethral folds do not extend beyond the coronary sulcus. An ectodermal epithelial cord grows through the glans and becomes the glandular urethra—which, with the already formed penile urethra, completes the penile urethra (see Chapter 37). Between the third and fifth months of fetal life, a skin fold at the base of the glans penis—the prepuce, or foreskin—enlarges to envelop the glans.

Anomalies
(Fig 39–2)

Total **absence of the penis** is a rare anomaly. However, the penis may remain a comparatively rudimentary structure; the condition is frequently seen in pseudohermaphroditism. A concealed penis or transposition of the penis and scrotum are rarely encountered. Failure of fusion or incomplete fusion of the urethral folds results in hypospadias of varying degrees. Because of the fusion of the urethral folds, the defect never extends to the urethral bulb.

⫸ *Hypospadias, a congenital deformity of the penile urethra, results from incomplete fusion of the urethral folds; it is usually accompanied by abnormal ventral curvature of the penis. The urethral meatus opens on the ventral surface of the penis; it may open as far dorsally as the perineum. If the anomaly extends toward the scrotum, the scrotum is bifid and resembles the labia majora of the female. With adequate surgical correction, the shaft of the penis can be straightened so that intercourse is possible. The urethra must be reconstructed so that it extends to the tip of the glans penis.*

If the genital primordia develop inferior to their normal position, the corpora cavernosa may form caudal to the outlet of the urogenital sinus, and the urethral groove is placed on the underside of the penis. Depending on the degree of the defect, there may be complete or an incomplete epispadias.

GROSS ANATOMY
(Figs 39–3 to 39–5)

The penis is a flaccid, tubular organ that hangs from the anterior and anterolateral surfaces of the pubic arch. When the penis is erect, it is roughly prismatic in shape.

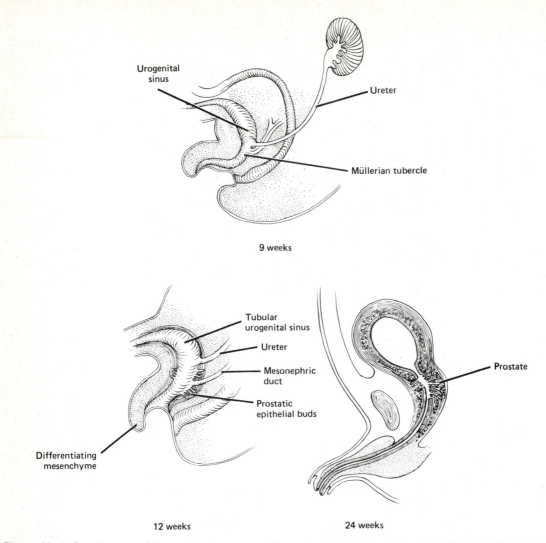

Figure 39–1. Development of the genitourinary tract. (Reproduced, with permission, from Tanagho EA, McAninch JW: *Smith's General Urology*, 12th ed. Appleton & Lange, 1988.)·

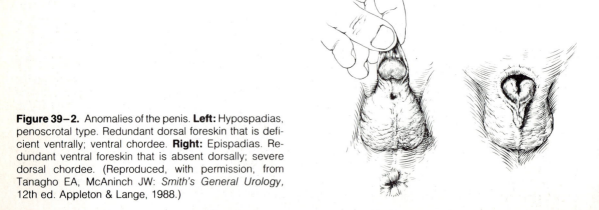

Figure 39–2. Anomalies of the penis. **Left:** Hypospadias, penoscrotal type. Redundant dorsal foreskin that is deficient ventrally; ventral chordee. **Right:** Epispadias. Redundant ventral foreskin that is absent dorsally; severe dorsal chordee. (Reproduced, with permission, from Tanagho EA, McAninch JW: *Smith's General Urology*, 12th ed. Appleton & Lange, 1988.)

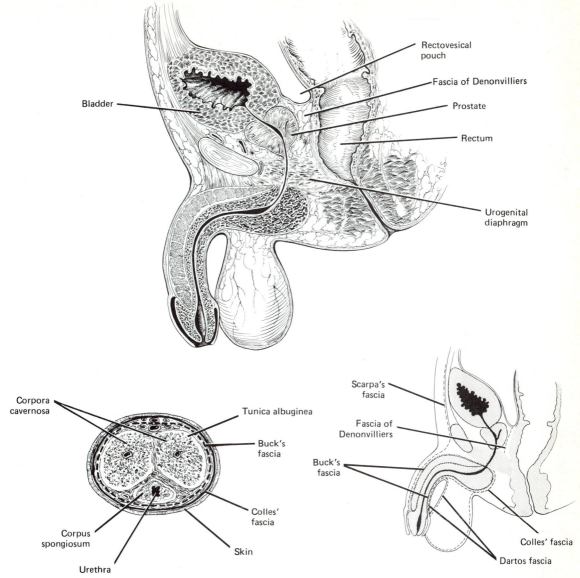

Figure 39–3. *Top:* Relations of the bladder, prostate, seminal vesicles, penis, urethra, and scrotal contents. ***Lower left:*** Transverse section through the penis. The paired upper structures are the corpora cavernosa. The single lower body surrounding the urethra is the corpus spongiosum. ***Lower right:*** Fascial planes of the lower genitourinary tract. (After Wesson.) (Reproduced, with permission, from Tanagho EA, McAninch JW: *Smith's General Urology,* 12th ed. Appleton & Lange, 1988.)

The penis consists of a fixed dorsal segment within the urogenital perineum and a mobile ventral segment suspended from the os pubis. The dorsal segment is called the root of the penis; the pendulous ventral segment is the penile body. At the narrowed, most ventral segment of the urogenital perineum, the 2 lateral corpora cavernosa penis and the central corpus spongiosum urethrae, which together form the root of the penis, unite to form the penis. The 2 corpora cavernosa fuse, lying side by side, and insert into the glans penis to form the superior (dorsal) surface of the organ. The thinner corpus spongiosum, contain-

ing the anterior urethra, lies below the fused corpora cavernosa and forms the inferior (ventral) portion. At the tip of the penis the corpus spongiosum swells to form the glans penis. The 3 segments of the penis are tightly bound together by dense fibrous tissue.

The glans penis resembles a cap as it sits tightly attached to the front of the corpora cavernosa. It is wider than the penile shaft and has a rounded proximal border, the corona glandis penis. Just proximal to the corona is a sulcus. At the tip of the glans is the urethral orifice.

The penile skin is thin, dark, and hairless and

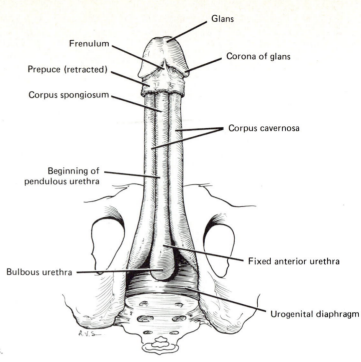

Figure 39–4. Ventral surface of the penis.

forms a double-layered hood over the glans penis, ie, the prepuce, or foreskin. At the level of the os pubis, the penile skin is continuous superiorly with the skin of the lower abdomen and inferiorly and posteriorly with the skin of the scrotum and the anterior perineum. The skin of the penis is loosely connected to the deeper parts of the organ.

The foreskin (prepuce) is normally quite easy to retract so that the glans penis can be inspected and cleansed. The inner (deep) surface of the foreskin contains lubricating sebaceous glands. The external urethral orifice is at the tip of the glans penis. The foreskin is attached to the underside of the urethral orifice by a fold of the duplicate foreskin, the frenulum of the glans penis. The skin of the glans is continuous with the mucous membrane of the urethral orifice and is also hairless.

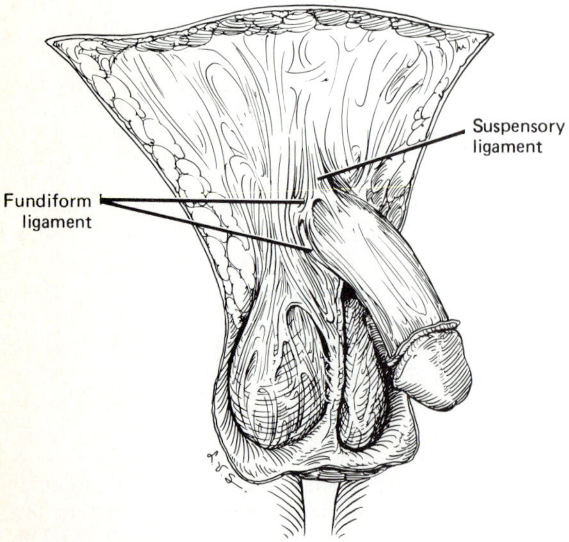

➡ ***Phimosis and meatal stenosis.** (Fig 39–6.) Phimosis (tight foreskin) is relieved by circumcision. Too small a uretheral orifice in infants (or occasionally adults) is relieved by meatotomy.*

Fascia & Ligaments

Just deep to the penile skin lie the superficial or subcutaneous penile fascia, an inferior midline extension of Scarpa's fascia of the ventrolateral abdominal wall. The subcutaneous fascia contains the tunica dartos, which is present not only in the penis but also occupies a subcutaneous position in the scrotum. After providing a layer to the penis and the scrotum, the fascia continues dorsally and becomes Colles' fascia as it enters the anterior perineum. The superficial fascia, as it covers the penis, is freely movable on the underlying tissues owing to a fascial cleft between it and the deep fascia.

The deep penile fascia (Buck's fascia) envelops the penile shaft as far anteriorly as the corona of

Figure 39–5. Suspensory and fundiform ligaments of the penis.

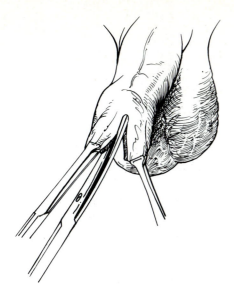

Figure 39–6. Dorsal slit for correction of phimosis. (Reproduced, with permission, from Mills J: *Current Emergency Diagnosis & Treatment,* 2nd ed. Lange, 1985.)

the glans penis. Dorsally, it envelops the 2 penile crura and the urethral bulb, and along with these structures it attaches to the ischiopubic rami and to the underside of the urogenital diaphragm.

➠ ***Buck's fascia in urinary extravasation.*** *(Fig 39–7.) Since Buck's fascia tightly encloses the deep penile tissue, hematomas, penile abscesses, and penile urinary extravasations such*

as may occur following rupture of the pendulous urethra are confined to the deep segment of the penis. However, in rupture of the membranous or fixed anterior urethra, urine enters the space between the superficial and deep penile fasciae. The space entered is continuous with the fascial space of the scrotum, the space superior to Colles' fascia in the perineum, and the space deep to Scarpa's fascia on the ventrolateral abdominal wall.

The 3 columnar bodies of the penis have readily distensible venous spaces that produce turgor and erection of the organ when suffused with blood. The venous spaces are surrounded by the third and deepest of the fascial coverings, a layer of dense fibrous tissue, the tunica albuginea.

The suspensory ligament of the penis, a fibrous band, runs from the superior border of the pubic symphysis and from the caudal end of the linea alba of the ventrolateral abdominal wall to the junction of the fixed and mobile segments of the penis. The fundiform ligament supports the penis in a slinglike fashion. It runs downward from the linea alba and blends with the superficial fascia on the proximal lateral and dorsal surfaces of the organ.

BLOOD VESSELS, LYMPHATICS, & NERVES (Fig 39–8)

Arteries

The 2 dorsal arteries of the penis are the terminal branches of the **internal pudendal artery.** They run forward in the urogenital perineum between the cor-

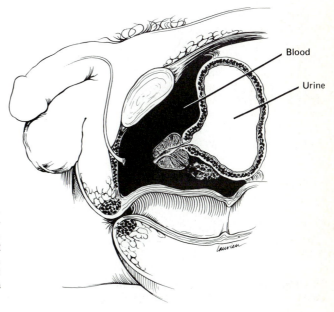

Blood

Urine

Figure 39–7. Injury to the membranous urethra. The prostate has been avulsed from the membranous urethra secondary to fracture of the pelvis. Extravasation occurs above the triangular ligament and is periprostatic and perivesical. (Reproduced, with permission, from Tanagho EA, McAninch JW: *Smith's General Urology,* 12th ed. Appleton & Lange, 1988.)

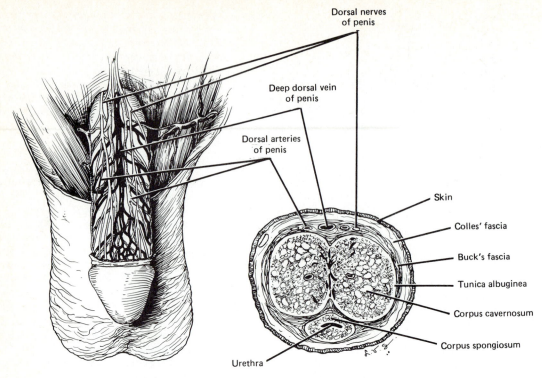

Figure 39–8. Blood vessels and nerves of the penis.

pora cavernosa of the fixed segment of the penis. Eventually the arteries reach the dorsal surface of the pendulous segment of the penis, where they lie deep to Buck's fascia, one on each side of the deep dorsal vein. The arteries penetrate the superior surface of the deep fibrous (Buck's) capsule to enter the deep cavernous portion of the organ.

Veins

The major veins of the penis, which return blood from its deep cavernous spaces, both lie in the midline of the dorsal surface of the penis. The large **superficial dorsal vein** lies between Buck's fascia and the superficial penile fascia, easily visible beneath the skin. The vein flows posteriorly, leaves the penis, and empties into the superficial external pudendal veins of the thigh. The **deep dorsal veins,** which are placed below Buck's fascia, run posteriorly in the midline between the 2 encircling borders of the suspensory ligament. They then pass to the region of the inferior pubic ligament, where they terminate by joining the prostatic venous plexus. The deep dorsal veins of the penis also connect with the vertebral venous flow.

➡ *Drainage of the deep penile dorsal vein into the vertebral venous pattern. Because the deep dorsal vein of the penis connects with the vertebral veins, metastases from cancer of the external genitalia may involve the vertebrae, brain,* *and skull somewhat in the same way as metastases from the prostate.*

Lymphatics

The penile lymphatics empty into channels that parallel the external pudendal vessels and terminate in the superficial inguinal and subinguinal lymph nodes. Lymphatics from the glans penis terminate in either the deep subinguinal or external iliac lymph nodes.

Nerves

Each of the 2 major nerves of the penis lies lateral to the dorsal arteries of the organ and deep to Buck's fascia. The nerves are terminal branches of the pudendal nerve and supply the penile skin, the corpora cavernosa, and the glans penis.

THE SCROTUM

GROSS ANATOMY
(Fig 39–9)

The scrotum, a pendulous sac between the upper inner surfaces of the thighs, is composed of skin

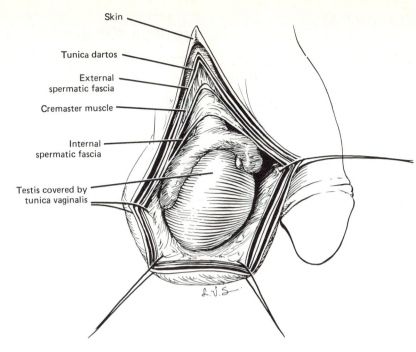

Figure 39–9. Layers of the scrotum.

and superficial fascia and contains the testes and the distal terminal portions of the spermatic cords. The fibrous subcutaneous median raphe incompletely divides the scrotum into right and left compartments and then moves superficially into the scrotal skin. It passes ventrally along the inferior surface of the skin of the penis and dorsally in the midline of the perineum to the anterior verge of the anus. The left lateral pocket normally hangs lower than the right to accommodate the longer left spermatic cord.

> ⟱ *Fluid in the scrotum in anasarca. Because the scrotum is freely suspended and because its tissues are lax and stretch easily, edema fluid secondary to cardiac and renal failure tends to collect within it. The physician must differentiate this fluid from scrotal swellings due to hernia or hydrocele.*

The scrotal skin is thin and usually darker than the skin of the adjacent perineum and upper thigh. The scrotal rugae vary in depth and number with age and with the environmental temperature. The rugae are connected to the subcutaneous thin, unstriped dartos muscle fibers that lie within the superficial fascia of the scrotum. The layers of skin and dartos muscle are separated by a well-defined fascial cleft from the 3 investing layers of the spermatic cord. Each of these layers is continuous with a corresponding layer of the ventrolateral abdominal wall, and

they cover the tests as it lies within the scrotal sac. The most superficial layer is the external spermatic fascia, a continuation of the external oblique fascia. It is a thin areolar fascia that lies just deep to the dartos muscle, upon which it glides with ease. The next deeper layer, the cremaster muscle and fascia, is derived from the internal oblique muscle. The loops of muscle fibers reach down to the upper third of the testis and draw the testis superiorly (cremaster reflex). The internal spermatic fascia, a continuation of the transversalis fascia, is the deepest of the 3 layers and closely invests the spermatic cord and the testis. The tunica vaginalis testis lies deep to the internal spermatic fascia. The tunica vaginalis has parietal and visceral surfaces that are separated by a potential space. The parietal layer lies deep to and is attached to the internal spermatic fascia. The visceral layer encloses both the epididymis and the testis proper. Normally, deep to the dartos muscle, all lining coats of spermatic cord and testis are tightly fused and difficult to dissect, appearing as a single fused layer.

> ⟱ *Transillumination in diagnosis of intrascrotal masses. Transillumination of an intrascrotal mass, preferably in a dark room, is an important diagnostic aid. Hydrocele causes the transilluminated intrascrotal mass to glow with a reddish color. Light will not penetrate a solid intrascrotal tumor, a segment of intestine, or a hematoma.*

multiple fibrous septa that run from the testicular surface into the deep areas of the gland.

⟹ *Hydrocele of tunica vaginalis testis. Hydrocele of the tunica vaginalis testis may present as a distinct entity or in association with single or multiple hydroceles of the spermatic cord or with an indirect inguinal hernia. Hydrocelectomy consists of evacuation of the encapsulated fluid and resection of as much as possible of the parietal serous surface of the tunica vaginalis testis without affecting testicular arterial circulation or venous drainage.*

Along the dorsal border of the testis, the tunica albuginea testis, which lies just deep to the tunica vaginalis testis, thickens to form a ridge, the **mediastinum testis.** From this ridge, fibrous septa reach into the testis and divide it into multiple lobules. The lobules contain the seminiferous tubules that run dorsally into the mediastinum testis to form the **rete testis,** a honeycomblike area of ducts. From the rete testis, 15–20 efferent ducts run from the upper pole of the testis to the head of the epididymis.

The epididymis adheres to the posterior border of the upper pole of the testis. The epididymis narrows from superior to inferior and consists of a head, body, and tail. The head, its broadest portion, sits like a cap on the upper posterior pole of the testis and is connected to it by many efferent testicular ducts. The body of the epididymis narrows as it descends along the posterior border of the organ. The body is separated from the testis by the epididymal sinus, or groove. The tail is the narrow inferior end of the epididymis and is attached to the lower posterior pole of the testis by loose areolar tissue. The canal of the epididymis begins in the head, where the efferent ducts of the testis unite to form a single duct. The canal coils within the epididymis in a tight springlike pattern that is 60–62 m long when uncoiled. The canal leaves the tail of the epididymis to run superiorly as the ductus deferens, an integral part of the spermatic cord. The ductus deferens carries spermatozoa from the testis to the prostatic urethra.

⟹ *Freeing the epididymis from the testis. One can easily detach the body and tail of the epididymis from the testis, but to free the epididymal head from the testis the efferent testicular ductules leading to it must be cut.*

⟹ *Torsion of the spermatic cord. Torsion of the spermatic cord—a surgical emergency—usually occurs just above the superior pole of the testis. If torsion is not reduced promptly, it can result in testicular necrosis and death. The spermatic cord is approached via a high scrotal incision, and the cord is untwisted. Because*

the cord and the attached testis are liable to twist again and because the cord and testis on the opposite side may do the same, both testes must be fixed to the midscrotal septum to prevent recurrence.

⟹ *Tuberculosis of the epididymis. Tuberculosis of the epididymis usually presents as a painless epididymal swelling. The prostate is always involved also, and usually other urogenital organs as well. Occasionally, tubercular epididymal disease will break through into the adjacent testis and result in a granulomatous testicular abscess.*

BLOOD VESSELS, LYMPHATICS, & NERVES (Fig 39–12)

Arteries

The testis is supplied by the testicular artery, a branch of the abdominal aorta that reaches the organ via the spermatic cord. The artery to the vas deferens, a branch of the superior vesical artery, rides on the serous surface of the vas deferens to the epididymis. The epididymis is supplied both by the testicular artery and by the artery to the vas. During the later decades of life, the testis picks up some arterial circulation from the vessels running to the adjacent scrotal areas.

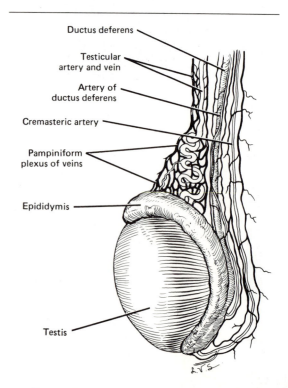

Ductus deferens

Testicular artery and vein

Artery of ductus deferens

Cremasteric artery

Pampiniform plexus of veins

Epididymis

Testis

Figure 39–12. Arteries and veins of the testis.

As a result, the spermatic cord may usually be divided without causing testicular necrosis and death.

Veins
(Fig 39–12)

Venous return from the testis ascends in the spermatic cord via 3 columns (anterior, middle, and posterior). The venous columns or cords surround the spermatic cord and by anastomosis form the complex pampiniform plexus of the spermatic cord. Venous flow from the right testis via the right testicular vein empties at an acute angle into the right side of the inferior vena cava below the level of the right renal vein. On the left side, venous drainage joins the left renal vein via the left testicular vein, which joins the inferior margin of the left renal vein at a right angle.

➥ *Varicocele. Varicocele is a condition in which the pampiniform plexus of veins, which envelops the spermatic cord, becomes varicose, ie, tortuous and thin-walled and of greatly increased girth. It occurs on the left side in 90% of cases, perhaps because the left testicular vein enters the left renal vein at a right angle so that increased pressure in the cava is transmitted directly to the left testicular vein via the left renal vein. On the right side, the right testicular vein joins the cava at an acute angle, so that an increase in caval pressure is not transmitted directly to the pampiniform plexus.*

Lymphatics

Lymphatic flow from the testis, epididymis, and spermatic cord is profuse, and the lymphatic channels are closely related to the venous channels of the spermatic cord. Lymph enters the deep inguinal ring and is distributed either to the external iliac nodes or to the lumbar nodes, which are placed close to the bifurcation of the abdominal aorta and to the beginning of the inferior vena cava. Testicular lymphatic flow continues superiorly from the primary nodal areas into higher retroperitoneal nodes lying both inferior and superior to the renal vessels.

➥ *Lymphatic spread of testicular tumors. Tumors of various cell types frequently appear in the testis and are most frequently seen in the young male. Because of the profuse venous and lymphatic drainage from the organ, spread of testicular tumors to the retroperitoneum occurs early and widely. The degree and extent of malignant spread can be monitored fairly accurately by retroperitoneal lymphangiography, CT scans, and ultrasound.*

➥ *Elephantiasis of the scrotum. Elephantiasis of the scrotum can result from obstruction of*

the scrotal lymphatic drainage. It may also occur secondary to filariasis. Scrotal edema can also occur secondary to radical resection of lymph nodes and lymph channels of the femoral and inguinal areas of the groin.

Nerves

The testis and epididymis are supplied by sympathetic fibers from the aortic and renal plexuses. The sympathetic fibers are carried inferiorly into the scrotum by the testicular artery and are then distributed to the testis and epididymis. Some fibers from the pelvic plexus (T10–12, L1) are brought to the testis and epididymis by the artery to the vas deferens. The genital branch of the genitofemoral nerve (L1, 2) supplies some sensory fibers to the tunica vaginalis testis.

II. INTRAPELVIC SEGMENT

EMBRYOLOGY

From the intermediate mesoderm are formed the wolffian (mesonephric) ducts, which run from the mesonephros to the cloaca. In the male there is both a mesonephric and a genital duct. The urogenital sinus is an entodermal bud derived from the ventral segment of the cloaca. The müllerian (paramesonephric) duct arises from an invagination of coelomic epithelium. It parallels and initially lies lateral to the wolffian duct and then crosses it ventrally to lie medial to it. When both mesonephric and paramesonephric genital ducts are present simultaneously, the genital duct system is in the indifferent stage.

The wolffian duct joins the urogenital sinus via its inferior extremity. The ureteral bud branches from the wolffian duct just above the urogenital sinus and runs superiorly. Distal to the budding of the ureteral bud, the wolffian duct becomes absorbed into the wall of the urogenital sinus.

Buds of endodermal origin protrude from the urethra below the entrance of the mesonephric duct into the urogenital sinus (from the prostatic urethra). In the male, the müllerian duct disappears almost entirely upon reaching the urogenital sinus. As the mesonephros degenerates, some tubules near the testis become the efferent ductules and open into the mesonephric duct, which becomes the duct of the epididymis. Distal to the epididymis, the mesonephros becomes surrounded by smooth muscle and becomes the ductus deferens. A growth from the terminal end of each mesonephric duct becomes the seminal vesicles. The segment of mesonephric duct between the vesicles and the urethra becomes the ejaculatory duct.

Adult Structures

(1) Epididymis, ductus deferens, seminal vesicles, ejaculatory ducts.

(2) Supramontal portion of the prostatic urethra.

(3) Inframontal portion of the prostatic urethra and membranous urethra.

(4) Prostate.

Anomalies

(1) Two anomalies: hypertrophy of the verumontanum and valves of the prostate urethra.

(2) Failure of complete division of the cloaca, with fistula formation between the rectum and the prostatic urethra.

(3) Accessory prostatic glands in subcervical or subtrigonal position.

(4) Müllerian duct cyst in the midline of the prostate dorsal to the prostatic urethra.

DUCTUS DEFERENS

GROSS ANATOMY

The ductus deferens (vas deferens) carries spermatozoa from the epididymis to the seminal vesicles and the prostatic ejaculatory ducts. Beginning in the scrotum as a continuation of the duct of the epididymis, the ductus deferens runs superiorly within the spermatic cord. It passes along the inguinal canal and eventually passes the deep inguinal ring as a component of the spermatic cord. At this point it leaves the spermatic cord and continues dorsally and medially to the posterior surface of the bladder fundus. From the bladder fundus, the ductus deferens runs caudally on the dorsal bladder surface to its junction with the seminal vesicle.

The ductus derferens is 40–45 cm long and quite tortuous within the scrotal sac. After entering the superficial inguinal ring, it straightens as it lies within the inguinal canal. On palpation, the ductus has a firm elastic feeling. It has an external areolar coat, a thick smooth muscular coat, and a narrow lumen lined with columnar epithelium. The thick muscular coat propels spermatozoa from the testis to the pelvic organs of reproduction.

⇒ *Sectioning of ductus deferens for male sterilization. The ductus deferens may be sectioned and both ends ligated to effect male sterilization. The procedure is usually done under local anesthesia at the superior end of the scrotal sac.*

⇒ *Congenital adhesions foreshorten ductus deferens in cryptorchidism. Many congenital ad-hesions that foreshorten the ductus deferens can be released—and the duct thereby lengthened—by means of the surgical procedure used in cryptorchidism. This enables the testis to be delivered down into the scrotum. Some of the tension on the shortened ductus can also be released by sectioning the inferior epigastric artery at the lower edge of the deep inguinal ring. The ductus, which is bowstringed over the artery, can be lengthened up to 1 cm by this procedure.*

⇒ *Injury to the ductus deferens. The ductus deferens is vulnerable to iatrogenic injury as it lies within the spermatic cord, both in the inguinal canal and in the upper scrotum. This is particularly true in male infants who suffer from congenital hernia or cryptorchidism. In these infants, the duct is extremely thin, small, difficult to locate, and easily sectioned during hernia repair or procedures for placement of the testis in the scrotal sac.*

PELVIC COURSE
OF THE DUCTUS DEFERENS
(Fig 39–13)

At the level of the deep inguinal ring, the ductus lies lateral to the inferior epigastric artery. After entering the deep ring, it crosses the external iliac vessels from lateral to medial. When it reaches the brim of the true pelvis, it moves caudally between the posterior peritoneum and the lateral pelvic wall. It then moves medially to the posterior surface of the fundus of the bladder, crosses the ureter ventrally from lateral to medial, and descends on the posterior bladder surface between the seminal vesicle and the ureter. Just below the fundus of the bladder, the ductus dilates into its ampullary portion. Just above the base of the prostate, the ampulla of the ductus deferens narrows into an isthmus and is joined laterally at an acute angle by the duct of the seminal vesicle; the 2 structures then form the prostatic ejaculatory duct. Riding on the ventral surface of the ductus deferens, from seminal vesicle to testis, is the small artery to the vas, a branch of the superior vesical artery.

BLOOD VESSELS, LYMPHATICS,
& NERVES

Blood supply to the ductus deferens is via a branch of the superior vesical artery. The ampullary portion of the ductus is supplied also by branches from the middle and inferior vesical arteries and the middle rectal artery. Venous drainage from the ductus is into the pampiniform, vesical, and prostatic venous plexuses.

The lymphatics of the ductus drain into the external iliac nodes.

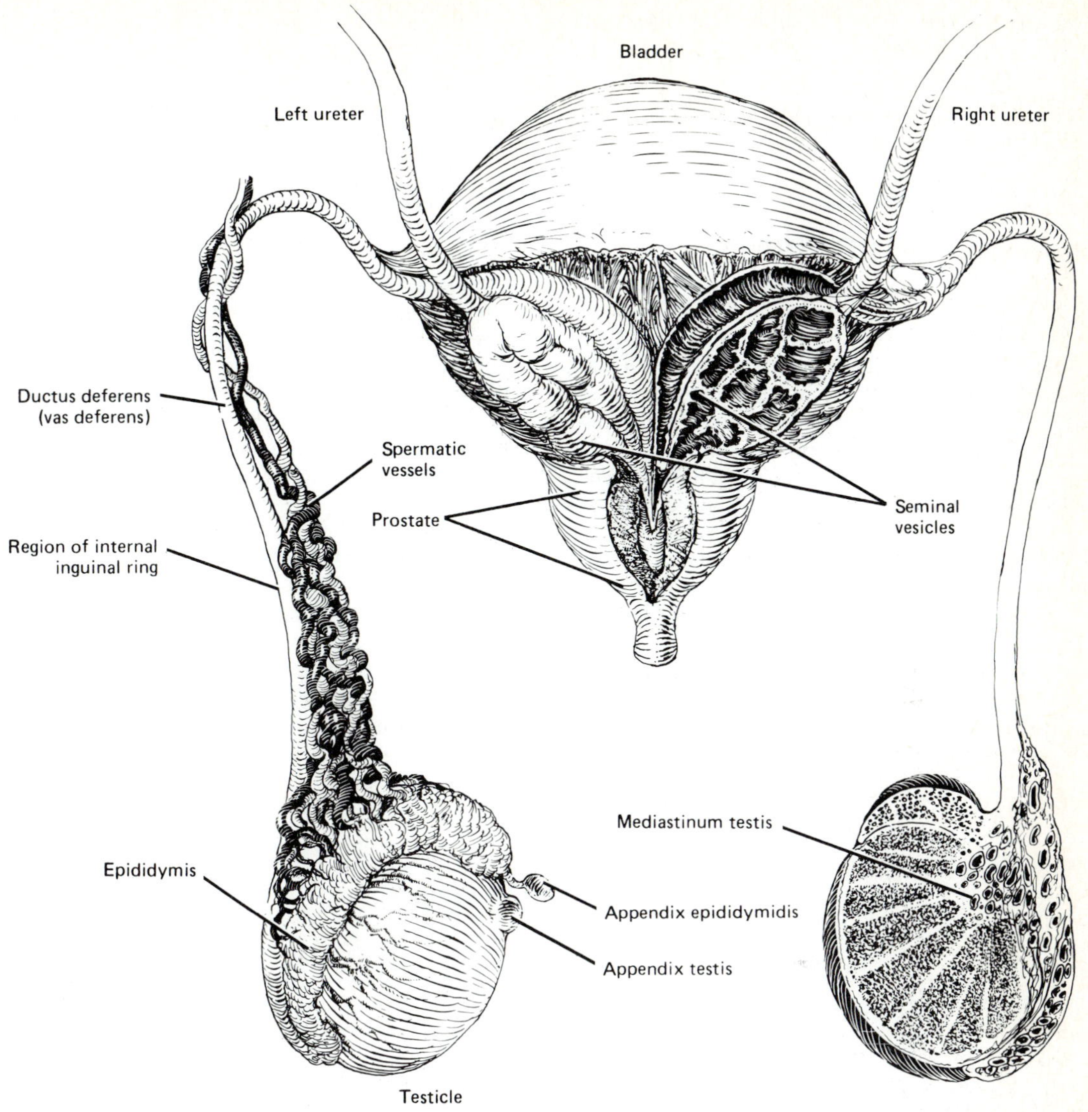

Figure 39–13. Relationships of the ductus deferens, seminal vesicles, prostate, and ureters to the posterior base of the bladder. Modified and reproduced, with permission, from Tanagho EA, McAninch JW: *Smith's General Urology,* 12th ed. Appleton & Lange, 1988.)

The nerves to the ductus are branches from the pelvic plexus.

THE SEMINAL VESICLES
(Fig 39–13)

The 2 seminal vesicles lie on the dorsal inferior surface of the bladder just superior to the base of the prostate. The vesicles secrete an alkaline liquid that makes up the bulk of the seminal fluid. The vesicles are bulbous sacs about 5 cm long; their surface is markedly lobulated. Ventrally, they adhere tightly to the anterior peritoneum of the rectovesical fossa. The degree of the peritoneal covering can be almost complete, but on occasion only the superior pole of the vesicle is covered by the peritoneum. The subperitoneal dorsal surface of the vesicles is related to Denonvilliers' fusion fascia, which separates the posterior wall of the vesicles from the ventral rectal wall. Just above the base of the prostate, each vesicle narrows to form a short terminal duct that joins the narrow terminal portion of the ductus deferens. The 2 ducts join at an acute angle to form the ejaculatory duct. The seminal vesicles have an external areolar coat, a thin 2-layered muscular coat, and an internal mucous coat of columnar epithelium containing goblet cells. The pelvic ureters lie medial and superior to the seminal vesicles just before the ureters pass into the posterior lateral bladder wall.

THE EJACULATORY DUCTS

The ejaculatory ducts begin just above the prostatic base at the junction of the ductus deferens and the seminal vesicles. They are 2 cm long and almost completely intraprostatic except at their level of formation. The ducts pierce the posteroinferior surface of the prostate and pass through the gland obliquely to empty into the prostatic urethra via narrow openings on the colliculus seminalis (verumontanum) on either side of the opening of the prostatic utricle. The course of the ejaculatory ducts within the prostate is obliquely ventral, caudal, and medial, as the 2 ducts converge toward the prostatic urethra.

Arterial supply, venous and lymphatic drainage, and nerve supply to the ducts are the same as for the prostate (see below).

THE PROSTATE
(Fig 39–14)

HISTOLOGY

The prostate consists of a fibromuscular tissue stroma that surrounds and supports the glandular prostatic structures. Septa from the true prostatic capsule run at right angles into the depths of the gland, dividing it into 40–50 separate lobules. The glandular tissue empties into 25–30 prostatic ducts that empty in turn into the prostatic sinuses on either side of the urethral crest on the posterior wall of the prostatic urethra.

GROSS ANATOMY

The prostate is a musculoglandular structure, roughly triangular in shape, with its apex directed toward the superior fascia of the urogenital diaphragm and its base lying against the posteroinferior surface of the bladder. The prostate lies entirely within the pelvis. It secretes a cloudy alkaline liquid that aids

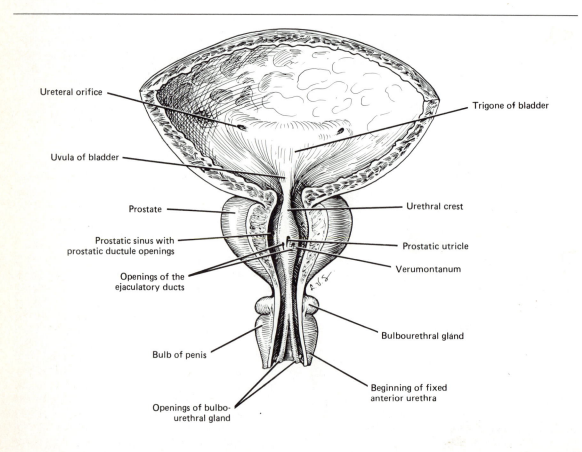

Ureteral orifice

Uvula of bladder

Prostate

Prostatic sinus with prostatic ductule openings

Openings of the ejaculatory ducts

Bulb of penis

Openings of bulbourethral gland

Trigone of bladder

Urethral crest

Prostatic utricle

Verumontanum

Bulbourethral gland

Beginning of fixed anterior urethra

the transport of sperm cells. The prostate surrounds the prostatic urethra.

➡ ***Common prostatic diseases.*** *Prostatitis, benign prostatic hypertrophy, and carcinoma of the prostate are the most common diseases affecting the prostate.*

The prostate is contained within 2 capsules. The true capsule, a fibrous layer of moderate thickness, is composed of intrinsic prostatic mesenchymal tissue and completely encircles the gland. The false capsule is a thickening of the extracellular connective tissue around the external surface of the gland. The false capsule shades into Denonvilliers' fusion fascia and also into the endopelvic lining fascia that surrounds the prostate and the urinary bladder.

➡ ***Bleeding associated with prostatectomy.*** *The periprostatic plexus of veins lies between the true and false capsules of the gland and makes prostatectomy an extremely vascular procedure. A third prostatic capsular structure associated with adenomatous enlargements of the gland can be called the pathologic prostatic capsule; it is formed of compressed peripheral prostatic glandular tissue, the compression resulting from the adenomatous enlargement of the gland. The compression capsule is left intact when the adenomatous gland is enucleated, because it prevents the surgeon from entering the venous spaces between the true and false capsules that both lie peripheral to the pathologic capsule.*

Lobes of the Prostate

The prostate is generally considered to have 5 lobes: 2 lateral, one anterior, one middle, and one posterior. The lateral lobes comprise over 50% of the gland substance.

A shallow median posterior groove, easily palpated on rectal examination, divides the prostate into its lateral lobes. The ejaculatory ducts enter the lateral lobes of the prostate just ventral to the dorsal border of the base of the gland and run obliquely ventrally, medially, and inferiorly to open on either side of the prostatic utricle. The lateral lobes surround the prostatic urethra and then fuse ventrally at the urethra to form the prostatic isthmus or anterior lobe. The anterior lobe is chiefly muscle and fibrous tissue and contains only a few adenomatous structures. The wedge of prostatic tissue that lies superior to the entrance of the ejaculatory ducts into the lateral lobes is called the middle lobe. That portion of the prostate dorsal and inferior to the entrance of the ejaculatory ducts is called the posterior lobe.

➡ ***Bladder neck distortion due to middle lobe enlargement.*** *Hypertrophy of the middle lobe in old age distorts and narrows the bladder neck.*

➡ ***Prevalence of cancer in the posterior lobe.*** *The posterior lobe frequently harbors the stony-hard nodules of prostatic cancer. When enlarged, the posterior lobe grows dorsally and superiorly and becomes easier to palpate through the anterior rectal wall.*

Relationships of the Prostate

Superiorly, the prostate appears to be a continuation of the bladder neck, the urethra entering the gland at bladder neck level; inferiorly, the gland rests upon the superior fascia of the urogenital diaphragm just superior to the sphincter of the membranous urethra, which lies within the deep perineal pouch. Ventrally, the anterior lobe of the prostate is separated from the dorsal surface of the symphysis pubica by extraperitoneal fat that fills the space of Retzius and the prevesical fascial cleft. The space of Retzius, lying just anterior to the prostate, contains a large venous plexus that can cause troublesome bleeding during retropubic prostatectomy. The 2 puboprostatic ligaments traverse the space of Retzius, passing from the prostatic apex dorsally to the dorsal surface of the pubic bones ventrally. Dorsally, the posterior surface of the prostate lies against the ventral surface of the rectum, separated from it by the fusion fascia of Denonvilliers. As a consequence of this relationship, one can palpate the dorsal surface of the prostate with a finger inserted in the rectum. Laterally, the most posterior portion of the prostate is related to the anteromedial fibers of the levator ani muscle; some fibers of the muscle (puboprostatic) insert into the lateral surface of the prostate capsule.

➡ ***Common approaches for prostatic surgery.*** *The prostate may be approached by the **suprapubic** route, in which an incision is made in the lower midline of the ventral abdominal wall; the space of Retzius is opened; and the urinary bladder is entered anteriorly in an extraperitoneal fashion. It may also be approached through the **retropubic** space, whereby the space of Retzius is invaded but the bladder is not opened. Or it may be approached **perineally** through an incision made in the urogenital triangle of the perineum just ventral to the perineal body and the anterior margin of the anus. This approach is used most frequently for advanced carcinoma of the prostate, with some capsular invasion but without marked fixation of the prostate to the surrounding tissues. Severing the rectal attachment to the central tendinous point of the perineum and the rectourethralis muscle allows the rectum to be retracted away from* *the urogenital triangle. The potential space between the 2 layers of Denonvilliers' fascia is opened, and the posterior surface of the prostate is then exposed.*

⫸ ***Prostatic trauma.*** *Disruption of the prostate and the prostatic urethra may follow perineal and abdominoperineal injuries. The attachments of the prostate to the os pubis, the superior fascia of the urogenital diaphragm, and the bladder neck may be partially or completely disrupted. The disruption can cause urine to leak into the extrapelvic cellular tissues, or it may result in formation of a pelvic hematoma. The released urine may flow ventrally into the space of Retzius. Rectal examination shows the disrupted prostate to be movable and to lie higher than is normally the case. Prostatic disruption may follow pelvic fractures or severe blows to the anterior perineum (straddle injuries, land mine explosions). Cystotomy should be done promptly. A urethral catheter should be placed in the bladder if that is possible. Urethral reconstruction and fixation of the prostate to the superior fascia of the urogenital diaphragm should be done later.*

The Prostatic Urethra

The prostatic urethra begins at the bladder neck and is the widest part of the urethra. The urethra runs inferiorly to the level of the superior fascia of the urogenital diaphragm where it becomes the membranous urethra. On the dorsal surface of the prostatic urethra, the urethral crest extends the entire length of the urethra. At the midpoint of the urethral crest are the colliculus seminalis (verumontanum) with the central opening of the prostatic utricle, the homolog of the vagina in the female, and the lateral openings of the 2 ejaculatory ducts. On either side of the colliculus seminalis are the many openings of the prostatic ducts. The colliculus seminalis is the homolog of the hymen in the female.

The glandular portion of the prostate consists of many follicular pouches lined with papillary excrescenses. The follicles develop into canals that join the prostatic excretory ducts. The canals are lined by columnar epithelium. Colloid masses—the amyloid bodies—are present in the prostatic tubules.

⫸ ***Endoscopy to visualize the periurethral prostatic segment.*** *The periurethral segment of the prostate can be seen with the urethroscope. Median bar and middle lobe prostatic enlargements are readily accessible to removal by the urethral resectoscope.*

⫸ ***Pressure of enlarged prostate on prostatic urethra.*** *Prostatic neoplasms can easily distort, completely occlude, or narrow the prostatic urethra.*

BLOOD VESSELS, LYMPHATICS, & NERVES

Arteries

The prostate receives blood from the inferior vesical artery, a branch of the anterior division of the internal iliac artery. The terminal prostatic arterial branches enter the gland laterally. The prostate is also minimally supplied by branches from the internal pudendal and middle rectal arteries.

Veins

Encircling the prostate is the prostatic plexus of veins, into which drains most of the venous flow from the gland. The plexus also receives venous blood from the dorsal vein of the penis. The prostatic venous plexus generally drains laterally into the internal iliac veins. A small amount of prostatic venous blood drains into a venous plexus just ventral to the lumbosacral vertebral bodies. This plexus connects with small vertebral veins lying within the neural canal.

⫸ ***Connection between prostatic venous blood and the vertebral veins of Bateson.*** *The vertebral veins, into which drains some prostatic venous blood, probably are avenues along which carcinoma of the prostate spreads to the bony vertebral bodies and on occasion to the brain.*

Lymphatics

The prostatic lymphatic channels, in conjunction with those from the seminal vesicles and the bladder neck, run primarily to the internal iliac and sacral lymph nodes.

Nerves

The prostate is supplied by the prostatic plexus of nerves that branches off from the hypogastric plexus.

The Female Genital System & Urethra

40

The female genital system (Fig 40–1) consists of an internal group of organs within the pelvis—the main subject matter of this chapter—and an external group below the level of the urogenital diaphragm within the perineum. The pelvic organs are the uterus, the ovaries, the uterine tubes, and the superior segment of the vagina. The perineal organs (described in Chapter 38) are the labia majora and minora, the vestibular bulbs, the greater vestibular glands, the clitoris, and the inferior segment of the vagina. The mid segment of the vagina lies between the superior and inferior fasciae of the urogenital diaphragm.

EMBRYOLOGY
(Fig 40–2)

Early in fetal life, the genital system is sexually undifferentiated (''indifferent stage''). Up to the sixth week, both males and females have 2 pairs of genital ducts: mesonephric (wolffian) ducts and paramesonephric (müllerian) ducts.

The testes and ovaries develop from 3 types of tissue: epithelium, adjacent mesenchyme, and the primordial germ cells.

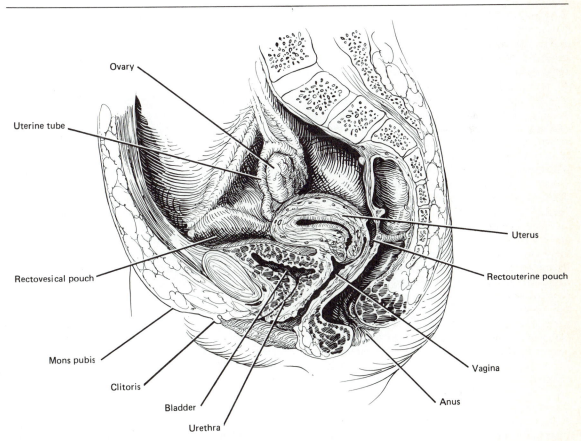

Figure 40–1. Midsaggital view of the female pelvic organs. (Modified and reproduced, with permission, from Benson RC: *Handbook of Obstetrics & Gynecology,* 8th ed. Lange, 1983.)

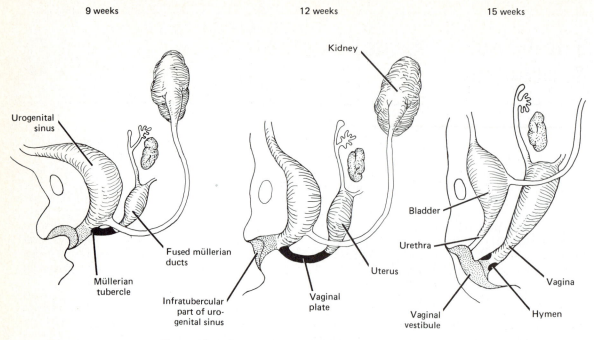

Figure 40–2. The urogenital system in the female embryo.

Female Ducts & Vagina

If the fetus is destined to become a female, only the müllerian ducts develop fully; the wolffian ducts regress, leaving behind only a few small atrophic remnants. The following events occur during müllerian duct development: (1) The superior segment of the duct opens into the coelomic cavity; (2) the mid segment crosses the wolffian duct horizontally; (3) the inferior segment joins the same segment of the contralateral duct; and (4) the dorsal wall of the urogenital sinus, from which part of the vagina develops, is reached by the inferior end of the müllerian ducts, establishing uterovaginal continuity.

In females, the mesonephric ducts mostly disappear and the paramesonephric ducts develop into the female generative tract. The superior unfused segment of the paramesonephric ducts becomes the uterine tubes, while the inferior fused segment forms the tissue from which the uterus and vagina will develop. Fusion of the distal ducts accounts for the presence of uterine epithelium and glands and the fibromuscular vaginal wall. The endometrial stroma and myometrium come from the surrounding mesenchyme. As a result of fusion of the distal segments of the 2 paramesonephric ducts, 2 lateral peritoneal folds appear and form the broad ligaments. The latter separate 2 compartments, the vesicouterine and rectouterine pouches. The mesenchyme just lateral to the uterus lying between the 2 layers of the broad ligament becomes the parametrium.

The epithelium of the inferior vagina develops from the endoderm of the urogenital sinus. The fibromuscular vaginal wall is derived from the uterovaginal primordium.

The Ovary

During the fifth fetal week, a condensed area of coelomic epithelium presents on the medial side of the mesonephros. Growth of the epithelium and the surrounding mesenchyme results in formation of the gonadal ridge. Strands of epithelium (primary sex cords), containing primordial germ cells from the yolk sac wall, grow into the mesenchyme, giving to the indifferent gonad an outer cortex and an inner medulla. The cortex becomes the ovary, and the medulla regresses.

One cannot distinguish the ovary per se until the tenth fetal week. The primary sex cords of the indifferent gonad move into the medulla and form a rete ovarii, but both degenerate and disappear. Soon after, a second wave of surface epithelium and primordial germ cells move into the underlying mesenchyme. During the 15th to 16th fetal weeks, primordial follicles, each containing a primordial germ cell, appear. The mesenchyme surrounding the follicles forms the stroma of the ovary and the follicular cells.

Anomalies
(Fig 40–3)

If the cranial portion of the wolffian system persists, it is found lying in the mesovarium as the epoophoron. If the caudal portion of the wolffian system persists, it is found in the vaginal wall as a cystic remnant (duct of Gartner).

Anomalies of the female reproductive system include double uterus with single or double vagina, single uterus with double vagina, bicornuate uterus, stenosis of the cervix or vagina, and complete absence of the uterus and vagina.

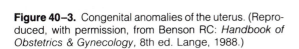

Uterus didelphys
bicollis

Uterus bicornis
unicollis

Uterus septus

Uterus subseptus

Uterus duplex bicornis
bicollis

Figure 40–3. Congenital anomalies of the uterus. (Reproduced, with permission, from Benson RC: *Handbook of Obstetrics & Gynecology*, 8th ed. Lange, 1988.)

GROSS ANATOMY

PERITONEAL LINING & LIGAMENTS OF THE FEMALE PELVIS (Fig 40–4)

The peritoneum of the ventrolateral abdominal wall is reflected onto the superior surface of the urinary bladder and then onto the ventral surface of the uterus to form the shallow vesicouterine pouch. The reflected bladder peritoneum covers the upper three-fourths of the anterior surface, the entire superior surface, and the superior two-thirds of the posterior surface of the uterus. Just above the posterior fornix of the vagina, the peritoneum continues onto the ventral surface of the rectum, forming the deep rectouterine pouch (pouch of Douglas).

⇒ *Digital, bimanual, and rectovaginal pelvic examinations. Important clinical information regarding the rectouterine pouch may be gained by vaginal, bimanual, rectal, or rectovaginal examination (Fig 40–5). These examinations enable the physician to diagnose masses, tenderness, and pelvic collections of blood or pus; to palpate pelvic organs that may have prolapsed into the rectouterine pouch; and to determine the presence or absence of peritoneal inflammation when tenderness is elicited on peritoneal pressure.*

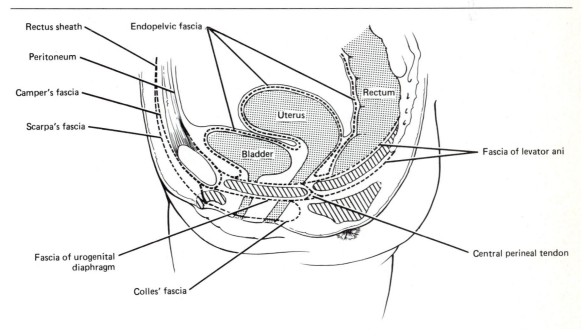

Rectus sheath

Endopelvic fascia

Peritoneum

Camper's fascia

Scarpa's fascia

Rectum

Uterus

Bladder

Fascia of levator ani

Fascia of urogenital
diaphragm

Colles' fascia

Central perineal tendon

Figure 40–4. Fascial planes of the female pelvis. (Modified after Netter. Reproduced, with permission, from Pernoll ML, Benson RC [editors]: *Current Obstetric & Gynecologic Diagnosis & Treatment*, 6th ed. Appleton & Lange, 1988.)

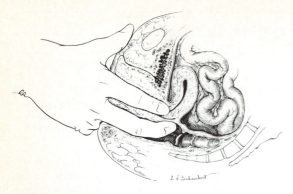

Figure 40–5. Rectovaginal examination. (Reproduced, with permission, from Pernoll ML, Benson RC: *Current Obstetric & Gynecologic Diagnosis & Treatment,* 6th ed. Appleton & Lange, 1988.)

Ligamentous Supports of the Female Pelvic Viscera (Figs 40–6 and 40–7)

The paired ligaments that support the female pelvic viscera are the broad ligaments, the suspensory ligaments of the ovaries, the round ligaments of the uterus, the uterosacral ligaments, the cardinal ligaments, and the ovarian ligaments. The muscles of the pelvic dia-

phragm (levator ani) and their fascial sheaths are the major uterine supports. Weakness of the diaphragm prevents the other supporting ligaments of the uterus from effective supportive function. The uterus also receives minor support from the vesicouterine, vesicorectal, and sacrogenital thickenings of the peritoneum.

A. The Broad Ligaments: Each of the 2 broad ligaments stretches transversely from the lateral pelvic wall to the lateral margin of the uterus. The broad ligaments are created by the embryonic medial movement of the paramesonephric ducts from their lateral pelvic position. During the movement, the ducts pull a double peritoneal fold from the pelvic wall to the midline of the pelvis. At the lateral borders of the uterus, the 2 peritoneal layers of each broad ligament separate to envelop the organ ventrally and dorsally. At the base of the broad ligament, the 2 layers diverge to cover the floor of the pelvis and the pelvic walls with peritoneum. At the upper uterine border, the 2 layers fuse and create a superior (apical) free border that tends to lie in a more ventral plane than the base of the ligament owing to the normal anterior angulation of the uterus. The uterine tube occupies the medial three-fourths of the superior surface of the broad ligament. The lateral one-fourth extends from the lateral fringed end of the uterine tube to the lateral pelvic wall. The lateral termination of the broad ligament continues onto the lateral pelvic wall

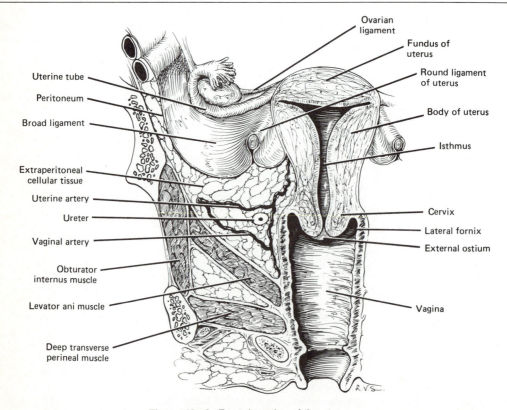

Figure 40–6. Frontal section of the uterus.

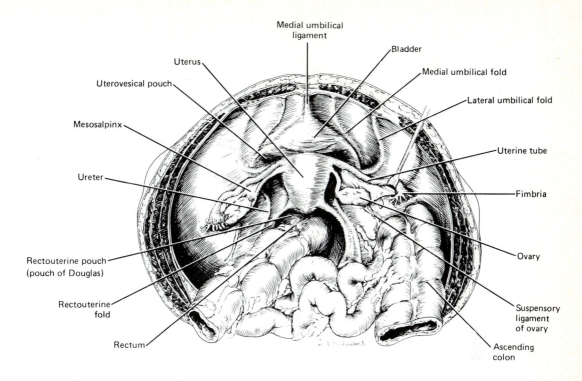

Figure 40–7. The female pelvic organs (superior view). (Reproduced, with permission, from Pernoll ML, Benson RC [editors]: *Current Obstetric & Gynecologic Diagnosis & Treatment,* 6th ed. Appleton & Lange, 1988.)

as the suspensory ligament of the ovary. Placed between the ventral and dorsal layers of the broad ligaments are loose areolar connective tissues (the parametrium), the round ligaments of the uterus, the uterine and ovarian vessels, the uterine tubes, the ovarian ligaments, the epoophoron, and multiple lymphatic vessels and nerve fibers. Two minor ligaments develop and depart from the broad ligament: a dorsal peritoneal fold, the mesovarium, which encloses the ovary and the ovarian ligament; and the mesosalpinx, which lies between the tube and the ovary.

The broad ligaments laterally and the uterus centrally together create a transverse partition across the female pelvis, separating the anterior (vesical) compartment of the pelvis from the dorsal (rectal) compartment. The broad ligament is thicker inferiorly at its pelvic attachment than superiorly at its free border.

B. The Suspensory Ligaments: The suspensory ligament of the ovary (infundibulopelvic ligament) runs from the lateral (tubal) end of the ovary to the lateral wall of the pelvis. The fold of peritoneum contains the ovarian artery and veins. The ligament passes superiorly and laterally from the ovary, ventral to the external iliac vessels. Terminally, the ligament blends with the posterior peritoneum covering the major psoas muscle.

C. The Round Ligaments: The round ligament of the uterus attaches to the superior lateral border of the uterus immediately inferior to the isthmus of

the uterine tube. It passes between the leaves of the broad ligament over the external iliac vessels and the inguinal ligament and enters the deep inguinal ring, runs the length of the inguinal canal, emerges through the subcutaneous inguinal ring, and terminates in the labia majora.

D. The Uterosacral Ligaments: The uterosacral ligaments are markedly thickened bands of subserous fascia that run from the sacral periosteum and fascia and terminate in the uterine cervix. The subserous fascial band is continuous with the cardinal ligament. The ligaments run along the lateral pelvic wall, causing a narrowing of the pelvic diameter anterior to the rectum. Lying inferior to the ligaments and between them is the rectouterine pouch (pouch of Douglas).

E. The Cardinal Ligaments: The cardinal ligaments are composed of a thickened subserous fascia on either side of the inferior half of the cervix and the upper half of the vagina. They pass across the floor of the vagina as an inferior extension of the broad ligament. Anteriorly, the ligament aids in support of the bladder; posteriorly, it joins with the uterosacral ligaments. The vaginal arterial branches of the uterine artery lie within the cardinal ligaments. On occasion, strands of smooth muscle are present in the ligament. The ligaments are important in support of the pelvic organs and in pelvic support following hysterectomy.

⇒ *Vulnerability of the ureters during hysterectomy. At the point where the ureters pierce the cervical ligaments, they become extremely vulnerable during those stages of total hysterectomy when the cardinal ligaments are severed and the uterine artery is secured and when the cardinal ligaments are brought together in the midline to suspend the upper vagina.*

F. The Ovarian Ligaments: The ovarian ligament is a fibromuscular cord that runs from the lower pole of the ovary to the lateral cornu of the uterus and attaches between the round ligament and the uterine tube. The ovarian ligament runs between the 2 peritoneal sheaths of the broad ligament and, together with the round ligament of the uterus, is the analog of the gubernaculum testis in the male.

I. THE UTERUS
(Figs 40–6 and 40–7)

The nulliparous uterus is a pear-shaped, muscular viscus, normally 7–8 cm long, 4–5 cm wide, and about 2 cm thick; it weighs 30–50 g. The uterus is divided into the fundus, body, isthmus, and cervix.

FUNDUS & BODY

The uterine fundus lies superior to the entrance of the uterine tubes into the lateral wall of the organ, and the body is inferior. The fundus is flattened ventrally and shows a convex curvature dorsally. Inferior to the tubal attachments, the ovarian ligaments attach to the dorsolateral surface and the round ligaments attach to the ventrolateral surface. Most of the ventral surface, the entire fundus, and the dorsal surface of the uterus is covered with peritoneum; the lateral surfaces are devoid of peritoneum, as they are related to the parametrial connective tissue that lies between the ventral and dorsal peritoneal layers of the broad ligament.

⇒ *Serous membrane covering of the anteroinferior surface of the uterus. The serosal covering of the anteroinferior surface of the uterus may usually be easily stripped from the uterus. The detached serosa is used for pelvic reperitonealization at the conclusion of hysterectomy. Care must be taken in its dissection ventrally not to perforate the bladder. Adequate mobilization of the bladder avoids the risk of ureteral injury when dividing the uterine vessels at hysterectomy.*

The ventral surface of the body of the uterus is normally anteflexed and rests on the superior surface of the empty urinary bladder. As the bladder fills, the uterus shifts from an oblique to an almost erect position. The dorsal surface of the body of the uterus faces the posterior pelvic cavity and the rectouterine pouch and is related to the sigmoid colon and the pelvic coils of the small bowel.

The uterus is lined by a mucosal layer, the **endometrium.** Lying external to the inner endometrial layer is a thick layer of smooth muscle, the **myometrium,** which is covered externally by a serosal layer, the **perimetrium.** The perimetrium (tunica serosa uteri) is firmly attached to the outer surface of the uterus except over the lower third of the anterior uterine surface and the dorsal surface of the uterus in the region of the supravaginal cervix. In these 2 areas, the serosal covering of the uterus is separated from the uterine muscular wall by loose areolar tissue and may be easily stripped from the organ. This allows the uterine serosa in these 2 areas to be dissected free easily during total hysterectomy.

ISTHMUS

The uterine body narrows, finally constricting into a waist, or isthmus. The uterine isthmus eventually merges into the cervix. The bladder peritoneum is reflected onto the ventral surface of the uterus at the midisthmic level.

CERVIX

The uterine cervix averages 2.5 cm in length. The caudal end of the cervix protrudes into the superior vagina. The terminal portion of the cervix presents an opening, the external os, that leads superiorly, through the cervical canal, to the internal os, which opens into the uterine cavity. The nulliparous external os is circular and narrow. The vaginal opening of the multiparous external cervical os is transverse, with a ventral and dorsal lip. The multiparous cervix tends to be patulous, while the nonpregnant cervix is firm and fibrous. The cervix softens in pregnancy and appears bluish in color rather than its normally pinkish hue. Ventrally, the parametrium separates the supravaginal cervix from the bladder. Laterally, the supravaginal cervix is related to the parametrium that reaches the lateral pelvic walls between the 2 peritoneal layers of the base of the broad ligament and to the cardinal ligaments of the uterus. The uterine arteries run medially toward the cervix in this parametrial tissue.

In the upper two-thirds of the cervical canal, the mucous membrane is of cylindric epithelium, ciliated type. In the lower third, the mucous membrane is composed of stratified squamous epithelium.

UTERINE CAVITY

The normal uterine cavity is triangular and, in nulliparas, about 6.5 cm long from external os to uterine fundus. At each lateral superior angle of the triangular cavity, the uterine tubes empty into the uterus. The uterine cavity narrows as it descends, and at about the level of the isthmus it enters the cervical canal via the internal os. It empties into the vagina at the external cervical os.

In the body of the uterus, the lining mucous membrane is pale red and consists of a single layer of high columnar ciliated epithelium.

➠ **Hysterectomy for uterine disease.** *Operations for treatment of uterine disease are common. Uterine tumors frequently call for removal of all or part of the uterus. During the late stages of pregnancy, several operative procedures upon the uterus may be carried out, eg, cesarean section, hysterectomy for a ruptured* uterus, *and hysterotomy for late (emergency) therapeutic abortion.*

➠ **Vaginal hysterectomy.** *Small uteri may be removed by the vaginal route. The procedure is often accompanied by perineal reconstructive surgery. Myomectomy (removal of fibromyomas) with preservation of the uterus can be safely performed and permits future childbearing.*

➠ **Cervical procedures performed vaginally.** *Cauterization of the cervix, dilation of the cervix, curettage of the uterus, removal of cervical polyps, and cervical biopsy are all performed by the vaginal route.*

POSITIONS OF THE UTERUS
(Fig 40–8)

In the presence of an empty bladder and rectum, the uterus usually assumes a horizontal position (ante-

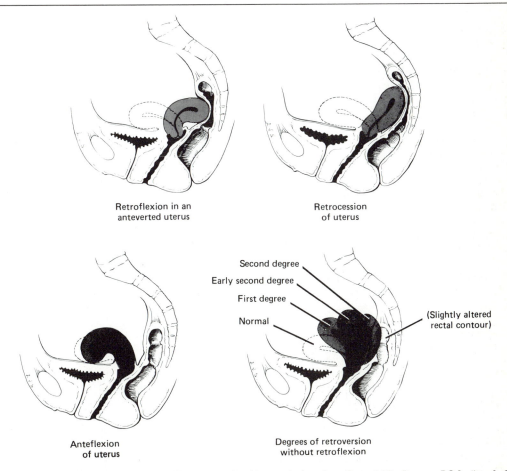

Retroflexion in an
anteverted uterus

Retrocession
of uterus

Anteflexion
of uterus

Second degree
Early second degree
First degree
Normal

(Slightly altered
rectal contour)

Degrees of retroversion
without retroflexion

Figure 40–8. Malpositions of the uterus. (Reproduced, with permission, from Pernoll ML, Benson RC [editors]: *Current Obstetric & Gynecologic Diagnosis & Treatment,* 6th ed. Appleton & Lange, 1988.)

flexion), its fundus pointing ventrally. The vaginal canal joins the cervical canal at an angle of approximately 85 degrees. With filling of the bladder, the uterus bends dorsally in the direction of the rectum, its angle of junction with the cervix gradually approaching 160–170 degrees.

➡ *Factors that cause variability in uterine position.* *The uterus normally lies in the mid segment of the pelvic cavity, but both its size and its position can vary markedly. Multiple pregnancies, endocrine dysfunction, menopausal atrophy, and the presence of uterine tumors can alter the size and position of the organ. Pressure against the uterus by the bladder or rectum or as a result of extrauterine pelvic disease frequently results in changed uterine position. Stretching of uterine supporting ligaments may displace the organ from its normal position.*

➡ *Causes of lateral deviation of the uterus.* *Lateral deviations of the uterus are usually caused by pressure from a tumor or an inflammatory mass in an adjacent organ or by traction exerted upon the uterus from an organizing or healing pelvic abscess or area of cellulitis.*

➡ *Posterior positioning of the uterine body.* *There are 2 posterior movements of the uterus. In retroversion, the long axis of the uterus is directed toward the hollow of the sacrum. The cervix, however, retains its normal position. In retroflexion, both the cervix and the uterus have moved posteriorly in the direction of the sacrum.*

➡ *Paucity of symptoms caused by uterine malpositions.* *In 80% of women, the uterine fundus is normally directed ventrally; in the remainder, so-called fundal retroposition occurs. In nulliparous women, the cervix is usually directed posteriorly toward the vaginal vault. In parous women, the cervix usually lies in the long axis of the vagina, reflecting either retrodisplacement of the body of the uterus or relaxation of the pelvic floor. When the round or transverse ligaments of the cervix show relaxation, the entire uterine body tends to move posteriorly.*

It is generally felt that no symptoms are caused by simple retroversions, anteversions, retroflexion, or anteflexion of the uterus in the absence of other pathologic changes. Surgery is not indicated for correction of these abnormalities.

RELATIONSHIPS OF THE UTERUS

The ventral surface of the body of the uterus is related to the posterior surface of the bladder, to the vesicouterine pouch, and to the free peritoneal cavity and its mobile loops of small bowel. The supravaginal portion of the cervix is related ventrally to the neck of the bladder and dorsally to the dorsal vaginal fornix; the intravaginal portion is related ventrally to the ventral vaginal fornix. Dorsally, the uterus is related to the rectouterine pouch, which contains the sigmoid colon and small bowel, and to the anterior surface of the rectum.

Laterally, the uterus is related to the parametrial tissues that lie between the leaves of the broad ligament. The supravaginal segment of the uterine cervix lies close to the pelvic ureters, which run anteriorly in the base of the broad ligament about 2.5 cm lateral to the cervix.

➡ *Relationship of uterine cervix to the pelvic ureters and posterior bladder.* *The position of the ureters in the lateral pelvic wall and their position adjacent to the uterine cervix as they course medially under the uterine vessels are important. Serious injury to genitourinary structures may occur during pelvic surgery. The relationship of the peritoneum on the anteroinferior surface of the uterus to the posterior bladder wall must be borne in mind so that the bladder will not be injured when the serous bladder flap is raised during hysterectomy.*

BLOOD VESSELS, LYMPHATICS, & NERVES

Arteries
(Fig 40–9)

The uterine and ovarian arteries are the chief sources of blood reaching the uterus.

The **uterine artery,** a branch of the anterior division of the internal iliac artery, reaches the body of the uterus at the uterine isthmus. The artery—accompanied by veins, nerves, and lymphatics—is embedded in the cellular areolar tissue (parametrium) lateral to the uterus. About 2 cm lateral to the uterine cervix, the pelvic ureter, passing from posterior to anterior, lies just inferior to the uterine artery. A branch from the uterine artery reaches the uterine wall at the uterine isthmus and divides into a large ascending branch and a smaller descending or vaginal branch that supplies the cervix and the upper and mid vagina. The ascending branch rises to the level of the junction of the uterine tube and the ovarian ligament with the uterus and terminates by anastomosing with the terminal or uterine branches of the ovarian artery.

The **ovarian artery** leaves the aorta just below the renal arteries. The vessel runs obliquely laterally and inferiorly, crosses the psoas muscles and the ureter, and reaches the brim of the true pelvis. There it turns medially, running first between the 2 layers of the suspensory ligament of the ovary, and then medially between the 2 layers of the broad ligament.

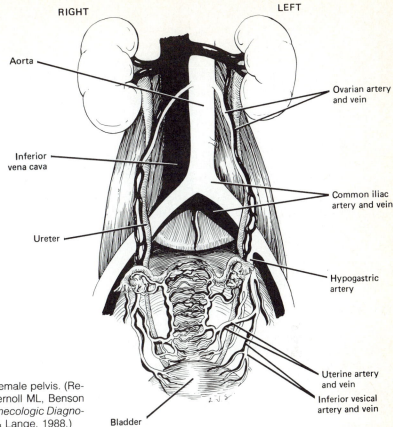

RIGHT   LEFT

Aorta

Ovarian artery
and vein

Inferior
vena cava

Common iliac
artery and vein

Ureter

Hypogastric
artery

Uterine artery
and vein

Inferior vesical
artery and vein

Bladder

Figure 40–9. Blood supply to the female pelvis. (Reproduced, with permission, from Pernoll ML, Benson RC [editors]: *Current Obstetric & Gynecologic Diagnosis & Treatment,* 6th ed. Appleton & Lange, 1988.)

The artery terminates on the superior lateral wall of the uterus by anastomosing with the ascending branch of the uterine artery. The ovarian artery supplies the ovary, the uterine tube, and the lateral superior surface of the uterus. As it enters the suspensory ligament of the ovary, it is closely related to the ureter lying in the ovarian fossa of the lateral pelvic wall.

Veins
(Fig 40–9)

The veins draining the uterus accompany the uterine arteries. The uterine veins communicate, via the pelvic plexus of veins, with the vaginal, vesical, and rectal veins. The right uterine veins enter the vena cava directly; the left uterine venous flow enters the left renal vein.

▪▪▶   *Clinical importance of broad ligament veins. The veins draining the uterus become part of the plexus of veins that lie in the broad ligament. The veins can become dilated and varicose. The broad ligament veins are often the sites of thrombus formation following pelvic surgery; thrombi from them frequently embolize via the inferior vena caval circulation. When surgery upon the vena cava is called for to prevent progression and recurrence of embolism, it is*

of great importance to ligate the left ovarian vein as well as the inferior vena cava, because the left vein enters the renal vein superior to the usual site of ligation of the inferior vena cava for thromboembolism.

Lymphatics
(Fig 40–10)

Uterine cancer is spread mainly by lymphatic channels. Lymphatic drainage consists of 3 systems: (1) lymph that drains from the uterine fundus and body, (2) lymph that drains from the cervix, and (3) lymph that drains from below the tubal insertions via the transverse lymphatic pedicle. Lymphatics from the uterine body and fundus leave via the 3 major lymphatic pedicles. The anterior lymphatic pedicle leaves the fundus by the round ligament and passes through the inguinal canal to the superior superficial inguinal lymph nodes. Via the utero-ovarian lymphatic pedicle, lymphatics from the uterine body and fundus join lymph vessels from the uterine tubes and the ovaries to empty into the nodes of the lumbar abdominal lymphatic chain.

Lymphatic drainage from the cervix is by 3 major pathways. The first pathway leads from the cervix to the external iliac nodes; the second pathway from the cervix into the internal iliac nodes; and the third

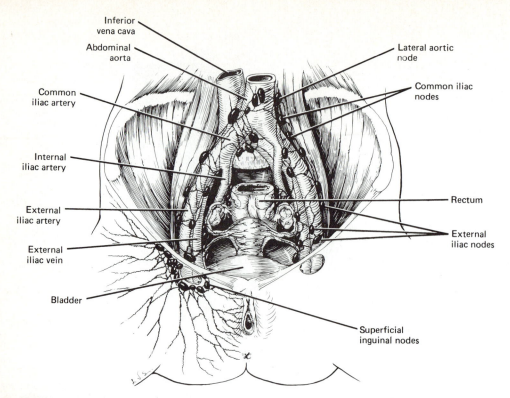

Figure 40–10. Lymphatic drainage of the female pelvis. (Reproduced, with permission, from Pernoll ML, Benson RC [editors]: *Current Obstetric & Gynecologic Diagnosis & Treatment,* 6th ed. Appleton & Lange, 1988.)

pathway from the cervix to lymph nodes near the promontory of the sacrum.

The transverse lymphatic pedicle carries lymphatic drainage from below the tubal insertions. The pedicle runs laterally to the external iliac nodes near the bifurcation of the common iliac artery.

Nerves
(Fig 40–11)

The uterus is supplied by nerves from the hypogastric and ovarian plexuses that lie on either side of the uterus at about the level of the supravaginal portion of the cervix. These plexuses consist of sympathetic, parasympathetic, and afferent fibers. The afferent fibers reach the spinal cord at the level of T11 and T12. The hypogastric and ovarian plexuses arise from the inferior segment of the pelvic autonomic plexus that is formed by the hypogastric plexus and by rami from the sacral division of the sympathetic chain.

II. THE OVARIES
(Fig 40–12)

The ovary is an oval organ, 3–4 cm long and weighing 2.5–3.5 g, attached to the broad ligament

by a small offshoot, the mesovarium. The ovary is the homolog of the testis in the male. It usually lies in the ovarian fossa, a shallow depression in the lateral wall of the pelvis, bounded superiorly by the external iliac vessels, posteroinferiorly by the ureter, and anteriorly by the pelvic wall attachment of the broad ligament. However, the ovary can be found in a variety of positions, including the rectouterine pouch, or even within the inguinal canal. A pathologically enlarged ovary may float free, high in the pelvic cavity, whereas an inflamed ovary may be bound tightly to any pelvic organ or to the pelvic walls. Lying in the mesosalpinx in close relationship to the ovary are the epoophoron and paroophoron. The epoophoron lies between the uterine tube and ovary. The paroophoron lies in the broad ligament between the uterus and epoophoron. Both are remnants of the embryonal mesonephric ductal system.

LIGAMENTS OF THE OVARY

The ovary has 3 ligaments of anatomic importance.

The **suspensory ligament** of the ovary (infundibulopelvic ligament) passes across the iliac vessels and the psoas muscles to the lateral pelvic wall. It carries the ovarian arteries, lymphatics, and veins.

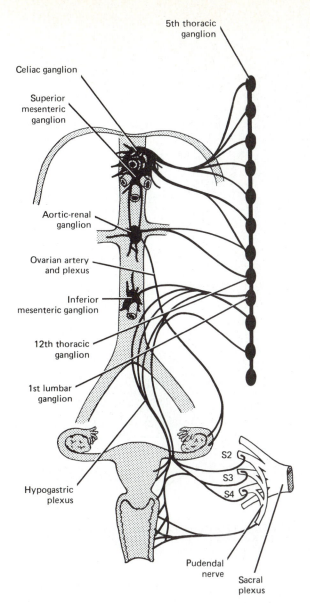

5th thoracic
ganglion

Celiac ganglion

Superior
mesenteric
ganglion

Aortic-renal
ganglion

Ovarian artery
and plexus

Inferior
mesenteric ganglion

12th thoracic
ganglion

1st lumbar
ganglion

Hypogastric
plexus

S2
S3
S4

Pudendal
nerve

Sacral
plexus

Figure 40–11. Innervation of the female genital tract.

The **ovarian ligament,** a round fibromuscular cord, runs from the inferior pole of the ovary to the lateral wall of the uterus, which it joins just inferior to the point of entrance of the uterine tube.

The **mesovarium** is a short serosal fold on the dorsal surface of the broad ligament. From this fold the ovarian vessels and nerves pass into the ovarian hilum. The free border of the fold is convex and faces toward the ureter. The ventral wall of the ovary is attached to the mesovarium; the dorsal ovarian wall is free.

RELATIONSHIP OF THE OVARIES

The lateral surface of the ovary is in contact with the parietal peritoneum lining the ovarian fossa. The fimbriated end of the uterine tube covers the medial ovarian surface. The superior surface of the ovary is overarched by the uterine tube. The free border of the ovary faces the pelvis.

BLOOD VESSELS, LYMPHATICS, & NERVES

The ovaries are supplied with arterial blood via the ovarian and uterine arteries, which anastomose at about the midpoint of the uterine tube. Venous return is via the pampiniform plexus, which eventually is consolidated into the ovarian vein. The right ovarian vein joins the inferior vena cava at an acute angle; the left ovarian vein joins the left renal vein at a right angle.

The ovarian lymphatics rise along with the ovarian artery to empty into the lateral aortic and preaortic nodes.

Nerve supply to the ovaries is from the hypogastric, pelvic, and ovarian plexuses.

III. THE UTERINE TUBES
(Fig 40–12)

The uterine tubes (fallopian tubes; oviducts) carry the discharged ovum from the ovary to the uterus. Each uterine tube occupies the medial four-fifths of the upper free border of the broad ligament. **The uterine tube opens into the free abdominal cavity through its lateral or abdominal ostium; its medial or uterine ostium connects with the uterine cavity.** The tube is 9–10 cm long. It is suspended from the mesosalpinx, which is derived from the broad ligament.

➭ *Importance in surgery of the relationship of the pelvic ureter to the infundibulopelvic ligament. The suspensory ligament of the ovary should not be transected too close to the peritoneum of the pelvic wall during pelvic surgery, because the ureter lies immediately below the peritoneum of the ovarian fossa. There is danger that the ureter may be transected, its course may be angulated acutely, or it may be tied off by the transfixion suture used for securing the suspensory ligament of the ovary.*

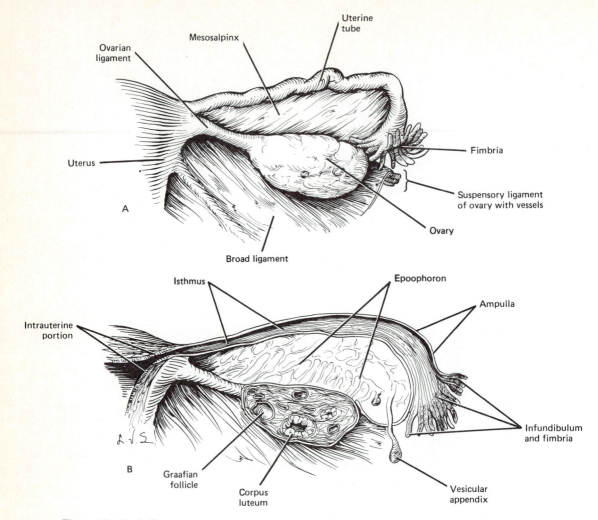

Figure 40–12. A: The ovary and uterine tube. **B:** Frontal section through the ovary and uterine tube.

DIVISIONS OF THE UTERINE TUBES

The uterine tube is divided into four segments: The **infundibulum,** the funnel-shaped lateral extremity of the uterine tube, opens into the free peritoneal cavity via the ostium. The ostium is fimbriated and closely applied to the medial surface of the ovary. The **ampulla,** the longest and widest segment of the tube, extends medially toward the uterus from the infundibulum. Its course is extremely convoluted. The **isthmus** is the short, thick tubal neck that extends medially from the ampulla. The **short interstitial segment** of the tube pierces the superior lateral uterine wall and connects the intrauterine tubal lumen with the uterine cavity.

⟹ *Tubal pregnancy. Occasionally, the fertilized ovum, which normally implants in the uterine endometrium (decidua), implants ectopically in the mucosa of the uterine tube. Abnormal implantation is usually due to distorting disease of the uterine tube that prevents normal migration of the ovum. The ovum is unable to grow normally within the tube, and the fetus may either abort early or grow and invade the tubal wall, with final rupture into the free pelvic cavity. Such a rupture usually causes massive intraperitoneal bleeding and calls for prompt surgical intervention. With increased medical surveillance early in pregnancy and more accurate blood and urine pregnancy tests, many tubal pregnancies are now being diagnosed and sur-*

gically treated before rupture. This permits conservative surgery and tubal preservation and reconstruction.

BLOOD VESSELS, LYMPHATICS, & NERVES

The uterine tubes are supplied by branches from the uterine and ovarian arteries, which anastomose along the tubal body. Venous return from the tube is into the uterine or the ovarian veins.

The tubal lymphatics run to the lumbar nodes via pathways accompanying either the uterine or the ovarian vessels.

The nerve supply to the tubes is from the ovarian and the uterine plexuses, with afferent fibers coming from T11, T12, and L1.

IV. THE VAGINA
(Figs 40–1 and 40–6)

The vagina is a canal that extends from the vulva to the cervix, thus connecting the pelvis with the urogenital perineum. The superior half of the vagina lies above the urogenital diaphragm and the levator ani complex and is therefore pelvic. The inferior half of the vagina is perineal (Chapter 38) as it lies inferior to those 2 muscular complexes.

The vaginal walls are normally flat and coapted but can be easily distended. The anterior vaginal wall is about 7.5 cm long and the posterior wall about 9 cm. The upper end of the vagina encircles the vaginal portion of the uterine cervix. The fornices are formed by projection of the cervix into the vagina. The dorsal fornix is deeper than the ventral fornix. Two lateral vaginal fornices connect the ventral and dorsal fornices. The vaginal direction roughly parallels that of the pelvic inlet, making an angle of about 90–100 degrees with the normal anteverted axis of the cervix.

➠ *Drainage of the peritoneal cavity via the posterior vaginal fornix. A pelvic abscess in the cul-de-sac can be drained through an incision made in the posterior vaginal fornix. The procedure is called a posterior colpotomy. Culdocentesis (aspiration of the cul-de-sac through the vagina) can be performed early to identify the type of fluid present in the peritoneal cavity (usually pus or blood).*

RELATIONSHIPS OF THE VAGINA

Ventrally and superiorly, the vagina touches the fundus of the empty bladder, being separated from it only by loose areolar tissue. Inferiorly and ventrally, the vagina adheres to the posterior wall of the urethra. Dorsally, from superior to inferior, the vagina is related to the rectouterine pouch, the rectovaginal septum, and the perineal body. Laterally, the vagina adheres to the fibers of the urogenital diaphragm, through which it passes, and to some fibers of insertion of the levator ani. The ureters lie just superior to the lateral fornices. Above the level of its vaginal relationship, the cervix is called the supravaginal cervix; below this level (the lower two-thirds), it is the vaginal portion of the cervix.

➠ *Repair of rectovaginal and vaginal vesicofistulae. Repair of fistulas between the vagina and the bladder and those between the rectum, the sigmoid, and the small bowel and the vagina are either closed via the vaginal or the combined vaginoabdominal approach.*

➠ *Gynecologic procedures performed via the vaginoperineal approach. Surgical procedures on the vagina, the cervix, or the uterus via the vaginoperineal approach include hysterectomy and repair of cystocele, rectocele, or urethrocele. The latter operations serve to strengthen the relaxed walls of the inferior pelvis and perineum in order to support the bladder, rectum, and urethra.*

BLOOD VESSELS, LYMPHATICS, & NERVES

The vaginal tissues receive arterial blood from branches of the internal iliac artery via the vaginal, uterine, internal pudendal, and middle rectal arteries. Venous return is through veins that parallel the arteries and empty into the internal iliac veins.

Lymphatic drainage leaves the vagina via 3 main routes: The upper vagina drains to the external and internal iliac nodes; the mid vagina drains into the internal iliac nodes; and the lower vagina drains into the superficial inguinal nodes.

The vaginal nerves are derived from the uterovaginal plexus.

V. THE FEMALE URETHRA
(Fig 40–1)

The female urethra is 3.5–4 cm long and averages 4.5 mm in diameter. In its descent, the urethra describes a wide curve that is concave ventrally. The urethra lies immediately ventral to the caudal half of the vagina and dorsal to the symphysis pubis. In the superior half of its curve, the urethra is separated from the vagina by a scanty layer of areolar tissue; in the inferior half, the urethra is actually embedded in the ventral vaginal wall.

As the urethra leaves the bladder, its walls are composed of oblique and longitudinal muscular fibers derived from the bladder neck musculature. Just inferior to the bladder neck, where the urethra pierces the urogenital diaphragm, it is surrounded by the sphincter of the membranous urethra, a voluntary muscle lying between the superior and inferior fasciae of the urogenital diaphragm. Despite this muscle, urinary continence in the female is mainly achieved by the thickened circular muscle fibers at the bladder neck. The urethra opens on the vestibule of the perineum just ventral to the vagina and about 2 cm dorsal to the clitoris. On either side of the urethral orifice are the openings of the paraurethral glands of Skene.

➠ *Infections of the female urethra. The short female urethra predisposes to infections of the urinary tract. The infections frequently start at the urethral orifice and ascend to bladder level. Sounding the urethra and catheterizing the bladder are simple procedures but can be followed by cystitis despite strict aseptic precautions.*

➠ *Stricture of the urethra. Urethral stricture in females is less common than in males. It may be due to a congenital defect or may follow infections.*

➠ *Inflammation of the paraurethral glands. The paraurethral glands may become chronically inflamed as a result of bacterial infections.*

➠ *Urethral caruncles. A reddish, vascular, benign tumor mass often develops on the posterior urethral lip. It can become friable and painful and may bleed at slight manipulation. If symptoms occur, it should be cauterized or removed surgically.*

BLOOD VESSELS, LYMPHATICS, & NERVES

The arterial supply to the urethra is via the pudendal and inferior vesicle arteries. Venous return is via the vaginal and vesicle plexus of veins, emptying eventually into the inferior vena cava.

The urethral lymphatics drain into the external iliac nodes.

The nerves to the urethra are derived from the pudendal nerves and the pelvic plexus.

Shoulder & Shoulder Joint

41

GROSS ANATOMY OF THE SHOULDER JOINT (Fig 41–1)

The shoulder joint is a bony junction of the ball-and-socket type, the rounded humeral head joining with the shallow glenoid cavity of the scapula. The joint is strengthened by tendons, ligaments, and muscles that help to prevent displacements of the humeral head. The acromial and coracoid processes of the scapula and the coracoacromial ligament provide a protective arch across the superior margin of the shoulder joint and help to prevent superior dislocation of the humeral head.

The shoulder joint allows for a wide range of movement: flexion, extension, abduction, adduction, lateral and medial rotation, and circumduction. These movements are possible because of the loose articular capsule surrounding the joint and the large size of the articular surfaces of the 2 adjoining bones. The **supraspinous, infraspinous, teres minor, and deltoid muscles** which lie superior to the shoulder joint, and the tendon of the **subscapularis muscle,** which lies ventral to the joint, comprise the rotator cuff

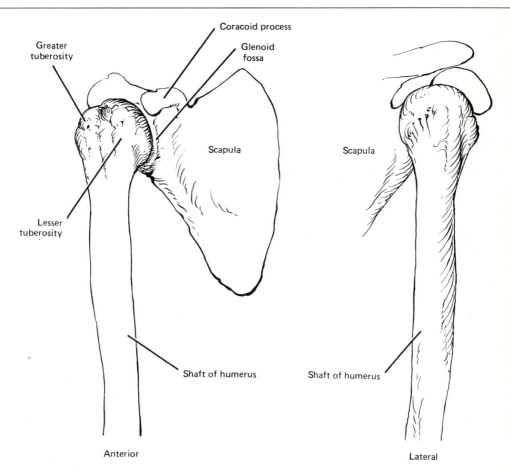

Figure 41–1. Anterior and lateral views of left shoulder joint.

525

group of shoulder area muscles responsible for abduction and internal rotation of the joint (Fig 41–2 and Tables 41–1 and 41–2).

➠ ***Rotator cuff disruption.*** *Complete or partial rupture of one or more of the muscles of the rotator cuff group gives rise to the* ***rotator cuff syndrome.*** *The syndrome is usually secondary to prolonged muscle wear and tear or to an acute fall on the outstretched arm and is manifested by severe limitation of shoulder joint motion in all directions, but chiefly abduction. The acute syndrome calls for prompt repair of the torn muscles and tendons about the joint. Chronic "wear and tear" injury is first treated conservatively. If such treatment fails, surgical repair is indicated to avoid a frozen adducted shoulder as the end result.*

Ligaments of the Shoulder Joint (Figs 41–2 and 41–3)

The major ligaments of the shoulder joint chiefly limit its degree of movement rather than hold its articular surfaces in close apposition. The 5 ligaments are the articular capsule and the glenoid cartilaginous labrum, together with the 3 joint ligaments that insert onto the humerus.

The **articular capsule** completely encompasses the joint cavity and is attached to its entire rim along the glenoid labrum. Inferiorly, the capsule is attached to the anatomic neck of the humerus. The capsule is loose and allows the 2 bones of the joint to separate as much as 3 cm, which allows for great freedom of joint movement but unfortunately also for frequent joint dislocations. The capsule is supported superiorly by the supraspinous tendon, inferiorly by the long head of the triceps muscle, dorsally by the tendons of the infraspinous and the teres minor muscles, and ventrally by the tendon of the subscapularis muscle. Openings in the capsular sac connect with 2 of the bursae about the joint. Another opening between the 2 humeral tubercles permits passage of the tendon of the long head of the biceps brachii. Still another opening, inferior to the coracoid process of the scapula, leads into a bursa inferior to the subscapularis tendon.

➠ ***Dislocations of the shoulder joint.*** *Dislocation is more common in the shoulder joint than in*

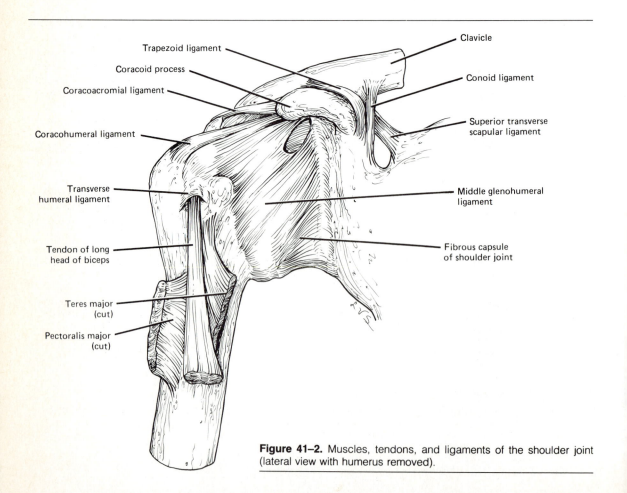

Figure 41–2. Muscles, tendons, and ligaments of the shoulder joint (lateral view with humerus removed).

Table 41–1. Muscles of the shoulder.

Muscle and Origin	Insertion	Innervation	Function
DELTOID Anterior border and upper surface of the lateral third of the clavicle; lateral margin and upper surface of the acromion; lower lip of the posterior border of the spine of the scapula.	Into the deltoid prominence on the middle of the lateral surface of the body of the humerus.	Axillary nerve (C5, 6).	Abducts the arm; clavicular and acromial portions flex the arm; spinous and adjacent acromial portions extend the arm; most of the ventral portion rotates the arm medially; most of the dorsal portion rotates the arm laterally.
SUBSCAPULARIS From the medial two-thirds of the scapular fossa and the lower two-thirds of the groove on the axillary border of the scapula.	The tendon of the muscle is inserted into the lesser tubercle of the humerus and into the anterior surface of the capsule of the shoulder joint.	Upper and lower subscapular nerves (C6, 7).	Rotates the arm medially; assists in flexion, extension, abduction, and adduction of the arm, depending upon arm position; draws the humerus toward the glenoid fossa.
SUPRASPINOUS From the medial two-thirds of the supraspinous fossa and from the supraspinous fascia.	Into the highest of the impressions on the greater tubercle of the humerus.	Suprascapular nerve (C5).	Initiates arm abduction; draws the humerus toward the glenoid fossa; acts as a weak lateral rotator and flexor of the arm.
INFRASPINOUS By fleshy fibers from most of the infraspinous fossa (medial two-thirds) and from the infraspinous fascia.	Into the middle impression on the greater tubercle of the humerus.	Suprascapular nerve (C5, 6).	Rotates the arm laterally; the upper segment of the muscle abducts the arm while the lower portion adducts it; draws the humerus toward the glenoid fossa.

any other major joint of the body. The shoulder joint capsule is supported ventrally and dorsally by a series of muscles and tendons and is reinforced superiorly by the coracoacromial arch. Inferiorly, the joint lacks such additional support. Consequently, the inferior area becomes the weakest point of the joint circumference. The head of the humerus therefore nearly always dislocates in an inferior direction. The subluxated humeral head is initially in the subglenoid area, pushing into the axilla ventral to the triceps muscle. Subsequently, the head may pass ventrally to a subcoracoid position (Fig 41–4 and 41–5) to be located inferior to the coracoid process deep to the pectoralis minor muscle. This is the most common final position of humeral head dislocations. In some anterior displacements, the head may subsequently slide to a subclavicular position or to a subacromial position, stretching or tearing the supraspinous tendon. The humeral head may occasionally assume a subspinous position, usually tearing the subscapularis muscle.

Most shoulder dislocations can be reduced by the Kocher method, which requires 3 movements:

(1) Traction is exerted upon the arm, which is abducted and externally rotated, thereby re-

Table 41–2. Muscles of the shoulder girdle.

Muscle and Origin	Insertion	Innervation	Function
TERES MINOR Dorsal surface of the upper two-thirds of the axillary border of the scapula; from 2 aponeurotic laminae, one separating it from the infraspinous and the other from the teres major muscles.	The upper fibers end in a tendon that inserts into the lowest impression on the greater tubercle of the humerus; the lowest fibers insert directly into the humerus below the impression on its greater tubercle.	Axillary nerve (C5).	Rotates the arm laterally; weak adduction of the arm; draws the humerus toward the glenoid fossa.
TERES MAJOR From the ovale area on the dorsal surface of the inferior angle of the scapula; from the fibrous septa lying between the teres major and teres minor and the infraspinous.	Into the crest of the lesser tubercle of the humerus; at the insertion, the tendon lies posterior to the tendon of the latissimus dorsi.	Lower subscapular nerve (C6, 7).	Adducts, extends, and medially rotates the arm.

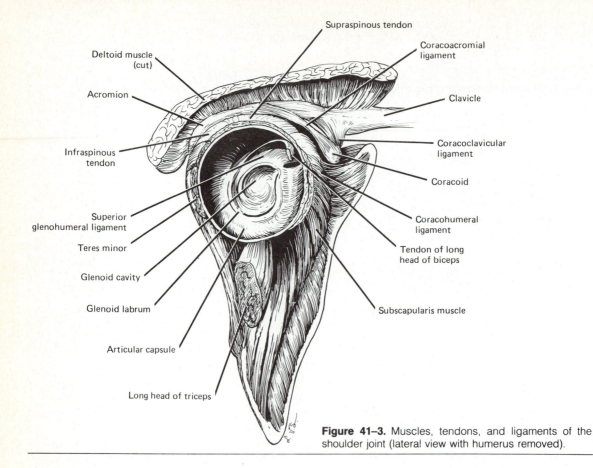

Deltoid muscle (cut)

Acromion

Infraspinous tendon

Superior glenohumeral ligament

Teres minor

Glenoid cavity

Glenoid labrum

Articular capsule

Long head of triceps

Supraspinous tendon

Coracoacromial ligament

Clavicle

Coracoclavicular ligament

Coracoid

Coracohumeral ligament

Tendon of long head of biceps

Subscapularis muscle

Figure 41–3. Muscles, tendons, and ligaments of the shoulder joint (lateral view with humerus removed).

lieving tension on the posterior scapular muscles and increasing the size of the capsular rent.

(2) With the elbow flexed and the arm externally rotated, the elbow is moved anteriorly and adducted, relaxing the tension on the capsule so that the humeral head can reenter its glenoid socket through the capsular tear.

(3) The arm is internally rotated with the patient's hand on the contralateral shoulder, thus bringing the humeral head into close apposition to the glenoid fossa.

Injuries associated with shoulder dislocations include tears of the musculotendinous rotator cuff; tears of the joint capsule, the glenoid labrum, and the glenohumeral ligaments; fractures of the greater tubercle of the humerus or of the glenoid rim; trauma to the ulnar nerve (usually in forward dislocations); trauma to the axillary nerve; and contusions, lacerations, and thrombosis of the axillary, posterior circumflex humeral, or subscapular vessels.

The **coracohumeral ligament** begins at the base of the coracoid process and passes obliquely to the greater tubercle of the humerus, at which point it blends with both the supraspinous tendon and the capsule of the joint. The ligament strengthens the superior segment of the shoulder joint capsule.

The **glenohumeral ligaments** are 3 thick fibrous bands that reinforce the joint capsule as they run from the glenoid rim to the lesser tuberosity and the anatomic neck of the humerus.

The **transverse humeral ligament,** a short, narrow fibrous band, runs from the greater to the lesser tubercle of the humerus. It roofs the intertubercular groove of the humerus, forming a cover for the slot in which lies the long head of the biceps brachii.

The **glenoid labrum** is a ring of fibrocartilage attached to the circumference of the glenoid cavity of the scapula. In cross section, the labrum is triangular, with its base attached to the bony glenoid rim and its thin apex facing outward. The labrum increases the depth of the glenoid cavity. It is joined to the long head of the biceps brachii by 2 fibrous bands that run from the tendon to the cartilaginous rim.

The tight junction of the tendons of the supraspinous, infraspinous, teres minor, and subscapularis muscles with the capsular ligament of the joint serve to make these muscles **accessory ligaments** of the joint.

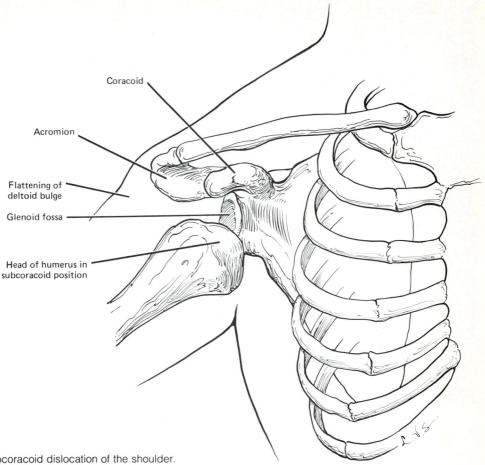

Coracoid

Acromion

Flattening of
deltoid bulge

Glenoid fossa

Head of humerus in
subcoracoid position

Figure 41–4. Subcoracoid dislocation of the shoulder.

Synovial Membrane

The synovial membrane of the shoulder joint passes from the edges of the glenoid cavity to cover the glenoid labrum. It lines the inner surface of the articular capsule and extends to the edge of the articular cartilage covering the humeral head. As the tendon of the long head of the biceps passes through the shoulder joint capsule, it is surrounded by a sheath of synovial membrane that covers the tendon within the intertubercular groove and descends to the surgical neck of the humerus. As a consequence, the tendon passes through the shoulder joint without actually being confined within the synovial cavity of the articulation.

Relationships of Shoulder Joint

The shoulder joint is closely related to a group of important structures: (1) superiorly, the bony arch of the coracoacromial complex; (2) inferiorly, the axillary nerve, the posterior humeral circumflex artery and vein, and the long head of the triceps brachii muscle; (3) ventrally, the subscapularis muscle, which is the only structure separating the shoulder joint from the axillary vessels and the nerves of the brachial

plexus as they lie in the neighboring axilla; and (4) dorsally, the covering deltoid muscle.

Bursae About the Shoulder Joint
(Fig 41–6)

There are 7 or 8 identified bursae about the shoulder joint, *2 of which are always present while others appear only occasionally.* The constant bursae are the one between the tendon of the subscapularis muscle and the joint capsule and the one between the undersurface of the deltoid muscle and the joint capsule. These 2 and the other bursae, when present, can cause shoulder pain and dysfunction of the shoulder joint if they become inflamed. The most common of the rarer bursae are the subacromial, subcoracoid, infraspinous, and subcutaneous subacromial bursae. The subscapular and infraspinous bursae normally communicate with the synovial cavity of the shoulder joint.

➡ *Calcareous deposits about the shoulder joint. Calcareous deposits occur frequently within the subacromial, subdeltoid, or subcoracoid bur-*

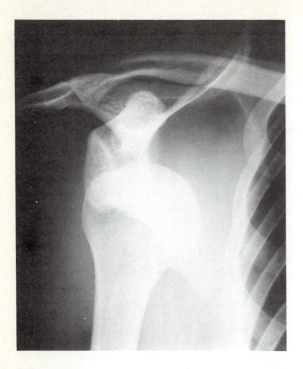

Figure 41–5. Anterior (subcoracoid) dislocation of the shoulder. (Reproduced, with permission, from Way LW [editor]: *Current Surgical Diagnosis & Treatment,* 7th ed. Lange, 1985.)

sae and within the tendons of the rotator cuff muscles. The calculi may be asymptomatic for varying periods but eventually cause severe shoulder pain and restricted shoulder motion. The calcareous areas are usually injected with a local anesthetic and aqueous hydrocortisone, which usually gives rapid symptomatic relief. Occasionally, surgical removal of large deposits is required.

Movements of the Shoulder Joint

A. Abduction and Adduction: The shoulder joint is abducted by the supraspinous and deltoid muscles and adducted by the pectoralis major, latissimus dorsi, subscapularis, and teres major muscles and by the weight of the arm.

B. Flexion: The joint is flexed by the pectoralis major, coracobrachialis, and anterior fibers of the deltoid and by the biceps brachii if the elbow is flexed.

C. Extension: The joint is extended by the teres major, latissimus dorsi, and posterior fibers of the deltoid and, if the elbow is extended, by the triceps.

D. Rotation: The joint is rotated medially by the pectoralis major, latissimus dorsi, teres major, subscapularis, and anterior deltoid fibers, and laterally by the infraspinous and teres minor and posterior fibers of the deltoid.

Movement of the shoulder joint is aided by move-

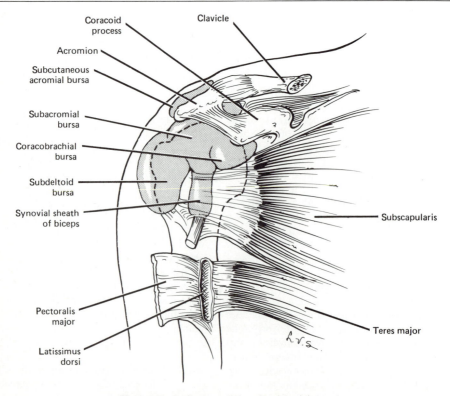

Figure 41–6. Bursae of the shoulder joint.

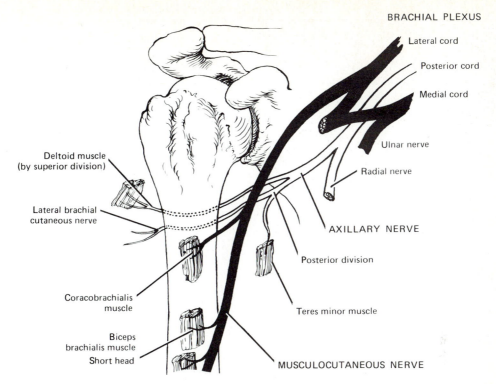

Figure 41–7. Innervation of the shoulder joint. (Reproduced, with permission, from Chusid JG: *Correlative Neuroanatomy & Functional Neurology,* 19th ed. Lange, 1985.)

ment of the scapula. Scapular movement at the acromioclavicular and sternoclavicular joints is quite limited. However, the scapula can move superiorly, inferiorly, anteriorly, and posteriorly upon the dorsal chest wall. As a result, the arm may be circumducted upon the chest wall. The movement of the scapula upon the chest wall plus the action of the shoulder joint allows the arm to be raised above the head.

Blood Vessels, Lymphatics, & Nerves

The shoulder joint receives arterial blood primarily from branches of the anterior and posterior circumflex humeral vessels. It also receives some blood from branches of the transverse scapular artery, a branch of the subclavian artery. Venous return from the shoulder joint roughly parallels the arterial supply and eventually reaches the superior vena cava.

Lymphatic drainage from the shoulder joint is mainly into the mid and lateral group of axillary nodes.

The joint is innervated by the axillary and suprascapular nerves. (Fig. 41–7).

*Operative approaches to the shoulder joint. There are 3 classic operative approaches to the shoulder joint: In the **anterior approach,** an incision is made in the deltopectoral groove and extended from the coracoid process to a point about 7.5 cm down the arm. The cephalic vein is retracted inferiorly, and the deltoid is retracted laterally. The joint capsule is then exposed by detaching the muscles attached to the greater and lesser tubercles.*

*In the **posterior (Kocher) approach,** the incision starts at the acromioclavicular joint and is extended posteriorly along the medial border of the acromion to the spine of the scapula, ending just above the posterior axillary fold. The deltoid is released from the scapular spine and retracted laterally. The posterior aspect of the joint capsule now comes into view, as do the infraspinous, teres major, and teres minor muscles and the long head of the triceps.*

*The **superior approach** is seldom used, since deltoid motion would be sacrificed. The incision is made along the dorsal border of the deltoid muscle.*

42

The Arm

I. THE HUMERUS

GROSS ANATOMY
(Figs 42–1 and 42–2)

The humerus is the longest and sturdiest of the 3 major bones of the upper extremity. It communicates superiorly via the shoulder joint with the scapula and inferiorly via the elbow joint with the radius and ulna. The most superior segment of the humerus is the head, which is connected by the neck to the shaft of the bone. The flattened distal end of the humerus is called the condyle.

Ossification of the humerus proceeds from 8 centers: one in the mid portion of the humeral body, one in the humeral head, one each in the greater and lesser tuberosities, one in each of the 2 epicondyles, one in the capitulum, and one in the trochlea. Ossification is completed by age 17–18 years.

The Humeral Head

The humeral head appears as almost a half-sphere. It presents 2 anterior protuberances: the **greater tuberosity** laterally and the **lesser tuberosity** medially. The head projects medially, superiorly, and slightly dorsally toward its articulation with the glenoid cavity of the scapula. At its inferior margin, the humeral head narrows slightly to form the anatomic neck of the humerus. Just inferior to the 2 humeral tuberosities, the head becomes markedly constricted at the **surgical neck,** a frequent fracture site. The anatomic neck is seldom fractured. The shoulder joint capsule attaches to the anatomic neck, and all fractures above the anatomic neck are thus intracapsular fractures.

The **greater tuberosity** lies lateral and inferior to the humeral head and lateral to the lesser tuberosity and gives insertion to the supraspinous muscle. The infraspinous and teres minor muscles attach successively to the greater tuberosity inferior to the supraspinous attachment.

The **lesser tuberosity** lies medial and inferior to the humeral head and is smaller but more protuberant than the greater tuberosity. The subscapularis muscle inserts into its anterior surface.

Between the 2 humeral tuberosities lies a deep furrow, the **intertubercular groove (sulcus),** which enfolds the tendon of the long head of the biceps brachii. The intertubercular groove continues about one-third down the anterior surface of the shaft of the humerus. The tendon of the latissimus dorsi muscle inserts into the medial margin of the most distal segment of the groove.

⮕ *Fractures of the superior end of the humerus. Anatomic neck fractures are intracapsular and relatively uncommon. The humeral shaft is usually impacted into the head of the bone. In fractures of the surgical neck, the superior end of the distal fragment is usually pulled into the axilla by the triceps, coracobrachialis, biceps brachii, and deltoid muscles (Fig 42–3). The proximal fragment is displaced medially by the pull of the pectoralis major, teres major, and latissimus dorsi muscles. Fractures of the surgical neck may involve the axillary nerve and the posterior humeral circumflex vessels in the quadrangular space.*

Fractures of the greater tuberosity of the humerus may result from a direct blow over the tuberosity or may occur secondary to the combined muscular pull of the supraspinous, infraspinous, and teres minor muscles, which insert on the tuberosity. Fractures of the lesser tuberosity are rare.

The Shaft of the Humerus

The superior half of the shaft of the humerus is well-rounded, but below the midpoint the shaft becomes a flattened prism until it blends with the condyle at the distal end of the bone.

The lateral border of the shaft runs from the greater tuberosity to the lateral epicondyle. The medial border runs from the lesser tuberosity to the medial epicondyle. The anterior surface of the bone is covered by the coracobrachialis, biceps brachii, and brachialis muscles. The posterior surface of the shaft appears to be twisted upon itself and is covered by the lateral and medial heads of the triceps muscle. The mid segment of the dorsal surface of the bone presents a shallow groove, the radial sulcus, in which lies the radial nerve.

The pectoralis major muscle inserts into the anterolateral surface of the humerus on the lateral lip of

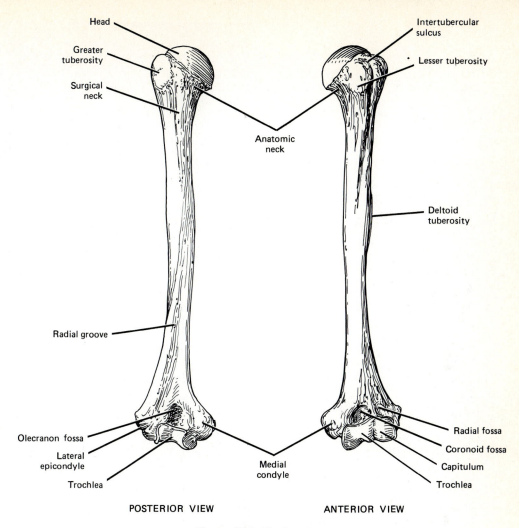

Figure 42–1. The humerus.

the intertubercular sulcus just inferior to the greater tuberosity. The deltoid muscle inserts into the deltoid tuberosity just inferior to the pectoral insertion. The anteromedial surface of the humerus receives insertion of the latissimus dorsi muscle proximally, and just distal to this insertion the teres major muscle inserts into the bone's anteromedial surface.

➤ *Fractures of the shaft of the humerus.* (Fig 42–4.) *In fractures above the deltoid attachment, the superior fragment is drawn medially by the pectoralis major, teres major, and latissimus dorsi muscles, and the lower fragment is pulled superiorly and laterally by the deltoid muscle. In fractures below the deltoid insertion, the superior fragment of the bone is drawn laterally by the deltoid and supraspinous muscles while the inferior fragment is drawn medially and superiorly by the pull of the triceps,* biceps, *and coracobrachialis muscles. Injury to the radial nerve and the deep brachial artery should be suspected in all cases of mid humeral shaft fracture. Below the insertion of the deltoid muscle, the radial nerve is held tightly against the posterior surface of the humerus, and a fracture may therefore be complicated by nerve injury. Radial nerve symptoms secondary to trauma in the mid humeral area are most often purely motor (wristdrop), since the sensory fibers of the nerve usually leave its main trunk before the nerve winds through the radial groove. In addition, late radial nerve deficit may occur during the process of fracture healing if the nerve is caught in the callus of the bone repair.*

➤ *Operative approach to the humerus.* An anterolateral approach is usual for humeral shaft exposure. The incision can be extended along

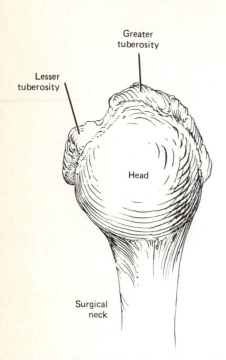

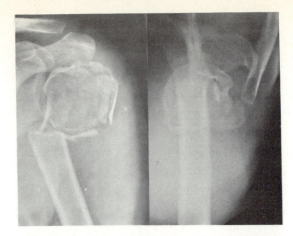

Figure 42–3. Comminuted fracture of the superior end of the humerus involving the surgical neck and greater tuberosity. The uninjured lesser tuberosity suggests that the articular fragment retains some blood supply. (Reproduced, with permission, from Way LW [editor]: *Current Surgical Diagnosis & Treatment,* 7th ed. Lange, 1985.)

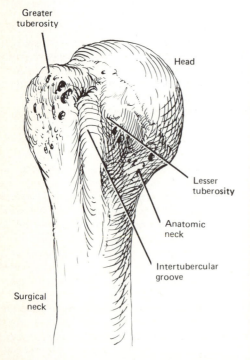

Figure 42–2. Head and neck of the humerus showing tuberosities.

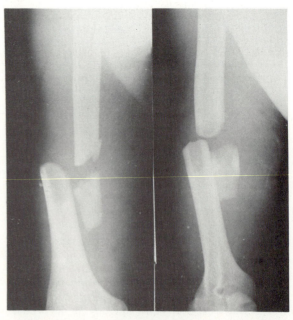

Figure 42–4. Comminuted fracture of the middle third of the humeral shaft complicated by immediate and complete paralysis of the radial nerve. (Reproduced, with permission, from Way LW [editor]: *Current Surgical Diagnosis & Treatment,* 7th ed. Lange, 1985.)

the entire length of the arm from the coracoid process of the scapula to the lateral border of the antecubital fossa.

The Condyle of the Humerus

The distal end of the humerus (the condyle) is wide and flat and angulates ventrally at about 45 degrees from the line of the shaft of the bone.

The humeral condyle presents a wide articular surface divided by a central ridge into lateral and medial compartments. Flanking each side of the articular surface is a projecting epicondyle.

The lateral segment of the humeral articular surface is the **capitulum.** It is a raised, smooth, oval surface that articulates with the fovea on the head of the radius. The capitulum projects ventrally and inferiorly. Just superior to the capitulum is a shallow depression, the **radial fossa,** which accepts the head of the radius when the forearm is flexed.

The **trochlea** is the medial segment of the inferior humeral articular surface. The ridgelike lateral border of the trochlea demarcates it from the capitulum. Superior to the dorsal surface of the trochlea lies the olecranon fossa, into which part of the olecranon process of the ulna fits when the arm is fully extended. Just superior to the ventral surface of the trochlea is a slight depression, the **coronoid fossa,** into which the coronoid process of the ulna fits when the forearm is flexed at the elbow joint. Both the coronoid and olecranon fossae are lined by the synovial membrane of the elbow joint.

The **lateral epicondyle** is a small, bony projection on the lateral side of the inferior articular surface of the humerus. It gives attachments to the radial collateral ligament of the elbow joint and to the tendons of origin of the supinator and extensor muscles of the forearm. The **medial epicondyle** is a more distinct tuberosity as it protrudes from the medial inferior articular surface of the humerus. Just posterior to the medial epicondyle lies the groove for the ulnar nerve. The medial epicondyle gives attachments to the ulnar collateral ligament of the elbow joint and to the pronator teres muscle; the common tendons of origin of many of the flexor muscles of the forearm arise from it.

➠ *Epicondylitis (tennis elbow). This syndrome is characterized by pain over the lateral humeral epicondyle and at the elbow secondary to chronic or repeated flexion and extension at the wrist. It usually follows prolonged rotary motion of the forearm. The lateral epicondyle is more commonly involved than the medial. Symptoms are due to inflammation of the origin of the common extensor muscle and occasionally to tear of the origin of the extensor carpi radialis brevis. Treatment usually consists of rest and analgesics followed by a program to strengthen the forearm extensor muscles. Injection of corticosteroids into the painful area may* help. *Refractory cases may require surgery on the involved epicondyle.*

➠ *Fractures of the distal end of the humerus. In falls upon the outstretched hand, force may be transmitted through the forearm to the distal end of the humerus, which is not strong, owing to the presence of the olecranon, radial, and coronoid fossae. As a consequence, epiphyseal displacement and intercondylar and epicondylar as well as supracondylar fractures are quite common.*

➠ *Trauma to the condyle of the humerus. Following arm trauma, a decrease in the degree of the ventral thrust of the condyle of the humerus should suggest supracondylar fracture. Displaced supracondylar fractures threaten the neurovascular status of the involved limb and may result in an unsightly deformity if reduction is not accurate. The wrist pulse and the function of the radial, ulnar, and median nerves should be checked immediately.*

In supracondylar fractures, the distal fragment is usually displaced posteriorly by the force of the blow, the combined action of the triceps, biceps, and brachialis muscles causing an overriding of the fragments. The supinating action of the biceps is lost, and the pronators tend to hold the elbow joint in full pronation. In supracondylar fractures, the sharp jagged edge of the proximal fragment is driven ventrally and may injure the brachial artery or the median or radial nerve. Nerve deficit in such cases appears either immediately or later during the period of formation of the healing callus.

Intercondylar fractures are supracondylar fractures that have advanced into the elbow joint in Y or T fashion. They are very hard to maintain in reduction. If the medial epicondyle is fractured, the ulnar nerve is liable to be injured.

In lower humeral epiphyseal separations (which occur mostly in children aged 4–10 years), the bony displacement is usually lateral and posterior.

II. THE ARM

GROSS ANATOMY

Boundaries, Fasciae, & Intermuscular Septa

The arm is bounded superiorly by the lower border of the teres major muscle and inferiorly by the 2 epicondyles of the humerus. The brachial fascia (the investing or deep fascia of the arm) is strong and membranous. Superficial to the investing brachial fascia is a poorly defined superficial fascia. Proximally, the deep fascia of the arm is continuous with the deltoid, axillary, and pectoral fasciae; inferiorly, it is continuous with the antebrachial fascia of the forearm. Between the epicondylar level and the deltoid attachment to the humerus are a pair of intermuscular septa that divide the arm into an anterior or flexor-supinator compartment and a posterior or extensor compartment. The **lateral intermuscular septum** runs from the investing fascia to the lateral supracondylar ridge of the humerus. The **medial intermuscular septum** runs from the investing fascia to the medial supracondylar ridge of the humerus. The posterior segment of the investing fascia is tightly attached to the underlying triceps muscle. A definite fascial cleft exists anteriorly in the arm between the biceps muscle and the investing fascia lying immediately anterior to the muscle.

Compartments of the Arm

The arm is divided into 2 compartments: anterior and posterior. The 3 muscles present in the **anterior compartment** are the coracobrachialis, the biceps brachii, and the brachialis (Table 42–1). These muscles make up the great bulk of the arm as they lie anterior to its lateral and medial intermuscular septa (Fig 42–5).

The nerves and major vessels of the anterior compartment of the arm run in the medial bicipital groove. They are the brachial artery and its associated veins and the musculocutaneous, median, and ulnar nerves.

The **posterior compartment** of the arm contains

Table 42–1. Muscles of the arm.

Muscle and Origin	Insertion	Innervation	Function
CORACOBRACHIALIS From the apex of the coracoid process along with the short head of the biceps and from the intermuscular septum between the 2 muscles.	Via a flat tendon into an impression into the middle of the medial surface of the body of the humerus between the origins of the triceps and brachialis muscles.	Musculocutaneous nerve (C6, 7).	Flexes and adducts the arm.
BICEPS BRACHII Arises via 2 heads: a short head via a tendon from the apex of the coracoid process, and a long head from the superior margin of the glenoid cavity. The tendon of the long head, enclosed in synovium of the shoulder joint, arches over the head of the humerus and descends in the intertubercular groove.	Via a flat tendon into the posterior portion of the tuberosity of the radius.	Musculocutaneous nerve (C5, 6).	Flexes the arm, flexes the forearm, supinates the hand; the long head draws the humerus toward the glenoid fossa, stabilizing the shoulder joint.
BRACHIALIS Arises from the distal half of the anterior aspect of the humerus, the origin extending down to 2.5 cm of the articular surface of the elbow joint. Arises also from the intermuscular septa.	Fibers converge into a thick tendon inserted onto the tuberosity of the ulna and onto the rough area on the anterior surface of the coronoid process.	Musculocutaneous nerve (C5, 6); also the radial nerve (C7, 8).	Flexes the forearm.
TRICEPS BRACHII The long head arises by a flattened tendon from the infraglenoid tuberosity of the scapula. The lateral head arises from the posterior surface of the body of the humerus near the insertion of the teres minor and from the lateral border of the humerus and the intermuscular septum. The medial head (deep) arises from the posterior surface of the body of the humerus distal to the groove for the radial nerve and from the medial border of the humerus and from the entire length of the intermuscular septum.	The triceps tendon starts at the middle of the muscle and is inserted into the posterior portion of the proximal surface of the olecranon. Some fibers continue farther inferiorly over the anconeus to blend with the deep forearm fascia.	Radial nerve (C7, 8).	Generally, extends the forearm; the long head of the triceps extends and adducts the arm.

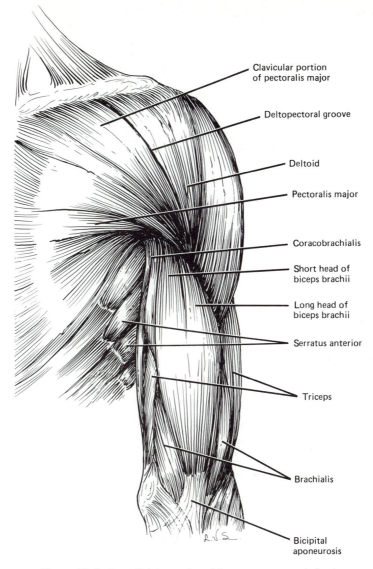

Clavicular portion
of pectoralis major

Deltopectoral groove

Deltoid

Pectoralis major

Coracobrachialis

Short head of
biceps brachii

Long head of
biceps brachii

Serratus anterior

Triceps

Brachialis

Bicipital
aponeurosis

Figure 42–5. Superficial muscles of the upper arm and chest.

only one muscle, the triceps brachii. It contains also the radial nerve. Lying between the superficial and deep fasciae covering the posterior arm compartment is the lateral brachial cutaneous nerve, closely related to the posterior edge of the deltoid muscle.

The triceps brachii has 3 heads of origin: long, lateral, and medial. The 3 heads join distally and insert into the olecranon process of the ulna. The triceps brachii runs the entire length of the dorsal surface of the humerus, its elongated tendon of insertion normally beginning at about mid arm level. The radial nerve supplies the triceps.

As the long head of the triceps descends, it creates the triangular and quadrangular spaces. The **quad-**

rangular space is bounded superiorly by the teres minor muscle, inferiorly by the teres major muscle, medially by the long head of the triceps, and laterally by the surgical neck of the humerus. Through the quadrangular space pass the axillary nerve and the posterior humeral circumflex vessels, both of which leave the axilla and pass dorsally just below the inferior attachment of the capsule of the shoulder joint (level of the anatomic neck of the humerus) (Fig 42–6). The base of the **triangular space** is formed by the long head of the triceps brachii, while the teres minor forms the superior arm of the triangle and the teres major its inferior arm. The triangular space transmits the circumflex scapular vessels.

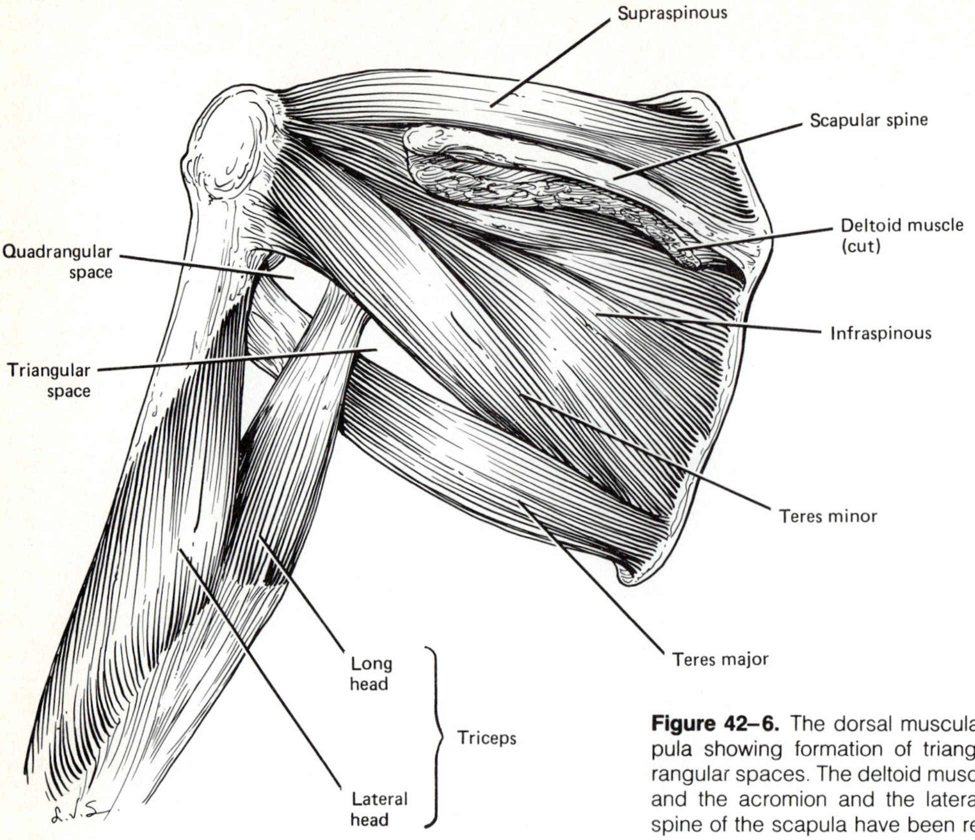

Figure 42–6. The dorsal musculature of the scapula showing formation of triangular and quadrangular spaces. The deltoid muscle has been cut, and the acromion and the lateral portion of the spine of the scapula have been removed.

BLOOD VESSELS, LYMPHATICS, & NERVES

Arteries (Fig 42–7)

The **brachial artery,** the major artery of the arm, has its origin in the axilla at the inferior margin of the teres major muscle. It terminates at the level of the elbow joint. The artery lies just deep to the ventral segment of the deep fascia of the arm. The artery is positioned ventrally upon the long head of the triceps brachii, then upon the medial head of the triceps brachii, and finally upon the insertion of the coracobrachialis and the body of the brachialis. At about mid arm level, the artery and its 2 accompanying veins are crossed from lateral to medial by the median nerve.

Branches of the brachial artery include the deep brachial artery, the nutrient artery of the humerus, the superior and inferior ulnar collateral arteries, and several small muscular branches. The **deep brachial artery** (arteria profunda brachii) leaves the main brachial trunk near the inferior border of the teres major muscle; it leaves the anterior compartment of the arm and enters the posterior compartment of the arm between the long and lateral heads of the triceps brachii muscle. The vessel then runs in the spiral radial groove along with the radial nerve; it gives off both muscular branches and nutrient branches to the humerus. The ascending branch of the deep brachial artery anastomoses with the posterior humeral circumflex branch of the axillary artery, thus setting up a collateral pathway between the axillary and brachial arteries. The **superior and inferior ulnar collateral arteries** both participate in the arterial anastomoses about the elbow joint whereby blood from the brachial artery joins with the distal radial and ulnar arteries.

The brachial artery terminates in the triangular antecubital fossa at the elbow joint level, where it divides into the radial and ulnar arteries. In the fossa, it is closely related to the median nerve, which lies medial to the artery, and to the tendon of the biceps brachii muscle, which is just lateral to the artery. The basilic vein lies medial to the artery in the antecubital fossa.

➠ ***Approach to brachial artery and median and ulnar nerves.*** *The operative approach is via an incision in the medial bicipital groove. The basilic vein is then retracted posteriorly and the medial border of the biceps brachii antero-*

laterally. This exposes the 2 nerves and the artery for a considerable length of their course.

Superficial Veins
(Fig 42–8)

Two important veins are situated between the superficial and deep fasciae of the arm. The **cephalic vein** runs superiorly in the lateral bicipital groove. It terminates by piercing the costocoracoid membrane in the deltopectoral triangle, entering the axillary vein just superior to the tendon of the pectoralis minor muscle.

The **basilic vein** runs superiorly in the medial bicipital groove. At a point about halfway between the elbow and shoulder, the basilic vein pierces the deep fascia of the arm and joins with the 2 brachial veins, the venae comitantes of the brachial artery, to form the axillary vein. There is a rich anastomosis between the veins of the superficial and deep areas of the arm.

➡ ***Preservation of cephalic vein.** In most operative procedures upon the axilla, it is important to locate and preserve the cephalic vein. **The vein is usually quite easily located at the point where it perforates the claviopectoral fascia just superior to the pectoralis minor tendon. In cases of transection, surgical ligation, or thrombosis of the axillary vein, the cephalic vein serves to empty venous blood returning from the forearm and arm into the axillary vein above the site of transection, thus serving as an important venous shunt.***

Lymphatics

The lymphatics of the arm are divided into 2 groups: superficial and deep. The superficial lymphatics are further divided into radial, median, and **ulnar** groups, which accompany the cephalic, median, and basilic veins, respectively. Some ulnar lymphatics

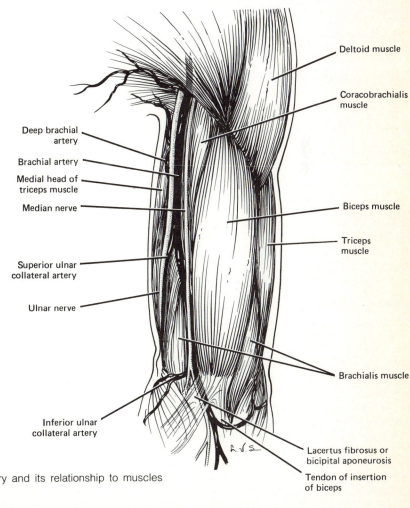

Figure 42–7. The brachial artery and its relationship to muscles and nerves of the arm.

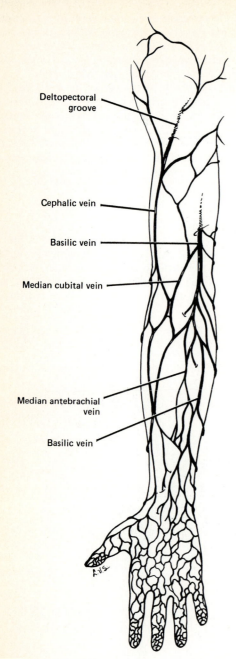

Deltopectoral groove

Cephalic vein

Basilic vein

Median cubital vein

Median antebrachial vein

Basilic vein

Figure 42–8. Superficial veins of the right upper extremity.

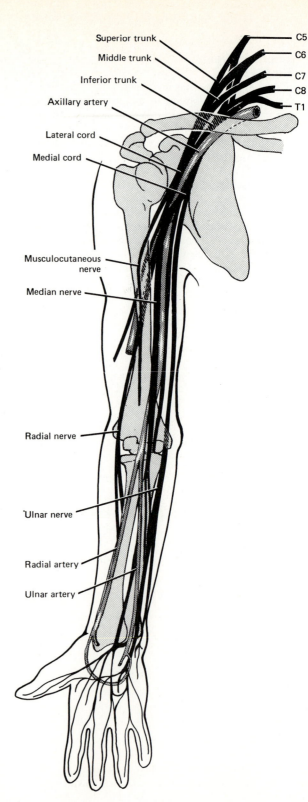

Superior trunk

Middle trunk

Inferior trunk

Axillary artery

Lateral cord

Medial cord

C5
C6
C7
C8
T1

Musculocutaneous nerve

Median nerve

Radial nerve

Ulnar nerve

Radial artery

Ulnar artery

Figure 42–9. The nerves in the right arm.

terminate in the supratrochlear nodes, but most ulnar lymph flow passes directly to the most lateral of the axillary nodes. Most of the radial lymphatics pass along the cephalic vein to the deltopectoral nodes. The deep lymphatics run with the deep blood vessels of the arm and end mainly in the most lateral group of the axillary nodes. There is considerable communication between the superficial and deep lymphatics.

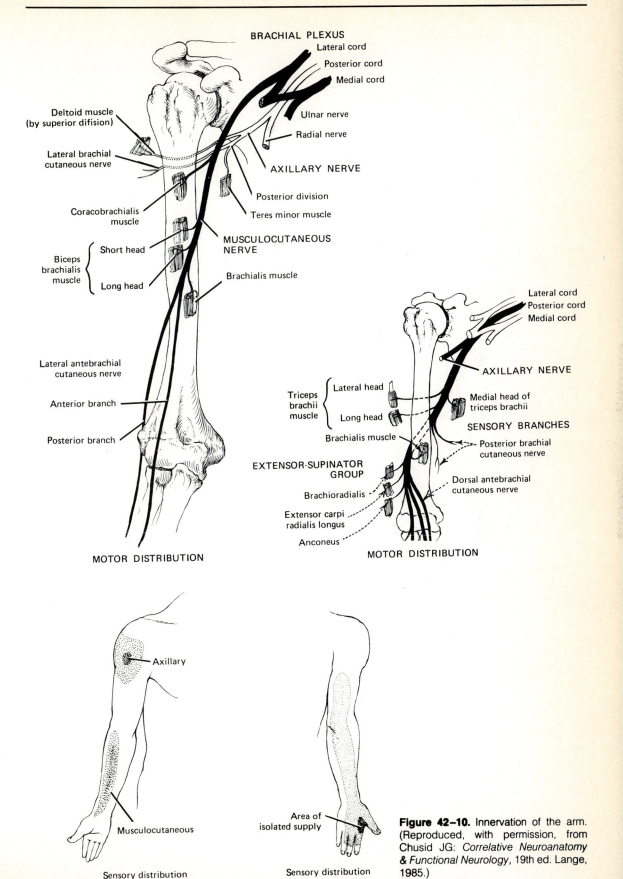

Figure 42–10. Innervation of the arm. (Reproduced, with permission, from Chusid JG: *Correlative Neuroanatomy & Functional Neurology*, 19th ed. Lange, 1985.)

⇒ *Lymphangitis. Infections originating on the radial side of the hand and forearm frequently produce epitrochlear adenopathy. However, there is adenopathy of the lateral axillary nodes in almost all acute hand and forearm infections. Axillary nodes may become tender and swollen and on occasion break down to form an axillary abscess. Red streaks along the arm and forearm signify lymphangitis.*

Nerves
(Figs 42–9 and 42–10)

The **musculocutaneous nerve** is derived from the lateral cord of the brachial plexus (C5–7). It pierces the coracobrachialis muscle high in the arm and then runs obliquely to the lateral side of the arm, lying between the biceps and brachialis muscles. Just above the elbow joint, it pierces the deep fascia lateral to the biceps brachii tendon and becomes superficial. The nerve then continues into the forearm as the lateral antebrachial cutaneous nerve (lateral cutaneous nerve of the forearm). In the arm, it innervates the coracobrachialis, biceps brachii, and the brachialis muscles.

The **median nerve** arises from 2 slips, one of which leaves the lateral cord and the other the medial cord of the brachial plexus in the axilla (C6–8, T1). It lies at first lateral to the brachial artery and, as it reaches the mid arm, crosses ventral to the brachial artery to lie just medial to it. At the level of the elbow joint, the median nerve lies medial to the brachial artery, deep to the bicipital fascia and separated from the elbow joint by the body of the brachialis muscle. There are no branches of the median nerve in the arm save for an occasional twig to the pronator teres.

The **ulnar nerve** arises from the medial cord of the brachial plexus distal to the point where the medial segment of the median nerve has left the cord (C8, T1). In the axilla, it lies deep to the median nerve, but in the inferior axilla and down to mid arm level, it lies medial to the brachial artery. At mid arm level, it pierces the medial intermuscular septum. In its continued descent in the posterior compartment of the arm, it comes to lie in the groove between the olecranon and the medial epicondyle of the humerus. It is accompanied at this level by the superior ulnar collateral artery. At elbow level, the nerve sits upon the posterior surface of the medial epicondyle of the humerus. At this level, it can be easily palpated and rolled against the bone as it lies on this segment of the lower humerus. It gives off no branches in the arm save for a small twig to the elbow joint.

The **radial nerve** and the deep brachial artery are the major nonmuscular structures that occupy the posterior compartment of the arm; they lie in the radial groove of the humerus. The radial nerve is derived from the posterior cord of the plexus at midaxillary level (C5–8). It descends from the axilla into the arm, lying first dorsal to the axillary artery and then dorsal to the brachial artery. It lies ventral to the tendons of the teres major and latissimus dorsi muscles. Accompanied by the deep brachial artery, the radial nerve crosses from the medial to the lateral side of the humerus in the radial groove on the dorsal surface of that bone. It then passes from dorsal to ventral, enters the anterior compartment of the arm by piercing the lateral intermuscular septum, and runs inferiorly between the brachialis and brachioradialis muscles. At the elbow it is placed on the ventral surface of the lateral epicondyle, where it divides into superficial and deep branches. The radial nerve gives off muscular branches to the triceps, anconeus, brachialis, brachioradialis, and extensor carpi radialis longus muscles; it also gives off 2 cutaneous branches: the posterior brachial cutaneous nerve to the arm and the dorsal antebrachial cutaneous nerve to the forearm.

⇒ *Surgical approach to the radial nerve. The radial nerve may be reached surgically by separating the lateral and long heads of the triceps muscle.*

⇒ *Vulnerability of the radial nerve. The close relationship of the radial nerve to the posterior mid shaft of the humerus and to the lateral humeral epicondyle makes it vulnerable to trauma at these levels.*

⇒ *Injury to median nerve in the arm. (Table 42–1.) When the median nerve is injured in the arm, there is no loss of power in any of the arm muscles. However, there is a loss of sensation over the lateral palm and over the thumb and the radial 2½ fingers. There is a loss of forearm pronation, wrist flexion, and finger flexion and of several thumb movements.*

⇒ *Injury to the ulnar nerve in the arm. (Table 42–1.) If the ulnar nerve is injured at arm level, there is a loss of wrist flexion and adduction, and the thumb and the ulnar 2 fingers show impaired movement.*

⇒ *Injury to the musculocutaneous nerve in the arm. (Table 42–1.) When the musculocutaneous nerve is injured, there is a loss of function of the coracobrachialis, biceps, and brachialis muscles.*

⇒ *Injury to the radial nerve in the arm. (Table 42–1.) When the radial nerve is injured in the arm, the following arm muscles are affected: the triceps brachii, the anconeus, the brachioradialis, the extensor carpi radialis longus, and the brachialis. Two cutaneous nerves—the posterior brachial cutaneous and the dorsal antebrachial cutaneous—are also affected.*

Elbow Joint

43

GROSS ANATOMY
(Figs 43–1, 43–2, & 43–3)

The elbow joint possesses a single synovial cavity that provides for 3 separate articulations between the arm and the forearm.

The 3 individual articulations are (1) the joint between the trochlea of the humerus and the trochlear notch of the ulna (hinge joint, or ginglymus); (2) the joint between the capitulum of the humerus and the concave superior surface of the radial head (ball-and-socket joint); and (3) the proximal radioulnar joint between the radial head and the radial notch of the ulna (pivot joint) (Figs 43–1 to 43–3).

The 3 separate joints are held together by an articular capsule that is thin anteriorly and posteriorly but thickens laterally and medially to form the ulnar (medial) and radial (lateral) collateral ligaments of the elbow joint. The medial and lateral epicondyles of the humerus, which do not articulate with any segment of the radius or ulna, are completely extracapsular. The anterior and posterior portions of the joint capsule are lax and allow for the hinge movements of flexion and extension at the elbow.

⇒ ***Effusions into the elbow joint.*** *Elbow joint effusions usually present posteriorly, since the joint capsule is weakest in that area and is not bolstered, as it is anteriorly, by muscles and deep fascia. The elbow joint is easily aspirated posteriorly with a needle inserted into the joint space from either side of the olecranon.*

Ligaments & Synovial Membrane of the Joint

The triangular **ulnar collateral ligament** is made up of 3 segments. The anterior band runs from the

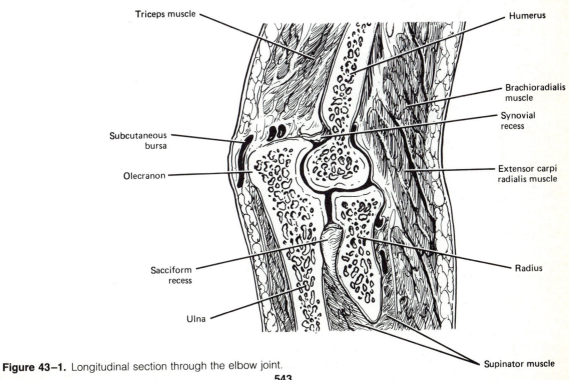

Figure 43–1. Longitudinal section through the elbow joint.

543

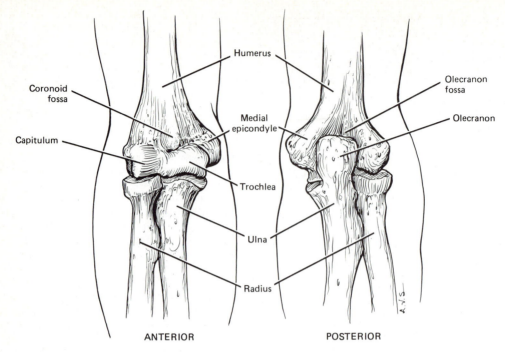

Figure 43–2. Anterior and posterior views of the bony articulation of the right elbow joint.

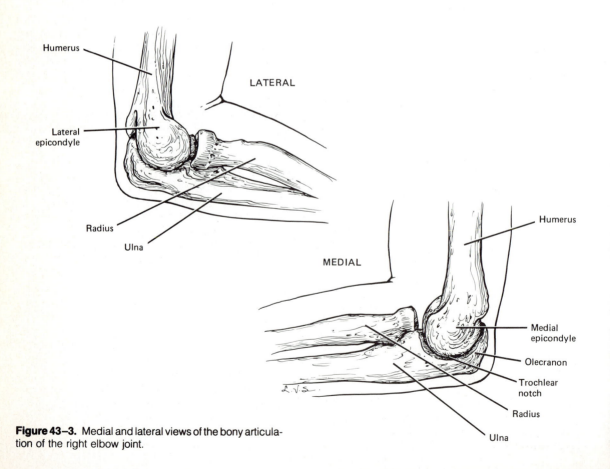

Figure 43–3. Medial and lateral views of the bony articulation of the right elbow joint.

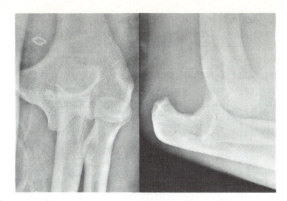

Figure 43–4. Complete posterior dislocation of the elbow joint without fracture or neurovascular injury. (Reproduced, with permission, from Way LW [editor]: *Current Surgical Diagnosis & Treatment,* 7th ed. Lange, 1985.)

The joint between the ulna and the humerus is a pure hinge joint and permits only flexion and extension. The elbow joint is flexed by the biceps brachii and brachialis muscles, with some assistance from the brachioradialis and the muscles that arise from the medial epicondyle of the humerus (see Table 44–1). The joint is extended by the triceps brachii and the anconeus, with minor help from the wrist and finger extensors.

The Annular Ligament

The annular ligament is an integral segment of the most superior junctions of the 3 levels of radioulnar articulation (proximal radioulnar joint, interosseous membrane of forearm, distal radioulnar articulation). The ligament is a strong fibrous band that surrounds the lateral two-thirds of the head of the radius, holding it firmly against the radial notch of the ulna. The ring about the radial head is completed medially by the radial notch of the ulna, to whose borders the annular ligament attaches. Superiorly, the annular ligament interdigitates with the ventral and dorsal supportive ligaments of the elbow joint. Running to the ulna and to the neck of the radius from the annular ligament is the short, square **quadrate ligament.** The deep surface of the annular ligament is covered by the synovia of the elbow joint.

The Synovia of the Elbow Joint

The complex nature of the elbow joint (3 joints in one), with its varied movements, calls for a large multilocular type of synovial membrane. Superiorly, the synovium begins at the joint surface of the humerus. From there, it passes inferiorly, laterally, and medially to line the 3 humeral fossae (coronoid, radial, and olecranon). It also lines the entire inner surface of the capsular ligament and dips inferiorly to interpose itself between the inner surface of the annular ligament and the radial head.

Elbow Joint Fat Pads

Three separate fat pads lie between the joint capsule and the synovium lining the elbow joint. They are placed in the 3 humeral fossae, the largest in the olecranon fossa. All 3 pads are compressed into their respective fossae during specific movements of the bones, muscles, and tendons that overlie them.

medial epicondyle of the humerus to the coronoid process of the ulna. The posterior band runs from the medial epicondyle to the olecranon. The oblique band is transverse between the coronoid process and the olecranon. The ulnar collateral ligament is close to the triceps and the flexor carpi ulnaris muscles and to the ulnar nerve.

The **radial collateral ligament** is not as well defined as the ulnar collateral ligament. It too is triangular and runs from the lateral epicondyle of the humerus to the annular ligament and to the edge of the ulna. The most distal fibers of the ligament are closely united with the tendon of origin of the supinator muscle.

➠ *Dislocations about the elbow joint. Dislocation of the elbow joint can involve one or both bones of the forearm and can occur dorsally, ventrally, laterally, or medially. One or both collateral ligaments and the elbow joint capsule are usually torn, and there may be an accompanying fracture of one of the humeral condyles. Posterior dislocations are the most common and usually follow a fall onto the outstretched hand (Fig 43–4). They are frequently accompanied by fracture of the radial head. If the coronoid process of the ulna is fractured along with the dislocation, the triangular relationship between the olecranon and the 2 humeral condyles is disturbed.*

Movements of the Elbow Joint

The elbow joint can perform flexion and extension at the humeroulnar and humeroradial joints and pronation and supination at the most superior of the 3 radioulnar articulations. Pronation and supination are aided by the mid and distal radioulnar articulations (see Chapter 44).

➠ *Effect of posterior dislocation of the elbow on the olecranon triangle. On the posterior surface of the elbow joint, lines joining the olecranon process and the 2 epicondyles of the humerus make up a triangle with the apex facing superiorly. If the supracondylar area of the humerus is fractured, the triangular relationship usually remains unchanged. However, with posterior dislocation of the elbow, the olecranon descends and comes to lie in the same horizontal plane as the 2 epicondyles.*

The Radial Capitulum Joint

The joint between the radial head and the capitulum of the humerus is primarily a gliding joint. Binding of the head of the radius to the radial notch of the ulna prevents lateral separation of the 2 bones, so that there is no lateral deviation of the radial head from its articulation with the humeral capitulum. The radial head is not in apposition to the capitulum in all movements of the joint, however, since the capitulum comprises only the anteroinferior surface of the lower end of the humerus.

➠ *Palpation of radial head on the posterior lateral elbow surface. Inspection of the posterolateral surface of the elbow when the arm is fully extended will show a depression just inferior to the lateral epicondyle. The depression marks the position of the head of the radius. Palpation of this area allows the examiner to feel the head of the radius as it rotates during pronation and supination. Pain on pressure over this area may indicate fracture of the radial head.*

The proximal radioulnar articulation allows only rotatory movements of the head of the radius within its osseofibrous ring. These rotatory motions are (1) pronation, effected by the pronator teres and pronator quadratus; and (2) supination, effected by the biceps brachii and the supinator. The ability of the elbow joint to flex and extend in combination with supination and pronation allows accuracy and efficiency of hand movement. Combined elbow and hand movement is best performed with the elbow joint in moderate flexion.

Relationships of the Elbow Joint

The important muscular and tendinous structures that embrace the elbow joint are (1) the brachialis muscle, which lies directly ventral to the joint; (2) the triceps brachii and anconeus, which lie directly dorsal to the joint; (3) the supinator and the common tendon of origin of the extensor muscles of the hand and wrist, which lie lateral to the joint; and (4) the common tendon of origin of the flexor muscles of the wrist and hand and the superior segment of the flexor carpi ulnaris, which lie medial to the joint.

Antecubital Fossa
(Fig 43–5)

The antecubital fossa is a shallow triangular depression just ventral to the elbow joint. The base of the triangle is a line drawn between the humeral epi-

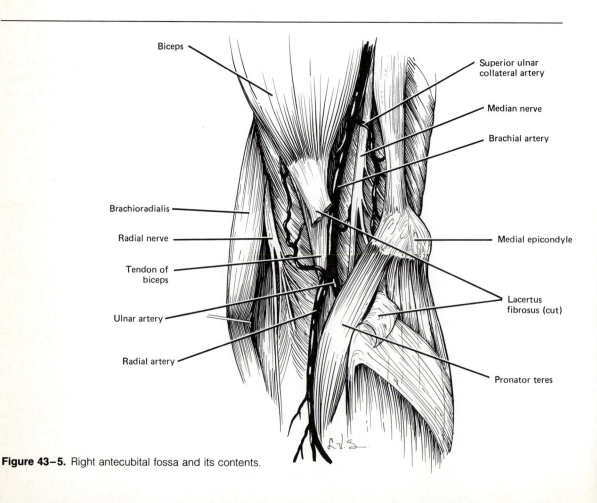

Figure 43–5. Right antecubital fossa and its contents.

condyles. The medial and lateral margins are formed by the pronator teres muscle medially and the brachioradialis muscle laterally. The floor of the fossa is formed by the brachialis and supinator muscles, which lie beneath the deep antebrachial fascia. Four or 5 superficial veins of the basilic and cephalic venous systems lie between the superficial and deep fasciae, which cover the fossa. Within the fossa lie the brachial artery, the origins of the radial and ulnar arteries, the terminal tendon of the biceps brachii, and the median nerve. A membranous band arising from the distal biceps brachii fibers often expands into a flat tendonlike structure that passes medially and distally to join with the deep forearm fascia. When present, the band lies in the mid portion of the antecubital fossa and is called the lacertus fibrosus (bicipital aponeurosis).

⇒ *Veins of the antecubital fossa. The veins in the antecubital fossa are subcutaneous in position and are easily aspirated for diagnostic purposes. The antecubital veins are the most common site in the body for injection of medications, blood, and other supportive fluids.*

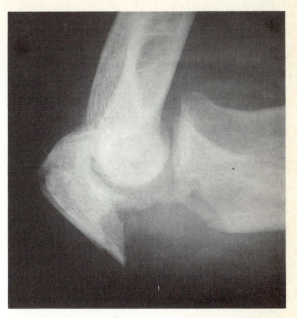

Figure 43–6. Fracture of the olecranon and anterior subluxation of the radius. (Reproduced, with permission, from Way LW [editor]: *Current Surgical Diagnosis & Treatment,* 7th ed. Lange, 1985.)

Olecranon Region

The olecranon, or posterior elbow region, is covered only by thin, soft tissues that allow for easy palpation of the bony structures, ie, the 2 epicondyles of the humerus, the olecranon, the superior dorsal segment of the ulna, the humeroradial joint, and the head of the radius. The ulnar nerve is palpable as it lies just medial to the paraolecranon groove. Owing to its superficial position, the ulnar nerve is easily contused or lacerated. Superficial to the bony olecranon and the tendon of the triceps muscle and just deep to the covering skin is the large olecranon bursa, a frequent site of bursitis. Following trauma or infection, the olecranon bursa frequently becomes a site of effusions and swellings. The skin over the posterior elbow region is thick but loose.

⇒ *Olecranon bursitis. Olecranon bursitis frequently accompanies gouty arthritis. Uric acid crystals are usually present in the bursal walls and cavity in such cases. Chronic recurrent olecranon bursitis due to any cause may call for surgical removal of the bursa. Aseptic olecranon bursitis is often present secondary to overuse of the elbow joint in industry and sports.*

⇒ *Fracture of the olecranon. (Fig 43–6.) Fractures of the olecranon are usually caused by forceful flexion of the elbow against the resistance of the triceps muscle. The fracture line is usually transverse, and the proximal frag-*

ment is pulled superiorly and separated from the distal ulna by the pull of the triceps muscle. Fractures of the head and neck of the radius or of the carpal navicular bone often accompany olecranon fracture. There may be signs and symptoms of ulnar nerve compression secondary to olecranon fractures.

BLOOD VESSELS & NERVES

The **brachial artery** lies in the center of the antecubital fossa deep to the skin and superficial fascia and lacertus fibrosus and medial to the cubital vein. At the level of the radial neck, the brachial artery divides into the radial and ulnar arteries. Two venae comitantes usually accompany the brachial artery at the level of the antecubital fossa. A rich arterial anastomosis about the elbow joint is derived from branches of the profunda brachii, from the radial and ulnar collateral branches of the brachial artery, and from the radial and ulnar arteries that reach the elbow area from the forearm.

When the lacertus fibrosus (aponeurosis) of the bicipital muscle is reflected, the brachial artery, the biceps brachii tendon, and the median nerve are seen lying just deep to the fascial structure (Fig 43–5). At the mid antecubital level, the brachial artery lies medial to the biceps tendon, while the median nerve lies medial to the brachial artery.

At the inferior end of the antecubital fossa, the

radial nerve lies lateral to the biceps tendon and medial to the brachioradialis muscle. If the brachioradialis is retracted laterally, the radial nerve can be seen dividing into deep and superficial branches. The brachial artery divides into a large ulnar and a smaller radial branch near the neck of the radius, which is about 3 cm distal to the cutaneous crease of the elbow.

The elbow joint receives its nerve supply from branches of the **musculocutaneous, ulnar, radial and median nerves.** Lying superficially in the antecubital area are minor branches of the lateral and medial antebrachial cutaneous nerves.

The Forearm

44

GROSS ANATOMY

The forearm extends from the elbow joint to the wrist joint between a transverse line connecting the 2 humeral epicondyles and the most distal of the volar cutaneous folds of the wrist.

BONES OF THE FOREARM
(Fig 44–1)

The ulna and radius are parallel bones to which the ventral and dorsal soft tissues of this segment of the upper extremity are attached.

1. ULNA
(Fig 44–2)

With the hand in the supine position, the ulna is the medial bone of the forearm.

The superior segment of the ulna is its widest and most solid area. The distal segment is considerably narrower and smaller.

The upper ulna has 2 hooklike processes—the olecranon and the coronoid—joined by an articular cavity, the semilunar or trochlear notch. On its inferior lateral surface just distal to the trochlear notch, the radial notch articulates with the medial surface of the head of the radius.

Olecranon

The olecranon is the dorsal superior end of the ulna. It fits into the olecranon fossa of the humerus during full forearm extension. The dorsal surface of the olecranon, with its covering bursa, makes up the posterior projection of the elbow joint and lies just beneath the skin. Consequently, the dorsal olecranon surface is easily palpable and visible. The anterior surface of the olecranon is concave and smooth, forming the superior segment of the semilunar notch.

Coronoid Process

The coronoid process of the ulna sits on the antero-superior surface of the bone. When the forearm is flexed, the point of the coronoid process tilts into the coronoid fossa of the humerus. The superior surface of the coronoid process is smooth and concave and continuous with the semilunar or trochlear notch.

Semilunar Notch

The semilunar notch, which articulates with the trochlea of the humerus, is the cavity formed by the junction of the olecranon with the coronoid process. On the lateral surface of the coronoid process is an oval facet, the radial notch, against which fits the head of the radius. The annular ligament of the elbow joint attaches to the edges of the radial notch.

Shaft of the Ulna

The shaft of the ulna decreases in girth from its superior to its inferior termination. The ulna has 3 borders and 3 surfaces. The anterior (volar) border separates the volar and medial surfaces; the sharp dorsal border separates the medial and dorsal surfaces; the external border, or interosseous crest, separates the volar from the dorsal surface of the bone. The interosseous membrane attaches to the interosseous crest. The concave volar surface of the ulna is broad superiorly and narrow inferiorly. The dorsal surface is also concave. The medial surface is concave superiorly and convex and subcutaneous in position inferiorly.

➡ *Isolated fractures of the ulnar shaft. Isolated fractures of the ulnar shaft are rare and are nearly always caused by a direct blow to the bone. Associated fracture of the head of the radius (Monteggia's fracture) should always be suspected and searched for in patients with ulnar shaft fractures.*

Distal End of the Ulna

The distal end of the ulna, unlike that of the radius, is small and delicate in appearance. It consists of the lateral ulnar head and a medial ulnar styloid. The rounded head articulates with a segment of the triangular articular disk distally and with the ulnar notch of the radius medially. The small, triangular ulnar styloid projects inferiorly. It is subcutaneous

Figure 44–1. Bones of the left forearm.

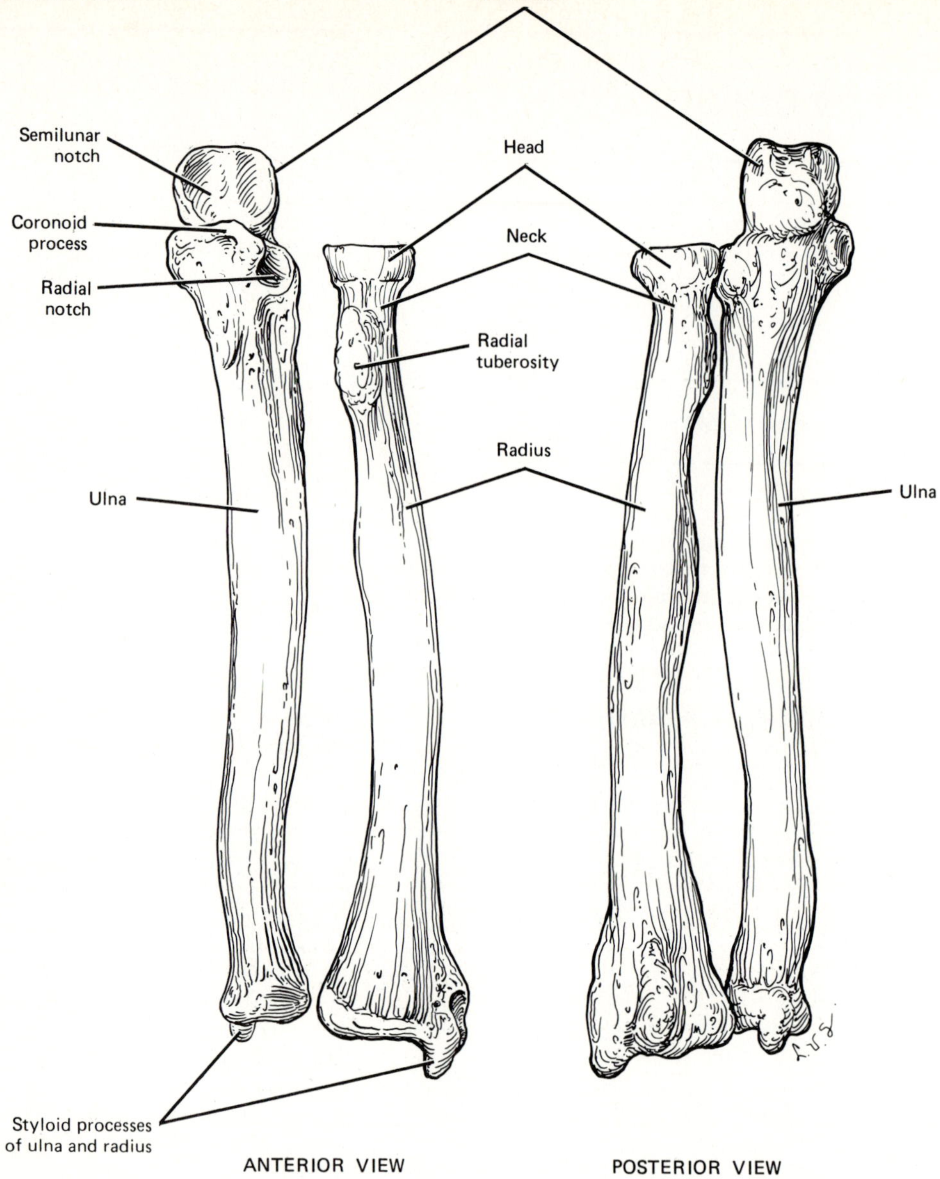

Olecranon

Semilunar notch

Coronoid process

Radial notch

Head

Neck

Radial tuberosity

Radius

Ulna

Ulna

Styloid processes of ulna and radius

ANTERIOR VIEW

POSTERIOR VIEW

in position and easily palpable when the hand is fully supinated. The triangular articular disk prevents the ulna from articulating directly with the wrist joint.

The styloid process of the ulna is nonarticular. The superior ulnar epiphysis is completely extracapsular and finally joins the body of the bone by about the 16th year of life. The inferior ulnar epiphysis is partly intracapsular and joins the body of the bone by about the 20th year.

➠ *Fractures of the ulnar styloid. Fractures of the ulnar styloid not associated with fractures of the lower end of the radius are usually caused by hyperabduction of the hand.*

2. RADIUS
(Fig 44–1)

The radius is the lateral bone of the forearm. While the ulna is thicker than the radius at the elbow joint, the radius is larger than the ulna distally, and it alone contributes to the wrist joint.

The radius may be divided into a head, a neck, and a tuberosity. The radial head is round and presents a depressed superior surface for articulation with the capitulum of the humerus. Next to its head, the radius narrows into its neck. The supinator muscle inserts into the dorsal surface of the radial neck.

Inferior and medial to the radial neck is the radial tuberosity. The tendon of the biceps brachii inserts

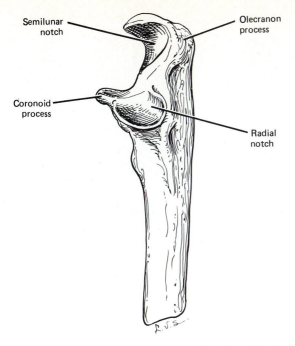

Figure 44–2. Proximal end of the left ulna (lateral view).

tral, dorsal, and lateral. The 3 edges are anterior, posterior, and the interosseous crest. To the latter is attached the interosseous membrane (Fig 44–3) that joins the shafts of the forearm bones. The dorsal surface of the radius is covered by the supinator muscle; the anterior surface of the bone is the site of origin of the flexor pollicis longus and gives insertion to the pronator quadratus inferiorly.

➠ *Fracture of the radial shaft. Fractures of the shaft of the radius are usually caused by a fall onto the hand or by a direct heavy blow to the side of the forearm. Fractures of the lower two-thirds of the radius are more liable to be of the compound type. Radial fracture displacement is nearly always due to muscular action and depends on the location of the fracture line. If the fracture line is above the prona-*

onto the posterior surface of this tuberosity. The radial head is held tightly against the radial notch of the ulna by the encircling annular ligament of the elbow joint.

➠ *Subluxation of radial head in children. In children up to age 5 years, the walls containing the annular ligament are vertical. A sudden jerk on a child's forearm may pull the radial head from the encircling annular ligament. The subluxation is easily reduced by putting the elbow joint into forced supination to ease the radial head back into the enclosing ligament.*

➠ *Fractures of the head and neck of radius. These usually result from a fall on the outstretched hand with the forearm partially pronated and flexed. Severe fractures call for removal of the radial head; the elbow joint still functions remarkably well following this procedure. In head and neck fractures of the radius, forced supination of the forearm is always limited and painful, as is pressure over the radial head. Severe fractures of the radial head and neck are frequently accompanied by posterior dislocation of the elbow joint.*

The distal segment of the radius is almost 3 times as wide as the radial neck. The radial shaft is slightly convex and roughly prismatic. Its 3 surfaces are ven-

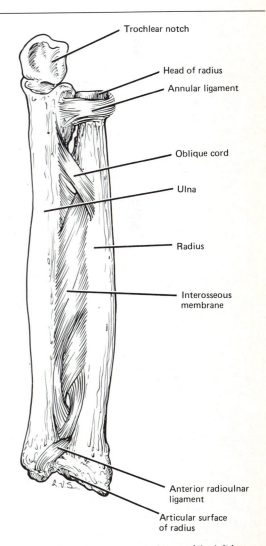

Figure 44–3. Interosseous membrane of the left forearm.

tor teres insertion and below the insertion of the biceps brachii, the proximal fragment will be supinated by the biceps and the distal fragment pronated by the pronator teres. If the fracture line is distal to the insertion of the pronator teres, the proximal fragment remains in situ through the counteraction of the biceps and pronator quadratus muscles.

The Terminal Segment of the Radius

The terminal segment of the radius is bulbous, roughly quadrilateral, and has 2 articular surfaces, one inferiorly with carpal articulation and one medially that accommodates inferior articulation of the radius with the ulna. The carpal articular surface, which lies against the proximal row of carpal bones, is smooth, concave, roughly triangular, and divided into 2 sockets by an anteroposterior central ridge. The lateral socket articulates with the scaphoid and the medial socket with the lunate bone.

The ulnar notch of the radius faces medially, is smooth and concave, and articulates with the head of the ulna. The base of the triangular articular disk is attached to a ridge between the carpal and ulnar articular surfaces of the radius.

⇒ *Fractures of the distal end of the radius. Fractures of the lower end of the radius are extremely common and usually result from a fall on the outstretched forearm with the hand pronated and the wrist extended. In Colles' fracture, the distal fragment is tilted dorsally and proximally, may be impacted, and may be associated with fracture of the ulnar styloid process (Fig 44-4). The proximal fragment may be driven deeply into the soft tissues of the palmar surface of the wrist, where it may exert pressure on the median nerve. It is important to check for median nerve deficit in all such fractures. If the median nerve is involved, the superficial thenar eminence muscles and the 2 radial lumbrical hand muscles will be involved.*

Nonarticular Surfaces of the Distal Radius

The 3 nonarticular surfaces of the distal end of the radius are volar, dorsal, and lateral. The volar nonarticular surface is smooth and is attached to the volar radiocarpal ligament. The dorsal nonarticular surface is the site of origin of the dorsal radiocarpal ligament and presents 3 channels for passage of the hand and wrist extensor tendons. From the lateral nonarticular surface protrudes a thick cone, the radial styloid. The tendon of the brachioradialis muscle inserts at the base of the radial styloid process, while at its apex attaches the radial collateral ligament of the wrist joint.

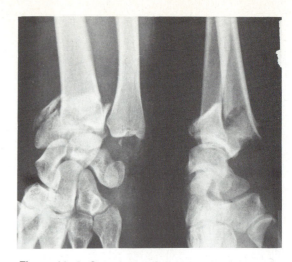

Figure 44-4. Comminuted Colles' fracture. Because of severe comminution, this fracture is unstable. (Reproduced, with permission, from Way LW [editor]: *Current Surgical Diagnosis & Treatment,* 7th ed. Lange, 1985.)

3. DISTAL EPIPHYSES OF THE RADIUS & ULNA

The ulna ossifies from 3 distinct centers: one for the shaft, one for the distal end of the bone, and one for the superior surface of the olecranon. The proximal ulnar epiphysis joins the shaft during the 15th and 16th years of life; the distal epiphysis joins the shaft in the 20th year, making it vulnerable to trauma and displacement.

The radius also ossifies from 3 centers: one for the shaft and one for each of the proximal and distal ends of the bone. The proximal epiphysis joins the radial shaft in the 17th year, whereas the distal epiphysis joins the shaft of the radius about the 20th year, making both the proximal and the distal radial epiphyses vulnerable to trauma and displacement.

⇒ *Separation of the epiphyses of the proximal and distal ends of the radius and ulna. In children and young adults, epiphyseal separation and displacements occurring at the distal end of the radius are common secondary to falls on the extended palm. Epiphyseal separations at the lower end of the ulna are rare. Displacements of the superior radial epiphysis (radial head) are fairly frequent.*

CONNECTIONS BETWEEN THE ULNA & RADIUS

In order to understand the complexities of pronation and supination of the forearm, a knowledge of the 3 connections between the radius and ulna is essential.

Proximally, the radius is connected to the ulna by the **pivot joint** between the radial head and the radial notch of the ulna. The encircling annular ligament holds the radial head tightly against the ulnar notch. The ligament is strengthened by fibers from the adjacent radial collateral ligament of the elbow joint. The deep surface of the annular ligament is lined by an extension of the synovial membrane of the elbow joint. The proximal radioulnar articulation allows for rotation of the radial head, and this movement assists markedly in pronation and supination of the forearm.

The second radioulnar articulation results from the presence of the **interosseous membrane,** a sheet of fibrous tissue that connects the entire length of the interosseous crest of the radius with the full length of the interosseous crest of the ulna (Fig 44–3). The membrane does not connect the most superior and inferior segments of the interosseous space of the forearm. Through the superior gap in the membrane pass the dorsal interosseous vessels. Just superior to its lower end is a circular opening for passage of the volar interosseous vessels to the dorsal surface of the forearm.

The **distal radioulnar articulation** is also a pivot joint formed by the head of the ulna and the ulnar notch on the end of the radius. Connecting the 2 articular surfaces are the palmar and dorsal radioulnar ligaments and the triangular articular disk. The articular disk lies in a transverse position and holds the inferior margins of the radius and ulna tightly together. The apex of the disk is concave and attaches to the styloid of the ulna; the base (its distal surface) is also concave and articulates with the medial superior half of the lunate and with the lateral superior surface of the triangular bone (os triquetrum). Movement of the distal radioulnar joint consists of rotation of the lower end of the radius about the head of the ulna, thus allowing pronation and supination of the forearm. The ulna is the more important bone at the elbow joint, whereas the radius is the more important bone at the wrist joint.

➡️ *Fractures of both bones of the forearm. In fractures of both bones of the forearm, the broken ends are usually drawn together by the supinators and pronators, with concurrent narrowing of the interosseous space (Fig 44–5). The distal fragments may be displaced laterally or anteroposteriorly with some overriding of the proximal and distal fragments and consequent shortening of the forearm. Combined fracture of the radius and ulna with concomitant tear of the connecting interosseous membrane usually calls for surgical reduction and fixation of the fragments. If there is an angular or rotational deformity, supination and pronation are usually impaired.*

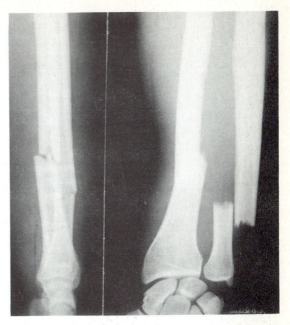

Figure 44–5. Fracture of the lower third of the shafts of the radius and ulna. (Reproduced, with permission, from Way LW [editor]: *Current Surgical Diagnosis & Treatment,* 7th ed. Lange, 1985.)

SOFT TISSUES OF THE FOREARM

1. COMPARTMENTS OF THE FOREARM

The forearm is divided into anterior and posterior compartments. The anterior compartment contains structures that lie ventral to the interosseous membrane and the forearm bones, primarily the flexor muscles of the wrist and hand. The posterior compartment contains structures that lie dorsal to the forearm bones and the interosseous membrane, primarily the muscles of the wrist and forearm.

The distal half of the forearm is noticeably thinner than the proximal half. This is because at the mid forearm the muscle bellies, both ventral and dorsal, have for the most part become tendons.

2. MUSCLES OF THE ANTERIOR COMPARTMENT OF THE FOREARM (Tables 44–1 and 44–2; Figs 44–6 and 44–7)

The muscle groups of the anterior (volar) compartment of the forearm are divided into 3 layers: superficial, medial, and deep. The superficial layer consists of muscles that have origin from the medial epicondyle of the humerus; they include the pronator teres, the flexor carpi radialis, the palmaris longus, and the flexor carpi ulnaris. Each of these muscles is supplied by the median nerve. The middle layer consists of

Table 44–1. Muscles of the forearm: Superficial anterior (volar) group.

Muscle and Origin	Insertion	Innervation	Function
PRONATOR TERES The humeral head arises just proximal to the medial epicondyle and from the common tendon of origin of the other superficial muscles; the ulnar head is a thin slip from the coronoid process of the ulna.	Ends in a flat tendon inserted into the midlateral surface of the body of the radius.	Median nerve (C6, 7).	Pronates the hand.
FLEXOR CARPI RADIALIS Arises from the medial condyle via the common flexor tendon, from the fascia of the forearm, and from the intermuscular septa.	Ends in a tendon (which makes up about half the length of the muscle) that runs through the volar carpal canal and is inserted into the base of the second metacarpal. It also sends a slip of insertion to the third metacarpal.	Median nerve (C6, 7).	Flexes the wrist and helps to abduct it radially.
PALMARIS LONGUS Arises from the medial epicondyle of the humerus via the common flexor tendon, from the intermuscular septa, and from the antebrachial fascia.	Ends in a narrow, flat tendon that inserts into the mid segment of the flexor retinaculum and into the palmar aponeurosis; on occasion, it sends a slip to the short thumb muscles.	Median nerve (C7, 8).	Flexes the wrist.
FLEXOR CARPI ULNARIS Has 2 heads of origin—one from the medial epicondyle of the humerus by the flexor common tendon and another from the medial edge of the olecranon of the ulna and from the proximal two-thirds of the posterior border of the ulna via an aponeurosis.	Via a tendon inserted into the pisiform bone and prolonged forward onto the hamate and the fifth metacarpal by ligamentous slips.	Ulnar nerve (C7, 8).	Flexes the wrist and helps to adduct the hand.
FLEXOR DIGITORUM SUPERFICIALIS Has 3 heads of origin. The humeral head arises from the common flexor tendon as well as from the ulnar collateral ligament of the elbow joint and from intermuscular septa. The ulnar head arises from the medial side of the coronoid process. The radial head arises from the oblique line of the radius, from the radial tuberosity to the level of the insertion of the pronator teres.	The muscle separates into 2 planes: superficial and deep. The superficial plane divides into 2 segments that give tendons to the middle and ring fingers. The deep plane gives off a slip that joins the tendon to the ring finger and then divides into 2 segments for tendons to the index and little fingers. Opposite the base of the proximal phalanx, each tendon divides into 2 slips to allow passage of the deep flexor tendon. The tendon then reunites and then separates again for insertion into the sides of the middle phalanx of the individual fingers.	Median nerve (C7, 8; T1).	Initially flexes the middle phalanx of each finger; with continued action, flexes the proximal phalanx and the wrist as well.

the flexor digitorum superficialis, which becomes tendinous in the lower third of the forearm. The deep layer of the ventral forearm muscles consists of the flexor pollicis longus, the flexor digitorum profundus, and the pronator quadratus, which lies slightly deeper than the 2 other muscles of the deep layer.

3. MUSCLES OF THE POSTERIOR COMPARTMENT OF THE FOREARM (Tables 44–3 and 44–4; Figs 44–8 and 44–9)

The posterior compartment contains both superficial and deep muscle layers. The muscles of the superficial layer are the brachioradialis, extensor carpi radialis brevis, and extensor carpi radialis longus. All lie lateral to the radial border of the antecubital fossa and are supplied by the main trunk of the radial nerve. The inner muscles of the superficial layer are the extensor digitorum and the extensor digiti minimi, supplied by the deep branch of the radial nerve. The deepest muscles of the superficial layer are the extensor carpi ulnaris, supplied by a branch of the deep radial nerve, and the anconeus, supplied by a branch of the radial nerve.

The deep layer of the posterior forearm muscles lies against the interosseous membrane. It is supplied

Table 44–2. Muscles of the forearm: Deep anterior (volar) group.

Muscle and Origin	Insertion	Innervation	Function
FLEXOR DIGITORUM PROFUNDUS Lies deep to the superficial flexors; arises from the proximal three-fourths of the volar and medial surfaces of the ulna; arises also from a depression on the medial side of the coronoid process and from the upper three-fourths of the dorsal border of the ulna and from the ulnar half of the interosseous membrane.	The muscle ends in 4 tendons that run deep to the tendons of the flexor digitorum superficialis. At the level of the base of the proximal phalanx, the tendons pass through openings in the tendons of the flexor digitorum superficialis and continue forward to be inserted into the bases of the distal phalanges.	Palmar interosseous branch of the median nerve and the ulnar nerve (C8, T1).	Flexes the distal phalanges of the 4 fingers and, by continuing the action, flexes the other phalanges and (slightly) the wrist.
FLEXOR POLLICIS LONGUS Arises from the grooved volar surface of the radius from below the tuberosity almost down to the pronator quadratus. Arises also from the adjacent interosseous membrane.	Via a flattened tendon passing deep to the flexor retinaculum to insert into the base of the distal phalanx of the thumb.	Palmar interosseous branch of the median nerve (C8, T1).	Flexes the distal phalanx of the thumb and, by continuing the action, flexes the proximal phalanx and the first metacarpal.
PRONATOR QUADRATUS From the pronator ridge on the distal segment of the palmar surface of the ulna; from the medial part of the palmar surface of the distal one-fourth of the ulna; and from the fascia covering the medial one-third of the muscle.	Into the distal one-fourth of the lateral border and the palmar surface of the radius. Deeper fibers insert just proximal to the ulnar notch of the radius.	Palmar interosseous branch of the median nerve (C8, T1).	Pronates the hand.

Table 44–3. Muscles of the forearm: Dorsal muscles, superficial group.

Muscle and Origin	Insertion	Innervation	Function
ANCONEUS Arises by a tendon from the dorsal part of the lateral epicondyle of the humerus.	Into the side of the olecranon and the proximal one-fourth of the dorsal surface of the body of the ulna.	Radial nerve (C7, 8).	Extends the elbow.
BRACHIORADIALIS From the proximal two-thirds of the lateral supracondylar ridge of the humerus and from the lateral intermuscular septum.	Ends in a flat tendon inserted into the lateral side of the base of the styloid process of the radius.	Radial nerve (C5, 6).	Flexes the elbow.
EXTENSOR CARPI RADIALIS LONGUS From the distal one-third of the lateral supracondylar ridge of the humerus and from the lateral intermuscular septum.	In the upper one-third of the forearm it ends as a flat tendon that inserts into the dorsal surface of the radial side of the base of the second metacarpal.	Radial nerve (C6, 7).	Extends and abducts the hand.
EXTENSOR CARPI RADIALIS BREVIS From the lateral epicondyle of the humerus, from the common extensor tendon, and from the antebrachial fascia.	Ends in a flat tendon close to the middle of the forearm that inserts into the dorsal surface of the base of the radial side of the second metacarpal.	Radial nerve (C7, 8).	Extends the hand.
EXTENSOR DIGITORUM COMMUNIS From the lateral epicondyle of the humerus, from the common extensor tendon, from the intermuscular septum, and from the antebrachial fascia.	Distally in the forearm, it divides into 4 tendons that diverge on the back of the hand to be inserted into the middle and distal phalanges of the 4 fingers. Two slips are inserted into the base of the middle phalanx, and a third slip is inserted into the dorsum of the distal phalanx.	Deep radial nerve (C7, 8).	Extends the phalanges and, by continuing the action, extends the wrist.

Table 44–3 (cont'd). Muscles of the forearm: Dorsal muscles, superficial group.

Muscle and Origin	Insertion	Innervation	Function
EXTENSOR DIGITI MINIMI By a thin slip from the common extensor tendon and from the intermuscular septa dividing it from adjacent muscles.	The tendon divides into 2 as it crosses the dorsum of the hand and then joins the expansion of the extensor digitorum tendon on the dorsum of the proximal phalanx of the little finger.	Deep radial nerve (C7, 8).	Extends the little finger.
EXTENSOR CARPI ULNARIS From the lateral epicondyle of the humerus by the common extensor tendon, from the deep fascia of the forearm, and by an aponeurosis arising from the dorsal border of the ulna.	Ends in a tendon that inserts on the tubercle on the ulnar side of the fifth metacarpal bone.	Deep radial nerve (C7, 8).	Extends and adducts the hand.

Table 44–4. Muscles of the forearm: Dorsal muscles, deep group.

Muscle and Origin	Insertion	Innervation	Function
SUPINATOR The muscle consists of 2 planes of fibers between which lies the deep branch of the radial nerve. Both planes arise in common from the lateral epicondyle of the humerus, the radial collateral ligament of the elbow joint, the annular ligament, the ridge on the ulna just below the radial notch, and the aponeurosis covering the muscle.	Superficial fibers surround the proximal part of the radius and insert into the lateral edge of its tuberosity and into its oblique line as far inferiorly as the insertion of the pronator teres. The deep fibers sling about the neck of the radius and attach to the posterior aspect of its medial surface. However, the greater portion of the deep fibers insert into the dorsal and lateral surfaces of the body of the radius halfway between the oblique line and the radial head.	Deep branch of the deep radial nerve (C6).	Along with the biceps, supinates the hand and forearm.
ABDUCTOR POLLICIS LONGUS Arises from the lateral part of the dorsal surface of the ulna distal to the anconeus insertion, from the interosseous membrane, and from the middle third of the dorsal surface of the body of the radius.	Ends in a tendon inserted into the radial side of the base of the first metacarpal; usually sends a slip to the trapezium.	Deep radial nerve (C7, 8).	Abducts the thumb and, if the action continues, abducts the wrist.
EXTENSOR POLLICIS BREVIS Arises from the dorsal surface of the body of the radius distal to the abductor pollicis longus and from the interosseous membrane.	Into the base of the proximal phalanx of the thumb.	Deep radial nerve (C7, 8).	Extends the proximal phalanx of the thumb and, if the action continues, adducts the hand.
EXTENSOR POLLICIS LONGUS Arises from the lateral side of the middle third of the dorsal surface of the body of the ulna distal to the origin of the abductor pollicis longus and from the interosseous membrane.	Ends in a tendon inserted into the base of the distal phalanx of the thumb.	Deep radial nerve (C7, 8).	Extends the distal phalanx of the thumb and, if the action continues, adducts the hand.
EXTENSOR INDICIS Arises from the dorsal surface of the body of the ulna below the origin of the extensor pollicis longus and from the interosseous membrane.	Opposite the head of the second metacarpal bone, its tendon joins the ulnar side of the extensor digitorum, which runs to the index finger.	Deep radial nerve (C7, 8).	Extends and slightly adducts the index finger.

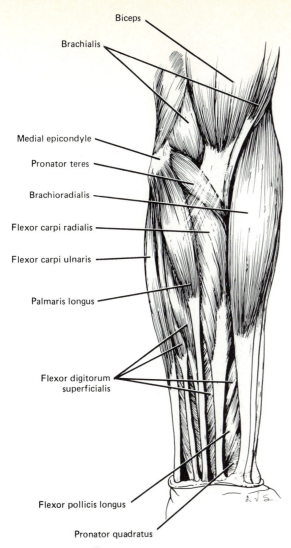

Biceps

Brachialis

Medial epicondyle

Pronator teres

Brachioradialis

Flexor carpi radialis

Flexor carpi ulnaris

Palmaris longus

Flexor digitorum
superficialis

Flexor pollicis longus

Pronator quadratus

Figure 44–6. Left anterior superficial muscles of the forearm.

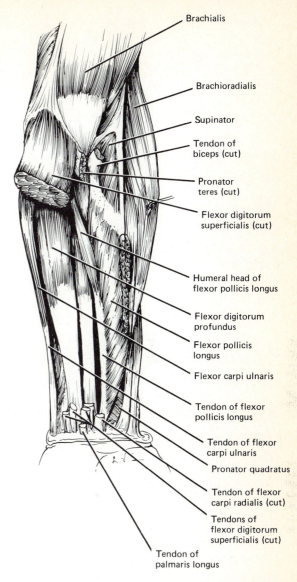

Brachialis

Brachioradialis

Supinator

Tendon of
biceps (cut)

Pronator
teres (cut)

Flexor digitorum
superficialis (cut)

Humeral head of
flexor pollicis longus

Flexor digitorum
profundus

Flexor pollicis
longus

Flexor carpi ulnaris

Tendon of flexor
pollicis longus

Tendon of flexor
carpi ulnaris

Pronator quadratus

Tendon of flexor
carpi radialis (cut)

Tendons of
flexor digitorum
superficialis (cut)

Tendon of
palmaris longus

Figure 44–7. Left anterior deep muscles of the forearm.

by the deep branch of the radial nerve. The muscles are the supinator, abductor pollicis longus, extensor pollicis brevis, extensor pollicis longus, and extensor indicis proprius.

➠ *Volkmann's contracture. Following extensive posttraumatic hemorrhage into either compartment of the forearm, whose limiting fasciae permit no blood to escape, ischemia in subsequent fibrous contracture of the long flexor or extensor muscles of the forearm can occur. The resulting muscular fibrosis secondary to the pressure of the enclosed hematoma is called Volkmann's ischemic contracture. It can be prevented by prompt incision of the restraining fascial septa. Such a procedure allows trapped blood to drain into an open area of the forearm.*

4. FASCIAE OF THE FOREARM
(Antebrachial Fascia)

The deep or brachial fascia of the arm continues into the forearm as a thick fibrous layer closely attached to the muscles that lie deep to it. Superiorly, the fascia is attached to the humeral epicondyles and to the olecranon; inferiorly, it is attached to the distal ends of the radius and ulna. It then continues farther inferiorly to blend with the fascia of the hand. The brachial fascia is attached to the posterior surface of the ulna and as a result isolates the flexor from the extensor compartment of the forearm. In the superior dorsal segment of the forearm, the fascia is

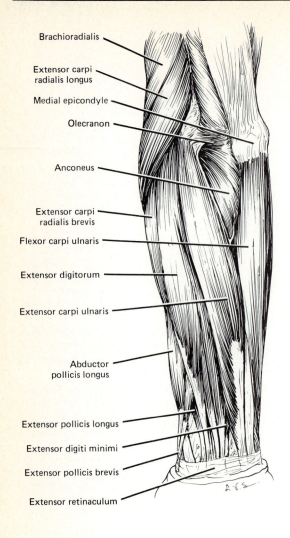

Brachioradialis

Extensor carpi
radialis longus

Medial epicondyle

Olecranon

Anconeus

Extensor carpi
radialis brevis

Flexor carpi ulnaris

Extensor digitorum

Extensor carpi ulnaris

Abductor
pollicis longus

Extensor pollicis longus

Extensor digiti minimi

Extensor pollicis brevis

Extensor retinaculum

Figure 44–8. Left posterior superficial muscles.

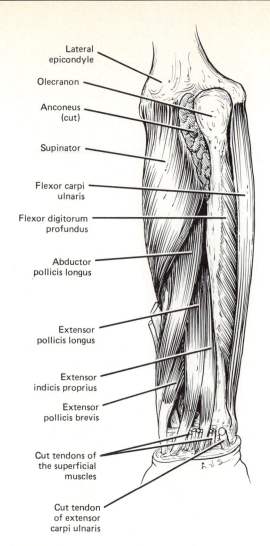

Lateral
epicondyle

Olecranon

Anconeus
(cut)

Supinator

Flexor carpi
ulnaris

Flexor digitorum
profundus

Abductor
pollicis longus

Extensor
pollicis longus

Extensor
indicis proprius

Extensor
pollicis brevis

Cut tendons of
the superficial
muscles

Cut tendon
of extensor
carpi ulnaris

Figure 44–9. Deep muscles of the left posterior surface.

strengthened by extensions of the triceps fascia. In the superior volar segment of the forearm, it is reinforced by the bicipital aponeurosis (lacertus fibrosus) and the tendon of the biceps brachii. At the level of the wrist, the forearm fascia thickens to form the volar and dorsal carpal ligaments. Strong intermuscular septa that arise from the deep surface of the brachial fascia separate the various forearm muscles and serve to create fascial clefts between the muscles themselves and between the muscles and the deep surface of the brachial fascia.

BLOOD VESSELS, LYMPHATICS, & NERVES

The major nerves and vessels of the anterior forearm lie ventral to the deep muscle layer of the anterior compartment. The major vessels and nerves of the posterior compartment of the forearm lie in the plane between the deep and superficial muscles.

Arteries
(Fig 44–10)

The radial and ulnar arteries—the terminal branches of the brachial artery—supply the anterior compartment of the forearm.

The **radial artery**—a terminal branch of the brachial artery—begins at the neck of the radius and descends in the forearm to the radial styloid. In the upper forearm, it lies deep to the brachioradialis muscle. In the inferior third of the forearm, it is covered only by skin and by the superficial and deep forearm fasciae. It gives off muscular, radial recurrent, superficial palmar, and palmar carpal branches. At the wrist joint, the vessel is so superficial that its pulsations are readily palpable and often visible. At wrist level it gives off its dorsal carpal and first dorsal metacarpal branches.

The **ulnar artery** begins in the forearm at the radial neck and lies on a deeper plane than the radial artery. In the upper arm, it is covered by the pronator teres, the flexor carpi radialis, the palmaris longus,

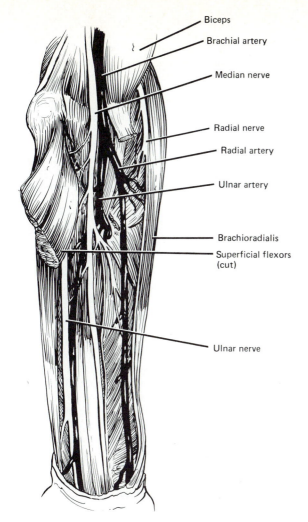

Biceps

Brachial artery

Median nerve

Radial nerve

Radial artery

Ulnar artery

Brachioradialis

Superficial flexors (cut)

Ulnar nerve

Figure 44–10. Arteries and nerves of the ventral surface of the left forearm.

and the flexor digitorum sublimis. At first, the median nerve lies medial to the artery; but in the mid forearm the nerve crosses the artery to lie lateral to it. In the lower third of the forearm, the ulnar nerve lies just medial to the artery. At wrist level, the artery is superficial, covered only by the skin and the volar carpal ligament, and is readily palpable. High in the forearm, the ulnar artery gives off the anterior and posterior recurrent branches, which contribute to the arterial anastomosis about the elbow joint. Just distal to the recurrent branches, the common interosseous branch is given off. This vessel, via its palmar and dorsal branches, is the major source of blood to the posterior forearm compartment. At wrist level, the ulnar artery gives off volar and dorsal carpal branches.

Veins

The **cephalic vein** on the radial side of the forearm carries blood from the lateral and dorsal surface veins of the hand. As it ascends in the forearm, it is joined by veins from both the anterior and posterior forearm compartments. Just before it reaches the antecubital fossa, it receives an anastomotic branch from the median cubital vein. The **basilic vein** arises in the medial segment of the dorsal venous plexus of the hand, ascends on the medial posterior surface of the forearm, and just below the elbow moves to the anterior surface of the forearm, where it is joined by the median cubital vein. The median antebrachial vein drains the palmar surface of the hand, runs superiorly along the anterior surface of the forearm, and ends by joining the median cubital vein.

The 2 major **deep veins** of the forearm closely accompany the radial and ulnar arteries. They are the superior continuations of the superficial and deep venous palmar arches. The deep ulnar veins are of larger caliber than the radial veins. The 2 deep veins of the forearm terminate in the antecubital fossa, where they join to form the brachial vein.

Lymphatics

The **superficial lymphatic vessels** of the forearm begin in lymphatic plexuses in the skin of the dorsal and palmar surfaces of the hand. At the level of the wrist, they divide into radial, median, and ulnar channels, which lie alongside the cephalic, median, and basilic veins, respectively. A few superficial lymphatics on the ulnar side of the forearm reach the supratrochlear nodes; however, most of the ascending lymphatic flow from the forearm passes directly to the most lateral axillary nodes. The superficial radial lymph channels, ascending along with the cephalic vein, usually end in the deltopectoral nodes from which the lymph flows either to the axillary nodes or to the lowest nodes of the cervical chain (supraclavicular nodes).

The **deep lymphatic vessels** of the forearm ascend alongside the major deep forearm vessels, divided into 4 groups related to the radial, ulnar, anterior, and posterior interosseous arteries, respectively. There are many connections between the superficial and deep forearm lymphatics. Most of the deep lymph eventually passes to the group of axillary nodes, related to the inferior edge of the ascending pectoralis major muscle (inferior subpectoral nodes).

Nerves
(Figs 44–10 to 44–12)

The **median nerve** serves the superficial group of flexor muscles on the lateral side of the forearm. The muscles are the pronator teres, flexor carpi radialis, palmaris longus, and flexor digitorum superficialis. By its anterior interosseous branch, the median nerve supplies the deep muscles of the anterior forearm compartment. These muscles are the flexor pollicis longus, flexor digitorum profundus (radial head only), and pronator quadratus.

The course of the median nerve in the forearm begins in the antecubital fossa, where it lies between the 2 heads of the pronator teres. High in the forearm, it gives off its muscular branches to the superficial

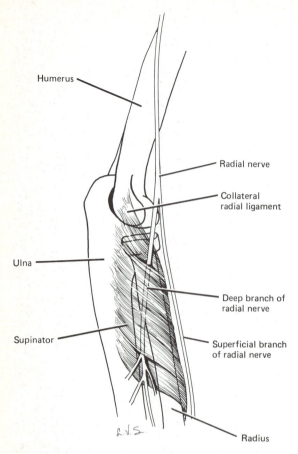

Figure 44–11. The supinator muscle and its relationship to the divisions of the radial nerve.

flexor group of the anterior forearm compartment and also some branches to the elbow joint. The anterior interosseous branch of the median nerve is given off in the proximal third of the forearm and proceeds dorsally to descend on the anterior surface of the interosseous membrane as far as the pronator quadratus muscle. It supplies the group of deep flexor muscles except for the medial half of the flexor digitorum profundus. The median nerve gives off no branches above the level of the elbow joint.

The major median trunk passes between the superficial and deep flexor muscles. Just before reaching the flexor retinaculum of the wrist, it becomes quite superficial between the flexor carpi radialis and flexor digitorum profundus tendons. At the wrist, it lies deep to the tendon of the palmaris longus.

At the elbow, the **ulnar nerve** lies dorsal to the medial epicondyle of the humerus. It then descends and moves ventrally. It enters the anterior compartment between the 2 heads of the flexor carpi ulnaris muscle. More distally, the ulnar nerve lies between the flexor carpi ulnaris and the flexor digitorum profundus. In the upper forearm, the ulnar nerve sends branches to the flexor carpi ulnaris and the ulnar portion of the flexor digitorum profundus. At the

wrist, it enters the carpal area deep to the volar carpal ligament but superficial to the transverse carpal ligament, where it lies medial to the ulnar artery. In the forearm, the ulnar nerve sends off articular branches to the elbow joint, muscular branches to the flexor carpi ulnaris and to the ulnar half of the flexor digitorum profundus, a palmar cutaneous branch, a dorsal branch, and a palmer branch that divides into a superficial and a deep branch.

The **radial nerve** (Fig 44–11) enters the antecubital fossa between the brachialis and brachioradialis muscles. It supplies the lateral group of forearm muscles, ie, the extensor group of the wrist and hand. Anterior to the lateral epicondyle of the humerus, the nerve passes through the lateral intermuscular septum and almost immediately divides into deep and superficial branches. The superficial branch, a sensory nerve, parallels the radial artery deep to the brachioradialis muscle. It pierces the deep fascia near the lower end of the forearm and divides into medial and lateral branches. The lateral branch supplies the skin of the back of the hand and the skin on the radial side and at the base of the thumb. The medial branch gives rise to the 4 dorsal digital nerves. These supply the medial side of the thumb, the lateral side of the index finger, the adjoining sides of the index and middle fingers, and the adjacent sides of the middle and ring fingers. The deep branch passes to the dorsal surface of the forearm via the lateral edge of the radius. It moves distally, situated between the deep and superficial layers of the dorsal forearm to the dorsum of the wrist, where it supplies the ligaments and joints of the wrist bones. The deep branch supplies all the muscles on the radial side and the dorsum of the forearm except the brachioradialis and the extensor carpi radialis longus.

➡ *Exposure of the radial nerve. The radial nerve is easily exposed in the upper segment of the forearm if the surgeon enters the plane between the brachialis and brachioradialis muscles.*

➡ *Radial nerve injury in the forearm. If the radial nerve in the forearm is injured or is affected by toxic neuritis (lead, methyl alcohol), the patient usually develops wristdrop (inability to extend the wrist even against gravity).*

➡ *Injury to the dorsal interosseous branch of the radial nerve. The most proximal segment of the dorsal interosseous branch of the radial nerve may be injured by fractures or dislocations of the radial head. The injury may cause weakness of the extensor carpi radialis brevis and the supinator muscle.*

➡ *Amputations. Elective forearm amputation is usually done close to the junction of the middle and lower thirds of the part. This gives a good length of forearm stump to fit well into a prosthesis.*

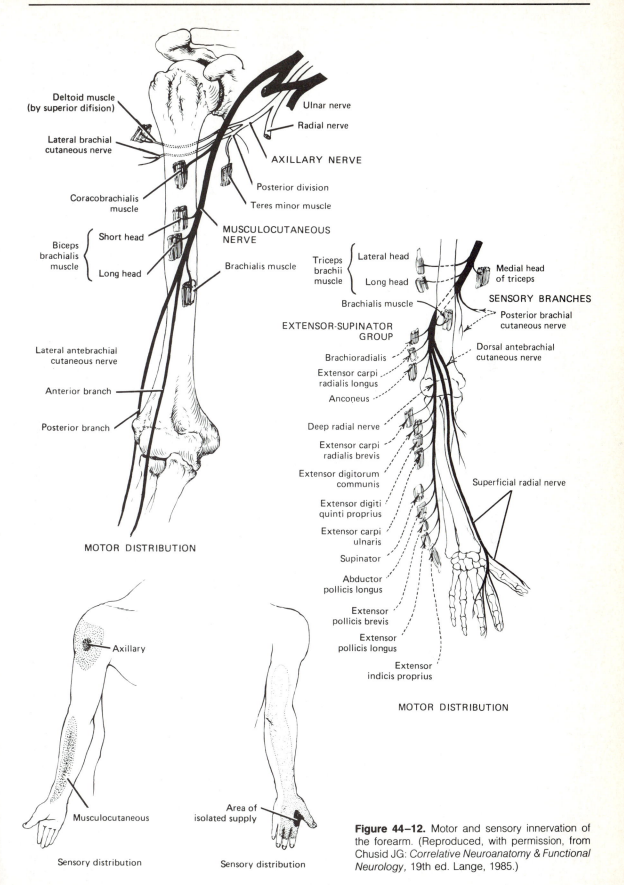

Figure 44–12. Motor and sensory innervation of the forearm. (Reproduced, with permission, from Chusid JG: *Correlative Neuroanatomy & Functional Neurology,* 19th ed. Lange, 1985.)

45

The Wrist

GROSS ANATOMY

BONES OF THE WRIST

The bony skeleton of the wrist is made up of the 8 carpal bones and the distal ends of the radius and ulna. The carpals may be divided into proximal and distal rows (Figs 45–1 and 45–2). In the proximal row, from lateral to medial, are the scaphoid (navicular), lunate, triquetrum, and pisiform. The scaphoid and the lunate articulate with the distal extremity of the radius, while the triquetrum is separated from the distal end of the ulna by the articular disk. The distal carpal row, from lateral to medial, is made up of the trapezium, trapezoid, capitate, and hamate. The distal row articulates proximally with the bones of the proximal carpal row and distally with the bases of the metacarpals. The irregular volar and dorsal surfaces of the carpal bones receive attachment of the maze of carpal ligaments. The carpal bones are composed of a central core of cancellous bone surrounded by a relatively thin shell of compact bone. In positions where a carpal bone abuts an adjacent carpal, the contiguous surface of each bone is quite smooth. Nonadjacent carpal surfaces are rough.

1. PROXIMAL CARPAL BONES

Scaphoid

The scaphoid bone (navicular bone; os scaphoideum, os naviculare) is the largest of the proximal carpal bones and articulates with 5 bones. Proximally, it is smooth and convex and articulates with the concavity of the distal end of the radius. Distally, the 2 smooth surfaces of the end of the bone articulate with the trapezium and trapezoid. The medial scaphoid surface is divided into 2 facets for articulation with the lunate and capitate bones. The radial collateral ligament of the wrist attaches to the lateral surface of the scaphoid; the palmar surface of the bone presents a tubercle that gives attachment to the flexor retinaculum.

➡️ ***Fractures of the scaphoid.*** *(Fig 45–3.) Fracture of the scaphoid is a common carpal bone injury, usually caused by a fall on the outstretched hand. Symptoms and tenderness and swelling over the "anatomic snuff box," the depressed area on the dorsoradial side of the wrist bounded laterally by the tendons of the abductor pollicis longus and extensor pollicis brevis and medially by the tendon of the extensor pollicis longus. Nonunion or delayed healing is relatively frequent with such fractures, because the nutrient artery to the bone is frequently transected at the fracture line. With delayed union, surgery is often needed. The fragments may be pinned together, or the bone may be drilled to increase circulation.*

Lunate

The lunate (os lunatum) is a crescent-shaped bone between the scaphoid and the triquetrum. Its convex proximal surface articulates with the concave articular surface of the radius; the distal surface of the lunate is concave and articulates with the heads of the capitate and hamate. Facets on the lateral and medial surfaces of the lunate articulate with the scaphoid and triquetrum, respectively. Its dorsal and volar surfaces are roughened at their points of ligamentous attachment. In all, the lunate articulates with 5 carpal bones.

➡️ ***Fractures and dislocations of the lunate.*** *Fractures of the lunate are rare and usually caused by a blow upon the palm with the wrist adducted. Lunate dislocations are the most common carpal bone dislocations. Lunate dislocation is always volar and usually results from a fall on the dorsiflexed hand. Pain over the bone and median nerve paresthesia frequently accompany lunate dislocation, as does apparent shortening of the third metacarpal. Rotary subluxation of the lunate is shown in Fig. 45–4.*

Triquetrum

The triquetrum (triangular bone, os triquetrum) is roughly pyramidal and articulates with 3 carpal bones. A circular facet on its midpalmar surface articulates with the pisiform bone. The proximal surface joins with the triangular articular disk of the wrist joint, which separates it from the ulna; the distal surface articulates with the hamate bone. The lateral

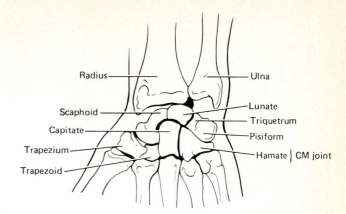

Figure 45-1. Bones of the wrist.

triangular surface articulates with the lunate; its medial surface gives attachment to the ulnar collateral ligament of the wrist joint.

Pisiform

The oval pisiform bone (os pisiforme) is the smallest of the wrist bones. It presents only one facet, which articulates with the triquetrum. The pisiform lies closer to the palmar surface of the wrist than any other wrist bone. To its rough palmar surface are attached the flexor retinaculum, the flexor carpi ulnaris, and the abductor digiti minimi muscles.

2. DISTAL CARPAL BONES

Trapezium

The trapezium (os trapezium) is situated on the radial side of the distal row of carpal bones. Its proximal surface articulates with the scaphoid, its distal surface with the base of the first metacarpal bone. Medially, the trapezium articulates with the trapezoid and with the base of the second metacarpal. In a deep groove on the palmar surface of the trapezium runs the tendon of the flexor carpi radialis. On the lateral side of its palmar surface are the attachments

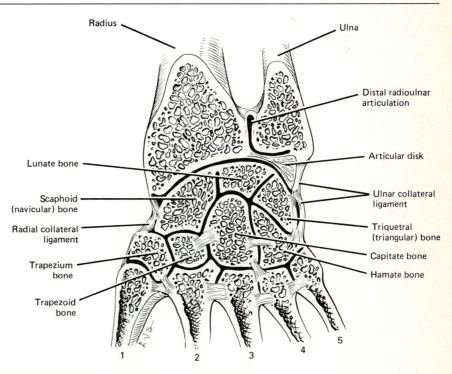

Figure 45-2. Articulations of the bones of the wrist.

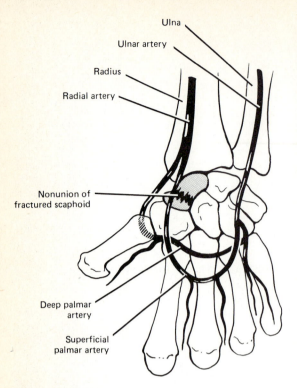

Figure 45–3. Fracture of the scaphoid (navicular) bone.

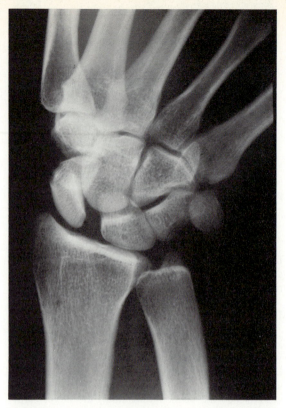

Figure 45–4. Rotatory subluxation. Note the triangular gap between the scaphoid and lunate. (Reproduced, with permission, from Way LW [editor]: *Current Surgical Diagnosis & Treatment,* 7th ed. Lange, 1985.)

of the opponens pollicis, the flexor pollicis brevis, the abductor pollicis brevis, and the flexor retinaculum.

Trapezoid

The trapezoid (os trapezoideum), the smallest of the distal carpal bones, is roughly pyramidal, with 4 articular facets. It articulates with the scaphoid proximally, the base of the second metacarpal distally, the trapezium laterally, and the capitate medially. The dorsal and volar surfaces of the bone are roughened for attachment of carpal ligaments.

Capitate

The capitate bone (os capitatum) has a central position and articulates with 7 bones of the wrist and hand. It is composed of a hemispherical head, a narrow neck, and a distal body. Its 7 articulations are as follows: (1) and (2) proximally with the concavity formed by the inferior surfaces of the scaphoid and lunate; (3), (4), and (5) distally with the bases of the second, third, and fourth metacarpals; (6) laterally with the trapezoid; and (7) medially with the hamate.

Hamate

The hamate (os hamatum) is the most medial of the distal row of carpal bones. It presents on its palmar surface an easily identifiable hook. The flexor retinaculum, the flexor carpi ulnaris, the flexor digiti quinti brevis, and the opponens digiti minimi attach to the hamulus. The hamate articulates with the lunate proximally, with the fourth and fifth metacarpals distally, with the triquetrum medially and superiorly, and with the capitate laterally.

CARPAL LIGAMENTS
(Figs 45–5 and 45–6)

The distal forearm articulates with the carpal area via 2 joints: the true wrist joint proximally and the midcarpal joint distally. The wrist joint is a compound articulation composed of the radiocarpal and distal radioulnar articulations. The wrist joint allows hand and wrist movements of flexion, extension, abduction, adduction, and circumduction. The radioulnar joint allows only pronation and supination (pivot joint).

The dorsal surface of the proximal row of carpal bones has attachments from 2 strong transverse ligaments that join the scaphoid with the lunate and the lunate with the triquetrum. The palmar surface of the proximal row has attachment from 2 less strong ligaments connecting the same bones as the dorsal ligament. Two thin interosseous ligaments also con-

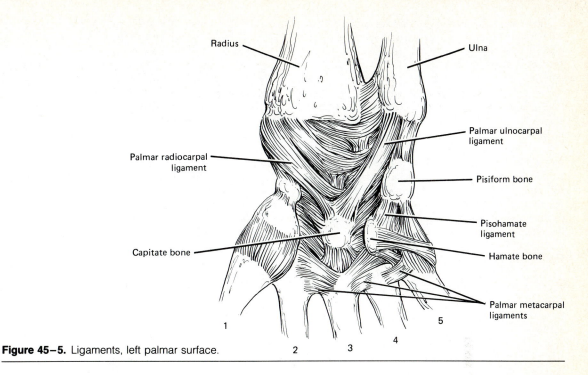

Figure 45–5. Ligaments, left palmar surface.

nect the scaphoid with the lunate and the lunate with the triquetrum. The distal carpal bones are also joined by transverse ligaments on their dorsal and palmar surfaces as well as by interosseous ligaments.

As the volar antebrachial fascia reaches the wrist, it forms a thick encircling cuff of fascia that holds the tendons tightly against the carpal bones.

On the volar surface of the wrist, a fascial thickening called the **flexor retinaculum** consists of 2 separate fascial strata: the palmar (volar) carpal ligament and the transverse carpal ligament. The palmar carpal ligament runs from the styloid process of the ulna to the styloid process of the radius, and deep to it lie the flexor tendons.

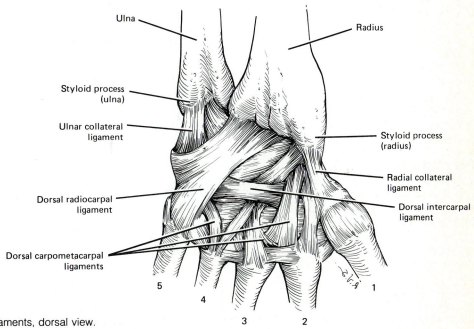

Figure 45–6. Ligaments, dorsal view.

The transverse carpal ligament arches over the palmar surface of the carpal bones, forming a canal through which pass the long flexor tendons and the median nerve. On the ulnar side of the wrist, it is fixed to the pisiform and the hook of the hamate; on the radial side, to the scaphoid tuberosity. Proximally, the ligament is closely allied to the palmar carpal ligament and to the deep surface of the palmar aponeurosis.

The **extensor retinaculum** lies on the dorsal surface of the wrist, and deep to it lie the extensor tendons. It is formed by a thickening of the dorsal division of the antebrachial fascia. Medially, the retinaculum is fastened to the ulnar styloid and to the pisiform and triquetrum. Laterally, it is attached to the lateral surface of the radius.

Radiocarpal Joint

The radiocarpal joint is condyloid in type. The distal end of the radius and the distal border of the articular disk together form a concave surface for the articulation. The convex aggregate of the superior surfaces of the scaphoid, lunate, and triquetrum fits neatly into this concavity. A well-fitting articular capsule plus the palmar and dorsal radiocarpal ligaments and the ulnar and radial collateral ligaments give stability to the joint. The palmar radiocarpal ligament extends from the distal end of the radius to the palmar surfaces of the 3 proximal carpal bones. The dorsal radiocarpal ligament stretches from the radius to the posterior surfaces of the scaphoid, lunate, and triquetrum.

The triangular fibrocartilaginous articular disk is the major structure uniting the distal ends of the radius and ulna. It is transverse, just distal to the head of the ulna and just superior to the triquetrum. It is connected by its base to the medial border of the ulnar notch of the radius, while its apex is attached to the base of the syloid process of the ulna. Its proximal surface articulates with the head of the ulna. The disk separates the cavity of the wrist joint from the cavity of the distal radioulnar joint.

The wrist joint permits all movements except rotation. The continuous superior surfaces of the bones in the distal row of carpal bones against the distal surfaces of the bones in the proximal row forms the **midcarpal joint.** At this level, flexion and extension are supplemented by a small arc of rotation.

Intercarpal Articulations

There are 3 categories of intercarpal articulations: (1) intercarpal articulations of the proximal carpal bones, (2) intercarpal articulations of the distal carpal bones, and (3) articulations between the individual carpal bones of both the proximal and distal rows are gliding joints supported by both palmar and dorsal interosseous ligaments.

Midcarpal Joint

The midcarpal joint is situated between the scaphoid, lunate, and triquetrum bones and the 4 bones of the distal row. It is supported by dorsal and volar carpal ligaments and by ulnar and radial collateral ligaments. The midcarpal joint is a complex of 3 separate joints: (1) the ball-and-socket joint between the head of the capitate and the superior surface of the hamate distally and the crescent-shaped cavity formed by the distal surfaces of the scaphoid and lunate proximally; (2) the lateral (radial) joint between the scaphoid, trapezoid, and trapezium; and (3) the medial (ulnar) joint between the hamate and triquetrum. The latter 2 joints are of the gliding type.

Flexion of the wrist is by the flexor carpi radialis, flexor carpi ulnaris, and palmaris longus. If the fingers are extended, wrist flexion can be accomplished by the flexor carpi radialis and flexor carpi ulnaris. If the fingers are flexed, wrist flexion is accomplished by the flexor digitorum superficialis and flexor digitorum profundus. Extension of the wrist is by the extensor carpi radialis longus, extensor carpi radialis

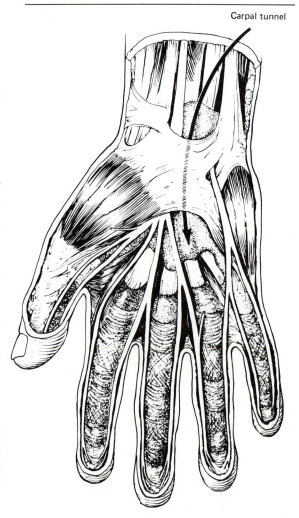

Carpal tunnel

Figure 45–7. Carpal tunnel. (Reproduced, with permission, from Way LW [editor]: *Current Surgical Diagnosis & Treatment,* 7th ed. Lange, 1985.)

brevis, and extensor carpi ulnaris. Adduction (ulnar flexion) of the wrist is by contractions of both the flexor carpi ulnaris and the extensor carpi ulnaris. Abduction (radial flexion) is by simultaneous contractions of the extensor carpi radialis longus, extensor carpi radialis brevis, and flexor carpi radialis.

BLOOD VESSELS, LYMPHATICS, & NERVES

The wrist joint and the intercarpal joints are supplied by the palmar and dorsal carpal branches of the radial and ulnar arteries. An additional arterial supply reaches the joints from the palmar and dorsal metacarpal branches of the radial and ulnar arteries, and a minor arterial supply also comes from branches of the deep palmar arch. Venous and lymphatic drainage from the wrist is into radial, median, and ulnar channels which, respectively, accompany the cephalic, median, and basilic veins in the forearm.

Nerve supply to the joints of the wrist area comes from the ulnar and dorsal interosseous nerves.

⇒ *Carpal tunnel syndrome. (Fig. 45–7.) At the wrist, the strong horizontal transverse carpal ligament bridges a tunnel whose dorsal relationship is the 2 rows of unyielding carpal bones. In this space are the median nerve and the flexor tendons of the hand. Conditions that decrease the anteroposterior diameter of the tunnel press upon the median nerve and the flexor tendons of the hand and can result in severe pain and disability in the wrist and hand.*

⇒ *Structures injured by wrist lacerations. Transverse laceration of the relatively superficial soft tissues at wrist joint level will endanger the following structures (from radial to ulnar): (1) the abductor pollicis longus, (2) the radial artery, (3) the tendon of the flexor carpi radialis muscle, (4) the median nerve, (5) the tendon of the palmaris longus muscle, (6) the ulnar artery and nerve, and (7) the tendon of the flexor carpi ulnaris muscle. If the laceration goes one layer deeper, it can cut the superficial row of flexor tendons to the fingers and the flexor pollicis longus.*

GROSS ANATOMY

BONES OF THE HAND
& THEIR ARTICULATIONS

The bony framework of the hand consists of the 5 metacarpals and the 14 phalanges. The 4 fingers have 3 phalanges each, the thumb only two.

1. METACARPALS
(Figs 46–1 and 46–2)

Each metacarpal is composed of a shaft, a head, and a base. The metacarpals are numbered 1–5 starting from the radial side of the hand. The medial and lateral surfaces of the metacarpals are bowed in the direction of the center of the bone, and the interosseous muscles attach to their borders. A palmar elevation separates the medial and lateral surfaces of the metacarpals. The distal two-thirds of the dorsal surfaces are smooth and flat and masked by the extensor tendons running toward the phalanges. On the dorsal surface of the metacarpals, a ridge separates 2 obliquely slanting surfaces to which the dorsal interossei attach. The metacarpal bases are squarish and concave, and they articulate both with the distal row of carpal bones and with the adjoining metacarpal bones. The metacarpal heads are convex and articulate with the concave bases of the proximal phalanges. Their bilateral tubercles provide attachment for the metacarpophalangeal collateral ligaments. The palmar surface of the metacarpal head has a midline groove for passage of the flexor tendons to the phalanges, while the extensor tendons lie directly upon the dorsal aspect of the metacarpal heads.

Individual Characteristics of the
5 Metacarpal Bones

The **first metacarpal** is the shortest and thickest of the 5 metacarpals. Its base articulates with the trapezium; its head is the widest of the metacarpal heads and it articulates with the proximal phalanx of the thumb.

The **second metacarpal** is the longest of the metacarpals. Its base is larger than the bases of metacarpals 3, 4, and 5. The base articulates with the trapezoid, trapezium, and capitate. On its ulnar side, the base articulates with the base of the third metacarpal. Its head articulates with the proximal phalanx of the index finger.

The **third metacarpal** has a concave carpal articular facet that joins only with the capitate. On the radial side, a facet articulates with the second metacarpal; on the ulnar side, 2 small articular surfaces join it to the fourth metacarpal. Its head articulates with the middle finger.

The **fourth metacarpal** has a 4-sided base that articulates proximally with the capitate and the hamate, radially with the third metacarpal, and medially with the fifth metacarpal. Its head articulates with the ring finger.

The **fifth metacarpal** articulates at its base with the hamate and on its radial basal border with the fourth metacarpal. Its head articulates with the little finger.

2. CARPOMETACARPAL
ARTICULATIONS
(Fig 46–3)

The carpometacarpal articulation of the thumb differs from the carpometacarpal junction of the 4 fingers. The proximal joint of the thumb, the articulation between the saddle-shaped distal surface of the trapezium and the base of the first metacarpal, allows for a wide range of thumb motions. At the carpometacarpal joint, the thumb can be flexed and extended, abducted and adducted. Circumduction and opposition movements may also be performed. The joint is supported by a thick but relatively loose capsule lined with synovial membrane.

The joints between the 4 remaining metacarpals and their adjacent carpal bones are all of the gliding type. They are supported by dorsal and palmar ligaments. In addition, interosseous ligaments connect the adjacent surfaces of the third and fourth metacarpals. The synovial cavity of the 4 medial carpometacarpal joints is prolonged distally to the carpometacarpal articulations as an offshoot from the intercarpal joint synovium. The fifth and fourth carpometacarpal joints allow the greatest degree of motion, whereas the third and second carpometacarpal joints have almost no motion. The bases of the metacarpals, except for the metacarpal of the thumb, join with the bases of the adjacent metacarpals via tiny articular surfaces. These small joints are strengthened by dorsal, palmar,

Figure 46–1. Bones of the right hand and wrist: palmar (volar) surface.

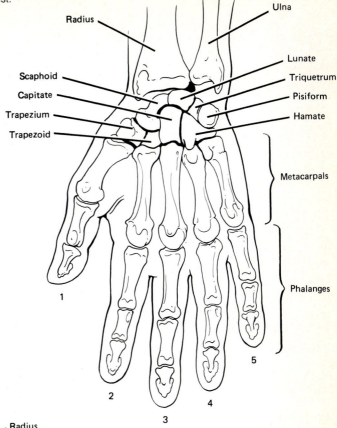

Figure 46–2. Bones of the right hand and wrist: dorsal surface.

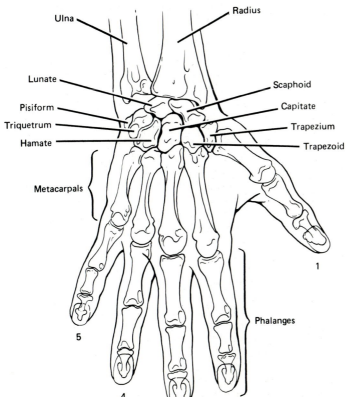

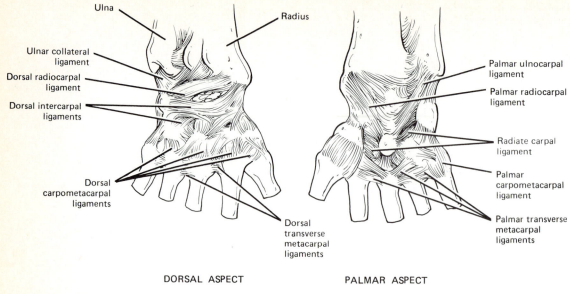

Figure 46–3. Carpometacarpal ligaments of the right hand.

and interosseous ligaments. The transverse metacarpal ligament, a thin fibrous strand on the palmar surface of the metacarpal heads, assists in joining the heads of metacarpals 3, 4, and 5.

⇒ *Fractures of the metacarpals. Bennett's intra-articular fracture is an impacted fracture of the metacarpal of the thumb. There is oblique separation of the palmar base from the dorsal base, which subluxates dorsally. Reduction of the fracture is achieved by pulling on the thumb and exerting palmar pressure on the metacarpal base. Fixation of the reduction is by use of a Kirschner wire. On occasion, surgical reduction is required.*

A spiral displaced fracture at the base of the fifth metacarpal should prompt the examiner to check the function of the first dorsal interosseous muscle to ascertain the integrity of the deep motor branch of the ulnar nerve, which may be traumatized in this fracture.

3. METACARPOPHALANGEAL ARTICULATIONS

The metacarpophalangeal articulations result from insertion of the round heads of the metacarpals into shallow concavities on the proximal ends of the proximal phalanges.

Articulation of the thumb is ginglymoid, whereas the metacarpophalangeal joints of the fingers are condyloid. Each metacarpophalangeal joint is reinforced by a palmar fibrocartilaginous ligament and lateral ligaments. The dorsal surface of each metacarpopha-

langeal joint of the fingers is covered by the fibrous expansion of the extensor tendon. The metacarpophalangeal joints of the fingers allow flexion, extension, abduction, adduction (through the action of the interossei), and circumduction. When the fingers are fully flexed, abduction and adduction in these joints cannot be carried out.

⇒ *Metacarpal and phalangeal fractures and small joint dislocations. Metacarpal and phalangeal fractures are common fractures and are often accompanied by dislocations of the metacarpophalangeal and interphalangeal joints. In fractures of the metacarpal shafts, the fragments are displaced dorsally, since the flexor muscles of the hand are stronger than the extensor muscles. In addition to dorsal angulation, the fragments tend to rotate. The forces responsible for angulation and rotation can best be countered by placing wrist and fingers in the position of optimum function (see below).*

4. PHALANGES

Each of the 14 phalanges of the hand consists of a body, a proximal end, and a distal end. The phalangeal body is convex dorsally and narrows distally. The 2 lateral surfaces of the middle phalanges have rough ridges that receive insertion of the flexor digitorum superficialis tendons. The distal or ungual phalanges are small; their palmar surface is flat and ends distally in a U-shaped elevation that supports the fingernail. The proximal phalanges of the 4 fingers articulate with their respective metacarpals and distally with the second row of phalanges. Since the thumb has only 2 phalanges, its proximal phalanx articulates with the short first metacarpal proximally and with the ungual phalanx distally.

➠ ***Reduction of phalangeal fractures.*** *In fractures of the proximal phalanx of the finger, the fragments are usually angulated toward the palmar surface of the hand by the combined pull of the palmar interosseous and lumbrical muscles upon the extensor tendon expansion. Reduction is achieved by relaxing the extensor muscles through flexion of the metacarpophalangeal and interphalangeal joints.*

Middle phalangeal fractures proximal to the attachment of the flexor digitorum superficialis tendon should be immobilized in an extension splint, since the palmar deformity is due to flexor pull. Middle phalangeal fractures distal to the attachment of the flexor digitorum superficialis tendon shows an extension deformity and should be immobilized in a flexion splint.

➠ ***Conservation of thumb.*** *Because so many skills depend on the strength, length, and motion of the thumb, the surgeon must preserve as much thumb length as possible. The thumb should always be placed in proper position for opposition to the fingers.*

5. INTERPHALANGEAL ARTICULATION

The articulations of the interphalangeal joints are ginglymoid (''hingelike''). Each interphalangeal joint has one palmar and 2 collateral ligaments. The extensor tendon expansions covering the dorsal surface of the interphalangeal joints act as their dorsal ligament. Flexion and extension of the interphalangeal joint are allowed. Extension is limited by the palmar and by lateral and medial collateral ligaments. Flexion can be performed to a considerable degree.

➠ ***Position of function.*** *In treating severe hand or wrist trauma, burns, or infections, the hand and wrist should be immobilized in the position of optimum function. Thus, if permanent partial or complete limitation of motion ultimately results, the extremity will retain as much useful function as possible. The elbow should be placed at a right angle, the forearm halfway between pronation and supination, the wrist extended 250–300 degrees, and the fingers flexed so that they almost touch the opposed tip of the thumb. There should be moderate flexion at the metacarpophalangeal joints and moderate digital flexion. The thumb should be slightly flexed and adducted. In this position, one can hold a pen and write.*

➠ ***Principles of care for hand burns.*** *Control of pain and swelling, prevention and control of infection, and prompt debridement and grafting are principles of care for hand burns. The hand should be mobilized as soon as consistent with healing.*

6. ACTION OF MUSCLE GROUPS ON LOWER FOREARM, WRIST, & HAND

The muscles that insert into or cover the carpal, metacarpal, and phalangeal areas frequently act together to achieve a single motion or series of motions. For example, wrist flexion is accomplished by the flexor carpi ulnaris, palmaris longus, and flexor carpi radialis muscles. The superficial and deep flexors of the fingers do not ordinarily flex the wrist but may do so if they are prevented from flexing the fingers. Similarly, the extensor carpi radialis longus and brevis and the extensor carpi ulnaris usually act as the primary extensors of the wrist (Fig. 46–4); but if the fingers are prevented from extending, the wrist will be extended by the extensor digitorum. Radial flexion of the wrist is a combined action of the flexor carpi radialis, the extensor carpi radialis longus and brevis, and the abductor pollicis longus. Ulnar flexion of the wrist is accomplished by the flexor carpi ulnaris and the extensor carpi ulnaris. The hand is pronated by the pronator quadratus and pronator teres muscles; it is supinated by the biceps brachii and by the supinator muscles.

SOFT TISSUES OF THE HAND

1. DORSUM OF THE HAND

Skin & Subcutaneous Tissues

The skin and subcutaneous tissues covering the dorsum of the hand differ markedly from the skin and subcutaneous tissues of the palm as regards their relationship to the structures lying deep to them. On the dorsum of the hand, the superficial tissues are so loosely applied to the underlying structures that they can be bluntly dissected free without difficulty and elevated from the dorsal deep fascia, which lies immediately deep to them. Looseness of the dorsal superficial tissues creates a space superficial to the deep fascia, the **dorsal subcutaneous space.**

The loose areolar tissue just deep to the skin of the dorsum of the hand contains many lymphatic channels, which drain the dorsum of the fingers and hand, the palmar surfaces of the fingers, the web spaces between the fingers, and the thenar and hypothenar eminences.

⇒ *Lymphedema on the dorsum of the hand. The marked lymphedema that usually appears on the dorsum of the hand secondary to infections on the palmar surface of the extremity shows the direction of lymph flow from the palmar to the dorsal hand surfaces. The physician should always search for a palmar lesion when dorsal lymphedema appears in order to avoid the mistake of incising the dorsal swelling thinking that it is the site of the primary infection.*

In addition to the multiple lymphatics, the dorsal subcutaneous space also contains many large veins and many superficial nerve fibers.

Dorsal Subcutaneous Fascia

The dorsal subcutaneous fascia has 2 layers. The superficial layer is thin and is directly connected to the superficial fascia of the forearm. The deep layer serves as a framework for the subcutaneous vessels and nerves.

Deep Fascia of the Dorsum of the Hand

The antebrachial fascia of the dorsum of the forearm invests the deep structures of the dorsum of the wrist and hand. At the wrist, the fascia is reinforced by the addition of fibrous bands, known as the **extensor retinaculum.** In the hand proper, the dorsal deep fascia fuses with the thenar and the hypothenar fascia of the palm. As a result, a closed

flattened space is formed, bounded superficially by the deep fascia of the dorsum of the hand, laterally and medially by the fusion of the deep dorsal fascia with the palmar fascia, and deeply by the fascia covering the dorsal interosseous muscles. This space is called the dorsal **subaponeurotic fascial cleft.** Passing through this cleft, just deep to the deep dorsal fascia, are the extensor tendons to the fingers. The cleft does not join with the forearm spaces, the palm of the hand, or the dorsal subcutaneous space.

⇒ *Infections of dorsal subaponeurotic fascial cleft. Infections in the space are limited to the deep dorsum of the hand and do not pass proximally into the forearm or distally into the fingers. Infections in this space are relatively rare.*

Dorsal Carpal Tunnels (Fig 46–5)

Deep to the extensor retinaculum but superficial to the dorsal surface of the carpal bones are 6 synovial tunnels for the passage of the extensor tendons as they move from forearm to wrist and hand. From lateral to medial, the 6 tunnels transmit (1) tendons of the abductor pollicis longus and extensor pollicis brevis, (2) tendons of the extensor carpi radialis longus and extensor carpi radialis brevis, (3) the tendon of the extensor pollicis longus, (4) tendons of the extensor digitorum and extensor indicis, (5) the tendon of the extensor digiti minimi, and (6) the tendon of

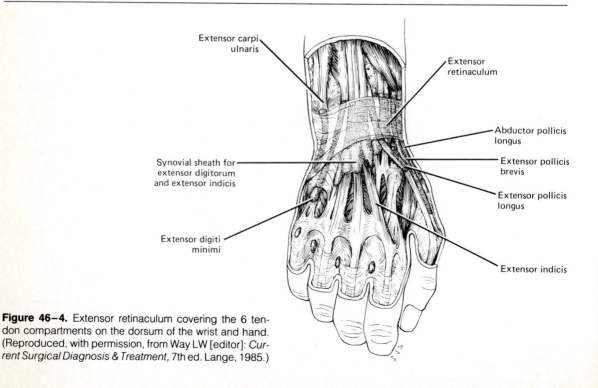

Figure 46–4. Extensor retinaculum covering the 6 tendon compartments on the dorsum of the wrist and hand. (Reproduced, with permission, from Way LW [editor]: *Current Surgical Diagnosis & Treatment,* 7th ed. Lange, 1985.)

the extensor carpi ulnaris. Each tunnel is composed of a separate synovial sheath that arises near the dorsal carpal ligament. The synovial sheaths mostly run distally as far as the bases of the metacarpals. Tunnels that transmit the extensor digitorum, extensor indicis, and extensor digiti minimi run to the middle third of the metacarpal shaft.

The extensor tendon compartment is closed at its borders by fusion of the deep investing fascia and the dorsal subaponeurotic fascia into a single membrane, which then fuses with the dorsal surfaces of the second metacarpal laterally and the fifth metacarpal medially. Distally, the 2 dorsally fused membranes fuse in the webs of the fingers; proximally, they fuse with the extensor tendon sheaths as they pass beneath the dorsal carpal ligament. The dorsal tendon compartment is separated from the subcutaneous fascia by the subcutaneous fascial cleft and from the dorsal interosseous fascia by the subaponeurotic fascial cleft.

2. PALMAR (VOLAR) SURFACE OF THE HAND

Superficial Fascia of the Palm

As the thin subcutaneous fascia leaves the wrist and enters the palm, it changes into a thick tough fascia that is superficial in both the palm of the hand and on the palmar surfaces of the digits. The palmar superficial or subcutaneous fascia contains a large amount of fat into which the underlying palmar aponeurosis sends off multiple vertical, fibrous septa toward the skin of the palm. They bind the skin together with the palmar aponeurosis and prevent the palmar skin from gliding upon the underlying tissues (Fig 46–5). These fibrous septa create many small, irregular fatty tissue islands in the subcutaneous tissues that reach to the dermis. The subcutaneous fascia adheres tightly to the underlying deep fascia over the entire palmar surface of the hand, particularly over the skin creases of the wrist, palm, and interdigital areas.

Deep Fascia of the Palm (Fig 46–6)

At the wrist, the deep fascia of the volar surface of the forearm thickens into a band, the flexor retinaculum, which holds the volar forearm tendons against the bones of the wrist. The flexor retinaculum is made up of the **volar carpal ligament** proximally and the **transverse carpal ligament** distally (Fig 46–7). The volar carpal ligament is a continuation of the investing fascia of the anterior forearm that thickens markedly at the wrist. The ligament is fixed to the styloid process of the radius laterally and the styloid process of the ulna medially. Deep to the volar carpal ligament run the flexor tendons plus the nerves and blood vessels to the wrist and hand. Distally, the volar carpal liga-

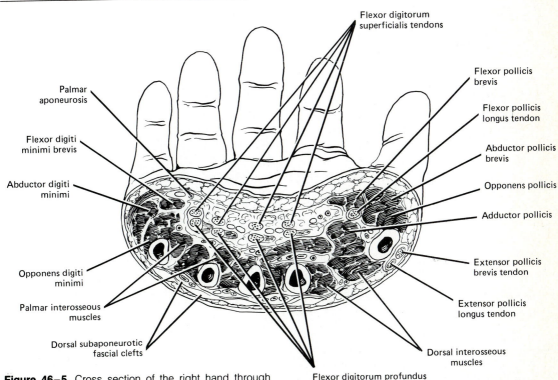

Figure 46–5. Cross section of the right hand through the metacarpals.

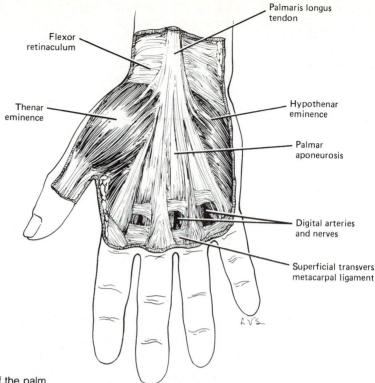

Flexor
retinaculum

Thenar
eminence

Palmaris longus
tendon

Hypothenar
eminence

Palmar
aponeurosis

Digital arteries
and nerves

Superficial transvers
metacarpal ligament

Figure 46–6. Superficial dissection of the palm.

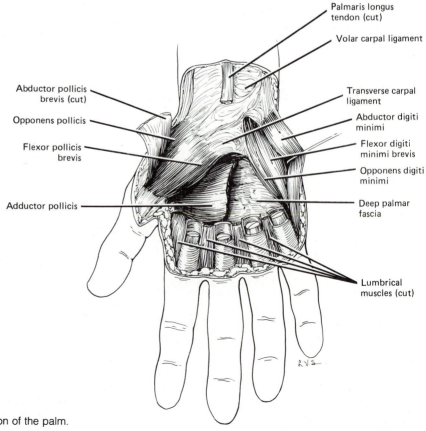

Palmaris longus
tendon (cut)

Volar carpal ligament

Abductor pollicis
brevis (cut)

Opponens pollicis

Flexor pollicis
brevis

Adductor pollicis

Transverse carpal
ligament

Abductor digiti
minimi

Flexor digiti
minimi brevis

Opponens digiti
minimi

Deep palmar
fascia

Lumbrical
muscles (cut)

Figure 46–7. Deep dissection of the palm.

ment blends with the transverse carpal ligament, and together they make up the flexor retinaculum. The **transverse carpal ligament** covers the concavity of the volar surface of the carpal bones and is thus the roof of a canal that introduces the long flexor tendons and the median nerve into the wrist and hand areas. It runs transversely from the pisiform and hamate bones medially to the scaphoid and trapezium laterally. Between the 2 ligaments are the ulnar artery and nerve as they move distally. The palmar aponeurosis attaches to the transverse carpal ligament via multiple obliquely placed fibers.

The deep fascia of the palm as it covers the thenar and hypothenar eminences is thinner than it is over the central palm, where it is reinforced by the overlying palmar aponeurosis.

➭ *Carpal tunnel syndrome. (Fig 46–8). Pressure on the medial nerve at volar wrist level may lead to chronic median nerve pressure neuritis. The syndrome usually results because the flexor tendons and the median nerve are encased in a rigid, unyielding tunnel bounded by the carpal bones dorsally and the thick transverse carpal ligament ventrally. Median nerve compression results in paresthesias over its area of sensory innervation of the hand and in weakness of the thenar muscles. If pressure on the median nerve leads to pain and disability, surgical decompression of the carpal tunnel area by transection of the transverse carpal ligament may give dramatic relief.*

Synovial Sheaths of the Palmar Tendons

About 2.5 cm proximal to the transverse carpal ligament, the superficial and deep flexor tendons of the volar surface of the wrist become encased in synovial sheaths that extend into the palm of the hand; the sheaths to the thumb and little finger extend out to the respective terminal phalanges instead of ending in the palm. The larger of the 2 sheaths, the ulnar bursa, extends to the mid palm and encloses the superficial and deep flexor tendons to the 4 fingers. The lateral segment of the ulnar bursa, which encloses the tendons for the little finger, continues from the mid palm to the volar surface of the little finger, running to the attachment of the deep flexor tendon into the terminal phalanx. At about the midpoint of the metacarpal area, the portion of the ulnar bursa that ensheathes the flexor tendons to the ring, middle, and index fingers narrows and terminates. From the line of the metacarpal heads, each of the flexor tendons to the ring, middle, and index fingers are covered by an individual synovial sheath that extends on those fingers to the insertion of the deep flexor onto the terminal digit.

The separate flexor synovial sheath to the thumb, the radial bursa, extends from a position about 2.5

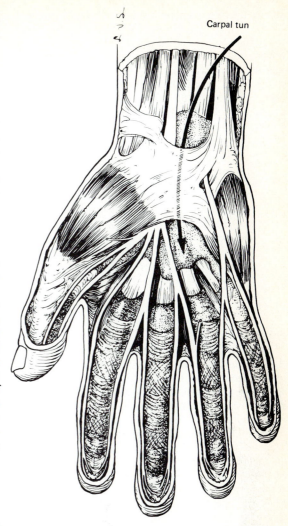

Figure 46–8. Carpal tunnel. (Reproduced, with permission, from Way LW [editor]: *Current Surgical Diagnosis & Treatment,* 7th ed. Lange, 1985.)

cm proximal to the volar crease of the wrist to the terminal phalanx of the thumb.

➭ *Atypical connection of radial and ulnar synovial sheaths. In about 10–15% of people, there is a communication between the radial and ulnar bursae, accounting for the occurrence of inflammation in both palmar bursae following inflammation of an individual synovial sheath.*

Palmar Aponeurosis (Fig 46–6)

The palmar aponeurosis is made up superficially of fibers that are the distal continuation of the palmaris longus tendon. At a deeper level, the aponeurosis is reinforced by transverse fibers that are a palmar extension of the palmar carpal ligament. These 2 segments of the palmar aponeurosis are tightly joined. The longitudinal fibers of the superficial layer divide into 5 bands, each of which runs to the base of a proximal phalanx, the bands covering the long flexor tendons to the digits. As each band terminates, the superficial portion attaches to the skin of the distal palm, while the deep portion attaches to the fibrous tendon sheath above which it lies. The fibers that attach to the skin terminate at the distal palmar crease.

⇒ *Dupuytren's contracture due to palmar fasciitis. Dupuytren's contracture may result from palmar fasciitis involving any digit or web space but usually those to the ring and little fingers. The skin over the area of fasciitis usually becomes raised and hard, and the involved fingers are drawn tightly toward the palm in varying degrees of flexion.*

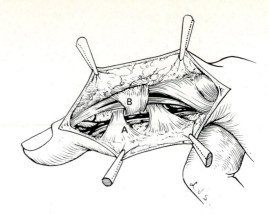

Figure 46–9. A: Cleland's ligament. **B:** Transverse retinacular ligament. (Reproduced, with permission, from Way LW [editor]: *Current Surgical Diagnosis & Treatment,* 7th ed. Lange, 1985.)

Flexor Tendon Sheaths

Distal to the metacarpophalangeal joints, the tendons of the deep and superficial flexors are encased in ligamentous tunnels called the digital fibrous tendon sheaths. Each tendon sheath is covered by a synovial sheath that lubricates the tendon. The **vincula tendinum digitorum manus,** a series of fibrous bands carrying minute vessels, connects the tendons of the deep and superficial flexors to one another and to the underlying phalanges. The **vincula brevia,** 2 for each finger, appear as semicircular fibrous expansions at the distal ends of the tendons. One expansion connects the superficial flexor tendon to the palmar surface of the proximal interphalangeal joint and to the head of the proximal phalanx; the other connects the deep flexor tendon to the palmar surface of the proximal interphalangeal joint and to the head of the middle phalanx. The **vincula longa** are 2 narrow pairs of fibrous bands. One pair in each finger connects the deep flexor tendon to the underlying superficial tendon; a second pair connects the superficial flexor tendon to the proximal phalanx.

The fibrous sheaths surrounding the flexor tendons prevent bowstringing and preserve the mechanical efficiency of the fingers as they flex toward the palm of the hand.

⇒ *De Quervain's tenosynovitis. In De Quervain's tenosynovitis (tenosynovitis stenosans), the pulley over the radial styloid that ensheathes the abductor pollicis longus and the extensor pollicis brevis closes tightly about the tendons. Inflammation and swelling prevent them from gliding freely within it. There is usually tenderness over the pulley, and the digit often locks in flexion. Injecting a corticosteroid into the tendon sheath usually gives relief. If conserva-*

tive treatment fails, the tendon must be released surgically.

Fascia of the Palmar Surfaces of the Fingers

Fascial bands bind the skin of the palmar surfaces of the fingers to the underlying bone. These bands aid in pinching and gripping and keep the skin from twisting around the finger. The bands are known as Cleland's and Grayson's ligaments (Fig. 46–9). The bands also serve to hold the flexor tendons against the concave surface of the arched interphalangeal joints, thereby increasing digital mechanical efficiency and strength.

Fascial Compartments of the Palmar Surface of the Hand

There are 4 fascial compartments within the palmar surface of the hand: thenar, hypothenar, central, and interosseous-adductor. These compartments are not to be confused with the palmar fascial clefts or spaces.

The **thenar compartment** makes up the bulk of the large radial eminence of the hand. Within it lie the flexor pollicis brevis, the abductor pollicis brevis, and the opponens pollicis, which together make up the superficial layer of short muscles of the thumb. The compartment is limited superficially by the investing layer of the deep fascia of the palm and by its deep continuation, the **thenar septum,** which separates the flexor pollicis brevis from the adductors of the thumb. The thenar compartment is well isolated from the remainder of the palm by the attachments of its limiting fascia. The limiting fascia is attached proximally to the carpal bones and to the transverse carpal ligament; distally, to the proximal phalanx of the thumb, where the muscles enclosed within the thenar compartment insert into the digit; dorsally, to the first metacarpal bone; and ventrally, to the adductor muscles. Also included within the thenar compartment are the metacarpal of the thumb, the superficial palmar branch of the radial artery, the palmar branch of the median nerve, and the radial bursa containing the flexor pollicis longus tendon.

The **hypothenar compartment** encloses the short muscles to the small finger and makes up the bulk of the hypothenar eminence. The hypothenar investing fascia and the hypothenar septum between the flexor digiti minimi and the third palmar interosseous muscle encompass the compartment. The limiting fascia attaches along the length of the fifth metacarpal bone.

The **central compartment** of the palm is separated by the thenar fascial system and by the hypothenar fascial system. It is contained superficially by the palmar aponeurosis and deeply by the fascial sheath that covers the deep surface of the long flexor tendons. Within the compartment lie the tendons of the superficial and deep flexor muscles, the lumbrical muscles, the superficial palmar arch, the superficial branch of the ulnar nerve, and the palmar branch of the median nerve. The tendon sheaths within the compartment run into the forearm. Distally, the contents of the compartment fuse gradually with the interdigital webs and with the individual fingers.

The **interosseus-adductor compartment** is formed by the presence of the interosseous muscles and the adductors of the thumb, which together form a barrier that separates the palmar from the dorsal compartments of the hand. The dorsal surface of the compartment is limited by the dorsal interosseous fascia, which adheres to the dorsal surfaces of metacarpals 2–5. The palmar surface of the compartment is limited by the palmar interosseous fascia on its ulnar side and by the fascia of the adductor muscles on its radial side. The dorsal and palmar interosseous fasciae join at the medial and lateral borders of the enclosed fascial space. Within this fascial space, which is closed proximally and distally by fascial attachments, lie the second, third, fourth, and fifth metacarpal bones, all of the interossei (volar and dorsal), the 2 adductor muscles of the thumb, the deep palmar arch, and the deep branch of the ulnar nerve.

Volar Fascial Spaces or Clefts

The thenar and midpalmar spaces lie deep to the flexor tendons but superficial to the adductor interossei compartment. The **thenar space** extends laterally from its attachment to the third metacarpal bone to the thenar septum and its first metacarpal attachment. It reaches from the transverse carpal ligament to a point about 1 cm proximal to the finger webs. The **midpalmar** space extends from the third metacarpal bone to the fifth and the hypothenar eminence and runs distally from the midcarpal ligament to reach the finger webs. The 2 volar spaces contribute to the ease of flexor tendon movement in those areas of the palm where the tendons have no covering synovial sheaths. The proximal end of the sheath to the index finger and the sheath of the first lumbrical muscle touch the thenar space; and the proximal ends of the flexor sheaths of the third, fourth, and fifth fingers and the sheaths of their neighboring lumbrical muscles touch the midpalmar space. In 10–15% of persons, the membrane dividing the 2 palmar spaces is an incomplete one, with a resultant communication between the 2 spaces.

➡ *Fascial spaces. The fascial spaces are potential areas for the gravitation of pus, blood, or serum after injury or infection in the palm of the hand. Infected collections in these spaces require surgical drainage.*

➡ *Infections that may rupture into the palmar spaces. Infections in the tendon sheaths of the index finger and thumb may rupture into the thenar space. Purulent tenosynovitis of the synovia of the middle, ring, and little fingers may rupture into the midpalmar space. In 10–15% of cases, infection can pass from one palmar space to the other with relative ease.*

The potential space on the volar surface of the wrist that lies deep to the tendons of the flexor pollicis longus and the flexor digitorum profundus but superficial to the pronator quadratus muscles is known as the subtendinous space of the wrist (Parona's space). The space frequently connects directly with the more distal thenar and midpalmar spaces, and as a consequence collections within the palmar spaces may extend into the lower volar forearm.

➡ *Infections of the hand. Infections that commonly involve the hand are (1) cellulitis with accompanying ascending lymphangitis; (2) subepithelial abscess; (3) infection in or around the nail bed (paronychia, eponychia, subungual abscess); (4) infections of the digital pulp; (5) infections of the web, midpalmar, thenar, and hypothenar spaces, with subsequent involvement of Parona's space; (6) infections of the dorsal subaponeurotic and dorsal subcutaneous spaces; (7) infectious tenosynovitis; and (8) infections of metacarpal bones and phalangeal joints. Infections of the hand secondary to human bites are notoriously hard to treat and often result in severe disability.*

3. MUSCLES OF THE HAND
(Tables 46–1, 46–2, and 46–3)

The extrinsic muscles of the hand are listed in Table 46–1 with their origins, insertions, actions, and nerve supply.

Supination of the hand is a combined action of the biceps brachii and the supinator. Hand pronation is a combined action of the pronator teres and pronator

Table 46–1. Muscles of the hand: Thenar muscles.

Muscle and Origin	Insertion	Innervation	Function
ABDUCTOR POLLICIS BREVIS The most superficial of the thenar muscles. It takes origin from the scaphoid, the transverse carpal ligament, and the trapezium.	On the radial side, the base of the proximal phalanx of the thumb inserts into the capsule of the metacarpophalangeal joint.	Median nerve (C8, T1).	Abduction of the thumb.
OPPONENS POLLICIS Lies deep to the abductor pollicis brevis. Takes origin from the trapezium and the flexor retinaculum.	Into the entire radial side of the thumb metacarpal.	Median and ulnar nerves (C8, T1).	Opposition of the thumb.
FLEXOR POLLICIS BREVIS A superficial segment takes origin from the flexor retinaculum and the trapezium; a deep segment takes origin from the trapezoid and capitate bones and from the palmar ligaments of the distal row of carpal bones.	Into the radial side of the base of the proximal phalanx of the thumb.	Ulnar and median nerves (C8, T1).	Flexion of the proximal phalanx of the thumb.
ADDUCTOR POLLICIS The oblique head of the adductor pollicis takes origin from the capitate bone, the bases of metacarpals 2 and 3, and the intercarpal ligaments. The transverse head takes origin from the distal two-thirds of the palmar surface of the third metacarpal.	Into the ulnar side of the base of the first phalanx of the thumb.	Deep branch of the ulnar nerve (C8, T1).	Adduction of the thumb.

quadratus. Adduction of the hand at wrist level is brought about by combined efforts of the flexor and extensor carpi ulnaris. Abduction at the wrist is the product of the combined action of the flexor carpi radialis, the extensor carpi radialis longus, and the extensor carpi radialis brevis. These 3 muscles, working together with the deep transverse metacarpal ligament, stabilize the hand at proximal metacarpal levels during flexion and extension of the fingers. Flexion of the wrist is by the combined action of the flexor carpi radialis, flexor carpi ulnaris, and palmaris longus. Extension of the wrist is by the combined actions of the extensor carpi radialis longus, extensor carpi radialis brevis, and extensor carpi ulnaris. The superficial and deep flexors of the fingers aid in wrist flexion if the digits are prevented from flexing. The extensor

Table 46–2. Muscles of the hand: Hypothenar muscles.

Muscle and Origin	Insertion	Innervation	Function
PALMARIS BREVIS From the transverse carpal ligament and the palmar aponeurosis.	Into the skin of the medial border of the hand.	Superficial branch of the ulnar nerve (C8, T1).	Moves skin of the medial side of the palm toward the mid palm.
ABDUCTOR DIGITI MINIMI From the pisiform bone and the tendon of the flexor carpi ulnaris and from the pisohamate ligament.	Separates into 2 tendons—one to the ulnar side of the base of the proximal phalanx of the little finger, and a second slip into the medial border of the extensor digiti minimi.	Deep branch of the ulnar nerve (C8, T1).	Abducts the little finger and flexes its proximal phalanx.
FLEXOR DIGITI MINIMI BREVIS From the hamulus (hook) of the hamate bone and the palmar surface of the flexor retinaculum.	Into the medial side of the base of the proximal phalanx of the small finger.	Deep branch of the ulnar nerve (C8, T1).	Flexes the little finger.
OPPONENS DIGITI MINIMI From the hamulus (hook) of the hamate bone and the flexor retinaculum.	Into the ulnar margin of the entire length of the fifth metacarpal.	Deep branch of the ulnar nerve (C8, T1).	Opposition of the fifth metacarpal.

Table 46–3. Muscles of the hand: Intermediate muscles.

Muscle and Origin	Insertion	Innervation	Function
THE LUMBRICALS Four small muscles arising from tendons of the flexor digitorum profundus. Lumbricals 1 and 2 arise from the lateral side and the volar surface of the index and middle fingers and tendons. The third lumbrical arises from adjoining sides of the tendons of the middle and ring fingers; the fourth arises from the adjoining sides of the tendons to the ring and little fingers.	Each muscle passes to the lateral side of the same finger and inserts into the dorsal tendinous expansion of the extensor digitorum at the level of the metacarpophalangeal joint.	Lumbricals 1 and 2 are innervated by the median nerve; 3 and 4 by the deep branch of the ulnar nerve (C8, T1).	Flexion of the metacarpophalangeal joint and extension of the middle and distal phalanges.
THE DORSAL INTEROSSEI Occupy spaces between the metacarpal bones. The 4 muscles arise from the adjoining sides of the metacarpals.	The dorsal interossei insert into the bases of the proximal phalanges and into the dorsal digital expansions.	Deep palmar branch of the ulnar nerve (C8, T1).	Abduction of the fingers, flexion of the metacarpophalangeal joints, and extension of the 2 terminal phalanges.
THE PALMAR INTEROSSEI Each of the 3 palmar interossei arises from an entire side of the metacarpal bone. The first arises from the ulnar side of the first metacarpal, the second from the radial side of the fourth metacarpal, and the third from the radial side of the fifth metacarpal.	The palmar interossei insert into the side of the base of the proximal phalanx and into the fibrous expansion of the extensor digitorum tendon of the same finger. The first inserts into the ulnar side of the index finger, the second into the radial side of the ring finger, and the third into the radial side of the little finger.	Deep palmar branch of the ulnar nerve (C8, T1).	Abduction of the digits, flexion of the metacarpophalangeal joints, and extension of the 2 terminal phalanges.

muscle to the digits may aid in extension of the hand at the wrist if the digits are not allowed to extend.

Intrinsic Muscles

The intrinsic muscles of the hand are those that make up the thenar and hypothenar eminences and the short muscles that lie close to the metacarpal bones between the eminences.

BLOOD VESSELS, LYMPHATICS, & NERVES

Arteries
(Fig 46–10)

The blood supply to the hand is conveyed by the radial and ulnar arteries. At wrist level, the **radial artery** is subcutaneous and lies on the volar surface of the distal end of the radius lateral to the flexor carpi radialis. At this location, the radial pulse is readily palpable. The artery then passes from the volar to the dorsal surface of the wrist between the tendons of the abductor pollicis longus and the extensor brevis of the thumb and the radial collateral ligament of the wrist. On the dorsum of the wrist, the artery lies first on the scaphoid and then on the trapezium. It then dives deep between the 2 heads of the first dorsal interosseous muscle. At this point, the tendon of the extensor pollicis longus crosses the artery. In the "anatomic snuff box," the artery is crossed by superficial branches of the radial nerve,

which run to the thumb and the first finger. At wrist level, the radial artery gives off its dorsal carpal and first dorsal metacarpal branches. On reaching the hand, it passes horizontally across the palm as far as the base of the fifth metacarpal, where it joins with the deep palmar branch of the ulnar artery to form the **deep palmar arch.** The deep palmar arch lies upon the proximal ends of the metacarpal bones and upon the palmar interossei and is deep to the lumbricals and the flexor tendons of the fingers. The palmar metacarpal arteries are given off from the deep palmar arch and run to the clefts of the fingers, where they join with the digital branches of the superficial palmar arch. The deep palmar arch is a smaller and less important source of blood to the distal hand than the superficial palmar arch.

The **ulnar artery** is the larger of the 2 terminal branches of the brachial artery. At the wrist, the ulnar artery is superficial, covered only by the skin of the volar surface of the wrist and by the palmar carpal ligament. At the wrist, it lies just lateral to the pisiform bone, rests upon the flexor retinaculum, and is just superficial to the ulnar nerve. Distal to the pisiform, the ulnar artery gives off dorsal and palmar carpal branches, which join with similar branches of the radial artery, and together the branches form an arterial circle about the carpal bones. Farther distally, the ulnar artery gives off its deep palmar branch, which forms the deep palmar arch with a branch of the radial artery. The major superficial trunk of the ulnar artery completes the superficial palmar arch

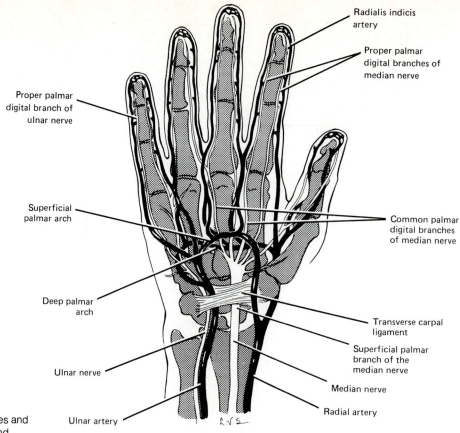

Figure 46–10. Arteries and nerves of the right hand.

by joining with the superficial palmar branch of the radial artery. The superficial palmar arch lies deep to the skin and the palmar aponeurosis but superficial to the flexor retinaculum, the tendons of the flexor digitorum superficialis, and the flexor to the fifth finger, the lumbricals, and the terminal branches of the median and ulnar nerves. The superficial palmar arch gives off 3 common palmar digital arteries, each of which divides into a pair of palmar digital arteries that run along adjacent sides of the 4 fingers deep to the corresponding digital nerves.

Veins
(Fig 46–11)

The major superficial veins lie subcutaneously on the superficial fascia of the dorsum of the hand, while the major deep veins lie in the palm in close relationship to the palmar arterial networks. The superficial venous system is accompanied by the lymphatics that drain the hand. Only a few superficial veins are present in the palm of the hand, between the skin and the palmar fascia. The loose subcutaneous tissues of the back of the hand and the fingers show well-marked dorsal venous arches. These arches are more prominent when the hand is in the dependent position. The arches receive the digital veins from the fingers and eventually join with the cephalic and basilic veins

on the radial and ulnar sides of the wrist, respectively. The deep venous return closely follows the palmar arterial pattern. The small digital veins drain the fingers and send blood into the superficial and deep venous arches that lie close to the superficial and deep arterial arches. Blood from the palmar venous arches then flows into the venae comitantes of the radial and ulnar arteries eventually to become the venae comitantes of the brachial artery at the elbow joint. There is free communication between the deep and superficial vein of the hand via multiple perforating veins.

Lymphatics

Lymphatic drainage from the hand closely follows the venous drainage pattern. Most of the lymph drainage from the phalangeal and web areas of the fingers and from the thenar and hypothenar eminences of the hand proceeds primarily toward the lymph channels that lie in the dorsal aponeurotic space of the hand. Hand lymph then continues superiorly via channels accompanying the basilic and cephalic veins, eventually to empty into the most lateral of the axillary nodes. The deep lymph channels in the palm of the hand join with the lymph channels accompanying the venous return from the palmar arches and follow the course of the basilic and axillary veins both to

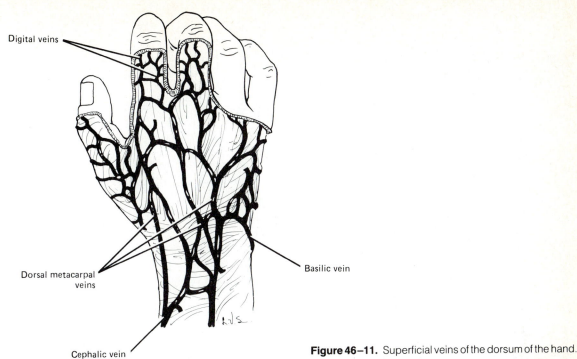

Digital veins

Dorsal metacarpal veins

Basilic vein

Cephalic vein

Figure 46–11. Superficial veins of the dorsum of the hand.

the axillary and to the deep chain of cervical lymph nodes.

⟹ ***Chronic infections resulting in axillary nodal involvement.*** *Chronic hand infections nearly always are accompanied by axillary lymphadenitis. The passage of infected lymph from hand to axilla is usually marked by red streaks along the course of the infected ascending lymph channel.*

Nerves
(Figs 46–8 and 46–12)

The 3 major nerves of the arm and forearm—radial, ulnar, and median—are responsible for sensation and motor power of the hand.

The **median nerve** supplies the radial side of the volar surface of the forearm and hand. In the wrist, the median nerve lies just deep to the tendon of the palmaris longus and slightly to its ulnar side. It passes through the flexor retinaculum tunnel, lying closer to the skin than the accompanying flexor tendons to the hand. When it leaves the flexor retinaculum tunnel, the median nerve divides into its terminal motor and sensory branches. The skin of the central palm and thenar eminence is supplied by the palmar branch of the median nerve. A short, stubby muscular branch is given off from the radial side of the median nerve to supply the abductor pollicis brevis, the opponens pollicis, and the superficial head of the flexor pollicis brevis.

⟹ ***Avoidance of motor branch of median nerve to thenar eminence.*** *To avoid injuring the motor branches of the median nerve to the muscles of the thenar eminence, palmar incisions along the ulnar border of the thenar eminence should not cross the midpoint of the first metacarpal bone.*

The midpoint of the first metacarpal bone marks the level of takeoff of the transverse course of the motor (recurrent) branch of the median nerve to the thenar eminence. The median nerve, after giving off its thenar eminence or recurrent median branch, continues distally into the palm and divides into the 3 palmar digital nerves: (1) The first common palmar digital nerve gives off 3 proper palmar digital branches; 2 of these supply the skin of the lateral and medial sides of the thumb, while the third sends a motor branch to the first lumbrical muscle and a sensory branch to the radial side of the index finger. (2) The second common palmar digital nerve sends a motor branch to the second lumbrical and then divides into sensory nerves that supply the adjoining sides of the index and ring fingers. (3) The third common palmar digital nerve sends sensory twigs to the adjoining surfaces of the middle and ring fingers. Rarely, it will send a motor twig to the third lumbrical muscle.

⟹ ***Thenar eminence denervation.*** *Surgical interruption of the course of the median nerve to*

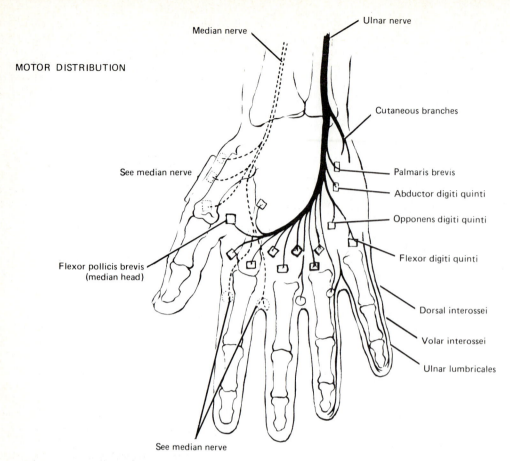

MOTOR DISTRIBUTION

Median nerve

Ulnar nerve

Cutaneous branches

See median nerve

Palmaris brevis

Abductor digiti quinti

Opponens digiti quinti

Flexor digiti quinti

Flexor pollicis brevis
(median head)

Dorsal interossei

Volar interossei

Ulnar lumbricales

See median nerve

SENSORY DISTRIBUTION

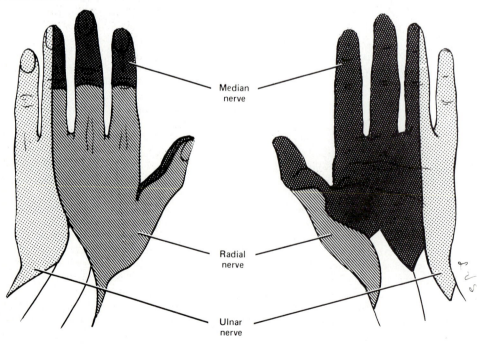

Median
nerve

Radial
nerve

Ulnar
nerve

Figure 46–12. Innervation of the hand. (Reproduced, with permission, from Chusid JG: *Correlative Neuroanatomy & Functional Neurology,* 19th ed. Lange, 1985.)

the thenar eminence will result in paralysis of the superficial muscles of the thenar eminence, markedly impairing flexion, abduction, and opposition of the thumb.

➡ *Median nerve section close to the wrist. If the median nerve is sectioned close to the wrist, where it parallels the palmaris longus tendon, a variable degree of hypesthesia or anesthesia in the areas supplied by its sensory divisions will result. Following a median nerve section at wrist level, the thenar eminence muscles will be paralyzed, making it difficult to place the thumb upon the tips of the fingers and to flex the index and middle fingers. Eventually, the thenar eminence will atrophy and appear less prominent.*

The **ulnar nerve** is the motor nerve of the muscles of the ulnar or medial segment of the hand and supplies sensation to the skin of the ulnar side of the palm and to the little finger and the ulnar side of the ring finger. The palmar cutaneous branch leaves the ulnar nerve in the mid forearm and runs with the ulnar artery into the palm of the hand. It innervates the ulnar side of the palm. The dorsal branch of the ulnar nerve leaves the main trunk of the nerve in the distal forearm and passes to the dorsum of the wrist, where it pierces the dorsal deep fascia and divides terminally into 2 dorsal digital nerves. The medial of these 2 nerves is sensory to the ulnar side of the little finger, while the lateral branch is sensory to the adjoining surfaces of the little and ring fingers. The palmar branch of the ulnar nerve enters the palm with the ulnar artery, lying upon the flexor retinaculum. Terminally, it divides into superficial and deep branches. The superficial branch is the nerve to the palmaris brevis and to the skin of the hypothenar eminence. It sends small sensory branches to the little and ring fingers. The deep branch is closely related to the deep palmar arch. Its initial branches are to the muscles of the hypothenar eminence. As it crosses the palm from the ulnar to the radial side, it gives motor branches to the third and fourth lumbricals and to all of the interossei, palmar and dorsal. It terminates in the thenar eminence by supplying the adductor pollicis and the deep head of the flexor pollicis brevis.

➡ *Section of ulnar nerve at forearm and wrist levels. If the ulnar nerve is severed or contused at the mid forearm, the patient will develop anesthesia (1) along the ulnar border of the hand, (2) over the palmar and dorsal aspects of the little finger, and (3) along the ulnar side of the ring finger. If the ulnar nerve is severed above the elbow, there is a loss of ulnar flexion of the wrist and of flexion of the distal phalanges of the ring and little fingers.*

There can be either complete or partial loss of abduction and adduction of the fingers. The thumb cannot be scraped across the distal palm and cannot make a circle with the little finger. The hypothenar eminence atrophies, and so do the dorsal projections of the interosseous muscles that normally fill in the gaps between the dorsal surfaces of the metacarpals.

➡ *Claw fingers. If the median and ulnar nerves are both severed in the forearm at a point distal to the takeoff of their motor branches to the finger, "claw fingers" will result. The deformity results because the extensor digitorum, innervated by the radial nerve, hyperextends the proximal phalanges, while the finger flexors, now unopposed by the denervated intrinsic hand muscles, flex the middle and terminal phalanges.*

In the proximal forearm, the **radial nerve** divides into superficial and deep branches. The superficial branch proceeds distally along the radial side of the forearm; crosses the dorsum of the wrist, where it pierces the deep fascia; and divides into lateral and medial branches. The lateral branch supplies the skin of the ball and lateral side of the thumb; the medial branch divides into 4 dorsal digital nerves. The first digital branch of the radial nerve runs to the medial side of the thumb; the second supplies the lateral side of the index finger; the third supplies the neighboring surfaces of the index and middle fingers; and the fourth supplies the neighboring surfaces of the middle and ring fingers. The deep branch of the radial nerve, called the dorsal interosseous nerve, reaches the back of the wrist deep to the extensor pollicis longus muscle. In the forearm, it gives off fibers that bring motor innervation to the extensor carpi radialis brevis and to the supinator. After the deep branch of the radial nerve passes through the supinator muscle, it passes dorsal to that muscle and gives off motor branches to the extensor digitorum, the extensor digiti minimi, the extensor carpi ulnaris, the 2 extensors of the thumb, the abductor pollicis, and the extensor indicis. All fibers given off from the radial nerve in the hand are sensory, since the motor fibers are all given off in the forearm.

➡ *Hypesthesia of the dorsum of the hand. If the radial nerve is severed at the level of the middle third of the humerus (in fracture of the mid humerus), hypesthesia of the dorsum of the forearm and the hand results. The hand is held in the "wrist drop" position. Adduction of the thumb combined with the flexed wrist makes flexion of the fingers difficult, and lateral movements of the whole hand are restricted. The proximal phalanges cannot be extended, and the thumb cannot be extended or abducted.*

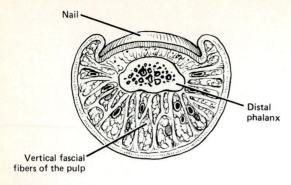

Figure 46–13. Cross section of the fingertip. (Reproduced, with permission, from *Current Surgical Diagnosis & Treatment,* 7th ed. Lange, 1985.)

Palpation of Structures at Volar Wrist Level

With the wrist flexed and the fist tightly clenched, one can palpate at volar wrist level the palmaris longus, the tendons of the flexor carpi radialis, the flexor carpi ulnaris, and the more superficial tendons of the flexor digitorum superficialis. Centrally on the volar surface of the wrist lie the so-called "median pair," the tendon of the palmaris longus and the median nerve. The nerve lies just dorsal and to the radial side of the tendon. On the radial side of the wrist, one can palpate the radial artery, the flexor carpi radialis, which lies to the ulnar side of the artery, and, at a deeper level, the tendon of the flexor pollicis longus. With the fist clenched and the wrist flexed, one can palpate the flexor carpi ulnaris tendon,

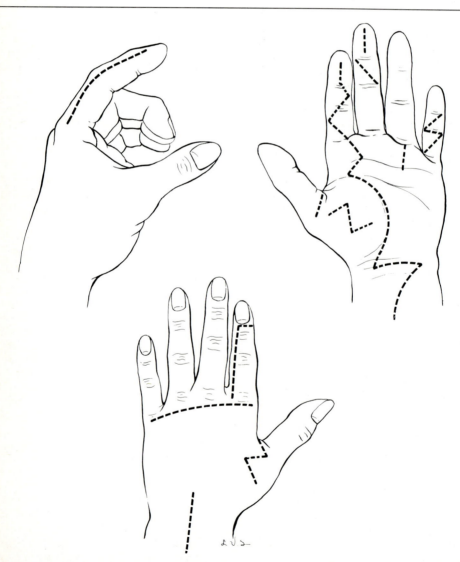

Figure 46–14. Proper placement of skin incisions for treatment of hand infections and injuries. (Reproduced, with permission, from *Current Surgical Diagnosis & Treatment,* 7th ed. Lange, 1985.)

the ulnar nerve, and the ulnar artery, which lie just to the ulnar side of the tendon.

▣➡ **Lacerations.** *Lacerations involving the tendon of the palmaris longus at the wrist frequently also involve the median nerve. Injury to one or more of the structures forming the "radial or ulnar triads" can readily involve the other structures of these groupings.*

SUPERFICIAL PULP SPACE OF THE FINGERS (Fig 46-13)

The palmar surfaces of the distal phalanges of the thumb and fingers are composed mainly of subcutaneous fatty tissue through which run multiple vertical fibrous septa. The septa pass from the skin to the periosteal surface of the underlying terminal phalanx. The subcutaneous fat and the fibrous septa are packed tightly into what amounts to a closed compartment, since the skin at the level of the flexor creases of the fingers is bound to the underlying flexor sheath.

▣➡ **Infected pulp space.** *The extremely tight crowding of the tissues in each digital compartment of the hand is responsible for the intense pain that accompanies an infected pulp space; there is no additional space into which the infected edematous tissues can expand.*

Since the blood vessels that supply the terminal phalanges must pass through the pulp space, they are prone to thrombosis in cases of pulp space infection. The thrombosis can lead *to secondary necrosis of the shaft of the terminal phalanx. The base of the distal phalanx seldom suffers necrosis secondary to pulp space infections, since its blood supply comes from a branch of the digital artery, which is given off at mid finger level and is consequently not liable to be affected by thrombosis.*

▣➡ **Principles of placement of skin incisions.** *(Fig 46–14.) Several important general anatomic principles govern the selection of sites for cutaneous incisions on the hand. Hand and finger incisions should always cross flexion creases in a Z fashion when such a crossing is necessary. Incisions on the lateral surfaces of the fingers, for drainage of suppurative tenosynovitis, should be placed at the dorsal limits of the finger creases to avoid the digital artery and nerves. Incisions should be placed on the radial side of the little finger and on the ulnar side of the index finger, so that the resultant scars will be less exposed to trauma.*

▣➡ **Paronychia.** *In treating paronychia, a dorsal incision on the distal phalanx should not be used; instead, the eponychium should be elevated from the nail edge and pus released. In more advanced and chronic cases, it may be necessary to remove the loosened nail root.*

▣➡ **Tumors of the hand.** *The commonest tumors found in the hand are ganglions or mucous cysts, inclusion cysts, posttraumatic neuromas, soft tissue giant cell tumors, giant cell tumors of bone, lipomas, neurofibromas, hemangiomas, actinic keratoses, and glomus tumors (which usually present deep to the fingernail).*

47

The Gluteal Region

GROSS ANATOMY

The gluteal region—the bulky superior posterior thigh—is of considerable anatomic interest. Deep to the great muscle mass in the area lie the following structures: the sacrotuberous and sacrospinous ligaments, the upper femur, the sacrum and coccyx, and parts of the ilium and ischium. There are also major nerves and vessels that supply the gluteal region, the perineum, and the lower extremity. Most of these vessels and nerves leave the posterior pelvis to appear high in the posterior thigh hidden by the gluteal musculature.

The gluteal region is bounded medially by the bony midsacral and midcoccygeal lines of the verte-bral column; laterally by a line dropped perpendicularly from the mid portion of the iliac crest; inferiorly by the prominent gluteal cutaneous fold; and superiorly by the iliac crest.

MUSCLES OF THE GLUTEAL REGION
(Fig 47–1 and Table 47–1)

The musculature of the gluteal region is divided into 3 layers.

Superficial Layer of Muscles

The superficial muscles of the gluteal region are the gluteus maximus and the tensor muscle of the fascia lata.

The **gluteus maximus** is a thick, coarsely fascicu-lated muscle whose fibers are directed inferiorly and

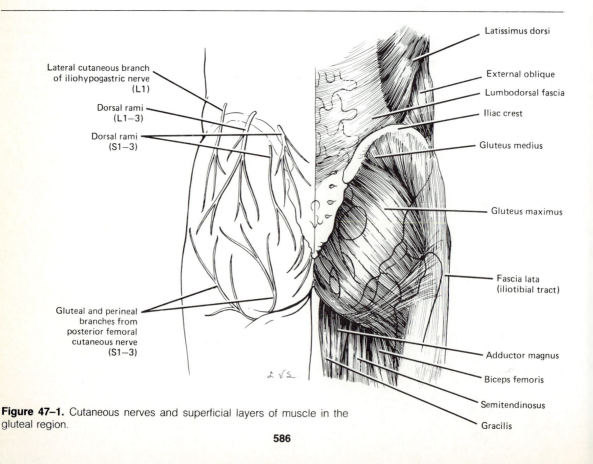

Figure 47–1. Cutaneous nerves and superficial layers of muscle in the gluteal region.

Latissimus dorsi

External oblique

Lumbodorsal fascia

Iliac crest

Gluteus medius

Gluteus maximus

Fascia lata (iliotibial tract)

Adductor magnus

Biceps femoris

Semitendinosus

Gracilis

Lateral cutaneous branch of iliohypogastric nerve (L1)

Dorsal rami (L1–3)

Dorsal rami (S1–3)

Gluteal and perineal branches from posterior femoral cutaneous nerve (S1–3)

Table 47–1. Muscles of the gluteal region.

Muscle and Origin	Insertion	Innervation	Function
GLUTEUS MAXIMUS The posterior gluteal line of the ilium. From the mid superior iliac crest, the posterior surface of the inferior sacral segment and the lateral coccygeal surface; from the sacrospinalis fascia, the sacrotuberous ligament, and the aponeurosis covering the gluteus medius.	Via a thick tendon into the iliotibial band of the fascia lata. Deeper muscle fibers insert into the gluteal tuberosity.	Inferior gluteal nerve (L5; S1, 2).	Extends and laterally rotates the thigh. Supports the knee when the joint is completely extended.
GLUTEUS MEDIUS From the external surface of the ilium between the iliac crest and the dorsal gluteal line. From the gluteal fascia, which covers the external surface.	Into an oblique ridge on the lateral surface of the greater trochanter of the femur.	Superior gluteal nerve (L5, S1).	Abducts the thigh. The anterior segment rotates the thigh medially.
GLUTEUS MINIMUS From the iliac surface and from the edges of the greater sciatic notch.	Via a tendon into the anterior border of the greater trochanter and into the hip joint capsule.	Superior gluteal nerve (L5, S1).	Rotates the thigh medially and abducts the thigh.
PIRIFORMIS Via slips from the anterior sacrum, the edge of the greater sciatic foramen, and the ventral portion of the sacrotuberous ligament.	Passes out through the greater sciatic notch and inserts via a tendon into the superior edge of the greater trochanter of the femur.	Branches from S1, 2.	Rotates the thigh laterally and abducts and extends the thigh.
OBTURATOR INTERNUS From the pelvic surface of the obturator membrane, the ramus of the ischium, the inner surface of the ilium and the anterolateral wall of the pelvis, and the inner surfaces of the superior and inferior pubic rami.	Into the medial surface of the greater trochanter superior to the intertrochanteric fossa.	Nerve to the obturator internus (L5, S1).	Rotates the thigh laterally. Extends and abducts the flexed thigh.
GEMELLUS SUPERIOR From the outer surface of the ischial spine.	Into the medial surface of the greater trochanter along with the obturator internus.	L5, S1 via a branch of the nerve to the obturator internus.	Rotates the thigh laterally.
GEMELLUS INFERIOR From the ischial tuberosity.	Into the medial surface of the greater trochanter along with the obturator internus.	L5, S1 via a branch of the nerve to the quadratus femoris.	Rotates the thigh laterally.
QUADRATUS FEMORIS From the lateral margin of the ischial tuberosity.	Into the quadrate line of the femur, which extends distally from the intertrochanteric crest.	Nerve to the quadratus femoris (L5, S1).	Rotates the thigh laterally.
OBTURATOR EXTERNUS From the bones around the medial side of the obturator foramen (pubis and ischium) and from the external surface of the obturator membrane.	Into the trochanteric fossa of the femur via a tendon that crosses the posterior femoral surface and the inferior segment of the hip capsule.	Obturator nerve (L3, 4).	Rotates the thigh laterally.

laterally. It takes its origin from the posterior gluteal line of the ilium, the dorsal surface of the sacrum, the lateral surface of the coccyx, the sacrotuberous ligament, the external fascia of the sacrospinalis muscle, and the fascia covering the underlying gluteus medius muscle. The superficial segment inserts via a broad tendon that crosses the greater trochanter of the femur to attach to the iliotibial band of the fascia lata of the thigh. The deeper hidden portion inserts into the gluteal tuberosity of the linea aspera of the

femur. A bursa separates the tendon of the gluteus maximus from the site of origin of the vastus lateralis muscle, and an inconstant bursa separates the deep surface of the gluteus maximus from the ischial tuberosity. A large loculated bursa separates the tendon of the muscle from the greater tochanter of the femur.

The gluteus maximus is the major anatomic structure that makes erect posture possible. It is a strong extensor of the thigh. Through its attachment to the iliotibial band, it helps hold the knee in full extension in the standing position. It is also a strong lateral rotator of the thigh, and its most inferior fibers tend to adduct the thigh. The gluteus maximus is supplied by the inferior gluteal nerve (L5; S1, 2).

▷ *Posterolateral exposure of the hip joint. (Fig 47–2.) A posterolateral approach is occasionally used for treatment of posterior hip dislocation and for reduction of a fracture-dislocation of the hip joint. The skin incision starts about 10 cm inferior to the greater trochanter of the femur and continues along the anterior border of the gluteus maximus, close to where it inserts into the fascia lata of the thigh. The incision is deepened and the muscle is reflected medially. The hip joint capsule is then exposed by cutting the tendons of the obturator internus, the gemelli, and the piriformis muscles. The surgeon then has good access to the posterolateral segments of the joint.*

The **tensor fasciae latae femoris** is a fusiform structure between the superficial and deep muscle layers of the fascia lata. It arises from the outer surface of the iliac crest, the anterosuperior iliac spine, and the fascia lata and inserts between the 2 surfaces of the iliotibial band of the fascia lata at the junction of the mid and superior thirds of the thigh. The most important function of this muscle and of the iliotibial band is stabilization of the extended knee. It does this by exerting tension on the iliotibial band of the fascia lata. The muscle also abducts the thigh and is a weak medial rotator of the thigh. It is supplied by a branch of the superior gluteal nerve (L4, 5).

Middle Layer of Muscles

The middle layer of muscles consists of the gluteus medius and piriformis muscles (Fig 47–3).

The posterior segment of the **gluteus medius** lies deep to the gluteus maximus; its anterior segment is separated from the skin and superficial fascia of the buttock by a gluteal aponeurosis. The muscle arises from the external surface of the ilium just inferior to the iliac crest and from the thick gluteal aponeurosis that encloses it. It inserts into the greater trochanter of the femur with a thick, flat tendon. A bursa separates the tendon from the greater trochanter. The gluteus medius abducts the hip and rotates it medially and fixes the pelvis during walking. It is supplied by branches from the superior gluteal nerve (L5, S1). The gluteal aponeurosis is part of the external fascia lata of the thigh. Between the crest of the ilium and the superior border of the gluteus maximus, this fascia is thick and well-formed.

The fan-shaped **piriformis** muscle arises from the

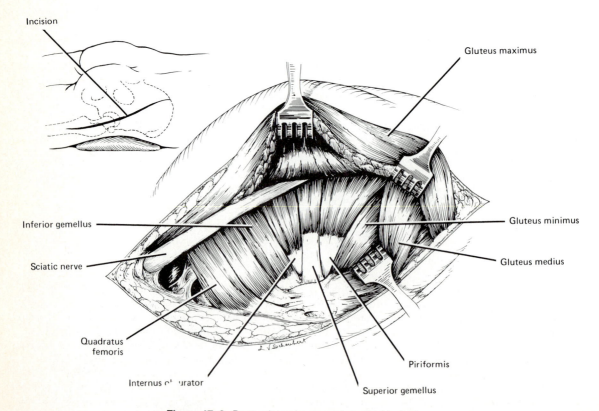

Figure 47–2. Posterolateral approach to the hip joint.

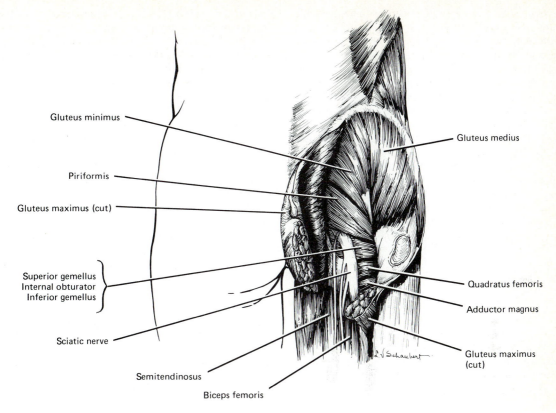

Figure 47–3. Middle and deep layers of musculature in the gluteal region.

ventral surfaces of vertebrae S2–4 and from the margins of the greater sciatic foramen. From its origin to its exit from the pelvis it forms part of the internal surface of the lateral pelvic wall. The muscle narrows as it leaves the pelvis through the greater sciatic foramen. It inserts onto the superior surface of the greater trochanter of the femur. It is supplied by branches from the first and second sacral nerves. The piriformis is principally an abductor and lateral rotator of the thigh. As it passes through the greater sciatic foramen, it divides the foramen into 2 apertures: the suprapiriformic and infrapiriformic spaces. The space inferior to the piriformis permits egress of the sciatic nerve, the inferior gluteal vessels and nerves, the posterior femoral cutaneous nerve of the thigh, the internal pudendal vessels, the pudendal nerve, and the nerves to the quadratus femoris and obturator internus. Superior to the piriformis, the superior gluteal vessels and nerve leave the pelvis through the greater sciatic notch.

Deep Layer of Muscles

The deepest and most ventral of the 3 muscle layers is composed of the gluteus minimus, the obturator internus, the obturator externus, the superior and inferior gemelli, and the quadratus femoris muscles.

The **gluteus minimus** is fan-shaped and lies deep to the gluteus medius. It arises from the external

surface of the ilium and from the edges of the greater sciatic notch. Its fibers converge and insert via a tendon that passes onto the anterosuperior surface of the greater trochanter of the femur. The tendon strengthens the anterior surface of the capsule of the hip joint. There is a bursa between the tendon of the muscle and its insertion into the trochanter. Along with the gluteus medius, the gluteus minimus abducts the femur. It assists in medially rotating the thigh, which is important in walking. The muscle also assists in keeping the pelvis fixed to the ipsilateral greater trochanter when the foot of the opposite side is lifted. This action prevents the pelvis from dropping down on the unsupported side. The muscle is supplied by a branch of the superior gluteal nerve (L4, 5; S1).

The **obturator externus** is a triangular muscle that overlies the external surface of the anterior pelvic wall. It arises from the bony medial edge of the obturator foramen, from the obturator membrane, from the pubis, and from the inferior ischial ramus. The muscle moves dorsolaterally, becomes tendinous, crosses the femoral neck, and terminates in the intertrochanteric fossa of the femur. It is a lateral rotator of the thigh and is supplied by the obturator nerve (L3, 4).

The **obturator internus** arises from the internal surface of the lateral pelvic wall. It covers most of the lateral and anterior walls of the true pelvis and almost completely surrounds the obturator foramen.

It arises also from the superior and inferior pubic rami, from the ischial ramus, and from the inner surface of the obturator membrane. From this broad base of origin, its fibers converge toward the lesser sciatic foramen and leave the pelvis through that aperture. Its fibers of insertion, consisting of 3 or 4 fibrous bands that lie on the deep surface of the muscle, make a right-angle turn in the space between the ischial spine and the ischial tuberosity, being separated from their bony surfaces by a bursa. The fibrous bands unite into a single tendon that passes across the hip joint to insert on the medial surface of the greater trochanter of the femur. The obturator internus rotates the hip laterally. With the thigh flexed, it also extends and abducts the hip. The muscle is supplied by the nerve to the obturator internus, derived from the sacral plexus (L5; S1, 2).

➤ *Obturator sign. An inflamed appendix or sigmoid diverticulum, a perforating sigmoid carcinoma, or an inflamed uterine tube or ovary may lie against the obturator internus fascia. The inflamed viscus may irritate the underlying obturator internus muscle and provoke some degree of spasm. Forced lateral rotation of the thigh will then be limited and painful.*

The 2 **gemelli muscles**—superior and inferior—are narrow muscular slips lying above and below the tendon of the obturator internus. The superior gemellus arises from the ischial spine; the inferior gemellus arises from the ischial tuberosity, and both coalesce with the tendon of the obturator internus. Both gemelli insert into the trochanteric fossa along with the obturator internus. The gemelli aid in lateral rotation of the thigh. The superior gemellus is supplied by a branch of the nerve to the obturator internus; the inferior gemellus is supplied by a branch of the nerve to the quadratus femoris.

The **quadratus femoris** is a thick square muscle that lies just inferior to the inferior gemellus. It arises from the external surface of the ischial tuberosity and inserts into the posterosuperior surface of the femur just inferior to the intertrochanteric crest. It is a powerful external rotator of the thigh. A bursa is often interposed between the muscle and the lesser trochanter of the femur. The muscle is supplied by the nerve to the quadratus femoris, arising from the sacral plexus (L4, 5; S1).

BLOOD VESSELS, LYMPHATICS, & NERVES

Arteries

The **superior gluteal artery** branches from the posterior division of the internal iliac artery. It runs briefly in the posterior pelvis between the descending lumbosacral trunk of the lumbar plexus and the highest sacral nerve (S1). It leaves the pelvis through the suprapiriformic space of the greater sciatic foramen and divides into its 2 terminal branches. The superficial branch supplies the gluteus maximus muscle and the cutaneous area over the dorsal surface of the sacrum. It has rich anastomoses with branches of the inferior gluteal artery. The deep branch rises beneath the deep surface of the gluteus medius muscle, where it divides into 2 terminal branches. The superior branch hugs the superior border of the gluteus minimus muscle as far as the anterosuperior iliac spine, where it joins with branches from the deep and superficial circumflex, iliac, and lateral femoral circumflex arteries. The inferior branch runs toward the greater trochanter. It supplies blood to all gluteal muscles and sends minor arterial branches to the hip joint.

The **inferior gluteal artery** is a branch of the anterior division of the internal iliac artery and a major source of arterial supply to the buttocks and upper posterior thigh. It runs posteriorly between nerve roots S1 and S2 and passes out of the pelvis via the infrapiriformic segment of the greater sciatic foramen. It lies deep to the gluteus maximus muscle, and in the upper posterior thigh it lies close to both the sciatic and the posterior femoral cutaneous nerves. It gives off visceral branches within the pelvis that supply the perirectal fat, the fundus of the bladder, the seminal vesicles, and the prostate. Within the pelvis, it supplies the piriformis and the muscles of the levator diaphragm. In the posterior thigh, it gives off important anastomotic branches that join with branches from the first perforating and medial and lateral femoral circumflex arteries to form the so-called cruciate anastomosis of the upper thigh. Some of its muscular branches join with branches of the obturator artery.

➤ *Role of gluteal arteries in anastomoses with branches of the femoral artery. Branches from the superior and inferior gluteal arteries anastomose with arterial branches from the circumflex femoral branches of the femoral artery, thus setting up an important arterial anastomotic linkage between the internal iliac and femoral arteries. This allows blood to be channeled to the buttock area from the femoral artery in cases of occlusion of the internal iliac artery with resultant relief of buttock muscle claudication. It also allows blood from the internal iliac artery to reach the thigh in cases of external iliac and upper femoral arterial blockage, thus helping to keep the lower limb viable.*

Veins

The superior and inferior gluteal veins are venae comitantes of the superior and inferior gluteal arteries. They enter the pelvic cavity via the greater sciatic foramen and eventually empty into the internal iliac vein. In the buttock area, the veins are large and multiple, but in the pelvis they become single veins.

➡ *Role of gluteal veins in buttock hematoma formation. Severe trauma to the buttock area usually results from a hard fall. Owing to the presence of several large veins between the gluteus maximus and gluteus medius muscles, trauma is frequently followed by formation of large deep hematomas (manifested by ecchymosis). Such hematomas are usually evacuated by aspiration or by incision and drainage.*

Lymphatics

Lymph from the buttocks and the upper thigh drain eventually into the internal iliac nodes within the pelvis, close to the internal iliac artery and its branches. The flow is then superior, into the lumbar and lower periaortic nodes.

Nerves

The lumbosacral, pudendal, and coccygeal plexuses send many of their terminal branches into the gluteal region.

The **sacral plexus** is derived from the anterior primary rami of L4, L5, and S1–4. A branch from L4 joins L5 to form the lumbosacral trunk, which is the most superior arm of the sacral plexus. The individual spinal nerves pass from within the bony spinal canal via the anterior sacral foramens, and just ventral to the piriformis muscle they form the complex sacral plexus. Branches from both the lumbosacral and sacral plexuses supply the gluteus muscles, the pelvic muscles, the muscles about the hip joint, the muscles of the posterior thigh, and all the musculature of the leg and foot. They also supply selected cutaneous areas of the posterior thigh, the buttock, and the leg and foot.

The buttock area is supplied mainly by the gluteal branches of the posterior femoral cutaneous nerve. The branches turn superiorly around the lower border of the gluteus maximus and become superficial, supplying the skin over the lower and lateral aspects of the buttock. They are derived from the dorsal divisions of S1–3. The remainder of the skin of the buttock is supplied by the posterior primary rami of L1–3 and S1–3.

Branches of the lumbar and sacral plexuses pass inferiorly into the lower pelvis and combine to form the large sciatic and smaller pudendal nerves. The motor and sensory nerves supplying the area about the hip joint, the upper posterior thigh, and the muscles of the pelvic diaphragm arise from branches of the lumbar and sacral plexuses.

The **pudendal nerve** arises from S2–4 and leaves the pelvis via the greater sciatic foramen along with the internal pudendal vessels. It passes between the piriformis and coccygeus muscles, then winds around the ischial spine and enters the perineum via the lesser sciatic foramen. In the perineum, the pudendal nerve occupies **Alcock's canal** along with the internal pudendal artery and vein. The canal is a fascial envelope developed from reduplication of the obturator internus fascia. Alcock's canal runs forward along the lateral

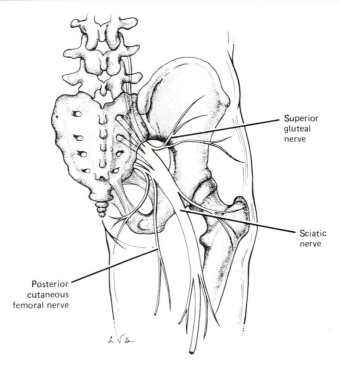

Superior gluteal nerve

Sciatic nerve

Posterior cutaneous femoral nerve

Figure 47–4. The sciatic nerve.

inferior wall of the inner surface of the perineum. In the posterior perineum, the pudendal nerve supplies the external sphincter ani and the skin of the anorectal perineum via the inferior rectal nerve. In the anterior perineum, its 2 terminal branches are the perineal nerve and the dorsal nerve to the penis or clitoris.

The **sciatic nerve** (Fig 47–4) is not only the largest of the terminal branches of the sacral plexus (L4, 5; S1–3), it is the largest nerve in the body. It emerges from the greater sciatic foramen just below the piriformis muscle and on the upper posterior thigh comes to lie under cover of the gluteus maximus muscle. The nerve ends by dividing into the tibial and common peroneal nerves, usually in the lower third of the thigh. However, the terminal bifurcation may occur in its intrapelvic course or in the greater sciatic foramen. In the superior segment of the thigh, the sciatic nerve lies upon the dorsal surface of the ischium between the ischial tuberosity and the greater trochanter of the femur. As it moves inferiorly, the nerve crosses the obturator internus, the gemelli, and the quadratus femoris. In the upper mid thigh, the nerve lies on the adductor magnus and deep to the long head of the biceps femoris. In the thigh, the sciatic nerve gives branches to both heads of the biceps femoris, the semimembranosus, the semitendinosus, and part of the adductor magnus muscle.

➠ *Precautions in giving injections into the gluteal region. The gluteal region is a frequent site of intermuscular injection. Injection should always be above a line extending from the posterosuperior iliac spine to the superior border of the greater trochanter of the femur, well above the level of the sciatic nerve. Complications of improper technique include hematoma or abscess formation, foreign body granulomas, sloughing of skin, and, on occasion, damage to the sciatic nerve. Oily, nonabsorbable substance should not be injected in this area. The depth of the injection varies depending upon the amount of subcutaneous fat in the gluteal region. The needle should ideally be placed just deep to the external sheath of the gluteus maximus.*

The Thigh & Hip Joint

48

The lower extremity serves both to support the body and to act as its primary means of locomotion. It is a composite of the thigh (discussed here), the leg (Chapter 50), and the foot (Chapter 52). Its bony components are the femur, the patella, the tibia, the fibula, the 7 tarsal bones, the 5 metatarsals, and the 14 phalanges. It is articulated by 3 major joints—the hip joint (discussed here), the knee joint (Chapter 49), and the ankle joint (Chapter 51)—and distal to the ankle it is joined by the intertarsal joints, the tarsometatarsal joints, the metatarsophalangeal joints, and the interphalangeal joints.

THE THIGH

THE FEMUR
(Fig 48–1)

The femur is both the longest and the sturdiest bone of the human body. Below its articulation with the pelvic bones, it inclines medially and inferiorly so that the knee joint is at the center of gravity of the skeleton. Medial inclination of the femur is more pronounced in females than in males because of the greater width of the female pelvis.

The femur is the first of the long bones to ossify. After puberty, the epiphyses unite in the following order: lesser trochanter, greater trochanter, head, and distal extremity, which does not unite until about the 20th or 21st year.

➡ *Measurement of femoral length in hip joint disease. Many disorders affecting the hip joint and femoral neck are associated with shortening of the lower extremity. This is measured by passing a tape from the anterosuperior iliac spine to the medial border of the patella and then to the tip of the medial malleolus of the tibia. The result is then compared with the contralateral limb. The angle at which the neck of the femur joins the femoral shaft should be measured also. The normal angle is about 130 degrees. If the angle is increased to 150–160 degees, coxa valga is present; if it is decreased to 90–110 degrees, coxa vara is present.*

Superior Segment of the Femur

The superior segment of the femur consists of a head, a neck, and a greater and a lesser trochanter. The rounded **femoral head** is completely covered with cartilage except for its central area, the **fovea capitis femoris,** the site of attachment of the ligamentum capitis femoris. The head of the femur articulates with the acetabular cavity of the pelvic girdle, the ball-and-socket articulation allowing for the multiple motions of the thigh upon the pelvis. (See Movements of the Hip Joint, below.)

The **neck of the femur** is roughly triangular. It connects the femoral head and the femoral shaft. With the thigh in a neutral position, the head and neck of the femur join its shaft at an angle of about 130 degrees, the so-called angle of femoral inclination. The angle of junction of the head and neck varies markedly with age. The femoral neck, as it leaves the upper end of the femoral shaft, projects in 3 planes: superiorly, medially, and dorsally. Since the femoral neck has a minor ventral thrust, a second angulation of the head and neck upon the femoral shaft results. This angle measures about 15 degrees and is called the angle of torsion or declination. The neck of the femur is wider laterally than it is medially, and its central area appears contracted.

➡ *Fractures of the femoral neck. (Fig 48–2.) The neck is the most frequently fractured segment of the femur because it is the narrowest and weakest portion of the bone and because with advanced age the neck becomes further weakened and brittle secondary to osteoporosis. The commonest femoral neck fractures are the subcapital, transcervical, and basilar neck fractures. Fractures of the trochanters also occur, alone or associated with other femoral fractures or with fractures of the pelvic girdle. Fractures of the intertrochanteric area (distal to the femoral neck) are also common in the elderly.*

➡ *Subcapital fracture of the femoral neck. Because subcapital fractures are completely intracapsular, the fracture may endanger the blood supply to the femoral head, since the capsular vessels carry the major portion of the blood supply to the head. If the blood supply entering the femoral head via the ligamentum capitis*

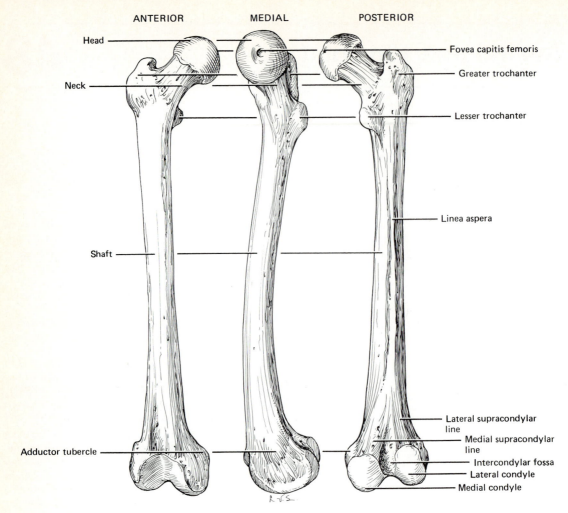

ANTERIOR   MEDIAL   POSTERIOR

Head

Neck

Shaft

Adductor tubercle

Fovea capitis femoris

Greater trochanter

Lesser trochanter

Linea aspera

Lateral supracondylar line

Medial supracondylar line

Intercondylar fossa

Lateral condyle

Medial condyle

Figure 48–1. The right femur.

femoris is inadequate to nourish the proximal fracture fragment, delayed healing of the fracture or avascular necrosis of the femoral head may result.

Transcervical femoral fractures. *A transcervical femoral fracture is an intracapsular break, the fracture line crossing the mid area of the neck of the bone. Since a large percentage of the blood supply to the femoral head and neck is from the medial and lateral femoral circumflex arteries, whose terminal course is within the joint capsule, a capsular tear frequently involves these vessels and can lead to delayed healing because of poor blood supply.*

Impaction of fractures of the femoral head and neck. *Fractures of the femoral head and neck are frequently impacted, the distal fragment overriding the proximal fragment. This may shorten the lower extremity slightly.*

The superior border of the femoral neck is relatively short and ends laterally in a vertical bony ridge, the greater trochanter. The concave inferior border of the neck is almost twice the length of the superior border and terminates in a bony projection, the lesser trochanter.

The actual fusion of the femoral neck with the femoral shaft occurs along a bony ridge, the intertrochanteric line, which extends from the greater to the lesser trochanter. The ridge is more prominent on the posterior than on the anterior surface of the femur.

The **greater trochanter** arises from the superior end of the junctional angle between the femoral neck and body. It has a convex, roughened lateral surface into which inserts the tendon of the gluteus medius. The medial surface is much shorter than the lateral surface, and at its base is a deep hollow, the trochanteric fossa; just anterior to the fossa, the obturator internus and the 2 gemelli insert. Into the superior border of the greater trochanter inserts the piriformis muscle. The inferior border of the greater trochanter,

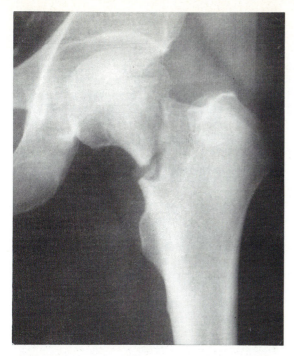

Figure 48–2. Fracture of neck of femur. (Reproduced, with permission, from Way LW [editor]: *Current Surgical Diagnosis & Treatment,* 7th ed. Lange, 1985.)

where its base joins the lateral shaft of the femur, is the site of origin of a portion of the vastus lateralis muscle. The anterior border of the greater trochanter is the site of insertion of the gluteus minimus, while its posterior border abuts the trochanteric fossa.

➠ *Fractures of the greater trochanter. Fractures of the greater trochanter usually result from a direct blow, a fall directly upon the trochanter, or a strong muscular pull upon the structure. Healing is usually rapid and complete following good anatomic reduction.*

The **lesser trochanter** faces dorsally as it projects from the base of the femoral neck. The roughened apex of the lesser trochanter is the site of insertion of the tendon of the iliopsoas muscle.

➠ *Fractures of the lesser trochanter. Fractures of the lesser trochanter usually result from a strong pull upon the trochanter by the iliopsoas muscle while the thigh is in hyperextension and abduction. Because of its deep position, the lesser trochanter is less likely to break as a result of a fall or direct blow.*

The **intertrochanteric crest** is an elevation on the posterior surface of the junctional area of the femoral neck and body. It runs in a curved line from the apex of the greater trochanter to the lesser trochanter.

➠ *Intertrochanteric femoral fractures. Intertrochanteric fractures of the femur are nearly always extracapsular. Since the fracture line is through well-nourished spongy bone and is extracapsular, healing is usually complete within 3–4 months.*

The **intertrochanteric line** runs obliquely from the greater to the lesser trochanter on the anterior surface of the junctional area of the femoral neck and the femoral shaft. Proximally, the line gives attachment to the iliofemoral ligament of the hip joint; distally, the superior segment of the vastus medialis muscle arises from the line.

The Shaft (Body) of the Femur

The shaft of the femur is an almost cylindric bowed bone which is wider both proximally and distally than it is centrally. Dorsally over the middle third of the shaft, the femur presents a vertical ridge, the **linea aspera.** Three smaller ridges diverge from the superior margin of the linea aspera. The roughened lateral ridge runs to the base of the greater trochanter, and the gluteus maximus inserts into it. The medial ridge terminates in the intertrochanteric line just below the insertion of the iliacus muscle. The central ridge runs to the inferior margin of the lesser trochanter. Inferiorly, the linea aspera splits into 2 supracondylar ridges. The depressed area between them is called the popliteal surface of the femur.

➠ *Fractures of the femoral shaft. (Fig 48–3.) Fractures of the shaft of the femur usually follow a direct blow. Displacement of fragments depends upon muscular pull, which varies at different levels. With fractures of the upper third of the shaft, the proximal fragment is pulled ventrally by the iliopsoas muscle, rotated laterally by the obturator and gemellus muscles, and abducted from the distal fragment by the gluteus medius muscle. In fractures of the middle third of the femur with disruption of the upper segment, both the gluteus maximus and gluteus medius muscles abduct the proximal segment, causing it to lie lateral to the distal fragment. Fractures of the lower segment respond to the strong pull of the adductor muscles, the proximal fragment being moved medial to the distal fragment.*

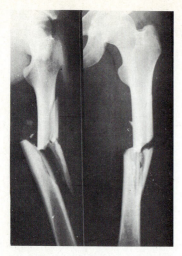

Figure 48-3. Fracture of shaft of femur. (Reproduced, with permission, from Way LW [editor]: *Current Surgical Diagnosis & Treatment,* 7th ed. Lange, 1985.)

Inferior Segment of the Femur

The distal segment of the femur is the broadest portion of the bone, and it consists of 2 large projections, the femoral condyles. The condyles protrude farther posteriorly than anteriorly. Anteriorly, the condyles are separated by a shallow depression, the patellar surface of the femur. Posteriorly, the condyles are separated by a deep recess, the intercondylar fossa. The medial condyle projects farther distally than the lateral one, but the lateral condyle is the larger one.

➡ *Fractures through the lower third of the femoral shaft. (Fig 48-4.) Fractures through the lower third of the femoral shaft can be supracondylar or intracondylar. With supracondylar fracture, the pull of the gastrocnemius displaces*

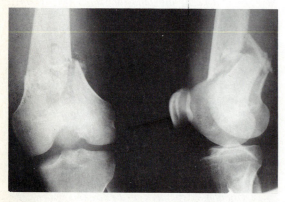

Figure 48-4. Fracture of lower part of femur. (Reproduced, with permission, from Way LW [editor]: *Current Surgical Diagnosis & Treatment,* 7th ed. Lange, 1985.)

the distal segment dorsally. This may traumatize the popliteal artery or vein, which lies close to the posterior surface of the femur at the fracture level. Intracondylar fractures are often of the T type, with resultant separation of the 2 distal articular surfaces of the femur. Improper or inadequate reduction of such a fracture may lead to deformity at the knee joint.

On the superior lateral border of each femoral condyle is a small elevation, the epicondyle. Both epicondyles give attachment to the collateral ligaments of the knee joint. The 2 cruciate ligaments of the knee joint are attached to the walls of the intercondylar fossa—the anterior cruciate to the lateral wall and the posterior cruciate to the medial wall. The anterior, inferior, and posterior surfaces of the femoral condyles are covered with cartilage for articulation with the tibia and its cartilaginous menisci. The lower anterior surface of the femur articulates with the patella.

FASCIAE OF THE THIGH

The **subcutaneous fascia** of the thigh is divided into a superficial adipose layer and a deep fibrous layer. Between the 2 layers of the subcutaneous fascia lie the greater saphenous vein, the superficial blood vessels and nerves of the thigh, and the superficial subinguinal lymph nodes.

The deep fibrous layer of the cutaneous fascia attaches to the fascia lata of the thigh just inferior to the inguinal ligament. In the medial superior thigh, it is adherent to the circumference of the fossa ovalis (the saphenous opening); a thin septum derived from the subcutaneous fascia, the **fascia cribrosa,** covers that oval opening. The septum is so named because veins, arteries, and lymphatics pass through it on their way to the deeper thigh structures. Between the deep surface of the subcutaneous thigh fascia and the ventral surface of the patella is a large bursa that frequently becomes inflamed (prepatellar bursitis).

The external investing layer of the deep thigh fascia is the **fascia lata** (Fig 48-5), which surrounds the thigh like a stocking. Laterally, the fascia lata is thick and strong; but anteriorly, the fascia is quite thin, so that the red muscle fibers lying deep to it can easily be seen through its covering membrane.

Medially, where the fascia lata covers the adductor muscles of the thigh, it is also quite thin except at knee level, where it is reinforced by fibers from the sartorius muscle.

The fascia lata is attached to the ischial tuberosity, the inferior ischiopubic ramus, the anterosuperior iliac spine, the inguinal ligament, and the pubic spine. Immediately inferior to the inguinal ligament, the fascia lata is reinforced by 3 abdominal fasciae: the deep layer of the superficial fascia of the abdomen

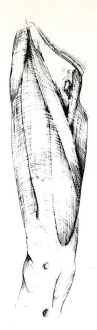

Figure 48–5. Fascia lata.

thick and presents an oval opening, the fossa ovalis (Fig. 48–6). (See section on femoral hernia in Chapter 23.) The lateral superior arc of the fossa ovalis has a thick, free crescentic margin (the falciform ligament of the fascia lata) that runs medially to attach to the pubic tubercle. The inferior arc of the fossa is thin and is separated from the lateral arc by a pad of fatty tissue.

The lateral segment of the fascia lata is extremely thick. Inserting into it are the gluteus maximus and tensor fasciae latae muscles. Superiorly, it attaches to the crest of the ilium and to the dorsal surface of the sacrum. As the fascia descends from there, it splits and ensheathes the gluteus maximus. Farther anteriorly, the fascia splits to enclose the tensor fasciae latae.

The posterior segment of the fascia lata covers the hamstring muscles and roofs over the popliteal fossa. It is formed by the junction of the 2 fascial sheaths which enclose the gluteus maximus.

Arising from the deep surface of the fascia lata and running to the linea aspera of the femur are 2 intermuscular septa. The lateral one separates the biceps femoris from the vastus lateralis. The medial one separates the adductors and the pectineus muscles from the vastus medialis.

(Scarpa's fascia); the transversalis fascia; and the iliacus fascia, which fuses with the fascia lata at the inguinal ligament. Inferior to the medial half of the inguinal ligament, the transversalis fascia and the iliacus fascia advance into the upper thigh as the ventral and dorsal sheaths of the femoral vessels and the femoral canal. As the fascia lata lies ventral to the femoral vessels and the femoral canal, it is quite

MUSCLES OF THE THIGH
(Fig 48–7)

The muscles of the thigh are arranged in 3 major groups: an anterior extensor group, a medial adductor

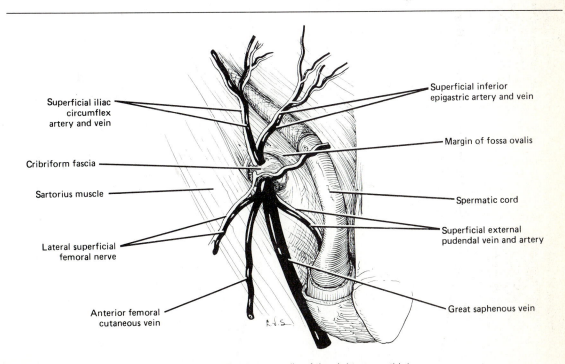

Figure 48–6. The fossa ovalis of the right upper thigh.

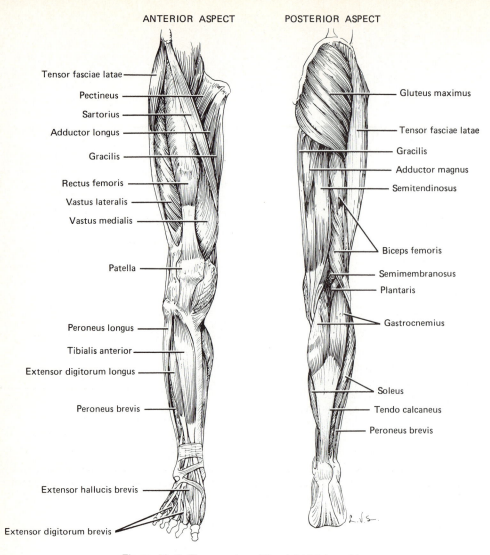

ANTERIOR ASPECT   POSTERIOR ASPECT

Tensor fasciae latae

Pectineus

Sartorius

Adductor longus

Gracilis

Rectus femoris

Vastus lateralis

Vastus medialis

Patella

Peroneus longus

Tibialis anterior

Extensor digitorum longus

Peroneus brevis

Extensor hallucis brevis

Extensor digitorum brevis

Gluteus maximus

Tensor fasciae latae

Gracilis

Adductor magnus

Semitendinosus

Biceps femoris

Semimembranosus

Plantaris

Gastrocnemius

Soleus

Tendo calcaneus

Peroneus brevis

Figure 48–7. The muscles of the right thigh and leg.

group, and a posterior flexor group. Generally, the anterior group is served by the femoral nerve, the medial group by the obturator nerve, and the posterior group by the sciatic nerve.

Anterior (Extensor) Group (Table 48–1)

The anterior group of thigh muscles is made up of the sartorius and the quadriceps extensor group (rectus femoris, vastus lateralis, intermedius, and medialis). All of the extensor muscles give stability to the knee joint. They tend to atrophy rapidly with disease, and following thigh and leg immobilization, early physiotherapy is required to restore their size, strength, and tone.

Medial (Adductor) Group (Table 48–2)

The medial group of thigh muscles all arise from one or more of the pelvic bones and insert onto either the medial or the posterior surface of the femur or tibia. They are the pectineus; the gracilis; the adductors longus, brevis, and magnus; and the obturator externus.

Posterior (Flexor) Group (Table 48–3)

The posterior group of muscles (the ''hamstrings'') are the biceps femoris, the semitendinosus, and the semimembranosus. All but the short head of the biceps arise from the ischial tuberosity and insert into either

Table 48–1. Muscles of the thigh: Anterior femoral muscles (anterior extensors).

Muscle and Origin	Insertion	Innervation	Function
RECTUS FEMORIS Anterior tendon of origin from the anteroinferior iliac spine. Reflected tendon of origin from the depression just superior to the acetabular rim.	Via a tendon into the base of the patella.	Femoral nerve (L2–4).	Extends the leg and flexes the thigh.
VASTUS LATERALIS The capsule of the hip joint, the femoral tubercle, the distal border of the greater trochanter, the anterior surface of the shaft of the femur medial to the greater trochanter; from the gluteal tuberosity, the proximal half of the lateral lip of the linea aspera, the fascia lata, and the lateral intermuscular septum. Origin is by a wide aponeurosis.	The lateral border of the patella, at which point it blends with the quadriceps femoris tendon.	Femoral nerve (L2–4).	Extends the leg.
VASTUS MEDIALIS The lower half of the intertrochanteric line, the medial lip of the linea aspera, the proximal two-thirds of the medial supracondylar line, the medial intermuscular septum, and the adductor magnus and longus tendons.	Via a tendon lying medial to the medial patellar border and to the medial border of the quadriceps femoris tendon. An expansion of this tendon runs to the knee joint capsule.	Femoral nerve (L2–4).	Extends the leg.
VASTUS INTERMEDIUS The anterior and lateral superior two-thirds of the body of the femur, the distal half of the linea aspera, and the distal third of the lateral intermuscular septum.	Forms the deep segment of the tendon of the quadriceps femoris.	Femoral nerve (L2–4).	Extends the leg.
ARTICULARIS GENU The distal one-fourth of the anterior surface of the femur.	Upper part of the synovial membrane of the knee joint.	Branch of the nerve to the vastus intermedius (L2–4).	Draws the synovial membrane of the knee joint proximally during extension of the leg.
SARTORIUS The anterior superior iliac spine and the iliac notch just inferior to the spine.	Ends in a tendon that dilates into a wide aponeurosis which inserts into the medial surface of the upper tibia. A segment of the inserting fascia blends with the fibers of the knee joint capsule.	Two branches from the femoral nerve (L2, 3).	Flexes the thigh and rotates it laterally. Flexes and medially rotates the leg.

of the 2 leg bones. The short head of the biceps arises from the lower half of the lateral lip of the linea aspera of the femur.

Femoral Triangle
(Table 48–4)

The femoral (Scarpa's) triangle (see also section on femoral hernia in Chapter 23) lies on the superior mid surface of the thigh. Its superior base is the inguinal ligament. The lateral side of the triangle is formed by the sartorius muscle and the medial side by the adductor longus. The floor of the area is formed by the iliopsoas muscle and the pectineus muscle. Superficially, the area contains the constant 3 small most superior branches of the femoral artery and vein, the termination of the long saphenous vein, the fossa ovalis, and the superficial subinguinal lymph nodes.

⟹ *Approaches to the most superior segment of the femur. Approaches to the femoral head, the femoral neck, and the trochanters may be by anterior, lateral, and posterior incisions. The anterior approach is via an incision that begins at the iliac crest and curves over the anterosuperior iliac spine to roughly parallel the upper femoral shaft. The incision ends at the upper one-fourth of the femur. The tensor fasciae latae are exposed and the upper fibers of the vastus lateralis are reflected dorsally to reveal the capsule of the hip joint, which lies just lateral to the rectus femoris muscle. An incision through the capsule then exposes the head of the femur and the acetabular rim.*

The lateral approach to the femoral neck and the greater trochanter is often used for

Table 48–2. Muscles of the thigh: Medial femoral muscles (medial adductors).

Muscle and Origin	Insertion	Innervation	Function
PECTINEUS The pectineal line, from the pubic bone anterior to the pectineal line and from the fascia that covers the muscle anteriorly.	Along the line leading from the lesser trochanter to the linea aspera.	Femoral nerve (L2–4) and accessory obturator nerve (L3).	Adducts, flexes, and rotates the thigh medially.
GRACILIS The lower half of the anterior surface of the symphysis pubica, all of the inferior pubic ramus, and part of the ramus of the ischium.	The medial surface of the body of the tibia inferior to the tibial condyle.	Obturator nerve, anterior division (L3, 4).	Adducts the thigh, flexes the leg, and rotates the leg medially.
ADDUCTOR LONGUS The anterior surface of the body of the pubis at the point where the pubic crest joins the pubic symphysis.	The medial lip of the linea aspera between the vastus medialis and the adductor magnus.	Obturator nerve, anterior division (L3, 4).	Adducts, flexes, and rotates the thigh medially.
ADDUCTOR BREVIS The external surface of the inferior pubic ramus between the gracilis and obturator externus muscles.	The proximal half of the linea aspera and between it and the lesser trochanter on the posterior surface of the femur.	Obturator nerve, anterior division (L3, 4).	Adducts, flexes, and rotates the thigh medially.
ADDUCTOR MAGNUS The ischial tuberosity, the edge of the inferior ischial ramus, and the anterior surface of the inferior pubic ramus.	Along a line from the greater trochanter to the linea aspera, the medial epicondylic ridge, and the adductor tubercle on the medial femoral condyle.	Obturator nerve, posterior division (L3), and the tibial nerve (L3, 4).	A powerful adductor of the thigh. The superior half rotates the thigh medially and flexes it. The inferior half extends the thigh and rotates it laterally.

Table 48–3. Muscles of the thigh: Posterior thigh muscles (posterior flexors).

Muscle and Origin	Insertion	Innervation	Function
BICEPS FEMORIS The long head arises from the lower medial segment of the ischial tuberosity and the sacro-tuberous ligament. The short head arises from the lateral lip of the linea as pera, the proximal two-thirds of the lateral supracondylar ridge, and the lateral intermuscular septum.	The lateral side of the head of the fibula. A small slip to the lateral tibial condyle.	The long head by the tibial division of the sciatic nerve (L5; S1, 2). The short head by the peroneal division of the sciatic nerve (L5; S1, 2).	Flexes the leg and then rotates it laterally. The long head extends the thigh and rotates it laterally.
SEMITENDINOSUS The lower medial segment of the ischial tuberosity, by a common tendon with the long head of the biceps femoris.	The medial posterior segment of the surface of the body of the tibia distal to the medial condyle and the deep fascia of the leg.	The tibial division of the sciatic nerve (L5; S1, 2).	Extends the thigh. Flexes and rotates the leg medially.
SEMIMEMBRANOSUS The upper lateral segment of the ischial tuberosity.	The posteromedial area of the tibial medial condyle. The popliteus muscle fascia and the posterior aspect of the lateral femoral condyle receive slips from the major area of insertion of the muscle.	The tibial division of the sciatic nerve (L5; S1, 2).	Extends the thigh. Flexes and rotates the leg medially.

Table 48–4. Muscles of the iliac region: Lateral superior thigh muscles.

Muscle and Origin	Insertion	Innervation	Function
PSOAS MAJOR From the base of the anterior surface of the transverse processes of vertebrae L1–5, the side of the bodies and intervertebral disks of T12–L5, and the tendinous arches on the anterior surfaces of L1–5.	Into the lesser trochanter of the femur.	Branches from L2 and L3.	Flexes the thigh and the lumbar vertebrae. Lateral flexion of the lumbar spine.
PSOAS MINOR From the lateral edges of the bodies of T12 and L1 and the intervening disk.	Into the pectineal line and the iliopectineal line. The lateral border inserts into the iliac fossa.	Branch from L1.	Flexes the pelvis and the lumbar vertebral column.
ILIACUS From the superior two-thirds of the iliac fossa, the inner lip of the iliac crest, the anterior sacroiliac and iliolumbar ligaments, and the dorsal sacral base.	Into the lateral edge of the psoas major tendon; with that tendon, inserts into the lesser trochanter of the femur.	Femoral nerve (L2, 3).	Flexes the thigh.
TENSOR FASCIAE LATAE From the anterior segment of the iliac crest, the anterosuperior iliac spine, and the deep surface of the fascia lata of the thigh.	Between the 2 layers of the iliotibeal band of the fascia lata.	Superior gluteal nerve (L4, 5).	Abducts and medially rotates the thigh and extends the knee.

fixation of femoral neck fractures. The incision extends from just superior to the greater trochanter down to the upper fourth of the femoral shaft. The tensor fasciae latae are incised, and the upper fibers of the vastus lateralis are separated. A finger is then inserted behind the rectus femoris muscle, and the femoral neck may then be palpated through the capsule of the hip joint.

The posterior approach to the hip joint is via a curvilinear inverted V-shaped incision, starting at the posterosuperior iliac spine and sweeping to the greater trochanter. The piriformis and obturator internus and externus are divided in order to visualize the femoral neck and hip joint.

⇒ ***Approach to the femoral shaft.*** *The femoral shaft may be approached by an anterior, lateral, posterior, or medial incision. The anterior approach is usually anteromedial, reaching the shaft between the vastus medialis and rectus femoris muscles. An anterolateral approach may be made by separating the rectus femoris from the vastus lateralis, with careful preservation of the vessels and nerves to the latter muscle. The posterior approach is via an incision made just lateral to the biceps femoris muscle, posterior to the lateral intermuscular septum. The medial approach is used in order to gain access to the distal femoral shaft. The posterior deep fascia is incised and the sartorius muscle is retracted posteriorly, while the vastus medialis and the tendon of the adductor magnus are retracted anteriorly.*

⇒ ***Amputations through the thigh.*** *Amputations through the thigh must seek to maintain a femoral stump of at least 7.5 cm to enable the thigh to function properly with a prosthesis. A longer stump is desirable. Supracondylar amputation avoids the undesirable bulbous distal segment of the femur. Gritti-Stokes amputation utilizes the patella as a weight-bearing cap placed over the end of the amputated femur. Guillotine amputation avoids opening muscle spaces in limbs that have infection distal to the area of amputation; it is the procedure of choice when gas gangrene and septic necrosis are present in tissues distal to the site of amputation.*

Adductor Canal

The adductor canal (Hunter's canal) begins at the femoral triangle and terminates at the superior border of the popliteal space at the distal border of the opening in the adductor magnus muscle. It lies in the middle third of the thigh. The sartorius and the vastus muscles form its anterior (roof) relationship. The posterior relationship (the floor of the canal) is made up of the vastus medialis, the adductor longus, and the adductor magnus muscles (Fig 48–8). Extending from the vastus medialis anteriorly to the adductor group of muscles posteriorly is a fascial membrane, the adductor membrane, which forms the medial wall of the canal. The canal proceeds inferiorly into the popliteal space. The termination of the canal is marked by an opening in the adductor magnus tendon, the adductor hiatus. The femoral artery and vein pass through the hiatus as they proceed from the anterior

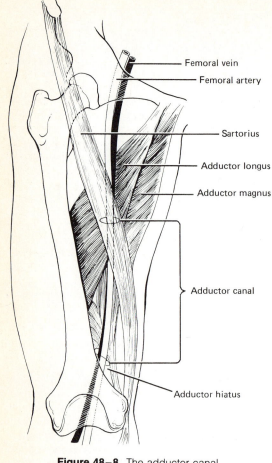

Figure 48–8. The adductor canal.

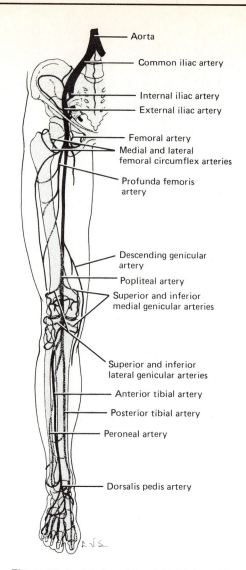

Figure 48–9. Arteries of the right thigh and leg.

to the dorsal thigh after running the entire length of the canal. Entering the canal but not leaving it via its terminal hiatus are the nerve to the vastus medialis and the saphenous nerve, both branches of the femoral nerve.

BLOOD VESSELS, LYMPHATICS, & NERVES

Arteries
(Fig 48–9)

The **femoral artery** reaches the thigh by passing deep to the midpoint of the inguinal ligament. Almost immediately upon reaching the anterosuperior surface of the thigh, it gives off 3 constant branches: the superficial inferior epigastric, the superficial external pudendal, and the superficial circumflex iliac arteries. These vessels, at their origin, lie on the deep surface of the fossa ovalis. The femoral artery also gives off small branches to the skin, muscles, and lymph nodes in the subinguinal area. Lying just lateral to the femoral artery in the femoral triangle is the femoral nerve and its upper thigh branches. In the femoral triangle, the femoral artery gives off from its lateral surface the **profunda femoris artery.** This large branch almost immediately passes dorsal to the femoral artery and comes to lie close to the medial surface of the femur. It supplies the muscles of the anterior and posterior surfaces of the thigh and also the femur via multiple perforating branches. It gives off the anastomotic medial and lateral femoral circumflex branches. The continuing femoral artery is often called the **superficial femoral artery,** which runs to the apex of Scarpa's triangle, where it enters the adductor canal, covered by the superficial and deep fascia of the thigh, the sartorius muscle, and the thick fascial roof of the adductor canal. At the level of the adductor hiatus, the femoral artery gives off the descending genicular artery, and then it becomes the popliteal artery.

➠ *Femoral artery in diagnostic studies. The femoral artery is often entered in order to insert a catheter for retrograde aortography or femoral arteriography, or to perform selective arteriography of the branches of the abdominal aorta. The femoral artery is also used as a source of arterial blood for blood gas studies. The vessel is usually entered just below the inguinal ligament at the base of the femoral triangle.*

➠ *Operative exposure of the femoral artery. This is accomplished via a vertical incision directly over the vessels, placed at a right angle to and just below the inguinal ligament. With the hip slightly flexed and externally rotated, the incision is extended inferiorly. The incision makes femoral arterial replacement via a bypass graft a reasonably easy procedure.*

➠ *The profunda femoris artery and arterial obliterative disease. The competency of the profunda femoris and of its multiple branches helps to assess the chances for success of an attempt to restore circulation to a poorly nourished lower limb. The runoff from the artery and its branches indicates that a bypass of the blocked femoral artery has a good chance of revascularizing the limb.*

The **obturator artery** supplies blood to the upper medial surface of the thigh. It branches from the anterior division of the internal iliac artery and leaves the pelvis via the obturator foramen along with the obturator nerve. It then divides into anterior and posterior branches. The posterior branch runs along the inferior ischial border, sends blood to the hip joint, and finally anastomoses with branches of the medial femoral circumflex artery. The anterior branch runs along the obturator membrane and gives off branches to the obturator externus, the pectineus, the 3 adductors, and the gracilis. It anastomoses with branches of the medial femoral circumflex artery. In 10–15% of people, the obturator artery arises either from the external iliac or the inferior epigastric artery. It runs to the obturator foramen, lies close to the crescentic border of the lacunar ligament, and thus becomes vulnerable in femoral hernia surgery.

There is excellent collateral circulation to the thigh in cases in which the external iliac or common femoral arteries are ligated or obliterated by disease. The medial and lateral circumflex branches of the deep femoral artery join with the descending branch of the inferior gluteal artery. The superior gluteal and iliolumbar branches of the internal iliac artery anastomose with the ascending branches of the 2 femoral circumflex arteries and the highest perforating branch of the deep femoral artery. The obturator artery anastomoses with the femoral circumflex arteries.

Veins
(Fig 48–10)

The **great saphenous vein,** the major vein draining the superficial tissues of the foot, leg, and thigh, runs just posterior to the medial condyle of the femur. It then lies between the superficial and deep layers of the superficial thigh fascia. Just inferior to the inguinal ligament, it perforates the fascia cribrosa, which roofs the fossa ovalis. The vein then joins with the superficial femoral vein to form the common femoral vein. In the thigh, it receives blood from the 2 femoral cutaneous veins, and in the fossa ovalis it receives blood from the 3 small veins that accompany the most superior 3 branches of the femoral artery. In the thigh it communicates with the superficial femoral vein via multiple short perforating veins.

The **obturator vein** accompanies the obturator artery in the superior medial thigh. It enters the pelvis through the obturator foramen and joins the internal iliac vein. On occasion it may join either the inferior

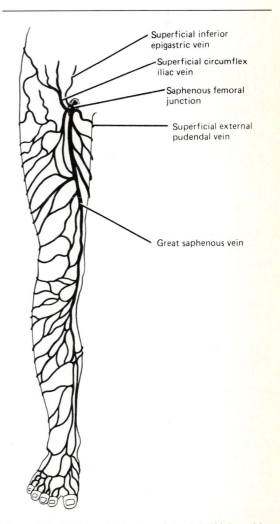

Superficial inferior epigastric vein

Superficial circumflex iliac vein

Saphenous femoral junction

Superficial external pudendal vein

Great saphenous vein

Figure 48–10. Superficial veins of the right thigh and leg.

epigastric or the external iliac vein rather than the internal iliac vein.

The **femoral vein** is the continuation of the popliteal vein. It parallels the descending course of the superficial and common femoral arteries. It receives the deep femoral vein, the 2 femoral circumflex veins, and the greater saphenous vein. Within the adductor canal, the femoral vein lies immediately dorsal to the femoral artery. This relationship persists in the femoral triangle. Then the vein comes to lie medial to and on the same plane as the femoral artery.

⟹ *Ligation of highest tributaries of the greater saphenous vein. If the superficial inferior epigastric, superficial external pudendal, and superficial circumflex iliac veins—high tributaries of the greater saphenous vein—are not diligently searched for, transected, and ligated in varicose vein ligation and stripping procedures, they may be a site of recurrence of varicosities.*

⟹ *Varicosities of the greater saphenous vein. The greater saphenous vein is often varicose in the thigh as well as in the leg. A large, tortuous, thin-walled vein in the medial aspect of the thigh with multiple dilated veins leading to it is an indication of venous disease in this vessel. There appears to be a strong hereditary factor.*

⟹ *Thrombophlebitis in the deep thigh veins. The deep veins of the thigh are frequently the site of thrombophlebitis and phlebothrombosis, usually secondary to lower extremity trauma or surgery upon any area of the body. The thrombotic disease may be asymptomatic until an embolus passes to the lung. Edema of the ankle and leg, calf or thigh tenderness, an increase in pulse rate, and low-grade fever should arouse suspicion, and radioisotope studies can help in localization of the site of the thrombotic process. Venography will provide definitive diagnosis.*

Lymphatics
(Fig 48–11)

The **superficial lymphatic channels** consist of a medial group, closely allied to the greater saphenous vein, which eventually empties into the superficial subinguinal nodes; and a lateral group, which ascends in the lateral thigh and then either crosses to join the medial group or empties directly into the superficial subinguinal nodes. The superficial lymphatics of the posterior thigh also drain into the superficial subinguinal nodes.

The **deep lymphatic channels of the anterior thigh** are closely related to the course of the femoral vein. They empty into the deep subinguinal nodes

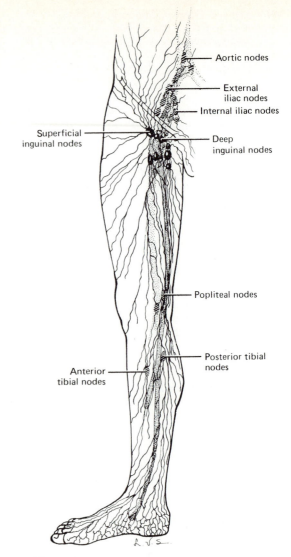

Figure 48–11. Lymphatics of the thigh and leg.

or on occasion directly into the external iliac nodes in the pelvis. The deep lymphatics of the posterosuperior thigh follow the course of the inferior gluteal vessels into the pelvis and empty into the internal iliac nodes.

Most of the lymph nodes of the thigh are in the subinguinal region.

The **subinguinal nodes** are divided into superficial and deep groups. With the saphenous vein and its branches, the superficial nodes, 6–30 in number, are located just deep to the superficial fascia of the thigh at the level of and superficial to the fossa ovalis. When many are present, the individual nodes are quite small. They receive lymph from 5 areas: the anterolateral abdominal wall, inferior to the umbilicus; the upper gluteal region; the external genitalia; the urogenital and anorectal perineum; and the entire lower extremity. There is frequently cross-midline drainage to the contralateral set of superficial subinguinal nodes. Generally, the nodes drain either to the external iliac group of nodes or to the deep inguinal nodes.

The **deep inguinal nodes** lie in the most superior part of the femoral triangle deep to the fossa ovalis. They form a continuous ascending chain along the femoral artery and vein. Distally, they may be found as low as the upper reaches of the adductor canal. The chain of deep subinguinal nodes runs superiorly deep to the inguinal ligament to join with the external iliac nodes. A constant node of the deep subinguinal chain lies in the femoral canal at the femoral ring. It is known as the node (or gland) of Cloquet. Communication between the superficial and deep inguinal nodes is via multiple small lymphatics that pierce the fascia cribrosa of the fossa ovalis.

➠ *Enlarged inguinal lymph nodes. When inguinal lymph node enlargement is present, the physician should consider the lower abdomen, the perineum, the external genitalia, the rectum, the lower back, and the lower extremity as possible sources.*

➠ *Differential diagnosis of enlarged subinguinal lymph nodes. Masses in the immediate subin-*

guinal region of the upper anterior thigh may pose a difficult diagnostic problem. The physician should consider a greater saphenous vein varix near the fossa ovalis, psoas abscess, femoral hernia, and suprainguinal adenopathy.

Nerves
(Figs 48–12 to 48–14)

Lying in the superficial tissues of the thigh are cutaneous nerves, most of which are branches of the lumbar plexus. These nerves include the **lateral femoral cutaneous nerve of the thigh** (L2, 3), which gives cutaneous sensation to the lateral thigh; the femoral branch of the **genitofemoral nerve** (L1, 2), which gives cutaneous sensation to the upper anterior thigh; and the **anterior cutaneous branches of the femoral nerve** (L2–4), one of which descends along

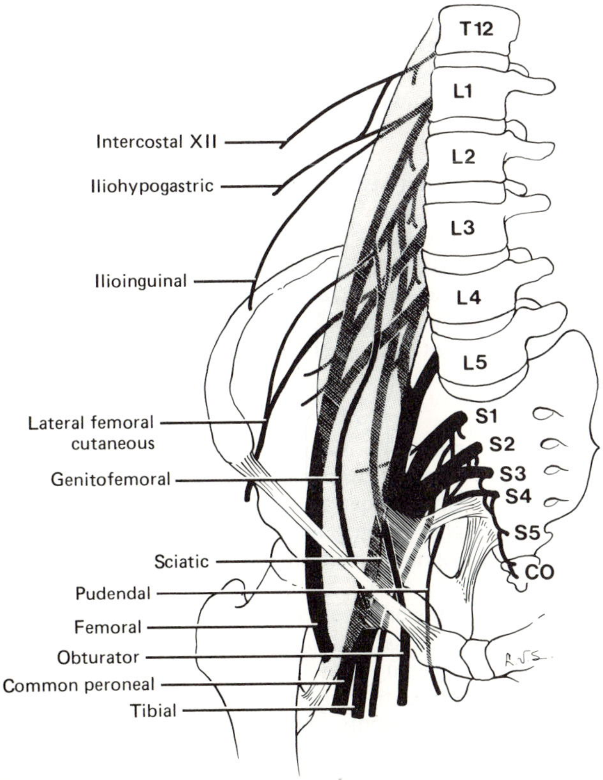

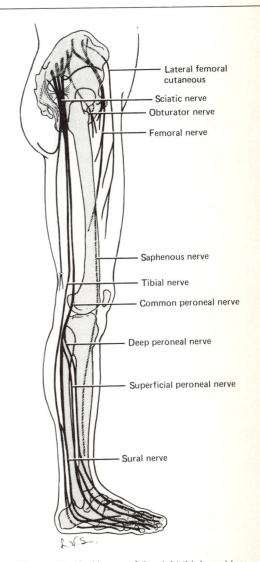

Figure 48–12. The lumbar and sacral plexus.

Figure 48–13. Nerves of the right thigh and leg.

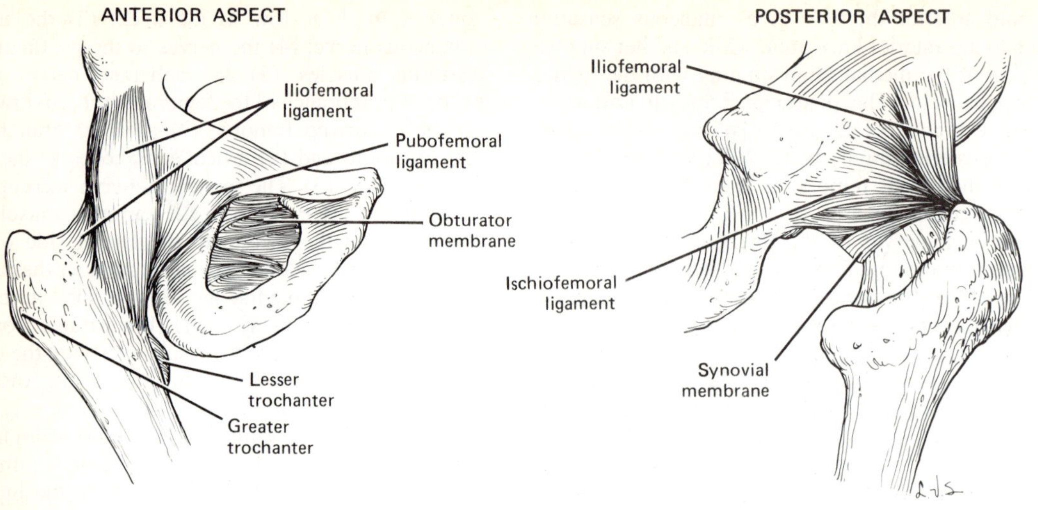

ANTERIOR ASPECT

POSTERIOR ASPECT

Iliofemoral
ligament

Pubofemoral
ligament

Obturator
membrane

Lesser
trochanter

Greater
trochanter

Iliofemoral
ligament

Ischiofemoral
ligament

Synovial
membrane

Figure 48–15. Ligaments of the right hip joint.

labrum and is closely related to the femoral neck. Anteriorly, it is attached to the intertrochanteric line; superiorly, to the base of the neck of the femur; posteriorly, to the femoral neck about 1 cm superior to the intertrochanteric crest; and inferiorly, to the distal segment of the neck close to the lesser trochanter. The capsule is strongest ventrally and proximally. Posteriorly, the capsule tends to hang loosely and is relatively thin. The capsule is supported by the iliofemoral, ischiofemoral, and pubofemoral ligaments. Anteriorly, the articular capsule is separated from the iliopsoas muscle by a bursa that on occasion connects with the cavity of the hip joint. The articular capsule covers only the proximal half of the posterior surface of the femoral neck.

The **iliofemoral ligament** (Y ligament of Bigelow) is an extremely strong band of fibers that lie immediately anterior to the hip joint and are bound tightly to the underlying joint capsule. Superiorly, the ligament attaches to the anteroinferior iliac spine. From this point the ligament runs laterally and inferiorly, dividing into 2 segments. One attaches to the lowermost part of the intertrochanteric line, the other to the most superior part of the same line. Between the 2 distal arms of the ligament, the articular capsule is quite weak.

The **ischiofemoral ligament** arises from the ischium, inferior and posterior to the acetabulum, and blends with the circular capsular fibers both anteriorly and posteriorly. It is roughly triangular.

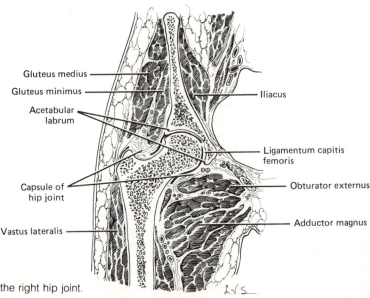

Gluteus medius

Gluteus minimus

Acetabular
labrum

Iliacus

Ligamentum capitis
femoris

Obturator externus

Capsule of
hip joint

Vastus lateralis

Adductor magnus

Figure 48–16. Coronal section through the right hip joint.

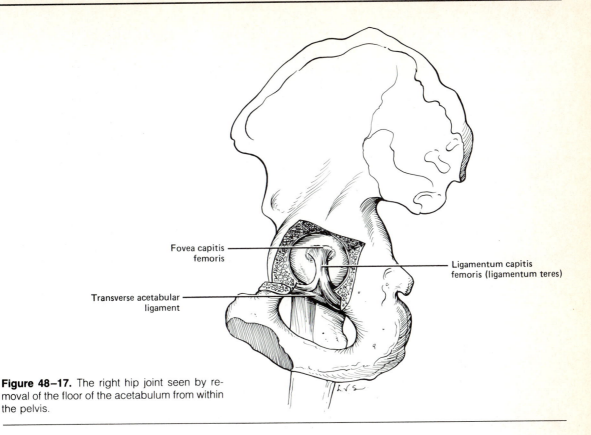

Fovea capitis femoris

Transverse acetabular ligament

Ligamentum capitis femoris (ligamentum teres)

Figure 48–17. The right hip joint seen by removal of the floor of the acetabulum from within the pelvis.

The **pubofemoral ligament** arises from the superior pubic ramus and the obturator crest and joins with the fibers of the iliofemoral ligament and with the joint capsule.

The **ligamentum capitis femoris,** or ligamentum teres, is a flattened band joined by its apex to the fovea capitis femoris and by its bifid base to the sides of the acetabular notch, where it blends with the transverse acetabular ligament (Fig 48–16). It is encased within the synovial membrane of the hip joint. As a joint ligament, it has limited function, tensing when the thigh is partially flexed and externally rotated and relaxing when the thigh is abducted.

The **acetabular labrum** is the partial circular fibrocartilage attached to the external circumference of the acetabulum superiorly and laterally, which deepens the acetabular cavity and protects its bony edges. It is of great importance in assisting the head of the femur to remain within the otherwise shallow acetabulum.

The **transverse acetabular ligament** is a fibrous band that bridges over the acetabular notch, the inferior deficient area of the acetabular labrum (Fig 48–17). It is a ligament, whereas the remainder of the labrum is fibrocartilage.

The capacious **synovial membrane of the hip joint,** starting at the acetabular labrum, envelops that portion of the femoral neck lying within the capsule of the hip joint (Fig 48–18). It lines the internal surface of the joint capsule, both surfaces of the acetabular labrum, and the fatty tissue at the base of the acetabulum; it also covers the ligamentum capitis as it passes to its insertion on the femoral head (Fig 48–19).

➡ *Dislocation of the hip joint. Femoral head dislocations are fairly uncommon, both because of the strong enclosing musculature and because of the capsular thickness and the strength of the intrinsic joint ligaments. Hip dislocations are classified according to the position of the femoral head after dislocation occurs: posterior, anterior, superior, inferior, and medial (intrapelvic).*

➡ *Avascular necrosis of the femoral head. (Fig 48–20.) Disruption of the ligamentum fovea capitis or interruption of the nutrient vessels running to the neck of the femur as a result of hip joint capsular tears may lead to avascular necrosis of the femoral head secondary to its impaired blood supply.*

➡ *Anterior dislocation of the hip joint. In anterior dislocation of the hip joint, the femoral head moves out of the acetabulum through a tear in the anterior segment of the capsule of the joint and passes medial to the strong iliofemoral ligament. The head comes to rest inferior to the os pubis, close to the obturator foramen.*

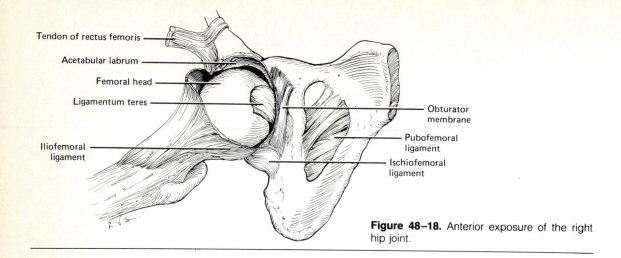

Figure 48–18. Anterior exposure of the right hip joint.

It may injure the adjacent femoral vessels. The patient is placed supine with the knee flexed, and the thigh is flexed. The thigh is then moderately abducted with traction, and the femoral shaft is gently rotated medially. This moves the femoral head from beneath the os pubis or the obturator foramen and brings it in line with the acetabulum for reduction.

▥▶ *Posterior dislocations of the hip joint.* Posterior dislocation of the hip joint tears the joint capsule posteriorly, the tear usually being about the size of the femoral head. In such cases, both the posterior acetabular rim and the ligamentum capitis femoris are likely to be ruptured. The femoral head usually comes to rest upon the ischium or upon the lower third of the ilium. With the patient lying supine, knee flexed, the thigh is flexed upon the abdo-

men and then adducted to deflect the displaced head from the acetabular rim. If the thigh is then rotated superiorly and medially, the femoral head is gradually restored to the acetabulum through the rent in the posterior capsule. Posterior dislocations are frequently accompanied by fracture of the posterior acetabular lip.

▥▶ *Medial or intrapelvic dislocation of the hip joint.* Medial or intrapelvic dislocation of the femoral head is always accompanied by fracture of the acetabular base. The dislocation usually results from application of strong force directly to the femoral head and neck. The accompanying acetabular fractures are usually multiple and radial. One or more of the acetabular fragments may be driven internally in the direction of the pelvis. Rectal and pelvic examinations help establish the degree of cen-

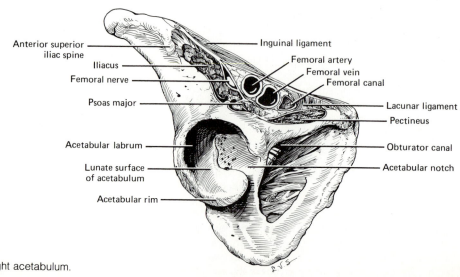

Figure 48–19. The right acetabulum.

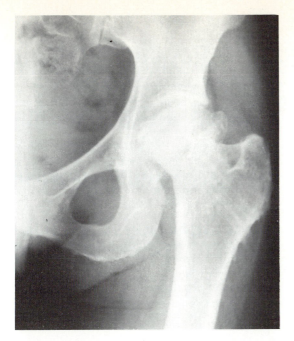

Figure 48–20. Avascular necrosis of the femoral head. (Reproduced, with permission, from Way LW [editor]: *Current Surgical Diagnosis & Treatment,* 7th ed. Lange, 1985.)

tral dislocation of the femoral head. In such dislocations, the bladder may be disrupted; the urine should be checked for blood, and cystograms should be taken. Reduction of central dislocation can usually be achieved by outward traction upon the upper thigh with concurrent downward traction upon the leg. Reduction is maintained with traction through a distal femoral or proximal tibial traction pin.

The hip joint is supplied by branches from the obturator, superior, and inferior gluteal arteries and by a branch from the medial femoral circumflex artery. It receives its nerve supply via articular branches from the sacral plexus. On occasion it receives a twig from the branch of the femoral nerve, which supplies the rectus femoris muscle.

The muscles that lie in relationship to the hip joint are of great clinical importance, particularly because they strengthen the joint but also because they must be considered in planning surgical approaches to the joint. Anterior to the joint are the psoas major and iliacus. Between these 2 muscles and the anterior segment of the joint capsule is a constant bursa. Posterior to the joint are the obturator externus, the 2 gemelli, the obturator internus, and the quadratus femoris. Lateral to the joint are the gluteus minimus and the reflected head of the rectus femoris. Medial to the joint are the pectineus and the obturator externus.

MOVEMENTS OF THE HIP JOINT

The hip joint may be flexed, extended, adducted, abducted, rotated, and circumducted. When the hip joint allows circumduction, the femur circumscribes a conical space. The distal end of the femur is the base of the cone, and the conical apex is the acetabular cavity. Two or more of these movements are often combined. For example, when the thigh is flexed or extended, the femoral head rotates within the acetabulum. This correlation of movements also takes place during abduction and adduction. Unlike the shoulder joint, where there is poor coaptation of the large humeral head to the small glenoid cavity, the head of the femur fits snugly into the acetabular cavity and its surrounding labrum and will remain in that position even after the capsular fibers of the joint are completely divided.

The hip is **flexed** by the iliacus, the psoas major, the tensor fasciae latae, the sartorius, the rectus femoris, the pectineus, the adductors longus and brevis, and the most anterior fibers of the gluteus medius and minimus.

Extension of the hip is carried out chiefly by the gluteus maximus with some assistance from the 3 hamstring muscles.

Adduction of the hip is performed by the 3 adductors, the gracilis, and the pectineus.

Abduction of the hip is performed by the gluteus medius and minimus.

Internal rotation of the thigh is performed by the gluteus minimus, the tensor fasciae latae, all 3 adductors, the pectineus, the psoas major, and the iliacus.

External rotation is performed by the gluteus medius, the piriformis, the 2 obturators and the 2 gemelli, the quadratus femoris, the sartorius, and the gluteus maximus.

Circumduction is accomplished by the combined action of the hip rotators, abductors, and adductors.

I. THE KNEE JOINT

GROSS ANATOMY
(Figs 49–1 and 49–2)

The knee joint, the largest joint of the body, executes a complex group of motions calling for flexion, extension, rotation, and fixation. The joint occupies a superficial position between the thigh and the leg, and its bony parts form a somewhat unstable articular mechanism. Stability is increased by the action of strong extrinsic ligaments and by the tendinous expansions of neighboring muscle groups.

The 2 condyles that make up the lower end of the femur articulate with the 2 tibial condyles and their covering menisci to establish the femorotibial articulation. The patella, a sesamoid bone situated in the inferior segment of the quadriceps femoris tendon, articulates with the patellar surface of the femur, which lies between the 2 femoral condyles on the anteroinferior surface of that bone.

The distal epiphysis of the femur, one of 5 femoral epiphyses, is the first to appear (in the ninth month of fetal life) and the last to be joined to the body of the femur (in the mid 20th year of life).

The knee joint is generally regarded as a ginglymus (hinge) joint, but it is actually a complex of 3 separate joints: (1) a condyloid articulation between each femoral condyle and the meniscus and the related condyle of the tibia, and (2) a single articulation of the partial arthrodial type between the dorsal surface of the patella and the femur. Some animals have knee joints with 3 separate synovial cavities, and in some early stage of phylogenetic development, humans may have had tripartite knee joints.

➠ *Relatively unstable articulation. Despite the presence of strong extrinsic and intrinsic ligaments supporting the joint and its close relationship to strong covering musculature, the knee joint is relatively weak and unstable, largely because of the inexact apposition of its bones.*

Injuries that involve one or more of the joint ligaments or cartilages are therefore often associated with injuries to the femur, tibia, or patella.

➠ *Quadriceps femoris and knee joint function. Unless the tone and strength of this muscle group are maintained, no reparative surgical procedure upon the knee joint structures will be completely satisfactory. Early physiotherapy to the quadriceps following knee joint surgery is thus of great importance.*

➠ *Genu valgum and genu varum. Irregular bony ossification and growth near the distal femoral epiphysis, with abnormal downgrowth of the medial femoral diaphysis, results in genu valgum (knock knee). The foot is everted and flattened (talipes valgus). The deformity can usually be corrected by femoral osteotomy. Genu varum (bowleg) usually occurs as a result of overgrowth of the entire distal femoral epiphysis. Both deformities may occur as manifestations of rickets; genu valgum may also occur as a complication of poliomyelitis.*

KNEE JOINT MOVEMENTS

The movements with the greatest range are flexion and extension, though with the knee in 60–90 degrees of flexion medial and lateral rotation are possible. Flexion and extension at the knee are accompanied by a shift of the axis around which these movements occur—anteriorly during extension and posteriorly during flexion.

At the conclusion of full extension, the knee is locked by medial rotation of the femur. When flexion is initiated from a position of full extension, the femur rotates externally to unlock the knee.

The **patella,** or kneecap, is a flattened, roughly triangular bone lying just anterior to the knee joint. Most anatomists describe it as a sesamoid bone, since it lies within the quadriceps femoris tendon. It is composed of thick cancellous bone covered by a thin but dense external lamina. Its ventral surface is slightly convex and is covered by a thin layer of fibrous tissue derived from the tendon of the quadriceps femoris muscle. This fibrous covering passes inferior to the patella to join with the fibers of the

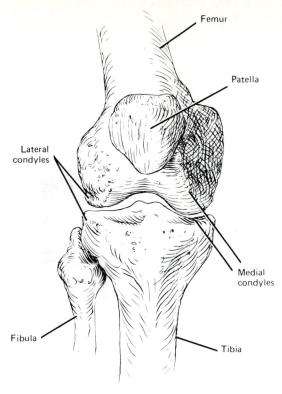

Figure **49–1.** Anterior view of right knee.

ligamentum patellae. The anterior surface of the patella is separated from the skin by a subcutaneous prepatellar bursa. The dorsal patellar surface is a smooth, almost circular area that articulates with the femur, divided into 2 segments by a vertical linear ridge. The lateral articular segment is the wider and deeper of the 2 posterior segments. Inferior to the articular surface of the patella is a roughened nonarticular area whose distal segment gives attachment to the ligamentum patellae. A plug of fatty tissue, the infrapatellar fat pad, separates the nonarticular distal posterior surface of the patella from the superior surface of the tibia.

➠ ***Osteochondritis of the cartilage on the dorsal surface of the patella.*** *Osteochondritis of the articular cartilage on the dorsal surface of the patella occurs frequently, and roughening of the cartilage interferes with knee joint movement and usually causes pain in the patellar area on movement of the joint. Chips of cartilage from the dorsal surface of the patella as well as from the articular surfaces of the femur are on occasion cast off into the knee joint cavity. This can result in painful internal derangements of the knee joint and "lock" the joint. "Locking" denotes inability to fully extend the knee. Even though locked, the knee usually can be flexed past 90 degrees.*

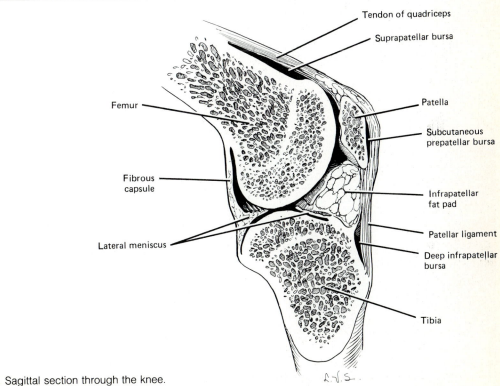

Figure **49–2.** Sagittal section through the knee.

➠ *Arthrography of the knee. The knee joint is usually aspirated or its cavity injected by placement of a needle just lateral or medial to the central infrapatellar area. Air or oxygen and contrast medium are injected into the joint, and x-rays are taken. X-rays are especially helpful in the diagnosis of meniscal tears.*

➠ *Test for knee joint effusion. Pressure upon the patella against the anterior surface of the femur will usually disclose the presence of joint effusion fluid. If there is an effusion, the patella seems to float upon the underlying femur.*

The patella protects the anterior segment of the knee joint and increases the mechanical efficiency of the quadriceps femoris muscle by increasing its angle of pull during quadriceps contraction. When the knee is fully flexed, the medial portion of the medial articular facet of the patella comes into opposition with the curved area on the edge of the medial femoral condyle. When the leg shifts from flexion to extension, the 3 horizontal facets on the posterior patellar surface, starting with the superior facet, are brought into apposition with the patellar area of the femur. When the leg is fully extended, the patella lies in a position that places it directly upon the terminal segment of the femur.

➠ *Patellar fractures. (Fig 49–3.) The patella may be fractured either alone or in combination with fractures of one or more of the other bones of the lower extremity. The fracture is usually of the simple transverse type, which can be repaired, but it may be comminuted and displaced, requiring complete removal of the bone (patellectomy) in order to permit full knee joint movement.*

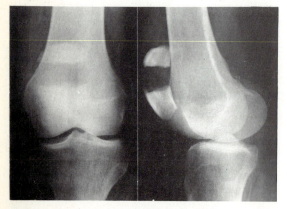

Figure 49–3. Transverse fracture of the patella. (Reproduced, with permission, from Way LW [editor]: *Current Surgical Diagnosis & Treatment,* 7th ed. Lange, 1985.)

LIGAMENTS OF THE KNEE JOINT
(Figs 49–4 and 49–5)

The 3 bones that make up the knee joint are bound together by a combination of 11 ligaments. The **articular capsule** (capsular ligament) is a thin sheet of fibrous tissue that loosely surrounds the joint. It is reinforced over almost its entire circumference by fibrous offshoots that arise from the tendinous structures adjoining the joint and by a reinforcing band running from the fascia lata of the thigh to the anterior segment of the capsule. Deep to the tendon of the quadriceps femoris, the capsule is missing; this allows the suprapatellar bursa to communicate directly with the knee joint. Posteriorly, the joint capsule is well supported by the oblique popliteal ligament.

The **patellar ligament** consists of the mid segment of the tendon of the quadriceps femoris muscle. The ligament is strong and dense and 7–10 cm in length. It is connected superiorly to the rounded apical superior surface of the patella and inferiorly to the protruding tibial tuberosity. Its deep surface is separated from the knee joint synovia by the infrapatellar fat pad, and the ligament is separated from the superior surface of the tibia by the deep infrapatellar bursa.

The **oblique popliteal ligament** arises from the superior border of the intercondylar fossa of the femur and inserts into the dorsal surface of the head of the tibia. The popliteal artery lies just dorsal to the ligament as the vessel passes into the upper leg.

The **arcuate popliteal ligament** is a short triangular band that leaves its base on the lateral condyle of the femur to run inferiorly and laterally toward its apex, which is attached to both the dorsal surface of the capsular ligament and the styloid process of the head of the fibula, to which it is joined by a pair of fibrous ligaments.

The **tibial collateral ligament** is wider and thinner than the fibular collateral ligament. It is attached superiorly to the medial condyle of the femur and inferiorly to the medial condyle and the superior medial surface of the tibia. The band is tightly connected to the medial border of the medial meniscus of the knee joint. The ligament lies in a more posterior position with regard to the vertical axis of the joint than does the fibular collateral ligament.

The **fibular collateral ligament** is attached superiorly to the dorsal surface of the lateral femoral condyle and inferiorly to the lateral side of the head of the fibula. It is masked by the covering tendon of the biceps femoris. Unlike the tibial collateral ligament, it is not attached to the adjacent meniscus of the knee joint.

The knee joint possesses 2 **cruciate ligaments** that cross in the fashion of the 2 arms of the letter X. Their names, anterior and posterior, are derived from their sites of attachment on the superior plateau of the tibia (Fig 49–5).

The **anterior cruciate ligament** is attached just anterior to the intercondylar eminence of the tibia, closely related to the anterior horn of the lateral menis-

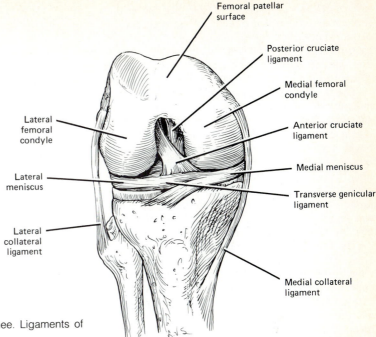

Figure 49–4. The fully flexed right knee. Ligaments of the knee joint.

cus. It inclines superiorly, laterally, and dorsally to attach to the medial side of the lateral condyle of the femur. Its inferior site of origin shows a minor attachment to the anterior margin of the medial meniscus.

The **posterior cruciate ligament** is shorter, straighter, and thicker than the anterior cruciate. It arises from the dorsal surface of the intercondylar fossa of the tibia and from the dorsal edge of the lateral meniscus. It passes superiorly, ventrally, and slightly medially to insert into the medial femoral condyle.

The **transverse ligament** connects the anterior margins of the 2 menisci.

The **coronary ligaments** are derived from the capsular ligament of the joint and serve to connect the edges of the menisci to the adjacent edges of the plateau of the tibia.

THE MENISCI
(Fig 49–5)

The menisci are 2 crescent-shaped fibrocartilages situated on the articular surfaces of the tibia. They deepen the tibial articular surfaces, and thus allow them to articulate more securely with the femoral condyles. This increases knee joint stability. The outer

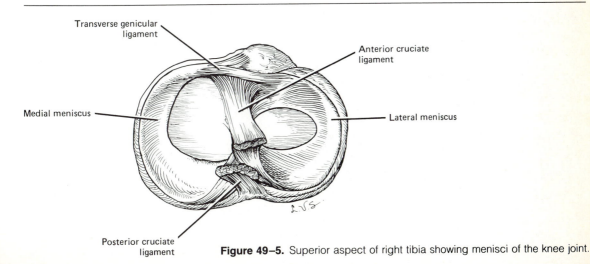

Figure 49–5. Superior aspect of right tibia showing menisci of the knee joint.

surface of each meniscus is thicker than the medial surface and is attached directly to the deep surface of the joint capsule. The inner (medial) border of each meniscus appears as an unattached thin edge. The superior surfaces of each meniscus are concave, while the inferior surface is flat on the tibial surface.

The **medial meniscus** is larger and forms about three-fourths of a circle. It is wider posteriorly than anteriorly. Its thin anterior horn is fixed to the anterior intercondylar fossa of the tibia, anterior to the origin of the anterior cruciate ligament. Its posterior horn is attached to the posterior intercondylar fossa of the tibia, just anterior to the attachment of the posterior cruciate ligament. The meniscus is tightly attached to the inner surface of the tibial collateral ligament, and injury to the ligament nearly always results in tears of the medial meniscus.

The **lateral meniscus** forms an almost complete circle and is smaller and more mobile than the medial meniscus. It is attached just beyond the intercondylar eminences of the tibia. Its anterior attachment blends with the anterior cruciate ligament, while the posterior attachment blends with the posterior cruciate ligament. It is separated from the fibular collateral ligament by the tendon of the popliteal muscle and as a consequence is less prone to injury in association with collateral ligament injury than is the medial meniscus. A strong fibrous band, the ligament of Wrisberg, is derived from its dorsal attachment. The band passes superiorly and laterally to attach to the medial condyle of the femur.

➠ *Sports injuries to the collateral ligaments and the menisci. Injury to the medial meniscus and to the attached tibial collateral ligament is the most common internal derangement of the knee joint. Injuries to the lateral collateral ligaments are less common and usually do not involve lateral meniscus injury. Simple suture repair usually is all that is needed in a lateral ligament tear.*

➠ *Pain on pressure over the lateral border of a meniscus. Spot tenderness when pressure is exerted upon the lateral border of a meniscus suggests injury to the underlying fibrocartilage. Arthrograms and direct arthroscopic visualization of the knee joint are of help both in diagnosis and in treatment.*

➠ *Serous or bloody effusions. Effusions following knee joint derangements may be evacuated (by aspiration) to allow for proper joint examination.*

➠ *Abnormal mobility. Lateral, medial, or anteroposterior abnormal mobility when the knee joint is forced into varus or valgus suggests contusion or tear of a collateral ligament. Abnormal dor-*

sal or ventral mobility following the diagnostic maneuver of ventral or dorsal thrust of the joint suggests cruciate ligament tear or weakness.

THE SYNOVIAL MEMBRANE OF THE KNEE JOINT

The synovial membrane of the knee joint is the most capacious and complex synovial joint of the body. Generally, the synovium of the knee joint lines the inner surface of the articular capsule except for an area dorsal to the tendon of the quadriceps femoris. In this subquadriceps position, the synovium presents as a large sac placed directly over the distal anterior segment of the femur, the sac usually communicating with a bursa between the quadriceps tendon and the femur. The synovial membrane attaches to the articular margins of the patella. Lateral and medial to the patella, the synovium spreads beneath the fascial terminations of the vasti; inferior to the patella, the synovium is separated from the patellar tendon by a large fat pad. From each of the lateral borders of the deep surface of the patella, a fold of synovium, the alar fold, projects into the cavity of the knee joint. The alar folds coalesce near the inferior margin of the joint to form a single patellar fold that passes inferiorly to attach to the intercondylar fossa of the femur. The synovial membrane attaches to the peripheral margins of the menisci. Since the synovium is reflected over only the anterior surfaces of the cruciate ligaments, these 2 structures do not lie within the synovial cavity of the joint.

BURSAE OF THE KNEE JOINT (Fig 49-6)

There are multiple areas of friction between the bones of the knee joint and its many surrounding muscles, tendons, and ligaments, and about 14 bursae of varying size placed about the joint assist in reducing wear and tear on the periarticular muscular and tendinous structures. These bursae range in size from the large subcutaneous bursa between the patella and the skin to multiple smaller bursae situated laterally and medially about the tibial and fibular collateral ligaments and the muscle bellies, tendons, and bony structures adjacent to these ligaments. The bursa between the quadriceps tendon and the lower end of the femur usually connects with the cavity of the knee joint.

➠ *Bursitis. The bursae around the knee joint often become inflamed secondary to infection or chronic mechanical irritation. The superficial prepatellar bursa is most commonly involved.*

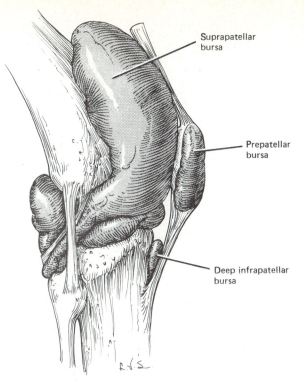

Figure 49–6. Bursae of the right knee joint.

RELATIONSHIPS OF THE KNEE JOINT (Figs 49–7 and 49–8)

The knee joint is related to the following structures: (1) ventrally, medially, and laterally, to components of the quadriceps femoris extensor apparatus; (2) laterally, to the biceps femoris tendon and the popliteal tendon; (3) medially, to the semimembranous, semitendinous, gracilis, and sartorius muscles; and (4) dorsally, to the popliteal vessels, the tibial and common peroneal nerves, the popliteal muscle, the 2 heads of the gastrocnemius muscle, the plantaris muscle, considerable fat, and a few scattered popliteal lymph nodes.

BLOOD VESSELS, LYMPHATICS, & NERVES (Figs 49–9 and 49–10)

Arteries & Veins

The knee joint is supplied by the descending genicular branch of the femoral artery, the multiple genicular branches of the popliteal artery, a descending branch of the lateral femoral circumflex artery, and ascending genicular branches from the anterior tibial artery. Venous return from the knee joint follows the arterial pathways to empty eventually into the common femoral vein.

Lymphatics

The lymphatics of the knee joint are situated mainly in the adjacent subcutaneous fascia. They proceed to join the superficial subinguinal group of nodes. There is a moderate degree of lymphatic drainage into the popliteal lymph nodes, whence the lymph passes alongside the femoral vessels to the deep inguinal nodes.

Nerves

The nerve supply to the knee joint is via branches of those nerves that supply the muscles around the joint and control their movements. They are derived from the obturator, femoral, and sciatic nerves. Since these same nerves also supply the hip joint, the clinician must be wary of referred pain from the hip joint to the knee secondary to hip joint disease.

➡ *Dislocations of the knee joint.* (*Fig 49–11.*) *Dislocation of the knee joint usually occurs only as a result of severe direct trauma. Subluxation occasionally occurs secondary to longstanding degenerative or infectious disease of the joint. The tibia may be dislocated ventrally, dorsally, or to either side, or it may be abnormally rotated upon the femur. The usual mechanism of knee joint dislocation is via hyperextension and torsion. Acute dislocation is frequently accompanied by injury to the vessels or nerves in the popliteal space.*

➡ *Surgical approaches to the knee joint. The knee joint is usually approached surgically by one of 3 classic incisions. The **median parapatellar approach** starts with a cutaneous incision that courses inferiorly along the medial border of the quadratus femoris, from the superior border along the medial border of the patella to the tibial tuberosity. The rectus femoris and vastus medialis muscles are separated, and the patella is retracted laterally. This exposes the joint capsule, which is then incised in order to gain entrance into the joint.*

*The **lateral parapatellar approach** starts at the proximal pole of the patella and curves around its lateral margin to the tibial tuberosity. It is easy to develop the incision down to the joint capsule and obtain good joint exposure.*

*The **posterior or popliteal approach** begins with an incision over the lateral border of the popliteal space. The incision is continued over the lateral head of the gastrocnemius. The 2 heads of the gastrocnemius are then carefully retracted so as not to injure vessels or nerves in the popliteal space. This incision is used in the treatment of popliteal aneurysms and for procedures aimed at relief of mid and lower leg vascular insufficiency.*

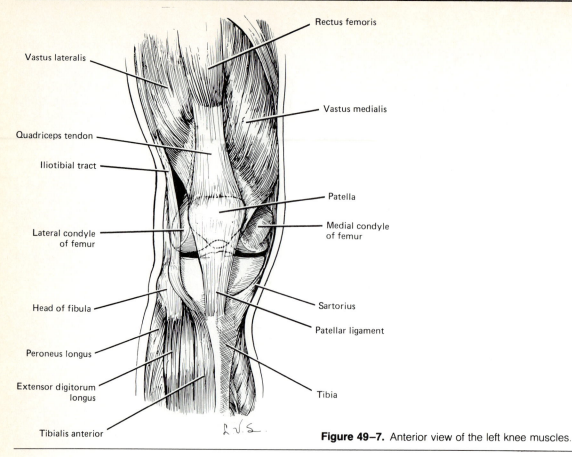

Rectus femoris

Vastus lateralis

Vastus medialis

Quadriceps tendon

Iliotibial tract

Patella

Lateral condyle
of femur

Medial condyle
of femur

Head of fibula

Sartorius

Peroneus longus

Patellar ligament

Extensor digitorum
longus

Tibialis anterior

Tibia

Figure 49–7. Anterior view of the left knee muscles.

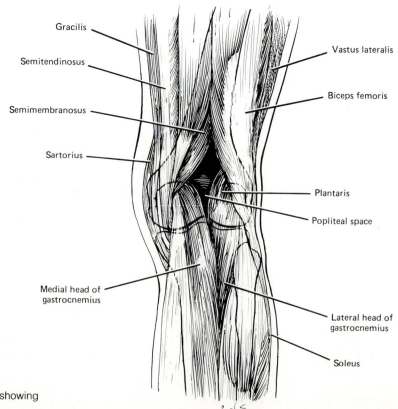

Gracilis

Vastus lateralis

Semitendinosus

Semimembranosus

Biceps femoris

Sartorius

Plantaris

Popliteal space

Medial head of
gastrocnemius

Lateral head of
gastrocnemius

Soleus

Figure 49–8. Right popliteal fossa showing
muscle relationships.

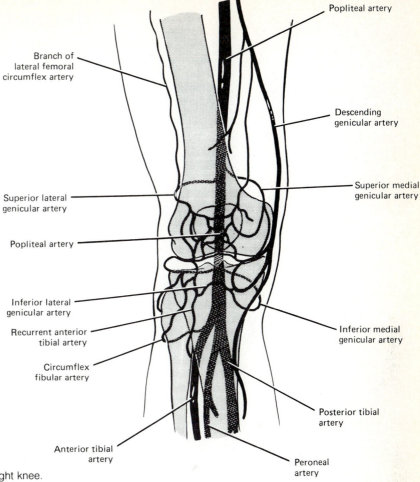

Figure 49–9. Arteries of the right knee.

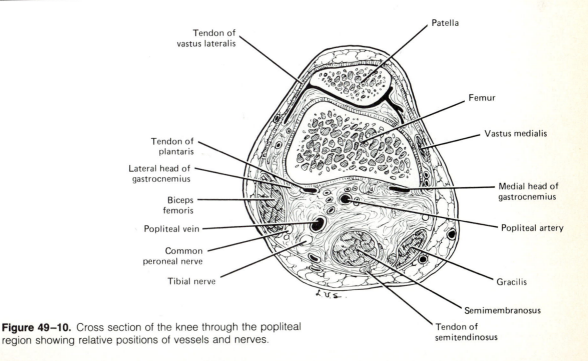

Figure 49–10. Cross section of the knee through the popliteal region showing relative positions of vessels and nerves.

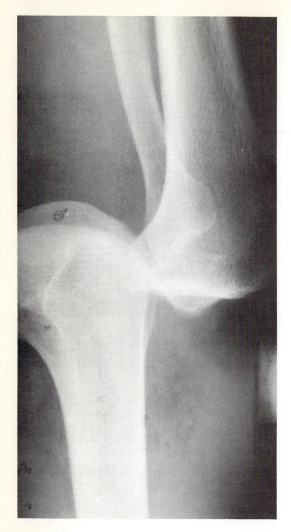

Figure 49–11. Complete closed dislocation of the knee joint in a 28-year-old man.

To approach the knee joint **posteriorly**, *an S-shaped incision is made beginning medially 8–10 cm superior to the flexion crease, proceeding transversely across the flexion crease and continuing laterally and inferiorly for 8–10 cm.*

➠ ***"Total knee" arthroplasty.*** *This consists of removing all intrinsic ligamentous and cartilaginous structures and replacing them with an artificial joint prosthesis. The procedure is indicated for patients with degenerative disease and posttraumatic arthritis.*

➠ ***The septic knee joint.*** *A septic knee joint may follow surgery upon the joint, infection around the joint, or blood-borne infection. Several bursae about the knee communicate with the knee joint, and infectious bursitis may spread to the*

knee joint. *Treatment consists of drainage and antibiotic drugs.*

➠ ***Tuberculosis of the knee joint.*** *Tuberculosis of the knee joint may follow infection of the joint via the bloodstream or may result from direct extension of tuberculosis from infection in the diaphysis of an adjacent bone. As a result of the chronic progressive granulomatous process in the joint, the knee assumes a fixed flexion deformity.*

➠ ***Arthroscopy in diagnosis and treatment of knee joint disease.*** *The arthroscope allows good visualization of the interior of the knee joint and provides access for correction of internal derangements without opening the joint widely. Its use in selected cases has cut down both hospital time and time of postoperative convalescence.*

II. THE POPLITEAL (POSTERIOR) KNEE REGION

GROSS ANATOMY (Fig 49–12)

The popliteal fossa, posterior to the knee joint, is composed of a superior femoral triangle and an inferior tibial triangle. It exhibits a floor, a roof, and lateral and medial boundaries.

Upon flexion of the knee, the popliteal space appears merely as a transverse hollow slit. In full extension of the knee, however, the diamond-shaped fossa becomes apparent, the area bulging dorsally because of the presence of fat lying just deep to its fascial roof.

➠ ***Palpation with the knee in semiflexion.*** *The contents of the popliteal fossa are palpated most effectively with the knee in semiflexion to relax the dense fascia roofing the area. Many disorders cause a swelling of the popliteal space, usually well contained by the strong roofing of popliteal fascia dorsally and by the femur and the tibia and fibula ventrally.*

The popliteal fossa is roofed dorsally by the deep strong fascia lata of the thigh, whose fibers are arranged in an almost circular pattern. The fascial roof

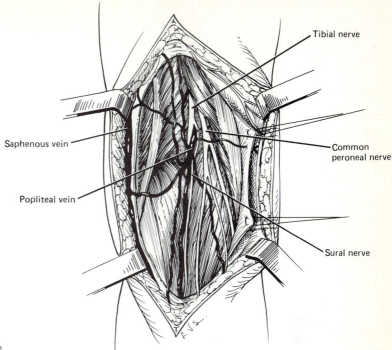

Figure 49–12. Popliteal knee region.

serves as a containing ligament for the hamstring muscles. The roof is pierced by the lesser saphenous vein as it turns ventrally, and the 2 converging heads of the gastrocnemius muscle cross the vein just before it empties into the popliteal vein deep within the fossa. The floor of the fossa is formed by the popliteal surface of the femur, the oblique popliteal ligament of the knee joint, the posterior segment of the knee joint capsule, and the popliteal muscle, with its strong covering fascia. The superior lateral boundary of the fossa is formed by the tendon of the biceps femoris muscle, while the superior medial boundary is formed by the tendons of the semimembranous and semitendinous muscles. The medial and lateral heads of the gastrocnemius muscle form the inferior medial and lateral borders of the area.

➭ *Popliteal cysts (Baker's cysts). Following a large knee joint effusion, the joint synovium occasionally herniates dorsally through the posterior segment of the joint capsule. In such cases, a fluctuant mass (Baker's cyst) becomes palpable deep to the roofing fascia of the area. Aspiration of the mass will show the presence of synovial fluid. Cysts impair flexion and extension and must be removed to restore full knee joint function.*

The popliteal muscle forms most of the inferior portion of the floor of the popliteal fossa. It is a narrow and roughly triangular band whose apex arises from the lateral condyle of the femur. The muscle inserts into the medial aspect of the posterior surface of the tibia. It is covered dorsally by a strong fascia derived from the tendon of the semimembranous muscle. The popliteal vessels lie upon the dorsal surface of the popliteal fascia covering the muscle. The popliteal artery bifurcates close to the lower border of the muscle.

BLOOD VESSELS, LYMPHATICS, & NERVES (Figs 49–10 and 49–12)

The popliteal fossa contains nerves, arteries, veins, considerable fat, and some lymph nodes.

Arteries

The **popliteal artery** leaves the adductor canal as the continuation of the femoral artery, and enters the popliteal space, lying halfway between the 2 femoral condyles. The artery runs the full length of the popliteal fossa to the lower border of the popliteal muscle, where it divides into the anterior and posterior tibial arteries. The popliteal artery is the deepest structure occupying the popliteal fossa. While passing inferiorly in the space, the artery gives off 5 genicular branches all of which enter into the arterial anastomoses between genicular branches of the popliteal, anterior tibial, lateral femoral circumflex, and femoral arteries. When the popliteal artery is ligated, blood is shunted to the lower limb from the femoral artery via the genicular anastomosis. The popliteal artery is separated from the bony dorsal surface of the femur and the posterior segment of the knee joint capsule by a thick pad of fat. Lying between the artery and the strong, thick popliteal fascia covering the dorsum of the popliteal space are its venae comitantes and the tibial nerve.

⟱ *Popliteal aneurysms. The popliteal space is a common site of popliteal arterial aneurysms. A pulsating popliteal mass with a palpable thrill and an audible bruit assists in diagnosis.*

⟱ *Popliteal arteriovenous fistula. Due to the proximity within the popliteal fossa of the popliteal artery and vein, posttraumatic arteriovenous fistulas between the 2 vessels can occur. They embarrass the circulation to the leg and foot and must be corrected by vascular surgery to provide adequate circulation to the inferior half of the lower limb. If present over a long period of time, they can contribute to cardiac decompensation.*

⟱ *Varix of the lesser saphenous vein in the popliteal space. The presence of a large varix of the lesser saphenous vein, close to its termination in the popliteal vein, must be considered in the differential diagnosis of a popliteal space mass.*

Veins

The **popliteal vein** begins at the lower border of the popliteal muscle as a result of the junction of the deep leg veins that accompany the anterior and posterior tibial arteries. It runs through the popliteal space to enter the adductor hiatus in the lower thigh and become the superficial femoral vein. The vein crosses the popliteal fossa from lateral to medial. Its main tributary in the fossa is the lesser saphenous vein. The popliteal vein and artery are bound together by a common fascial covering. The popliteal vein lies at first superficial and central to the artery but later it comes to lie medial to and on the same plane as the artery. The common fascial envelope must be dissected free in order to separate the 2 vessels from each other when vascular surgery is performed in the area.

The **lesser saphenous vein** runs from the ankle to the knee superficial to the deep fascia of the mid posterior calf. It enters the popliteal space by piercing the covering dorsal fascia. The vein divides into 2 branches; one branch enters the space to join the popliteal vein, while the second branch runs medially to join with the greater saphenous vein. A valve is always present in the lesser saphenous vein just proximal to its entrance into the popliteal vein.

Lymphatics

Lymphatic drainage into the popliteal space from the leg, ankle, and foot terminates in a group of nodes that lie deep to the covering fascia of the area. The popliteal efferents bring lymph from the knee joint, the skin of the lateral aspect of the leg and foot, and from some deep areas of the foot. The efferent lymphatics from the popliteal nodes accompany the popliteal vessels and then the femoral vessels. They terminate eventually in the deep subinguinal lymph nodes.

Nerves

The **tibial nerve,** the larger division of the sciatic nerve, lies in a relatively superficial position in the popliteal fossa. It enters the space at its superior apex, lateral to the popliteal vessels, and then runs to the lower border of the space, in a plane superficial to both the popliteal artery and vein. As the nerve runs inferiorly, it crosses both major vessels from lateral to medial. It supplies the 2 gastrocnemius heads, the popliteus, the soleus, and the plantaris. Since only one branch of the nerve comes off its medial side while it is traversing the popliteal space, the medial side is preferred for dissection of the nerve. The sural nerve leaves the tibial nerve in the popliteal fossa and runs inferiorly on the superficial surface of the calf muscles to supply the skin of the dorsum of the leg. The nerve lies close to the course of the lesser saphenous vein.

The **common or lateral peroneal nerve** is the other terminal branch of the sciatic nerve. Usually given off in the thigh—but occasionally in the superior triangle of the popliteal fossa—it enters the fossa lateral to the tibial nerve and moves farther laterally as it descends. It leaves the lateral margin of the fossa between the medial edge of the biceps femoris tendon and the lateral head of the gastrocnemius. It reaches the fibular head and then twists around the neck of that bone. It ends beneath the deep surface of the peroneus longus muscle by dividing into the superficial and deep peroneal nerves. It gives off no muscular branches in the popliteal fossa, but it sends small branches to the knee joint. The common peroneal nerve gives off the lateral cutaneous nerve of the calf and the sural anastomotic nerve. The common peroneal nerve is vulnerable to trauma because of its superficial position at the neck of the fibula. The sural anastomotic nerve joins the sural nerve and gives sensory innervation to the lateral aspect of the dorsum of the foot.

⟱ *Tibial nerve pain with popliteal aneurysms. The tibial nerve lies just superficial to the popliteal vessels, and a popliteal aneurysm, as it enlarges, may stretch the nerve. Pain in such* cases is usually referred down the dorsal surface of the calf of the leg.

⟹ ***Lateral peroneal nerve and trauma to the head and neck of the fibula.*** *In its superficial position at the head and neck of the fibula, both the common peroneal nerve and its lateral branch are particularly vulnerable to direct blows upon the upper lateral leg that drive the nerve against the bony fibula. Posttraumatic nerve palsy may result. Fractures of the neck and head of the fibula may involve the lateral peroneal nerve in the callus of their repair, also causing peroneal nerve palsy ("footdrop").*

50

The Leg

GROSS ANATOMY

THE TIBIA
(Fig 50–1)

The tibia, the second-longest bone of the body, is situated on the medial side of the leg. It consists of a central body and 2 expanded ends. The superior end articulates with the femur; the inferior end forms the superior medial segment of the ankle joint mortise as it articulates with the talus.

The widened superior end of the tibia shows a medial and a lateral condyle, and the superior surface of each is covered by an articular facet. The medial facet is oval, while the lateral facet is round. The mid segment of each facet articulates with the adjacent femoral condyle, and laterally it gives attachment also to a cartilaginous meniscus of the knee joint. Between the 2 articular surfaces of the tibia is the intercondylar eminence, which is crested both laterally and medially by a tubercle. Lying both anterior and posterior to the eminence are shallow pits for the attachments of the cruciate ligaments and for attachment of the menisci to the tibial condyles.

The ventral proximal surface of the tibia has a quadrangular elevation, the tibial tuberosity, to which the patellar ligament is attached. A bursa just superior to the tuberosity lies between the patellar ligament and the anteroposterior surface of the tibia. The center of the surface of the medial tibial condyle exhibits a transverse notch for attachment of the semimembranous tendon. The medial edge of the medial tibial condyle gives attachment to the tibial collateral ligament. Posteriorly and superiorly, the lateral tibial condyle shows a flattened facet with which the head of the fibula articulates.

➠ ***"Plateau" fractures of the superior end of the tibia.*** *Fractures of the superior segment of the tibia often show a depression of one of the fragments of the superior tibial margin ("plateau fracture"). The depressed fragment must be properly reduced in order to preserve the anatomic transverse level of the tibial articulating surface without which the normal range of knee joint movement is markedly restricted.*

➠ ***Osgood-Schlatter disease.*** *Chronic epiphysitis of the tibial tuberosity is an occasional occurrence in young adults. There is pain in the upper anterior leg and tenderness on pressure over the tuberosity. It is only moderately disabling and usually corrects itself by age 20. X-ray shows a poorly attached superior tibial epiphysis.*

The shaft of the tibia has 3 borders and 3 surfaces. The anterior border is easily palpable in an immediate subcutaneous position. The anterior border begins at the inferior margin of the tibial tuberosity, and it terminates by becoming the anterior margin of the medial malleolus. The deep fascia of the leg attaches to the anterior tibial border. The medial border of the tibia is rounded and most easily palpable over the mid portion of the shaft. It begins at the border of the medial condyle and runs inferiorly to the posterior margin of the medial malleolus. The tibial collateral ligament inserts into the superior segment of the medial border of the tibia, and the soleus and flexor digitorum longus arise in part from its mid third. The lateral border of the tibia is quite thin. It gives attachment to the interosseous membrane. It begins at the facet for the superior tibial fibular articulation, and in its downward course it splits into 2 divisions to form a roughened triangular area into which the interosseous ligament inserts.

The medial surface of the tibia is quite wide. Its superior third lies deep to a fascial sheet that develops from a junction of the tendons of the sartorius, gracilis, and semitendinosus muscles. The lower two-thirds of the medial tibial surface is subcutaneous.

The lateral surface of the tibia is not as wide as the medial surface, and its superior half shows a depressed area covered by the tibialis anterior muscle. Proximally, the posterior tibial surface shows the elevated soleal line. The popliteal muscle inserts into an area just superior to the line, and segments of the soleus, flexor digitorum longus, and tibialis posterior arise from the line. The inferior third of the posterior surface is rounded and is covered by the flexor muscles of the foot.

The distal end of the tibia is less massive than the proximal end. The medial surface of the tibia terminates distally as a thick triangular bony protuberance, the medial malleolus. The medial surface of the malleolus is rounded and easily palpable, since

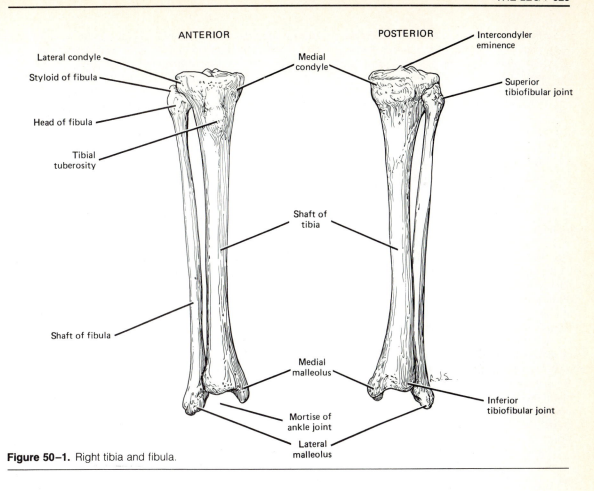

ANTERIOR

POSTERIOR

Lateral condyle

Styloid of fibula

Head of fibula

Tibial
tuberosity

Medial
condyle

Intercondyler
eminence

Superior
tibiofibular joint

Shaft of
tibia

Shaft of fibula

Medial
malleolus

Inferior
tibiofibular joint

Mortise of
ankle joint

Lateral
malleolus

Figure 50–1. Right tibia and fibula.

it is subcutaneous. The deltoid ligament of the ankle joint is attached to the inferior surface of the medial malleolus, and the posterior malleolar border contains a groove for the passage toward the foot of the tendons of the flexor digitorum longus and the tibialis posterior muscles. The lateral inferior surface of the tibia is concave, and its most inferior segment articulates with the fibula.

The distal end of the tibia articulates directly with the talus, forming the medial segment of the ankle joint mortise. The anteroinferior surface is smooth superiorly but roughened inferiorly, where it gives attachment to the articular capsule of the ankle joint. The anteroinferior surface is closely related to the extensor muscles of the foot, which pass directly anterior to it. The posteroinferior surface of the tibia is grooved for the passage of the tendon of the flexor hallucis longus.

⇒ *Open fractures of the tibia and fibula. Since both bones lie close to the skin, fractures are often of the open type, with consequent possibility of infection and delayed union.*

THE FIBULA
(Fig 50–1)

The fibula, situated lateral to the tibia, is a much smaller and more delicate bone. It appears just below the level of the knee joint, in which its superior surface plays no part. Its superior part lies on a slightly more posterior plane than the tibia, but farther distally it reaches the same plane as the tibia, and this relationship is maintained as the fibula forms the lateral segment of the ankle joint mortise.

Proximally, the fibula consists of a head, a neck, and a styloid process. The medial surface of the head has a facet for articulation with the lateral tibial condyle. Projecting from the lateral side of the head of the fibula is the short apical styloid process, to which are attached both the tendon of the biceps femoris and the fibular collateral ligament of the knee joint. One can palpate the head of the fibula just below the lateral aspect of the knee joint, and the common peroneal nerve may be rolled against the fibular head.

⇒ *Fractures of the fibula with common peroneal nerve involvement. The fibula is most often fractured just above the ankle joint; the second most common site of fracture is just below the knee joint. Fractures in the vicinity of the fibular head may involve the common peroneal nerve directly, or it may become involved in the callus of healing. The common peroneal nerve may be injured when blunt trauma compresses the nerve against the underlying fibula. Peroneal palsy ("footdrop") may also be caused by too tight an elastic bandage or plaster cast improperly applied to the head of the fibula.*

The neck of the fibula is a narrow portion distal to the head.

The shaft of the fibula presents 3 surfaces separated by 3 bony crests. In the proximal third of the shaft of the fibula, the medial crest is paralleled by the interosseous crest, which is the fibular attachment of the interosseous membrane. The interosseous crest terminates just proximal to the articular facet of the lateral malleolus of the fibula.

The lateral malleolus is the bulbous lower end of the fibula. Medially and anteriorly, it presents an oval facet for articulation with the talus. Laterally, the malleolus forms the lateral segment of the mortise of the ankle joint into which the talus fits. On the tibial side of the lower end of the fibula a roughened curved surface serves as attachment for the tibiofibular ligament.

➡ ***Reduction of bone fragments in leg fractures.*** *Unreduced angulation of bony fragments may shift the weight-bearing axis so that undue stress is exerted upon both the knee and the ankle on the involved side. Over a period of time, these people often also develop evidence of both hip and lower back stress.*

TIBIOFIBULAR ARTICULATIONS

The tibia and fibula are joined by 3 separate areas of union: (1) the superior tibiofibular articulation, (2) the interosseous membrane, and (3) the inferior tibiofibular articulation.

The **superior tibiofibular articulation** is a bony junction of the gliding type between the lateral condyle of the tibia and the fibular head. The 2 bones are joined by means of oval facets covered with cartilage and held together by an articular capsule and by both anterior and posterior joint ligaments.

The **interosseous membrane,** which connects the mid segments of the 2 bones, runs from the interosseous crest of the tibia to the interosseous ridge of the fibula. It also divides the muscles of the dorsal and ventral surfaces of the leg. It is a thin membrane with oblique fibers which reaches almost to the proximal tibiofibular joint. This creates a circular hiatus superior to the interosseous membrane which allows

for passage of the anterior tibial vessels into the anterior compartment of the limb. Ventral to the interosseous membrane are the tibialis anterior, extensor digitorum longus, extensor hallucis longus, and peroneus tertius muscles; the deep peroneal nerve; and the anterior tibial vessels. Dorsal to the interosseous membrane are the tibialis posterior and flexor hallucis longus muscles. Distally, at the ankle joint, the membrane is continuous with the interosseous ligament of the tibiofibular syndesmosis.

The **inferior tibiofibular joint** is of a fibrous type, or a syndesmosis articulation. It is formed by the convex distal end of the fibula and the concave distal surface of the tibia. The 2 linked rough bony surfaces are joined by interosseous ligaments. The syndesmosis is supported by multiple small ligaments that surround the bony junction and, together with the interosseous ligaments, normally hold the 2 surfaces tightly together.

➡ ***Importance of interosseous membrane in treatment of fractures of both bones.*** *Fractures of the tibia or fibula (or both) often occur as a result of motorcycle and skiing accidents. Fracture of only one bone rarely results in deformity, since the 2 bones are joined together by the interosseous membrane, so that the unfractured bone acts as a splint. Fracture of both bones usually occurs at about the same level. The fracture lines in such cases are usually transverse, and the fractures are frequently comminuted. If one of the bones is fractured at a level different from the other, some leg shortening usually results. The shortening in such cases is difficult both to reduce and to hold in reduction because of the pull, transmitted through the interosseous membrane, of one bone upon the other. As a consequence, following reduction, the bones frequently are held in place by pinning, wiring, or plating.*

➡ ***Leg amputations.*** *Leg amputation may be done as treatment for spreading gas gangrene; for extensive, severe, crushing trauma to the limb; for severe vascular obliterative disease; and for malignant tumor. The ideal site for leg amputation is 13–18 cm below the knee joint. A stump of this size permits fitting of a prosthesis that will allow good lower limb leverage.*

SURFACE ANATOMY OF THE LEG

The surface anatomy of the leg is of clinical interest because its visible or palpable bony eminences and tendinous structures serve as landmarks for diagnosis and treatment of lower limb disorders.

The **patellar tendon** is visible and palpable in the midline of the upper anterior surfaces of the leg.

The **calcaneal (Achilles) tendon** is readily seen and palpated above the heel, the bulge of the posterior calf muscles lying immediately superior to it.

⟹ *Rupture of calcaneal tendon. Traumatic rupture of the calcaneal tendon is a disabling injury calling for immediate surgical tendoplasty to avoid permanent foot and ankle malfunction. As a result of the rupture, the foot is held in plantar flexion and the patient is unable to dorsiflex at the ankle joint with any power. Healing is slow, and athletes must endure a period of disability of 6–9 months even when prompt repair has been done.*

Both the **head** and the **lateral malleolus of the fibula** are readily seen and palpated on the superior and inferior lateral surfaces of the leg, respectively.

The lower third of the **shaft of the fibula** lies just deep to the skin and subcutaneous tissues.

The **tibial tuberosity** is palpable and often visible in the midline of the upper third of the leg.

The **medial and lateral tibial condyles** are easily palpated on the superior aspect of the leg.

The **inferior terminal projection of the tibia,** the **medial malleolus,** and the **anteromedial surface of the tibial shaft** are easily palpable through the skin and subcutaneous tissue of the anterior and medial segments of the leg.

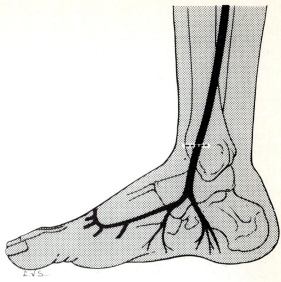

Figure 50–2. Anatomic relationships of saphenous vein. (Reproduced, with permission, from Dunphy JE, Way LW [editors]: *Current Surgical Diagnosis & Treatment,* 5th ed. Lange, 1981.)

SOFT TISSUES OF THE LEG

Subcutaneous Structures

The cutaneous nerves of the leg and the greater and lesser saphenous veins lie just deep to the superficial leg fascia.

The **greater and lesser saphenous veins** (Fig 50–2) begin in the large and complex venous plexuses situated superficially on the dorsum of the foot. The greater saphenous vein passes directly over or slightly anterior to the medial malleolus, then along the medial aspect of the leg, just medial to the anteromedial border of the tibia, close to the saphenous nerve. It passes across the medial aspect of the knee joint and onto the medial surface of the thigh. The lesser saphenous vein leaves the foot and ascends posterior to the lateral malleolus of the fibula, then into the mid portion of the posterior calf and eventually pierces the deep popliteal fascia to join the popliteal vein. The superficial tissues of the leg also present multiple connections between the greater and lesser saphenous veins. These connecting veins, along with the 2 major saphenous veins, enlarge and become thin-walled, tortuous, and visible in varicose vein disease of the lower extremity.

⟹ *Use of the greater saphenous vein for infant transfusions. The greater saphenous vein, with*

its constant position just anterior to the medial malleolus, is the most common site for transfusion of blood and injection of fluids in infants and children. It is also used for intravenous infusions in adults when the veins of the forearm and arm are small or thrombosed; when a needle placed in the antecubital fossa would interfere with operative procedures on the upper extremity; or when burns of both arms prevent use of antecubital fossa veins.

⟹ *Varicosities of the greater and lesser saphenous veins. Varicosities of saphenous veins of the leg and thigh are quite common. Communicating veins also frequently become varicose and lose their valvular competency. At operation, it is important to remove these communicating veins along with the major and minor saphenous trunks.*

⟹ *Chronic ulceration from varicosities of the saphenous venous system. The cutaneous and subcutaneous areas at and immediately above the ankle joint are frequent sites of chronic ulcerations secondary to varicose vein disease. These areas tend to develop ulcerations as a result of severe varicosities of the greater saphenous venous system, both with and without concomitant venous disease of the deep veins of the leg. Chronic leg ulcerations are often present in arteriosclerotic obliterative disease of the leg and in long-standing severe diabetes, associated with vascular disease of the lower extremity.*

⮕ **Use of saphenous veins as vein grafts.** *Both the greater and lesser saphenous veins may be removed and used as venous grafts in vascularization procedures upon the heart.*

Deep Leg Fascia
(Fig 50–3)

The deep fascia of the leg entirely encases the limb's muscles and tendons and its 2 bones. Superiorly, the deep fascia is continuous with the fascia lata of the thigh. Posteriorly and superiorly, as it descends, it roofs over the popliteal fossa and is called the popliteal fascia. Anteriorly, it joins with the periosteum covering the anterior surface of the tibia and the head and lateral malleolus of the fibula. At the ankle joint, the fascia blends with both the flexor and extensor retinacula. It sends a fascial partition (deep transverse fascia) deep into the limb to attach to the deep surface of the fibula, with resultant division of the posterior leg into 2 compartments: superficial and deep. The tibia and the interosseous membrane separate the extensor muscles of the anterior compart-ment of the leg from the deep muscles of the posterior leg compartment. Two short but sturdy fibrous septa—the anterior and posterior intercrural septa—on the lateral side of the leg run from the fibula to the deep surface of the deep fascia and encase the peroneus longus and peroneus brevis muscles, effectively separating these 2 muscles from the muscles of the anterior and posterior leg compartments.

⮕ **Compartment syndrome.** *Division of the leg into 3 compartments by the tibia and the multiple enclosing fascial walls may lead to the compartment syndrome. Increased pressure from bleeding into a closed compartment eventually causes severe ischemic damage to muscles, nerves, and blood vessels which lie within the compartment. This syndrome should be carefully watched for in patients with lower extremity injuries so that the containing fascia can be incised.*

The junction distally of the deep fascia of the leg with the flexor and extensor retinacula of the ankle joint is of great mechanical importance. The

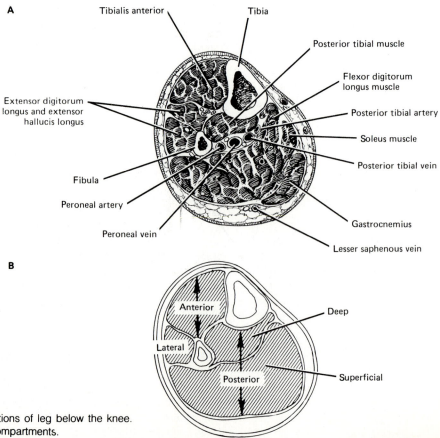

Figure 50–3. Cross sections of leg below the knee. **A:** muscles. **B:** fascial compartments.

2 retinacula closely bind the assorted tendons, which pass across the ankle joint, to the underlying bony tissues of the joint. Accordingly, the retinacula keep the tendons from bowstringing during dorsiflexion and plantar flexion.

Contents of the 3 Major Compartments of the Leg (Tables 50–1 and 50–2; Figs 50–3 to 50–6)

A. Lateral (Peroneal) Compartment: The lateral compartment of the leg contains only 2 muscles: the peroneus longus and the peroneus brevis. Both muscles evert and plantar-flex the foot and are supplied by the superficial peroneal nerve, a branch of the common peroneal nerve.

The common peroneal nerve usually arises in the popliteal space as a branch of the sciatic nerve. It leaves via the lateral border of the space, winds around the neck of the fibula, and enters the lateral leg compartment. It then divides into a recurrent geniculate branch (the lateral sural cutaneous nerve), a deep peroneal or anterior tibial branch, and a superficial peroneal branch, which, in addition to supplying the 2 peroneal muscles, innervates the skin of the lateral side of the leg and the dorsum of the foot. Because of its relatively superficial position as the nerve winds about the neck of the fibula, it is susceptible to injury in approaches to lateral fibula and in blunt trauma to the leg.

B. Anterior (Extensor) Compartment: The anterior compartment contains 4 muscles, all of which dorsiflex the foot: tibialis anterior, extensor digitorum longus, peroneus tertius, and extensor hallucis longus. The long extensors serve also to extend the metatarsophalangeal and interphalangeal joints. The deep peroneal nerve, along with the anterior tibial artery and its accompanying veins, makes up a neurovascular bundle that begins high in the leg between the tibialis anterior medially and the extensor digitorum longus laterally. The neurovascular bundle lies on the interosseous membrane, and distally it is crossed by the extensor hallucis longus tendon.

The deep peroneal nerve, sometimes called the anterior tibial nerve, arises from the common peroneal nerve soon after that nerve has entered the lateral compartment of the leg. It leaves the lateral compartment and enters the anterior compartment, in which it courses inferiorly dorsal to the extensor digitorum longus, closely accompanied by the anterior tibial

Table 50–1. Muscles of the leg: Anterior and lateral compartment muscles.

Muscle and Origin	Insertion	Innervation	Function
Anterior compartment muscles			
TIBIALIS ANTERIOR From the lateral condyle and the superior half of the lateral surface of the tibia, the interosseous membrane, and the intermuscular septum dividing it from the extensor digitorum longus.	The medial and plantar surface of the first cuneiform and the base of the first metatarsal.	Deep peroneal nerve (L4, 5).	Dorsiflexes and inverts the foot.
EXTENSOR DIGITORUM LONGUS From the lateral condyle of the tibia, the superior three-fourths of the fibula, the anterosuperior segment of the interosseous membrane, the anterior crural intermuscular septum, and the septum between it and the tibialis anterior.	Divides into 4 slips that run anteriorly on the dorsum of the foot to insert into the distal and middle phalanges of the 4 lateral toes.	Deep peroneal nerve (L4, 5; S1).	Extends the phalanges of the lateral toes and dorsiflexes the foot.
EXTENSOR HALLUCIS LONGUS From the anterior surface of the middle third of the fibula and the middle third of the adjacent interosseous membrane.	The base of the distal phalanx of the great toe.	Deep peroneal nerve (L4, 5; S1).	Extends the phalanges of the great toe and dorsiflexes and inverts the foot.
PERONEUS TERTIUS From the distal third of the anterior surface of the fibula and the interosseous membrane.	The dorsal surface of the base of the fifth metatarsal.	Deep peroneal nerve (L4, 5; S1).	Everts and dorsiflexes the foot.
Lateral compartmental muscles			
PERONEUS LONGUS From the head and the superior two-thirds of the lateral surfaces of the fibula. A few fibers arise from the lateral tibial condyle and from the adjacent intermuscular septa.	The lateral side of the base of the first metatarsal and the lateral side of the medial cuneiform.	Superficial peroneal nerve (L4, 5; S1).	Everts and plantar-flexes the foot.
PERONEUS BREVIS From the inferior two-thirds of the lateral surface of the fibula and from the adjacent intermuscular septa.	Into the tuberosity at the base of the fifth metatarsal.	Superficial peroneal nerve (L4, 5; S1).	Everts and plantar-flexes the foot.

Table 50–2. Muscles of the leg: Superficial and deep posterior compartment muscles.

Muscle and Origin	Insertion	Innervation	Function
Superficial group			
GASTROCNEMIUS			
The medial head: the popliteal surface of the femur proximal to the medial condyle and from the adjacent area of the femur. The lateral head: the proximal posterior part of the lateral surface of the lateral femoral condyle and the lateral supracondylar ridge.	The mid posterior surface of the os calcis (calcaneus) via the tendo calcaneus along with the soleus tendon.	Tibial nerve (S1, 2).	Plantar-flexes the foot and flexes the leg.
SOLEUS			
From the posterior surface of the head of the fibula and the proximal one-third of the posterior fibular shaft, the fibrous arch between the tibia and fibula, the popliteal line of the tibia, and the middle third of the medial border of the tibia.	Along with the gastrocnemius muscle tendon (tendo calcaneus) into the middle of the posterior surface of the os calcis.	Tibial nerve (S1, 2).	Plantar-flexes the foot.
PLANTARIS			
From the lateral supracondylar ridge of the femur superior to the lateral head of the gastrocnemius and from the oblique popliteal ligament of the knee joint.	The posterior surface of the os calcis via the tendo calcaneus.	Tibial nerve (S1, 2).	Flexes the leg and plantar-flexes the foot.
Deep group			
POPLITEUS			
From the lateral aspect of the lateral condyle of the femur, the oblique popliteal ligament of the knee joint, and the outer margin of the lateral meniscus.	The popliteal fascia and into the dorsal surface of the tibia above the popliteal line.	Tibial nerve (L4, 5; S1).	Flexes the leg, rotates the femur laterally when the tibia is fixed, draws the posterior part of the lateral meniscus posteriorly, and plantar-flexes the foot.
TIBIALIS POSTERIOR			
From the middle third of the posterior surface of the tibia, the medial surface of the proximal four-fifths of the fibula, and the posterior surface of the interosseous membrane.	The tubercle of the navicular bone and (by fibrous septa) to the plantar surfaces of the second and third cuneiform bones, the cuboid bone, the bases of the second, third, and fourth metatarsal bones, and the sustentaculum tali of the os calcis.	Branch of the tibial nerve (L4, 5).	Inverts and plantar-flexes the foot.
FLEXOR DIGITORUM LONGUS			
From the middle third of the posterior surface of the body of the tibia and from the fascia covering the tibialis posterior muscle.	Divides into 4 tendons that insert into the bases of the distal phalanges of the lateral 4 toes.	Tibial nerve (S2, 3).	Flexes the phalanges of the lateral toes. Plantar-flexes and inverts the foot.
FLEXOR HALLUCIS LONGUS			
From the posterior surface of the distal two-thirds of the fibular shaft, the adjoining intermuscular septum, the inferior one-fourth of the interosseous membrane, and from fascia overlying the tibialis posterior muscle.	The base of the distal phalanx of the great toe.	Tibial nerve (S2, 3).	Flexes the phalanges of the great toe. Plantar-flexes and inverts the foot.

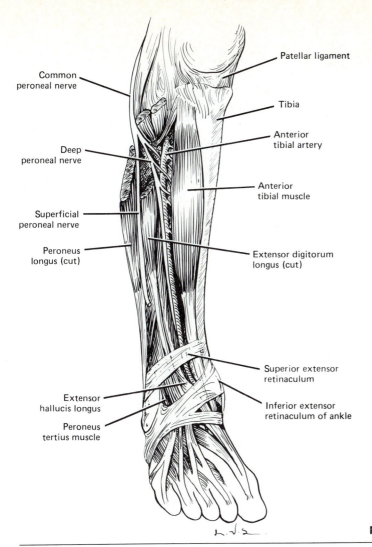

Common peroneal nerve

Deep peroneal nerve

Superficial peroneal nerve

Peroneus longus (cut)

Extensor hallucis longus

Peroneus tertius muscle

Patellar ligament

Tibia

Anterior tibial artery

Anterior tibial muscle

Extensor digitorum longus (cut)

Superior extensor retinaculum

Inferior extensor retinaculum of ankle

Figure 50–4. Dissection of anterior right leg.

artery. The nerve innervates the 4 muscles of the compartment and sends twigs to the ankle joint. It lies upon the interosseous membrane until it leaves the distal segment of the anterior compartment to pass onto the dorsum of the foot along with the dorsalis pedis artery. It divides into a lateral branch, which supplies the extensor digitorum brevis; and a medial branch, which provides the dorsal digital nerves that supply the adjacent sides of the first and second toes.

The anterior tibial artery originates at the lower border of the popliteal muscle, from the popliteal artery. It passes into the anterior compartment of the leg at the top of the interosseous membrane between the 2 heads of the tibialis posterior muscle. It descends along with the deep peroneal nerve, at first deep to the anterior surface of the interosseous membrane, gradually becoming more superficial. Just superior to the ankle joint, it lies on the anterior surface of the tibia and then passes onto the dorsum of the foot (dorsalis pedis artery), where it is easily

palpable. The quality of the pulse at this level provides a clue to the adequacy of the circulation in the distal segment of the lower limb. It gives off posterior and anterior tibial recurrent branches and fibular, muscular, and anterior medial and anterior lateral malleolar branches. It participates also in the arterial anastomoses around the knee and the ankle joints.

C. Posterior (Flexor) Compartment: The 3 superficial muscles are the gastrocnemius, the soleus, and the plantaris, all 3 joining distally to form the strong calcaneal tendon (triceps surae), which inserts onto the posterior surface of the calcaneus (os calcis). The superficial muscles of the posterior compartment are primarily flexors of the knee and plantar flexors of the foot, and all are supplied by the tibial nerve. The calcaneal tendon descends from the mid leg and becomes progressively narrower, only to widen again just before it inserts into the posterior surface of the calcaneus. The tendon is separated from the posterosuperior segment of the calcaneus by a bursa, a common

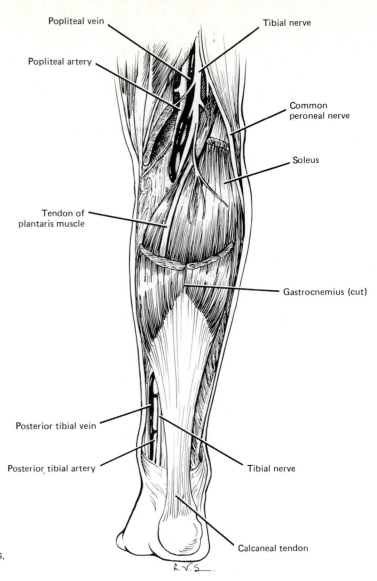

Figure 50–5. Superficial muscles, vessels, and nerves of the leg (posterior view).

site for acute or chronic bursitis. The superior portion of the calcaneal tendon is covered by fibers of the soleus muscle.

The 4 deep muscles of the posterior compartment of the leg are separated from the superficial muscles by the deep transverse fascia. The muscles are the popliteus, the flexor hallucis longus, the flexor digitorum longus, and the tibialis posterior. The popliteus is mainly a knee joint flexor. The flexor hallucis longis is the flexor of the large toe and also helps to plantar-flex and to invert the foot. The flexor digitorum longus flexes the toes, tends to approximate the arches of the foot, and supports the arch of the foot. The tibialis posterior plantar-flexes the foot as well as inverting it. This group of muscles are all innervated by the tibial nerve.

➠ *Surgical approaches to the leg compartments. All 3 of the compartments of the leg must on occasion be opened surgically. The compartments are usually approached directly by a posterolateral, anterior, or medial incision depending upon the area to be explored or treated.*

BLOOD VESSELS, LYMPHATICS, & NERVES

Arteries

The major arteries of the leg are the anterior tibial, posterior tibial, and peroneal. The **posterior tibial artery** is one terminal branch of the popliteal artery, arising close to the lower border of the popliteal mus-

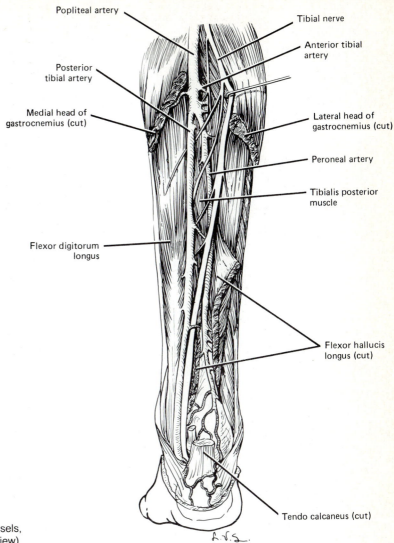

Figure 50–6. Deep muscles, vessels, and nerves of the leg (posterior view).

cle. The artery continues inferiorly, slanting gradually in a medial direction toward the tibial side of the leg. It lies close to the posterior tibial nerve. The flexor hallucis longus lies lateral to the artery, and the flexor digitorum longus lies medial to it. Just superior to the ankle joint, the posterior tibial artery and nerve lie deep to the fascia covering the posterior tibial muscle. If one relaxes this fascia by inverting the foot, the pulse of the posterior tibial artery is palpable about 1 cm posterior to the medial malleolus. At the level of the flexor retinaculum of the ankle, it divides into the medial and lateral plantar arteries. In the leg, the posterior tibial artery sends off muscular and nutrient tibial branches.

The **peroneal artery,** the largest branch of the posterior tibial artery, is given off about 3 cm below the distal edge of the popliteus and descends along the medial margin of the fibula. It sends branches to muscles in both the lateral and posterior leg com-

partments. It either lies in a fascial envelope between the flexor hallucis longus and tibialis posterior or within the flexor hallucis longus muscle. It terminates on the lateral surface of the calcaneus as the lateral calcaneal artery.

The **anterior tibial artery** is described in the preceding section on compartments of the leg.

➭ *Arterial bypass surgery in the leg. Iliopopliteal, femoral popliteal, or femorotibial bypass grafts are on occasion valuable procedures in restoring circulation to the leg and foot. Their success depends to a large extent upon the adequacy of the vascular bed of the lower leg and its collateral runoff. The bypass procedure to the leg vessels is generally not as successful as the iliofemoral or iliopopliteal bypass in the thigh.*

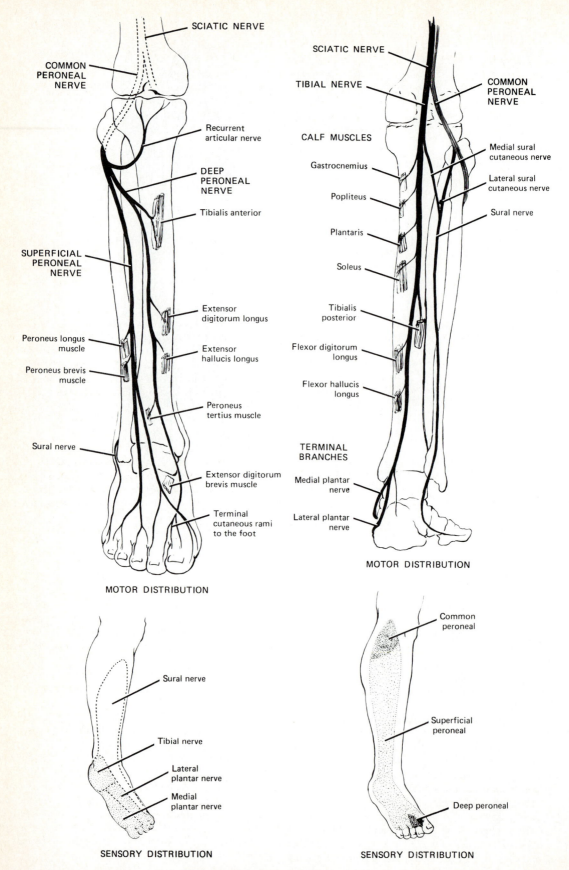

Figure 50–7. Innervation of the lower leg.

Deep Veins

The deep veins of the lower leg generally run alongside the major deep arteries. The posterior tibial veins run with the posterior tibial artery. The peroneal veins usually empty into the posterior tibial veins. The anterior tibial veins, which are the superior continuation of the venae comitantes of the dorsalis pedis artery, run superiorly between the tibia and fibula, crossing over the superior border of the interosseous membrane, and joining with the posterior tibial vein to empty into the popliteal vein.

⇒ *Thrombophlebitis of the deep veins of the leg. The deep veins of the leg are a frequent site of phlebothrombosis or thrombophlebitis. The thrombotic phenomena occur spontaneously in some systemic diseases and also secondary to accidental or surgical trauma, particularly to the lower abdomen, the pelvis, and the lower extremity. Postoperative immobility is a common cause of deep vein thrombosis. The deep leg veins are frequently a source of systemic venous emboli. Systemic venous emboli seldom leave the superficial saphenous system to reach the inferior vena cava. They frequently leave the deep veins of the leg, thigh, pelvis, and perineum to reach the inferior vena cava and eventually the right heart to cause pulmonary embolism.*

Lymphatics

The **superficial lymphatics** lie in the subcutaneous tissues near the greater and lesser saphenous veins. The medial group, which accompanies the greater saphenous vein, is larger and comprises more vessels than the group running with the lesser saphenous vein. The medial superficial lymphatics empty into the superficial subinguinal nodes. A lateral group of superficial lymphatics runs superiorly from the fibular side of the foot to accompany the small saphenous vein and empty into the popliteal nodes.

The **deep lymphatics** of the leg are relatively few in number. They run superiorly alongside the deep blood vessels. There are 3 major groups of deep lymphatics—anterior tibial, posterior tibial, and peroneal—and there are usually 3–5 channels accompanying each of the 3 major arterial vessels. The deep lymphatics empty into the popliteal lymph nodes.

Nerves
(Fig 50–7)

The tibial nerve supplies the muscles of the posterior compartment of the leg. It usually first appears deep to the long head of the biceps femoris as a terminal branch of the sciatic nerve. It then passes through the middle of the popliteal fossa, lying just deep to the roofing popliteal fascia. It runs across the popliteal muscle and gives off cutaneous and articular branches. The tibial nerve then descends between the 2 heads of the gastrocnemius and passes deep to the soleus muscle in order to reach the deep group of posterior compartment muscles. It lies medial to the calcaneal tendon in the lower leg until it reaches the flexor retinaculum, where it divides into the medial and lateral plantar nerves. It gives off articular branches to the knee and ankle joints, muscular branches to the muscles of the posterior compartment, the medial sural cutaneous nerve, the sural nerve, the medial calcaneal nerve, and the medial and lateral plantar nerves. (The common peroneal nerve and the deep peroneal nerve are described in the section on compartments of the leg.)

GROSS ANATOMY
(Figs 51–1 and 51–2)

The leg is connected to the foot by a hinge (ginglymus) joint whose superior components are the distal end of the tibia, the tibial malleolus, the fibular malleolus, and the inferior transverse ligament. The inferior components of the joint are the superior convex surface and the medial and lateral facets of the talus bone. Together, the superior joint components form a mortise into which both the upper surface of the talus and the lateral and medial talar facets fit in snug fashion.

SURFACE ANATOMY
OF THE ANKLE JOINT

The lateral malleolus of the fibula extends about 1 cm farther distally and slightly farther posteriorly than the medial malleolus of the tibia. However, the lateral malleolus is less prominent than the medial malleolus, and the medial malleolus is easier to examine. Two hollow areas lie in relationship to the malleoli. The first of these lies just anterior to the lateral malleolus and lateral to the tendon of the peroneus tertius. The second area lies between the medial malleolus and the tendon of the tibialis anterior. Because of their subcutaneous position, fluid within the joint causes noticeable swelling over these 2 areas.

The line of the ankle joint can usually be identified about 1 cm superior to the tip of the medial malleolus. The calcaneal tendon stands out and lies posterior to the surface of the ankle joint. Lateral and medial to the calcaneal tendon are 2 hollows between the tendon and dorsal to the 2 joint malleoli.

The tendons of the extensor muscles, which pass distally to the foot, lie on the ventral surface of the ankle joint, and are easily seen when the foot is forcibly dorsiflexed. Posterior to the medial malleolus, the posterior tibial artery and the flexor digitorum tendons are palpable, while posterior to the lateral malleolus the tendons of the peroneus longus and brevis muscles are palpable. Between the medial malleolus and the calcaneus lies the deltoid ligament, which roofs a canal for the tendons of the flexor

digitorum longus, the flexor hallucis longus, and the tibialis posterior muscles. The anterior tibial artery lies on the midventral surface of the ankle joint, and immediately distal to the joint it becomes the dorsalis pedis artery which is easily palpable on the dorsum of the foot.

➠ *Aspiration of ankle joint effusions. Ankle joint effusion may develop as a result of chronic postural strain or acute or chronic arthritis of the joint, or it may be secondary to direct or indirect trauma to the joint. Since the anterior surface of the joint is very close to the skin and subcutaneous tissue—even more so upon plantar flexion of the foot—it is easy to aspirate the ankle joint, determine the type of fluid present, or inject an anti-inflammatory substance directly into the joint cavity.*

➠ *Early treatment of bloody effusion of the ankle joint. Blood effusions of the ankle joint frequently follow trauma to the joint or adjacent bony areas. If possible, the joint should be aspirated as soon as the diagnosis of effusion is made. The aspiration helps to speed healing and prevent posttraumatic disability.*

DEEP FASCIA

The deep fascia that covers the external surface of the ankle joint is both thick and resistant and is continuous superiorly with the deep fascia of the leg and inferiorly with the fascia of the foot. On the anterior, lateral, and medial surfaces of the ankle, the deep fascia thickens into several distinct bands both superior and inferior to the ankle joint. These bands (1) tend to support the joint; (2) participate in the formation of osseoaponeurotic passages through which tendons, nerves, and vessels pass from leg to foot; and (3) keep the tendons in close contact with the bones of the joint, thereby preventing bowstringing. Two of the bands lie anteriorly: the **transverse crural** and the **cruciate ligaments (superior and inferior extensor retinacula).** The laciniate ligament, or flexor retinaculum pedis, lies medial to the joint, while laterally there are the superior and inferior peroneal retinacula.

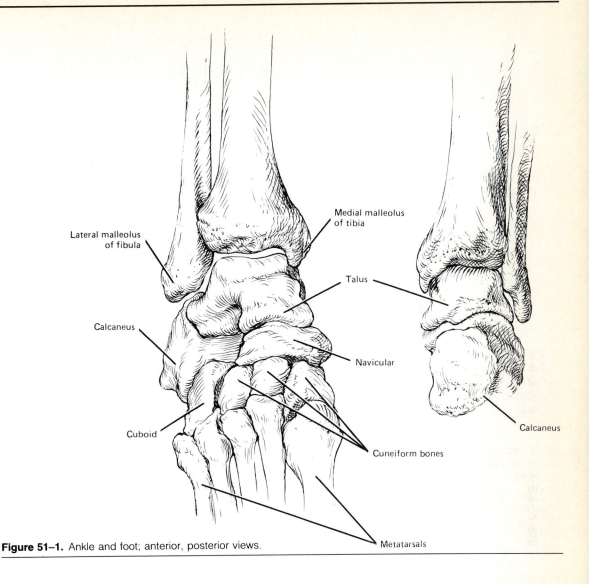

Figure 51–1. Ankle and foot; anterior, posterior views.

THE ANKLE JOINT LIGAMENTS & THE ARTICULAR CAPSULE
(Figs 51–3 and 51–4)

The 3 bones of the ankle joint are bound tightly together by the articular capsule, which is divided into 4 segments: medial, lateral, anterior, and posterior. The capsule is attached superiorly to the articular edges of the tibia and both malleoli and to the talus inferiorly.

The anterior segment of the articular capsule is quite thin and lies just deep to the tendons of the extenders of the toes, the tibialis anterior, and the peroneus tertius and to the deep peroneal nerve, the anterior tibial artery and vein. The posterior segment of the articular capsule is also quite thin and blends with the inferior transverse ligament, which connects the tibia and fibula distally. Laterally and medially, the capsule is thickened. The anterior and posterior

thinness of the capsule facilitates the movements of flexion and extension. The medial and lateral collateral ligaments of the ankle joint lend strength.

The **deltoid ligament** is a very strong fibrous band that serves as the major medial ligament of the ankle joint. It is made up of a superficial and a deep layer of fibers arranged in the shape of a pyramid. Superiorly, the apex of the triangular ligament is attached to the medial malleolus of the tibia. The more anterior of the superficial fibers of the ligament run to the tuberosity of the navicular; the middle group of fibers insert into the calcaneus; and the posterior superficial fibers run to the medial surface of the talus. The deep fibers of the ligament are attached to the medial malleolus superiorly and to the medial surface of the talus inferiorly. Lying just superficial to the ligament are the tendons of the tibialis posterior and the flexor digitorum longus.

The **lateral ligament** of the ankle joint is actually

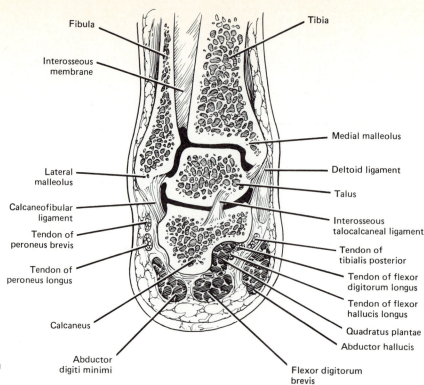

Figure 51–2. Coronal section through the ankle joint.

a combination of 3 ligaments: the anterior and posterior talofibular ligaments and the calcaneofibular ligament. The **anterior talofibular ligament** is a short fibrous band that runs from the lateral malleolus to the talus, where it attaches anterior to the lateral articular facet. The **posterior talofibular ligament** runs from the fibular malleolus to a tubercle on the posterior talar surface. The **calcaneofibular ligament** is a thin fibrous band that runs from the lateral malleolus to a tubercle on the lateral surface of the calcaneus. Superficial to the calcaneofibular ligament are the tendons of the peroneus longus and brevis.

A synovial membrane lines the entire inner surface of the capsule of the ankle joint. It extends superiorly between the tibia and fibula to the lower end of the interosseous membrane. Ventrally and dorsally, the

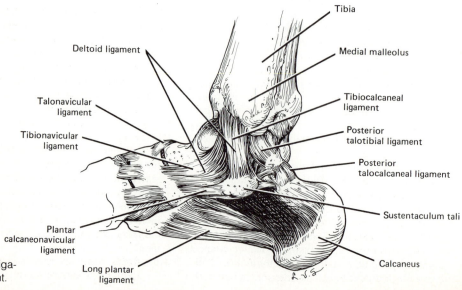

Figure 51–3. Medial ligaments of the ankle joint.

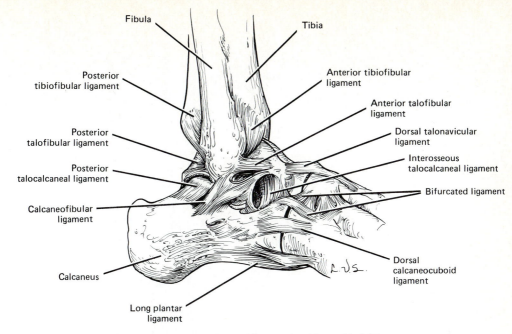

Fibula

Tibia

Posterior
tibiofibular ligament

Anterior tibiofibular
ligament

Anterior talofibular
ligament

Dorsal talonavicular
ligament

Posterior
talofibular ligament

Interosseous
talocalcaneal ligament

Posterior
talocalcaneal ligament

Bifurcated ligament

Calcaneofibular
ligament

Dorsal
calcaneocuboid
ligament

Calcaneus

Long plantar
ligament

Figure 51–4. Lateral ligaments of the ankle joint.

synovial membrane is loose, so that an effusion within the joint will distend the membrane in those 2 directions.

The strength and stability of the ankle joint are due mainly to its strong supporting ligaments, the support of the subjacent tendons and the excellent coaptation of the structures that make up the mortise-like arrangement of the bones of the joint. The roof of the joint is formed entirely by the tibia, while the malleoli of both the tibia and the fibula cling firmly to the lateral and medial sides of the talus, preventing all but the slightest lateral or medial movements of the ankle joint. The joint is strengthened also by the inferior transverse ligament, a thick fibrous connection between the tibia and the fibula. It stretches transversely across the posterior surface of the joint from the lateral malleolus to the dorsal margin of the articular surface of the tibia. The ligament protrudes farther inferiorly than the tibia and fibula and thus contributes to the surface with which the talus articulates.

➡ *Chronic ankle strain. Since the ankle joint must support the entire weight of the body in the upright position, it is frequently the site of chronic strain brought on by an abnormally inverted foot; disturbances of the muscular or nervous system affecting the lower trunk or the lower limbs; chronic arthritis of the spine, hip, knee, or ankle; and osteoporosis of the lower extremity. Ankle strain is usually reflected by the presence of abnormal tenderness over the medial or lateral collateral ligaments of*

the joint or in the plantar fascial areas of the foot (longitudinal arch).

➡ *Integrity of the ankle mortise. Fractures of one or more of the bones about the ankle joint frequently complicate severe acute ankle sprains. The medial and lateral malleoli are the bony areas most often fractured in such cases; consequently, severe fracture involving these areas of bone may disrupt the integrity of the joint mortise. Permanent ankle instability and arthritis ensue if the joint mortise is not properly restored.*

➡ *Inversion and eversion ankle injuries. Sprains are probably the most common trauma affecting the ankle joint. They usually result from forced eversion or inversion of the foot. With such a sprain there may be either complete or partial tearing of joint ligaments. Complete ligamentous tears often result in joint instability. The tear of a ligament with a concomitant bony chip fracture at the site of the origin or insertion of the ligament is known as a sprain fracture. Most sprains are of the inversion type with a concomitant tear of the lateral collateral ligament. Eversion sprains with a tear of the medial collateral ligament also occur often. Point tenderness over the involved ligament and its sites of attachment plus some resultant ankle instability are usually present in severe sprains.*

➡ *Ankle dislocations. Dislocation of the ankle joint secondary to tearing of one or more of*

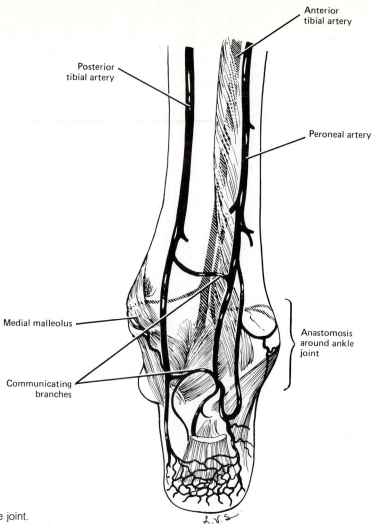

Figure 51–5. Arteries related to the ankle joint.

the joint ligaments is relatively uncommon. Dislocations may be dorsal, ventral, medial, lateral, or superior. Lateral and medial luxations occur along with tibial and fibular malleolar fractures and secondary to Pott's fracture. Dorsal displacement is the most common dislocation and results from extreme plantar flexion of the foot. Such a dislocation results in a shortened foot and a very prominent heel.

▮▶ *Fracture-dislocations of the ankle.* These are illustrated in Figures 51–6 and 51–7.

RELATIONSHIPS OF THE ANKLE JOINT

The ankle joint is related to several important structures. Anterior to the joint lie the tendons of the tibialis anterior, extensor hallucis longus, extensor digitorum longus, and peroneus tertius muscles. The anterior tibial vessels and the deep peroneal nerve also lie anterior to the joint. Posterior to the joint lie the tendons of the tibialis posterior and the flexor digitorum longus; medial to the ankle joint lie the posterior tibial vessels, the tibial nerve, and the flexor hallucis longus tendon; and lateral to the joint lie the tendons of the peroneus longus and brevis, which course behind the lateral malleolus.

▮▶ *Amputation through the ankle joint.* Amputation through the ankle joint is known as the Syme procedure. This operation consists of surgical disarticulation of the ankle joint and resection of both the tibial and the fibular malleoli and the articular surface of the tibia. Because the imperfect end-bearing stump that results is difficult to fit with a prosthesis, this type of lower leg amputation is seldom used today.

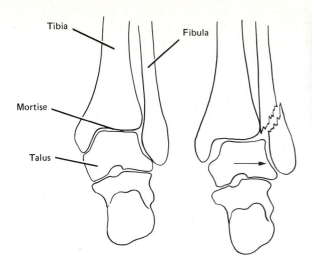

Figure 51–6. Fracture-dislocations of the ankle. Drawing of mortise view x-ray of the ankle showing fracture-dislocation of the lateral malleolus with lateral displacement of the talus. (Reproduced, with permission, from Mills J, Ho MT, Trunkey DD [editors]: *Current Emergency Diagnosis & Treatment*. Lange, 1983.)

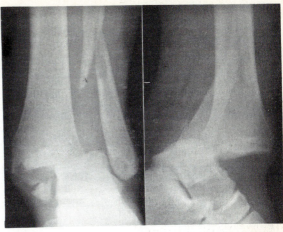

Figure 51–7. Fracture-dislocation of the ankle. Antero-posterior (left) and lateral (right) x-ray views of closed fracture of the lower fibular shaft and medial malleolus with dislocation of the inferior tibiofibular and ankle joints. (Reproduced, with permission, from: Way LW [editor]: *Current Surgical Diagnosis & Treatment*, 7th ed. Lange, 1985.)

MOVEMENTS OF THE ANKLE JOINT

Normally, when the torso is positioned vertically, the foot is held at right angles to the lower extremity.

The ankle joint allows but 2 movements: dorsiflexion (extension) and plantar flexion (flexion). The range of motion varies from 45 to 90 degrees. A small amount of side-to-side movement is made possible by stretching of the ligaments of the talofibular syndesmosis and slight bending of the fibula rather than by movement within the joint mortise. Since the superior articular surface of the talus is wider ventrally than dorsally, in order to dorsiflex, a wider space is needed between the 2 malleoli, this space being obtained by minor rotation of the distal end of the fibula plus relaxation of the ligaments of the talofibular junction. When the foot is inverted or everted, movement of the joint takes place at the level of the intertarsal joints rather than at the hinge of the ankle joint. Inversion may be increased in range if the foot is plantarflexed. The posterior calf muscles raise the heel from the ground, while the 4 anterior crural muscles raise the foot from the ground and dorsiflex the foot at the ankle.

BLOOD VESSELS & NERVES

Blood is supplied to the ankle joint by branches from the peroneal artery and the anterior and posterior tibial arteries (Fig 51–5). Nerve supply is via the saphenous branch of the femoral nerve and from branches of the anterior tibial nerve and the deep peroneal nerves.

BONES OF THE FOOT
(Figs 52–1 and 52–2)

For descriptive purposes, the bones of the foot are divided into 3 groups: the hindfoot (talus, calcaneus), the mid foot (navicular, cuboid, cuneiforms), and the forefoot (metatarsals and phalanges).

THE TARSUS

The tarsus is made up of 3 rows of bones: a dorsal row consisting of the talus and the calcaneus; a middle row that contains a single bone, the navicular; and a ventral row consisting of the 3 cuneiforms and the cuboid.

Talus

The talus (astragalus, or ankle bone) lies directly inferior to the tibia and rests upon the superior surface of the calcaneus. It is held firmly in position by its articulation with the lateral and medial malleoli. The weight of the tibia rests directly upon it. The **anterior portion** of the talus (the head) articulates with the navicular via a large convex oval facet. The narrow **central portion** of the bone (the neck) lies between the head and the body. Multiple ankle joint ligaments are attached to the lateral and medial neck surfaces. The **posterior segment** of the talus (the body) is held firmly in the grasp of the 2 malleoli, since its superior surface articulates with the tibia and its lateral and medial surfaces articulate with the malleolus of the fibula and of the tibia, respectively. The inferior surface of the body of the talus rests both upon the calcaneus and on the spring ligament of the foot.

➡ *Fractures and dislocations of the talus. Major fractures of the talus usually involve either the body or the neck. In fractures of the body of the talus, the proximal fragment is apt to be dislocated from both the ankle joint and the subtalar joint. Occasionally, dislocation of both the subtalar and the talonavicular joints may occur. With talonavicular dislocation, the tendon of the posterior tibial muscle may be caught within the talonavicular joint and requires open reduction.*

Calcaneus

The calcaneus (os calcis) is also called the "heel bone." Its anterior segment is arched superiorly, and upon it rest the body, neck, and head of the talus. Its posterior third is the heel. It is prominent dorsally and easily palpable. The posteroinferior surface of the calcaneus is covered by the thick fibrous tissue pad of the heel. Its posterior surface gives attachment to the calcaneal tendon, and over the superior posterior surface of the bone the calcaneal tendon is separated by a bursa from the calcaneal heel. Anteriorly, the calcaneus articulates via a large facet with the cuboid bone. Laterally, the calcaneus lies in a superficial subcutaneous position and is palpable along its entire length. Medially, the calcaneus presents a markedly concave surface. From this surface there projects a horizontal ridge called the sustentaculum tali, which is palpable about 2 cm directly inferior to the medial malleolus. The calcaneus serves as the final transmitter of the body weight onto the ground.

➡ *Calcaneal disabilities. The skin over the posterior surface of the calcaneus is a common site of decubiti ("pressure sores"), and consequently it must be protected in bedridden patients. Calcaneal bony spurs may cause severe pain upon pressure. Fractures of the calcaneus are usually due to direct trauma, eg, a fall from a height directly onto the heel. Such fractures are frequently comminuted and impacted. Comminuted fractures often involve the subtalar and calcaneocuboid joints. Persistent pain in the area of the subtalar joint may require a joint arthrodesis for relief. If the calcaneocuboid joint is also involved, a triple arthrodesis may be required for relief of pain.*

Navicular
(Os Naviculare)

The navicular bone lies on the medial side of the foot. it articulates with the talus posteriorly and with the 3 cuneiform bones anteriorly. Medially, the navicular presents a tuberosity that is palpable about 2.5 cm inferior to the medial malleolus halfway between the heel and the proximal portion of the metatarsal of the great toe. The tuberosity gives insertion to the tendon of the posterior tibial muscle. Multiple foot ligaments attach to the roughened plantar and dorsal surfaces of the navicular. Occasionally, a small

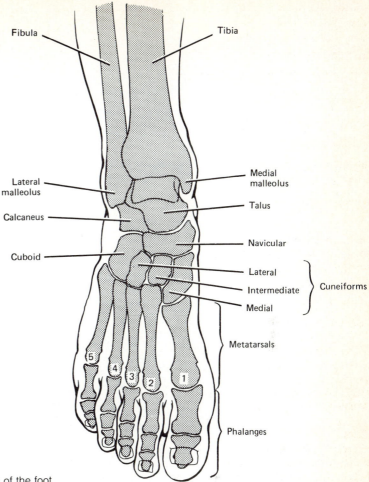

Figure 52–1. Anterior view of the bones of the foot.

segment of the lateral surface of the bone will articulate with the cuboid.

→ ***Fractures of the navicular.*** *Minor avulsion fractures of the tarsal navicular bone may accompany severe midtarsal sprain. Major navicular fractures occur in the mid portion of the bone and are usually impacted.*

Cuboid

The cuboid articulates posteriorly with the calcaneus, anteriorly with the fourth and fifth metatarsals, and medially with the lateral cuneiform. Rarely, it also articulates with the navicular. Multiple ligaments attach to the irregular dorsal surface of the cuboid. The deep flexor surface of the bone shows a deep oblique concavity that holds the tendon of the peroneus longus muscle.

Cuneiforms

The **medial and lateral cuneiforms** each articulate with the intermediate cuneiform. The **intermediate cuneiform** is shorter than the other 2 cuneiforms, and the base of the second metatarsal articulates laterally and medially with the medial and lateral cuneiforms as well as with the intermediate cuneiform. The **lateral cuneiform** articulates with the navicular, the intermediate cuneiform, the cuboid, and the second, third, and fourth metatarsals. The intermediate cuneiform articulates with the medial and lateral cuneiforms, the navicular, and the second metatarsal. The **medial cuneiform** articulates with the navicular, the intermediate cuneiform, and the first and second metatarsals.

→ ***Fractures of the cuboid and cuneiform bones.*** *Because of their protected position in the mid tarsus, isolated fractures of the cuboid and cuneiform bones seldom occur.*

THE METATARSALS

The 5 metatarsal bones are so numbered that bone No. 1 is the most medial and bone No. 5 the most

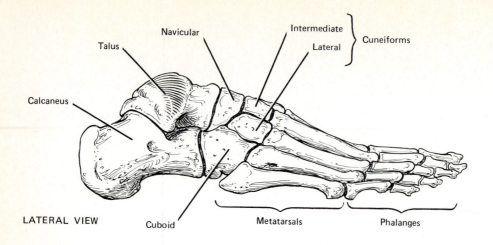

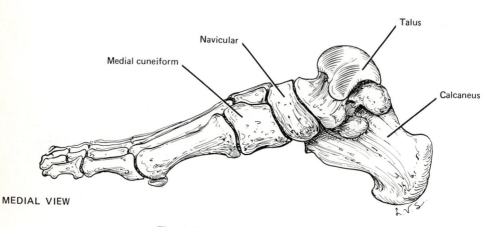

Figure 52–2. Bones of the foot.

lateral. Each metatarsal bone is divided into a distal head, a central body, and a proximal base. Proximally, metatarsals 1, 2, and 3 articulate with the 3 cuneiforms, while the proximal portions of the fourth and fifth metatarsals articulate with the cuboid. The proximal lateral sides of the metatarsals articulate also with the medial sides of the adjacent metatarsals. The metatarsal heads articulate with the proximal phalanges of the foot and are rounded, with an anterior convexity. The metatarsal bodies have a concavity facing the sole of the foot and running in the long axis of the foot. The first metatarsal is the shortest, and the second metatarsal is the longest. The base of metatarsal No. 5 lies proximal to the joint lines of the other 4 metatarsals and projects laterally as the styloid process, an easily palpable bony tuberosity on the midlateral surface of the foot. This makes the fifth metatarsal more vulnerable to trauma than any of the others.

➡️ *Fractures of the metatarsal. (Fig 52–3.) Fractures of the metatarsals and tarsometatarsal dislocations are usually caused either by direct crushing blows or by indirect torsion injuries to the forefoot. They are often accompanied by soft tissue lesions, the commonest being subfascial hematomas. Fatigue fractures of the metatarsal shafts (stress fracture, march fracture) occur in young adults not used to vigorous and excessive walking or running. X-rays may not show this fracture until healing callus has appeared.*

PHALANGES

The individual bones of the toes are called the phalanges. The great toe (the hallux) possesses only 2 phalanges; the other 4 toes have 3 phalanges. The

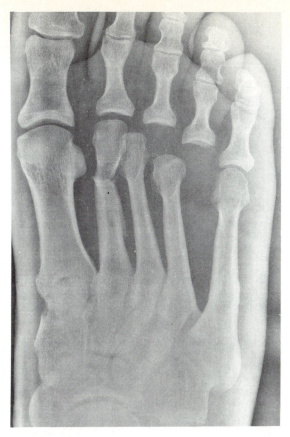

Figure 52–3. Closed fracture of the shaft of the second metatarsal and dislocations of the third and fourth metatarsophalangeal joints. (Reproduced, with permission, from Way LW [editor]: *Current Surgical Diagnosis & Treatment,* 7th ed. Lange, 1985.)

proximal phalanx of each toe articulates via the metatarsophalangeal joint with its corresponding metatarsal head. The mid phalanx articulates with the other 2 phalanges via its proximal and distal interphalangeal joints. The distal phalanx articulates only with the mid phalanx. The phalanges of the toes are shorter than those in the fingers.

⇒ *Phalangeal fractures. Fractures of the toe phalanges are very common and usually caused by the violence of crushing or stubbing. Comminuted fracture of the proximal phalanx of the great toe is the most disabling of these fractures.*

SESAMOID BONES

About 25–30% of normal feet possess accessory bones, the sesamoids. They usually occupy well-defined locations. They are nearly always present bilaterally, and both feet must be x-rayed to avoid confusing the sesamoids with fracture fragments. The most constant position of the sesamoids (often 2) is in the tendons of the flexor hallucis brevis at the level of the metatarsophalangeal joint of the great toe. Sesamoids are occasionally found also over the metatarsophalangeal joints of the second and fifth toes and rarely at the interphalangeal joint of the great toe. On rare occasions, sesamoids are present in the tendon of the peroneus longus, the tibialis anterior, and the tibialis posterior.

⇒ *Fractures of great toe sesamoid. Fractures of the sesamoid bone of the great toe may result from crushing injury. If it does not heal properly, the sesamoid must be excised to diminish pain.*

JOINTS OF THE TARSUS

INTERTARSAL JOINTS

The intertarsal articulations are those that join the bones of the posterior half of the foot.

There are 2 joints between the talus and the calcaneus. The posterior joint is the **subtalar articulation,** between the posterior calcaneal facet on the undersurface of the talus and the facet on the superior surface of the calcaneus. The 2 bones making up the subtalar joint are connected by an articular capsule and surrounded by multiple collateral ligaments. The subtalar articulation allows only a side-to-side gliding motion.

The **talocalcaneonavicular** joint is formed by the articulation of the rounded head of the talus with the concavity formed jointly by the posterior surface of the navicular, the anterior articular surface of the calcaneus, and the proximal edge of the plantar calcaneonavicular ligament. This joint has only 2 supporting ligaments, and dislocation of the navicular and calcaneus from the talus occasionally occurs. The joint is capable of both a marked gliding motion and a small amount of rotatory motion.

The **calcaneocuboid articulation** is the junction of the anterior calcaneal surface with the posterior surface of the cuboid. The capsular ligament of this joint is reinforced inferiorly by the long and short plantar ligaments. Together the talocalcaneonavicular and calcaneocuboid joints form the **transverse tarsal joint,** which allows both inversion and eversion of the foot.

The **cuneonavicular joint** is formed by the 3 cuneiforms anteriorly and by the anterior portion of the navicular bone posteriorly. The capsular ligament of this joint is strengthened by dorsal and plantar ligaments. Only gliding movements are possible at this joint.

The **cuboideonavicular articulation** connects the cuboid to the navicular bone and permits only slight gliding movements. The **intercuneiform** and **cuneocuboid articulations** also allow only a slight gliding movement.

➧ *Midtarsal dislocations. Midtarsal dislocations may occur at the level of the cuneonavicular and the calcaneocuboid joints, or they may occur through the talocalcaneonavicular and the calcaneocuboid joints. Such dislocations usually follow torsion injury to the forefoot and are accompanied by fractures of adjacent bones.*

The cuboid metatarsal joints are between the cuboid posteriorly and the 2 lateral metatarsal bases (4 and 5) anteriorly. Only slight gliding movements occur except in the talocalcaneonavicular articulation, where greater gliding movement is possible.

TARSOMETATARSAL JOINTS

The tarsometatarsal joints are formed by union of the bases of the 3 medial metatarsals (1, 2, and 3) with the anterior surfaces of the 3 cuneiform bones. The fourth metatarsal unites with both the lateral cuneiform and the cuboid, while the fifth metatarsal unites only with the cuboid. All of the tarsometatarsal joints are strengthened by dorsal, plantar, and interosseous ligaments. The only movement possible in these joints is a very slight gliding of the bones one upon the other.

➧ *Tarsometatarsal dislocations. Tarsometatarsal dislocations usually involve the 4 lateral metatarsals, since the first metatarsal has a strong ligamentous support at its base. They are usually caused by direct injury to the joint but may also result from undue stress applied through the forefoot. Such fractures and accompanying dislocations can cause prolonged foot distress. Operative stabilization is often required to prevent long-term disability.*

METATARSOPHALANGEAL JOINTS

The metatarsophalangeal joints are formed by articulations between the metatarsal heads and the bases of the proximal phalanges. The capsular ligament of these joints is thickened both laterally and on the plantar surface of the joint to give strength and stability. The joints allow flexion, extension, abduction, and adduction and are of the condyloid type.

➧ *Amputations. Amputation of the entire foot or part of the foot may be done because of the chronic painful foot disability that results from vascular disease of diabetes mellitus, or because of cancer. The Lisfranc amputation is carried out at the level of the tarsometatarsal articulations; the Chopart resection is done at the midtarsal level between the talus and navicular medially and the calcaneus and the cuboid laterally. On occasion, the entire foot or part of it is so destroyed that it requires amputation because it cannot provide proper weight bearing.*

➧ *Hallux valgus. Hallux valgus is a common deformity of the metatarsophalangeal joint of the great toe. The toe gradually adducts toward the midline of the foot, and a bursa over the head of the first metatarsal becomes painfully inflamed (bunion). Resection of the painful protuberant bursa and correction of adduction of the great toe relieves pain and corrects the deformity. The metatarsal must often be aligned to correct "splayed foot."*

INTERPHALANGEAL JOINTS

The interphalangeal joints lie between the phalanges of the toes. They are strengthened by 2 collateral ligaments and by a plantar ligament. These ligaments are thickenings of the articular capsule of the joints. The interphalangeal joints permit only flexion and extension.

MOVEMENT OF THE FOOT

The major movements of the foot at the ankle joint are inversion and eversion. These movements take place at the talocalcaneal and midtarsal articulations. The other tarsal joints allow only slight gliding motion and add little to overall foot motion. Inversion of the foot is accomplished by the combined action of the tibialis anterior and posterior with some help from the long extensor and long flexor tendons to the great toe. Eversion is accomplished by the peronei.

WEIGHT BEARING

In the erect position with the weight resting on the foot, the body weight is supported mainly by the metatarsal heads and by the heel. Some of the weight is borne by the lateral margin of the foot and the tips of the toes.

➡ ***Causes of abnormal foot positions.*** *The normal position of the foot is maintained by interaction of the various muscle groups in the foot. Paralysis, weakness, or spasticity of one or more muscle groups leads to foot deformity. A deformity during childhood may become a fixed deformity in adulthood either because of muscle contracture or because of abnormal development of the foot during its period of growth.*

➡ ***Deformities of the foot.*** *The most common foot deformities are (1) talipes equinus, in which the foot points downward and is fixed in plantar flexion; (2) talipes calcaneus, in which the heel points downward with the foot fixed in dorsiflexion; (3) talipes varus, in which the entire foot deviates medially, the movements and fixation occurring at points distal to the ankle joints; (4) talipes valgus, in which the deviation of the foot is lateral; (5) pes planus (flat foot), due to flattening of the longitudinal arch; and (6) talipes cavus, in which there is deepening of the longitudinal arch. The various foot malpositions often occur in combination, the most common being talipes equinovarus, the clubfoot of children. Other foot deformities are due to osteochondritis of the navicular bone (Kohler's disease) or of the second metatarsal head (Freiberg's disease). The second and third digits may be affected by the hammer toe deformity.*

➡ ***Foot disability following trauma.*** *Loss of inversion and eversion of the foot (secondary to rheumatoid or traumatic arthritis or to the late complications of severe tarsal bone fractures) may cause marked disability, particularly on hilly or uneven ground.*

ARCHES OF THE FOOT

LONGITUDINAL ARCHES

The bones of the foot with their connecting ligamentous bands form 2 longitudinal arches; medial and lateral. The medial arch is composed of the calcaneus, the talus, the navicular, the 3 cuneiforms, and the 3 medial metatarsals. The talus occupies the apex of the medial arch. The lateral arch is composed of the calcaneus, the cuboid, and the 2 lateral metatarsals, the calcaneus making up the apex of the arch.

The foot with its 2 longitudinal arches performs a dual physiologic role: (1) It provides a relatively rigid support for the body in the erect position, and (2) it acts as a spring in locomotion. In the standing position, both longitudinal arches tend to lie more inferior because of the transmitted weight of the body, and the ligaments connecting the bones of the arches become tense to anchor the body. Initiating locomotion takes the weight off the lateral arches; the interosseous ligaments relax, and the bones of the arches unlock and thus give to the foot its springlike action.

The longitudinal arches are maintained in place by 3 factors: the interlocking of the component bones of the arch, the action of the foot ligaments, and the action of muscles related to the positioning of the arches. If the longitudinal arch is flattened, it results in a pronated or flat foot. Such feet can cause not only foot disability but also leg cramps, knee pain, and hip and lumbosacral disability.

TRANSVERSE ARCHES

Two transverse arches are present in the foot. The more anterior of these 2 arches is formed by the heads of the metatarsals; the posterior transverse arch is formed by the navicular and cuboid bones. Both transverse arches are convex toward the dorsum of the foot and concave toward the foot's plantar surface. The transverse arches are supported by ligaments and by the tendons of adjacent muscles. If the anterior arch collapses, pressure is exerted by it against the plantar nerves and vessels, causing nerve pain and on occasion some degree of vascular insufficiency distal to the arch. Such cases are known as Morton's metatarsalgia.

MAJOR FOOT LIGAMENTS (Fig 52–4)

There are 4 major sets of foot ligaments. The primary function of each is to strengthen and thus maintain proper posture of the arches of the foot: (1) The dorsal, plantar, and interosseous ligaments support the transmetatarsal arch; (2) the plantar calcaneonavicular ligament (so-called spring ligament) of the foot runs from the sustentaculum tali of the calcaneus to the tuberosity of the navicular and in so doing supports the talus; (3) the short plantar ligament runs from the plantar surface of the calcaneus to the cuboid; and (4) the long plantar ligament stretches from the plantar surface of the calcaneus to an insertion into the bases of the second, third, and fourth metatarsals. The long plantar ligament lies superficial to the short plantar ligament.

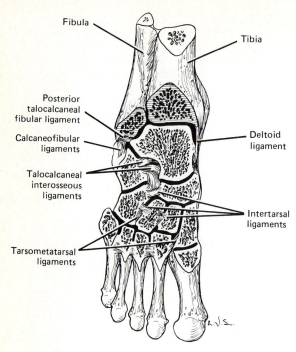

Figure 52–4. Frontal view of the right foot.

anterior and posterior, the flexor hallucis longus, and the small intrinsic foot muscles (Fig 52–4).

The peroneus longus tendon crosses the foot horizontally from lateral to medial, lying in a tunnel formed by the cuboid bone and the long plantar ligament. It inserts into the lateral side of the base of the first metatarsal and into the lateral side of the first cuneiform bone, and it forms a supportive sling for the mid portion of the medial longitudinal arch. The **tendon of the tibialis anterior** is inserted into the medial side of the first metatarsal and into the medial cuneiform, and this helps support the medial longitudinal arch. The medial longitudinal arch is strengthened also by the flexor hallucis longus, whose tendon passes under the sustentaculum tali of the calcaneus. The tibialis posterior, whose fibers are inserted into the tuberosity of the navicular, gives support to the spring ligament of the foot. The transverse arches of the foot are supported by the interosseous, plantar, and dorsal ligaments and by the peroneus longus tendon.

ASPECTS & SURFACES OF THE FOOT

LATERAL & MEDIAL ASPECTS

The lateral aspect of the foot presents a tuberosity at the base of the fifth metatarsal, a good landmark for disarticulation of the tarsometatarsal joint. The lateral margin of the foot is flat and rests upon the ground along its entire length. The medial aspect arches superiorly and rests upon the ground only at the heel and the head of the first metatarsal. The tuberosity of the navicular is palpable and occasionally visible 2 cm anterior to the medial malleolus. It is an excellent landmark for injection of the tibialis posterior tendon.

DORSAL SURFACE

1. SKIN

The skin of the dorsal surface of the foot is thinner and less sensitive than the skin on the plantar surface. The subcutaneous tissue is very loose deep to the dorsal skin. Edema of the foot is always most marked over this surface. In the standing position, the distal veins over the dorsum remain distended and form a transverse arch. The greater and lesser saphenous veins arise from the 2 ends of this arch. The extensor tendons to the toes as they run anteriorly to their insertions are visible and palpable through the thin skin. The extensor hallucis longus tendon medially

PLANTAR FASCIA

The 4 groups of ligaments of the foot are helped in strengthening the foot arches by the presence of plantar fascia, a thickening of the deep fascia of the sole of the foot. The plantar fascia arises from the undersurface of the calcaneus and runs forward to attach to the deep series of short transverse ligaments that join the metatarsal heads. It then extends forward into the plantar surface of each toe, where it forms fibrous flexor sheaths. The plantar or deep fascia of the foot lies superficial to the vessels, nerves, muscles, and tendons of the plantar surface of the foot. It is relatively weak medially and laterally and very strong centrally.

MUSCLES & TENDONS
(Figs 52–5 and 52–6)

Several muscles are intimately related to the arches of the foot and are of help in their support. These muscles also serve the mechanical actions of the foot in both locomotion and in stability. The major muscles so concerned are the peroneus longus, the tibialis

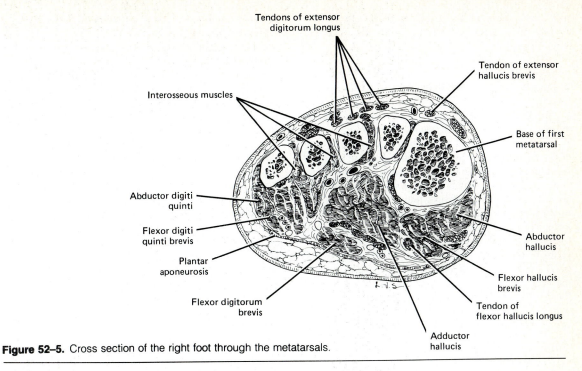

Tendons of extensor
digitorum longus

Tendon of extensor
hallucis brevis

Interosseous muscles

Base of first
metatarsal

Abductor digiti
quinti

Flexor digiti
quinti brevis

Plantar
aponeurosis

Abductor
hallucis

Flexor hallucis
brevis

Tendon of
flexor hallucis longus

Flexor digitorum
brevis

Adductor
hallucis

Figure 52–5. Cross section of the right foot through the metatarsals.

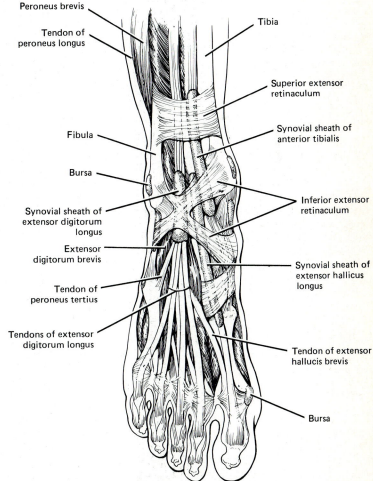

Peroneus brevis

Tibia

Tendon of
peroneus longus

Superior extensor
retinaculum

Fibula

Synovial sheath of
anterior tibialis

Bursa

Inferior extensor
retinaculum

Synovial sheath of
extensor digitorum
longus

Extensor
digitorum brevis

Synovial sheath of
extensor hallicus
longus

Tendon of
peroneus tertius

Tendons of extensor
digitorum longus

Tendon of extensor
hallucis brevis

Bursa

Figure 52–6. Tendons, sheaths, and muscles of the dorsum of the right foot.

and the 4 twigs of the extensor digitorum longus tendon more laterally are both visible and palpable (Fig 52–5).

2. MUSCLES, LIGAMENTS, & TENDONS

Just distal to the ankle joint, the deep fascia of the dorsum of the foot thickens to form 2 ligaments. These ligaments are the extensor and the peroneal retinacula, and they hold the long extensor tendons and the tendons of the peronei close to the underlying bony structures around the anterior surface of the ankle joint. As the extrinsic muscles on the dorsum of the foot pass from their site of origin in the leg to their sites of insertion in the foot, they lie ventral to the ankle joint and deep to the extensor retinaculum. From medial to lateral, they are the tendons of the tibialis anterior, the extensor hallucis longus, the extensor digitorum longus, and the peroneus tertius. Farther laterally are the tendons of the peroneus longus and brevis, which pass posterior to the lateral malleolus. The deep flexor muscles arising in the posterior

compartment of the calf pass posterior to the medial malleolus and with their accompanying vessels and nerves proceed into the plantar surface of the foot. They are neither visible nor palpable.

There is only one intrinsic muscle of the dorsum of the foot: the extensor digitorum brevis. It arises on the calcaneus and passes anteriorly to insert into the tendon of the extensor digitorum longus, which in turn is attached to the middle and distal phalanges. It is a supplementary extensor of the toes.

3. BLOOD VESSELS & NERVE

Arteries (Fig 52–7)

The anterior tibial artery continues into the dorsum of the foot as the dorsalis pedis artery. It passes between the tendons of the extensor hallucis longus and the extensor digitorum longus. The vessel is normally palpable just distal to the ankle joint and indicates the arterial vascular sufficiency of the foot. The dorsalis pedis gives off a medial and lateral tarsal

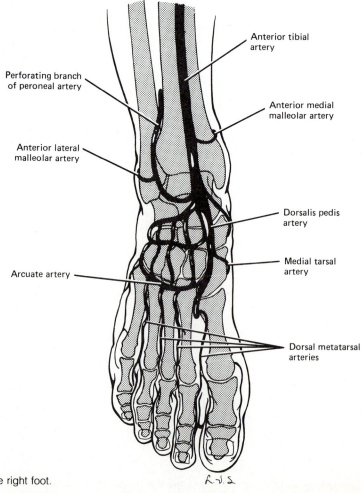

Figure 52–7. Arteries of the dorsum of the right foot.

branch; and at the base of the first metatarsal, the arcuate artery arises from it. The second, third, and fourth metatarsal vessels arise from the arch of the arcuate artery. The dorsalis pedis artery ends in the first interosseous space by forming the first metatarsal artery and by sending a branch into the plantar surface of the foot that assists in formation of the plantar arterial arch.

Veins

The digital veins of the dorsum of the foot receive some blood from the plantar cutaneous arch via the interdigital webs. The common digital veins are thus formed, and at the level of the metatarsal heads they form the dorsal venous arch. Blood from the arch empties into an irregular subcutaneous venous network on the dorsum of the foot, proximal to the arch. The dorsal network receives blood from the superficial veins of the plantar surface of the foot via lateral and medial veins and eventually empties into the greater and lesser saphenous veins.

Nerves
(Fig 52–8)

Sensation for most of the dorsal surface of the foot is supplied by the medial and intermediate dorsal cutaneous nerves, branches of the superficial peroneal nerve.

PLANTAR SURFACE

The plantar surface of the foot is in many respects similar to that of the palm of the hand. Four major differences must be stressed: (1) In the plantar aspect of the foot there is no opponens for the large toe; (2) there are differences in innervation of the lumbrical muscles; (3) the interossei of the foot act centrally on the second toe, whereas in the hand they act on the middle finger; and (4) the foot has an extra intrinsic muscle (quadratus plantae).

1. SKIN

The skin over the major weight-bearing areas of the foot is markedly thickened (heel, lateral foot surface, undersurface of ball of great toe). Sweat glands are numerous in the plantar skin, and the skin of the entire sole of the foot is quite sensitive.

1. PLANTAR FASCIA

The plantar fascia has 3 major divisions: (1) medial, which overlies the intrinsic muscles of the great toe; (2) lateral, which covers the muscles of the little toe; and (3) the plantar aponeurosis, which runs from the calcaneus to the bases of the 5 toes and inserts both into the deep skin areas over the metatarsal heads and into the tendon sheaths of the flexor tendons to

the digits. Arising from the plantar aponeurosis are 2 incomplete vertical septa that tend to divide the sole of the foot into 3 chambers: the medial chamber, which contains the intrinsic muscles of the great toe; the lateral chamber, which contains the intrinsic muscles of the little toe; and the middle compartment, which contains the long tendons and intrinsic muscles to the toes.

3. MUSCLES & TENDONS
(Table 52–1; Fig 52–9)

The intrinsic muscles and long flexor tendons of the toes on the plantar aspect of the foot are in layers.

The first and most superficial layer of muscles of the abductor hallucis, the abductor digit quinti, and the flexor digitorum brevis. The muscles in this layer assist in support of the longitudinal arches of the foot.

The second layer of muscles and tendons consists of the 4 lumbricals and the quadratus plantae muscles and the tendons of the flexor digitorum longus and flexor hallucis longus. The lumbricals arise from the flexor digitorum longus tendons and run to the medial side of the respective proximal phalanges. The quadratus plantae is a supporter of the longitudinal arch. It arises on the calcaneus and inserts into the tendon of the flexor digitorum longus.

The third muscle layer is made up of the flexor hallucis brevis, the adductor hallucis, and the flexor digiti quinti.

The interosseous muscles make up the fourth and deepest layer of the muscles of the plantar surface of the foot. The group consists of 4 dorsal muscles and 3 plantar ones. The dorsal interossei arise by dual heads from adjoining sides of the metatarsal bones and insert into the proximal phalangeal bases. The plantar interossei arise from the medial sides of metatarsals 3, 4, and 5 and insert into the medial borders of the proximal phalanges of toes 3, 4, and 5, respectively.

4. BLOOD VESSELS, LYMPHATICS, & NERVES

Arteries & Veins
(Fig 52–10)

Arterial blood is brought to the plantar surface of the foot by the medial and lateral plantar arteries and the terminal branches of the posterior tibial artery. Venous return from the plantar aspect of the foot follows the arterial pattern. There are abundant venous anastomoses between the veins of both the plantar and dorsal areas of the foot. The superficial veins of the plantar surface form an arch at the bases of the toes. The blood from the arch drains via lateral and medial veins into the dorsal foot veins. While most of the plantar surface veins join the dorsal network, there is some drainage proximally on the sole

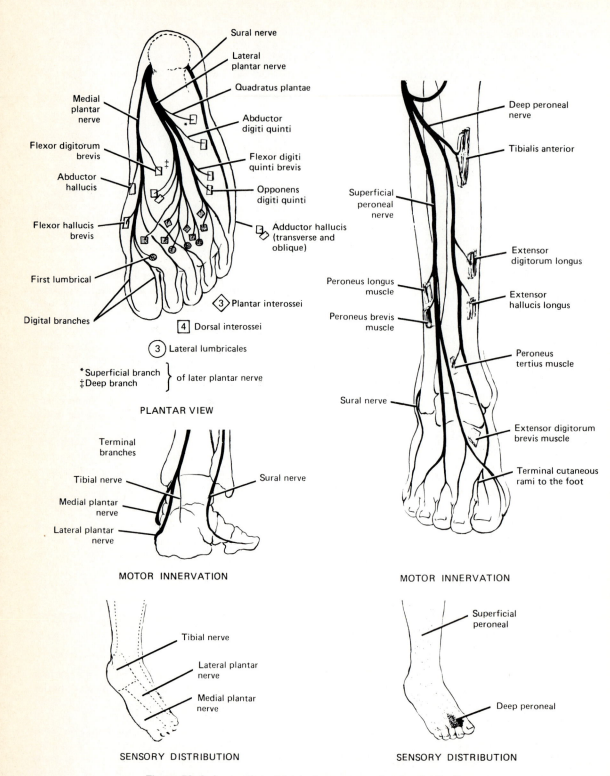

Figure 52–8. Innervation of the foot; sensory and motor distribution.

Table 52–1. Muscles of the foot.

Muscle and Origin	Insertion	Innervation	Function
Dorsal foot muscle			
EXTENSOR DIGITORUM BREVIS From the distal and lateral edges of the calcaneus, the lateral talo-calcaneal ligament, and the inferior extensor retinaculum.	Ends in 4 tendons. The most medial inserts into the dorsal surface of the base of the proximal phalanx of the great toe; the lateral 3 insert into the lateral sides of the tendons of the extensor digitorum longus to the second, third, and fourth toes.	Deep peroneal nerve (S1, 2).	Extends the proximal phalanges of the great toe and the 3 adjacent toes.
Plantar foot muscles			
1. First layer			
ABDUCTOR HALLUCIS From the medial process of the calcaneal tuberosity, the flexor retinaculum, and the plantar aponeurosis.	Inserts along with the medial tendon of the flexor hallucis brevis into the medial side of the base of the proximal phalanx of the great toe.	Medial plantar nerve (S2, 3).	Abducts the great toe.
FLEXOR DIGITORUM BREVIS From the medial process of the calcaneal tuberosity, the plantar aponeurosis, and adjacent intermuscular septa.	Divides into 4 tendons, one for each of the 4 lateral toes. At the base of the first phalanx, each tendon divides into 2 to allow passage of the flexor digitorum longus tendons. The tendons then unite and then divide again to insert into the sides of the mid segment of the second phalanx.	Medial plantar nerve (S2, 3).	Flexes the middle phalanges of the 4 lateral toes.
ABDUCTOR DIGITI MINIMI From the lateral process of the calcaneal tuberosity, the undersurface of the calcaneus, and the plantar aponeurosis.	On the lateral side, inserts into the base of the proximal phalanx of the fifth toe along with the flexor digiti minimi.	Lateral plantar nerve (S2, 3).	Abducts the fifth toe.
2. Second layer			
QUADRATUS PLANTAE OR FLEXOR DIGITORUM ACCESSORIUS Arises by 2 heads: a medial or muscular head from the medial surface of the calcaneus and a lateral or tendinous head from the lateral border of the inferior calcaneal surface.	Tendon of flexor digitorum longus.	Lateral plantar nerve (S2, 3).	Flexes the terminal phalanges of the 4 lateral toes.
FOUR LUMBRICALS Arise from tendons of the flexor digitorum longus. The first lumbrical, arising from the most medial tendon, has one head; the other 3 arise from the adjacent tendons and thus have 2 heads of origin.	The tendons pass medial to the 4 lesser toes and insert into the fibrous expansions of the extensor digitorum longus.	First lumbrical by the medial plantar nerve (S2, 3). Other 3 by the lateral plantar nerve (S2, 3).	Flex the proximal phalanges and extend the middle and distal phalanges of the 4 lateral toes.
3. Third layer FLEXOR HALLUCIS BREVIS Arises by a tendon from the undersurface of the cuboid, from the adjacent part of the lateral cuneiform, and from the tendon of the tibialis anterior.	Divides into 2 segments that insert into the medial and lateral edges of the proximal phalanx of the great toe.	Medial plantar nerve (S2, 3).	Flexes the proximal phalanx of the great toe.
ADDUCTOR HALLUCIS Arises via 2 heads: an oblique head from the base of the second, third, and fourth metatarsals and from the tendon of the peroneus longus; and a transverse head from the plantar metatarsophalangeal ligaments of toes 3, 4, and 5 and from the transverse metatarsal ligament.	The transverse head inserts along with the oblique head into the lateral side of the base of the first phalanx of the great toe.	Lateral plantar nerve (S2, 3).	Adducts the great toe.

Table 52–1 (*cont'd*). Muscles of the foot.

Muscle and Origin	Insertion	Innervation	Function
FLEXOR DIGITI QUINTI BREVIS From the base of the fifth metatarsal and from the sheath of the peroneus longus.	The lateral side of the base of the proximal phalanx of the fifth toe.	Lateral plantar nerve (S2, 3).	Flexes the proximal phalanx of the fifth toe.
4. Fourth layer **DORSAL INTEROSSEI** Each of the 4 muscles arises by 2 heads from adjacent sides of the metatarsal bones.	Tendons insert into the bases of the proximal phalanges and into the expansions of tendons of the extensor digitorum longus. The first inserts into the medial side of the second toe and the remainder into the lateral sides of toes 2, 3, and 4.	Lateral plantar nerve (S2, 3).	Abduct the toes. Flex the proximal and extend the distal and middle phalanges.
PLANTAR INTEROSSEI Each of the 3 muscles arises from bases and medial sides of the bodies of metatarsals 3, 4, and 5.	Into the medial sides of the bases of the proximal phalanges of the same toes and into the expansions of tendons of the extensor digitorum longus.	Branches of the lateral plantar nerve (S2, 3).	Adduct the toes. Flex the proximal and extend the distal and middle phalanges.

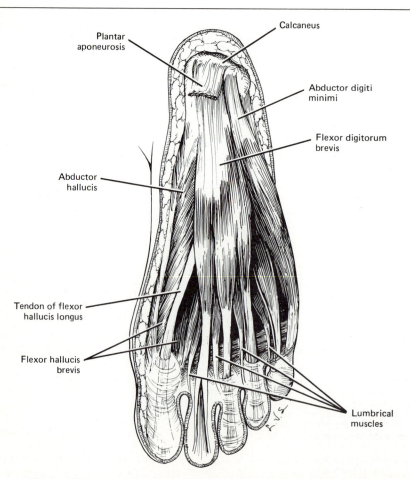

Figure 52–9. Muscles and tendons of the plantar region of the left foot.

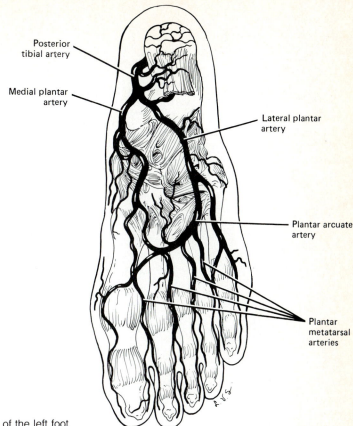

Figure 52–10. Arteries of the plantar region of the left foot.

of the foot into a plantar cutaneous venous network that drains chiefly into the deep leg veins.

Lymphatics

The deep lymphatics of both the plantar and dorsal foot areas follow the deep arterial and venous patterns, emptying first into the popliteal nodes and then into the deep inguinal or external iliac nodes.

➠ *Lymphangiography of the lower extremity. In performing lower limb lymphangiography, a lymphatic channel on the lateral side of the medial venous arch on the dorsum of the foot is dissected out; a small-bore needle is inserted into the vessel, and radiopaque material is injected. The procedure helps in visualizing the lymphatics of the foot, leg, thigh, and inferior retroperitoneum. It can aid in developing a plan for the treatment of cancer of the lower kin's disease. Pertinent information regarding the status of the retroperitoneal lymph nodes and channels can be obtained. However, it has been largely supplanted by CT scan.*

➠ *Infections of the foot. Foot infections are common, though less so than hand infections. They may be approached and drained with knowl-* edge of the 3 median fascial spaces on the plantar surface and the 2 fascial spaces on the dorsum of the foot. On the plantar surface of the foot, spaces exist (1) between the plantar aponeurosis and the flexor digitorum brevis; (2) between the flexor digitorum longus and associated lumbricals and the oblique head of the adductor hallucis; and (3) between the oblique head of the adductor hallucis and the second and third metatarsal bones and their adjoining interosseous muscles. The 3 plantar fascial spaces are best incised and drained along the medial side of the foot so as not to leave a painful scar in a weight-bearing area. The incision is made along the medial side of the first metatarsal and developed between that bone and the flexor hallucis longus tendon. The 2 spaces on the dorsum of the foot are easily drained directly.*

Nerves

The sole of the foot is innervated by the lateral and medial plantar nerves and also by terminal branches of the tibial nerve. The lateral plantar nerve, derived from S1 and S2, is the major nerve to the intrinsic foot muscles.

Index

Note to the reader: Terms in this index are listed mainly under nouns rather than under descriptive adjectives. For example, the carotid artery is listed under the heading Arter(ies), carotid, not under Carotid artery. Page numbers followed by *(i)* indicate that the item is found in an illustration only; page numbers followed by a *(t)* indicate that the item is found in a table.

Receptaculum chyli, 321(i), 322
injury to, 322
Recess
intersigmoid mesenteric, 374
pineal, 23
sphenoethmoidal, 70
Rectosigmoid, 378, 379(i)
arteries supplying, 383(i)
diseases of, 378
embryology of, 378
position of, 378
trauma to, 388
Rectum, 378–387
anomalies of, 378
arteries supplying, 382–383, 384(i)
curves of, 380
digital examination of, 381–382
diseases of, 385
embryology of, 378
ligaments of, 382
surgical mobilization of, 382
location of, 379–380
lymphatics draining, 385–386
mucosal coat of, 382
muscles of, 382
nerves of, 386–387
peritoneal covering of, 379
relationships of, 380–382
serous layer of, 382
submucosal layer of, 382
trauma to, 388
veins draining, 383–386
wall of, structure of, 382
Reflux, urinary ureteral, 452
Rete testis, 504
Reticular formation, in spinal cord, 111
Retina, 87(i), 88(i), 91
disorders of, 91
Retinaculum
extensor
of hand, 572
of knee, 614–615, 636
of wrist, 566
flexor, of wrist, 565
Retinopathy, diabetic, 91
Retromandibular space, 47–48
Retroperitoneum, 317–325
arteries supplying, 318–319
lymphatics draining, 320–322
nerves of, 322–325
pancreas related to, 427
veins draining, 319–320
Rhinorrhea, cerebrospinal fluid, 11
Rhinoscopy, posterior, 69
Rhombencephalon, 18
anomalies of, 18
Rib cage, 191
Rib(s), 191–195
accessory, 183
anomalies of, 183
articulations of, 193–194
cervical, 174, 175(i)
clinical syndrome caused by, 174
embryology of, 183
first, 191
fractures of, 193
fractures of, 193
complications of, 193
cords of brachial plexus injured by, 173–174

Rib(s) (cont'd)
fractures of (cont'd)
flail segment of, 193
pleural disease secondary to, 219
groove on, 191
metastases to, 193
periosteum of, 191–193
spaces between. See Intercostal spaces.
typical structure of, 191, 192(i)
Ridge(s)
infraorbital, 40
superciliary, 40
Rima glottidis, 146
Ring
bony pelvic, 458
fracture of, 458
inguinal, deep, 288(i), 289, 293
Root(s)
of lungs, 262
of spinal nerves, 115–116
anterior, 116
posterior, 116
Rotator cuff, 525–526
disruption of, 526
Rotator cuff syndrome, 526
Rub, pleural friction, 214, 215(i)
Rugae, gastric, disease causing changes in, 332

Sac
lacrimal, 86
lesser, relationship of to posterior surface of stomach, 331
pericardial, 235
drainage of, 235, 236(i)
yolk, and embryology of gastrointestinal tract, 277
Saccule, of ear, 80–81
Sacral canal, 102
Sacral gap, 102
Sacrum, 101–103, 360, 461(i)
alae of, 101
anterior foramens in, 102
apex of, 101
arteries supplying, 106
auricular surfaces of, 101
base of, 101
fractures of, 103, 460
lateral crest of, 102
median crest of, 102
pelvic surface of, 101
Salivary glands, 60(i), 61(i). See also specific glands.
calculi in, impaction of, 59
sublingual, 60
duct draining, 61
and spread of intraoral infection, 60
submandibular gland tissue related to, 127
submandibular, 127–128
duct of, 60, 61(i), 127
removal of in radical neck dissection, 158
sublingual gland tissue related to, 127
submandibular lymph nodes related to, 128

Scala
media, of ear, 81–82
vestibuli, of ear, 81(i)
Scalene biopsy, of internal jugular lymph nodes, 229
Scalenus anticus syndrome, 174
Scalp, 1–2
connective tissue of, 2
trauma to, 2
epicranial aponeurosis (galea) of, 2
hemorrhage of, 2
loose connective tissue of, 2
muscles of, 2
pericranium of, 2
and closure of cranial defects, 2
repair of wounds of, 2
sebaceous cysts of, 2
skin of, 2
trauma to, 2
Scapula, 189–191
angles of, 190
bony processes of, 190
borders of, 189–190
congenital elevation of, 190
fractures of, 190
cords of brachial plexus injured by, 173–174
ligaments of, 190–191
movement of, 190–191
right, posterior view of, 189(i)
surfaces of, 190
Schlemm, canal of, 90
Sclera, 87(i), 88–89
Scoliosis, abnormalities of thoracic cage caused by, 184–185
Scrotum, 500–502
arteries supplying, 502
elephantiasis of, 505
fluid in, in anasarca, 501
layers of, 501(i)
lymphatics draining, 502
masses in, transillumination in diagnosis of, 501
nerves of, 502
skin of, 501
veins draining, 502
"Seatbelt fractures," 100
Seizures, temporal lobe tumors causing, 20
Sella turcica, 11
Semicircular canals, 80
Seminal vesicles, 507–508
Septum
atrial, defects of, 232
interventricular
defect of, 232
development of, 232
lateral intermuscular, of arm, 536
medial intermuscular, of arm, 536
nasal, 66, 69
deviation of, 69
thenar, of hand, 576
of tongue, 62–63
transversum, and embryology of gastrointestinal tract, 275–277
Sheath
anterior rectus, 292
axillary, 210
of common carotid artery, 151
femoral, transversalis fascia and, 294